Handbook of Behavioral Assessment *edited by Anthony R. Ciminero, Karen S. Calhoun, and Henry E. Adams*

Counseling and Psychotherapy: A Behavioral Approach *by E. Lakin Phillips*

Dimensions of Personality *edited by Harvey London and John E. Exner, Jr.*

The Mental Health Industry: A Cultural Phenomenon *by Peter A. Magaro, Robert Gripp, David McDowell, and Ivan W. Miller III*

Nonverbal Communication: The State of the Art *by Robert G. Harper, Arthur N. Weins, and Joseph D. Matarazzo*

Alcoholism and Treatment *by David J. Armor, J. Michael Polich, and Harriet B. Stambul*

A Biodevelopmental Approach to Clinical Child Psychology: Cognitive Controls and Cognitive Control Theory *by Sebastiano Santostefano*

Handbook of Infant Development *edited by Joy D. Osofsky*

Understanding the Rape Victim: A Synthesis of Research Findings *by Sedelle Katz and Mary Ann Mazur*

Childhood Pathology and Later Adjustment: The Question of Prediction *by Loretta K. Cass and Carolyn B. Thomas*

Intelligent Testing with the WISC-R *by Alan S. Kaufman*

Adaptation in Schizophrenia: The Theory of Segmental Set *by David Shakow*

Psychotherapy: An Eclectic Approach *by Sol L. Garfield*

Handbook of Minimal Brain Dysfunctions *edited by Herbert E. Rie and Ellen D. Rie*

Handbook of Behavioral Interventions: A Clinical Guide *edited by Alan Goldstein and Edna B. Foa*

Art Psychotherapy *by Harriet Wadeson*

Handbook of Adolescent Psychology *edited by Joseph Adelson*

Psychotherapy Supervision: Theory, Research and Practice *edited by Allen K. Hess*

Psychology and Psychiatry in Courts and Corrections: Controversy and Change *by Ellsworth A. Fersch, Jr.*

Restricted Environmental Stimulation: Research and Clinical Applications *by Peter Suedfeld*

Personal Construct Psychology: Psychotherapy and Personality *edited by Alvin W. Landfield and Larry M. Leitner*

Mothers, Grandmothers, and Daughters: Personality and Child Care in Three-Generation Families *by Bertram J. Cohler and Henry U. Grunebaum*

Further Explorations in Personality *edited by A.I. Rabin, Joel Aronoff, Andrew M. Barclay, and Robert A. Zucker*

Hypnosis and Relaxation: Modern Verification of an Old Equation *by William E. Edmonston, Jr.*

Handbook of Clinical Behavior Therapy *edited by Samuel M. Turner, Karen S. Calhoun, and Henry E. Adams*

Handbook of Clinical Neuropsychology *edited by Susan B. Filskov and Thomas J. Boll*

The Course of Alcoholism: Four Years After Treatment *by J. Michael Polich, David J. Armor, and Harriet B. Braiker*

Handbook of Innovative Psychotherapies *edited by Raymond J. Corsini*

The Role of the Father in Child Development (Second Edition) *edited by Michael E. Lamb*

Behavioral Medicine: Clinical Applications *by Susan S. Pinkerton, Howard Hughes, and W.W. Wenrich*

Handbook for the Practice of Pediatric Psychology *edited by June M. Tuma*

Change Through Interaction: Social Psychological Processes of Counseling and Psychotherapy *by Stanley R. Strong and Charles D. Claiborn*

Drugs and Behavior (Second Edition) *by Fred Leavitt*

(*continued on back*)

HANDBOOK OF CHILD PSYCHIATRIC DIAGNOSIS

Handbook of Child Psychiatric Diagnosis

Edited by

CYNTHIA G. LAST

MICHEL HERSEN

For your references !!

1989

WILEY

A WILEY-INTERSCIENCE PUBLICATION

JOHN WILEY & SONS

New York • Chichester • Brisbane • Toronto • Singapore

To my husband, Barry M. Rubin
C. G. L.

To my parents, Leon and Betty Hersen
M. H.

Library of Congress Cataloging in Publication Data:

Handbook of child psychiatric diagnosis / edited by Cynthia G. Last,
  Michel Hersen.
      p.   cm.
   Includes bibliographies.
   ISBN 0-471-84887-5
   1. Mental illness—Diagnosis.   2. Child psychopathology—
Classification.   I. Last, Cynthia G.   II. Hersen, Michel
   [DNLM: 1. Mental Disorders—classification.   2. Mental Disorders—
diagnosis.   3. Mental Disorders—in infancy & childhood.   WS 350
H2358]
RJ503.5.H37 1988
618.92′89075—dc19
DNLM/DLC
for Library of Congress   88-17079
                                                              CIP

Printed in the United States of America
10 9 8 7 6 5 4 3 2 1

Contributors

Alan A. Baumeister, Ph.D., Assistant Professor of Psychology, Louisiana State University, Baton Rouge, Louisiana

Alfred A. Baumeister, Ph.D., Professor of Psychology, Human Development, and Special Education, Harvey Branscomb Distinguished Professor, Vanderbilt University, Nashville, Tennessee

Richardean Benjamin, Ph.D., Post-Doctoral Fellow in Psychiatric Epidemiology, University of Pittsburgh School of Medicine, Pittsburgh, Pennsylvania

Daniel J. Burbach, Ph.D., Assistant Professor, Department of Psychiatry, Duke University Medical Center, Durham, North Carolina

Sheila Cantor, M.D., Assistant Professor, University of Manitoba, Winnipeg, Manitoba, Canada (deceased)

John Chaney, M.A., Graduate Research Assistant, Department of Psychology, University of Missouri, Columbia, Missouri

Anthony Costello, M.D., Professor of Psychiatry, Director, Division of Child and Adolescent Psychiatry, University of Massachusetts, Worcester, Massachusetts

Elizabeth J. Costello, Ph.D., Assistant Professor of Child & Adolescent Psychiatry & Epidemiology, Duke University Medical Center, Durham, North Carolina

Daniel M. Doleys, Ph.D., Director, Pain and Rehabilitation Center, Brookwood Medical Center, Birmingham, Alabama

Mina K. Dulcan, M.D., Associate Professor of Psychiatry, Chief, Child and Adolescent Psychiatry, Emory University, Atlanta, Georgia

M. Jerome Fialkov, M.D., Department of Psychiatry, Sharon General Hospital, Sharon, Pennsylvania

Greta Francis, Ph.D., Assistant Professor of Psychiatry and Human Behavior, Department of Psychiatry and Human Behavior, Bradley Hospital, East Providence, Rhode Island

Paul E. Garfinkel, M.D., F.R.C.P., Professor and Vice-Chairman, Department of Psychiatry, University of Toronto, Toronto, Ontario, Canada

David S. Goldbloom, M.D., F.R.C.P., Assistant Professor, Department of Psychiatry, University of Toronto, Toronto, Ontario, Canada

Gregory Hanna, M.D., Assistant Professor of Psychiatry, Biobehavioral Sciences, University of California at Los Angeles, Los Angeles, California

Michel Hersen, Ph.D., Professor of Psychiatry and Psychology, University of Pittsburgh School of Medicine, Pittsburgh, Pennsylvania

Alan E. Kazdin, Ph.D., Professor of Child Psychiatry and Psychology, University of Pittsburgh School of Medicine, Pittsburgh, Pennsylvania

Martin B. Keller, M.D., Associate Professor, Harvard Medical School, and Director of Outpatient Research, Massachusetts General Hospital, Boston, Massachusetts

David J. Kolko, Ph.D., Associate Professor of Child Psychiatry, University of Pittsburgh School of Medicine, Pittsburgh, Pennsylvania

Cynthia G. Last, Ph.D., Assistant Professor of Child Psychiatry, University of Pittsburgh School of Medicine, Pittsburgh, Pennsylvania

Melvin Lewis, M.D., Professor of Pediatrics and Psychiatry, Yale University, New Haven, Connecticut

James McCracken, M.D., Assistant Professor of Psychiatry, Behavioral Sciences, University of California at Los Angeles, Los Angeles, California

Edward M. Ornitz, M.D., Professor of Mental Retardation and Child Psychiatry, University of California at Los Angeles, Neuropsychiatric Institute, Los Angeles, California

Helen Orvaschel, Ph.D., Associate Professor and Director of Child Psychology, Medical College of Pennsylvania, Philadelphia, Pennsylvania

Lizette Peterson, Ph.D., Associate Professor, Department of Psychology, University of Missouri—Columbia, Columbia, Missouri

Judith L. Rapoport, M.D., Chief, Child Psychiatry Branch, National Institute of Mental Health, Bethesda, Maryland

Judith J. Regan, M.D., Assistant Clinical Professor, Vanderbilt University, Nashville, Tennessee

William M. Regan, M.D., Assistant Professor, Vanderbilt University, Nashville, Tennessee

Donald K. Routh, Ph.D., Professor, Department of Psychology, University of Miami, Coral Gables, Florida

Neal D. Ryan, M.D., Assistant Professor of Child Psychiatry, University of Pittsburgh School of Medicine, Pittsburgh, Pennsylvania

Frances M. Sessa, B.A., Research Analyst, Massachusetts General Hospital, Boston, Massachusetts

Cyd C. Strauss, Ph.D., Assistant Professor of Child Psychiatry, University of Pittsburgh School of Medicine, Pittsburgh, Pennsylvania

Michael Strober, Ph.D., Associate Professor of Psychiatry, Biobehavioral Sciences, University of California at Los Angeles, Los Angeles, California

Paul V. Trad, M.D., Director, Child and Adolescent Outpatient Unit, New York Hospital—Cornell University Medical Center, Westchester Division, White Plains, New York

Lawrence Vitulano, Ph.D., Assistant Clinical Professor, Yale University, New Haven, Connecticut

Richard Wolff, Ph.D., Assistant Clinical Professor of Child and Health Development, George Washington University School of Medicine and Health Sciences, Bethesda, Maryland

Sula Wolff, F.R.C.P., F.R.C.Psych., Honorary Fellow, University of Edinburgh, Edinburgh, Scotland

Kenneth J. Zucker, Ph.D., Assistant Professor, University of Toronto, Toronto, Ontario, Canada

Series Preface

This series of books is addressed to behavioral scientists interested in the nature of human personality. Its scope should prove pertinent to personality theorists and researchers as well as to clinicians concerned with applying an understanding of personality processes to the amelioration of emotional difficulties in living. To this end, the series provides a scholarly integration of theoretical formulations, empirical data, and practical recommendations.

Six major aspects of studying and learning about human personality can be designated: personality theory, personality structure and dynamics, personality development, personality assessment, personality change, and personality adjustment. In exploring these aspects of personality, the books in the series discuss a number of distinct but related subject areas: the nature and implications of various theories of personality; personality characteristics that account for consistencies and variations in human behavior; the emergence of personality processes in children and adolescents; the use of interviewing and testing procedures to evaluate individual differences in personality; efforts to modify personality styles through psychotherapy, counseling, behavior therapy, and other methods of influence; and patterns of abnormal personality functioning that impair individual competence.

IRVING B. WEINER

Fairleigh Dickinson University
Rutherford, New Jersey

ix

Preface

Publication of DSM-III and, more recently, that of DSM-III-R generally have been considered to be major steps forward in the classification of childhood psychiatric disorders. Since the original publication of DSM-III in 1980, an enormous amount of research activity has focused on the new (or revised) child psychiatric categories. In response to this research activity, we conceived of the *Handbook of Child Psychiatric Diagnosis* as a means of consolidating these research findings into one state-of-the-art volume.

The handbook is divided into four parts. In Part 1 (Overview) general issues pertinent to child and adolescent diagnosis are covered, including the historical perspective, the current nosological system for diagnosing childhood psychopathology, and the issues of diagnostic reliability and validity. Part 2 (Specific Diagnoses) includes 18 chapters focusing on the DSM diagnostic categories. These chapters are research based and summarize the most recent empirical findings for each disorder. Chapters in Part 2 are presented in a format similar to that employed in DSM: (1) Definition; (2) Historical Background; (3) Clinical Picture; (4) Associated Features; (5) Course and Prognosis; (6) Impairment; (7) Complications; (8) Epidemiology; (9) Familial Pattern; (10) Differential Diagnosis; and (11) Clinical Management: Research Findings. In addition, the final section of each chapter discusses in detail the modifications in diagnostic procedures and diagnostic criteria contained in the recently published DSM-III-R.

Part 3 (Special Topics) of the handbook includes four chapters that focus on several salient issues currently facing the field of child diagnosis. These include developmental issues, structured diagnostic interviews for use with children, the role of epidemiology in child diagnosis, and the relationship between psychiatric diagnosis and behavioral assessment. Finally, Part 4 (Future Directions) contains a chapter delineating the path of the future in childhood diagnosis.

Throughout this handbook our contributors have pointed out the differences between DSM-III-R and its predecessor, DSM-III. Differences for some diagnoses are negligible, while for others the changes in the revision are pronounced. However, the research supporting the diagnostic reliability and validity of the specific categories and subcategories is almost entirely based on DSM-III. Indeed, we now have almost a decade of research documenting both the positive and the negative features of the nosological scheme.

It will be several years before we see a similar amount of research for DSM-III-R. Unfortunately, one of the problems with the DSM is that the categories tend to be determined à priori, with research conducted later. An exception to this is our own empirical work on the overanxious category in children, which as a result has been retained in DSM-III-R.

We also should note that DSM-III-R has not yet been fully accepted universally. This seems to be the case for several reasons. First, many psychiatric settings are still following DSM-III for classification purposes. Second, many third-party payers, in similar fashion, are still adhering to reimbursement on the basis of DSM-III. Third, in the transition between DSM-III and DSM-III-R, there still are many funded federal research grants dealing with categories provided in DSM-III, especially in the longitudinal studies. And fourth, as already noted, the bulk of the empirical literature is concerned with DSM-III.

Many people have contributed their time and effort to this volume. First and foremost we thank our eminent contributors for sharing their expertise with us. Second, we are most appreciative of the technical assistance of Kim Sterner, Jenifer McKelvey, Mary Joe Horgan, and Mary H. Newell. Finally, we thank Herb Reich, our editor at John Wiley, for his support and forbearance in the face of the inevitable delays.

CYNTHIA G. LAST
MICHEL HERSEN

Pittsburgh, Pennsylvania
January 1989

Contents

HANDBOOK OF CHILD PSYCHIATRIC DIAGNOSIS

PART 1

Overview

CHAPTER 1

A Historical Perspective on Views
of Childhood Psychopathology

MELVIN LEWIS AND LAWRENCE VITULANO

An overview of the history of child and adolescent psychiatry reveals astonishing changes in our viewpoints of childhood psychopathology. By and large, six major perspectives can be discerned: descriptive, nature–nurture, psychoanalytic, biological, developmental, and interactional. Usually one or another of these perspectives is dominant at a particular moment in history. Sometimes the change from one perspective to the next is precipitated by the genius of a new conceptual approach, sometimes by the discovery of a technological advance, and sometimes by the prevailing economic and political climate. Occasionally we seem to go in circles or swing like a pendulum from one extreme to another. Yet on the whole the increase in our knowledge of psychopathology is immense and has perhaps increased exponentially in recent years. We will attempt here to view historically these six perspectives and the consequent changes that have occurred in our knowledge and viewpoints on psychopathology in childhood and adolescence.

Description and Measurement

When child psychiatry as a professional field began to emerge in the late nineteenth and early twentieth centuries the most impressive studies on childhood psychopathology were found in the work done on mentally retarded children. Studies by such pioneers as Lightner Witmer (see Sears, 1975) at the University of Pennsylvania, H. H. Goddard (1912) in Vineland, New Jersey, and Walter Fernald in Boston made great strides in describing, defining, and measuring the kinds and degrees of mental retardation in children. And, as so often happens in the history of ideas, the investigators made good use of tests that had serendipitously been developed elsewhere, in this case by Binet and Simon for schoolchildren in Paris. This early goal of describing, defining, and measuring represents an important basic theme in the history of the conceptualization and subsequent scientific study of childhood psychopathology.

The Nature–Nurture Controversy

Very shortly after this early work on retarded children, what were to become classical studies of juvenile delinquents began to appear. William Healy (see Sears, 1975), a neurologist at the Juvenile Psychopathic Institute in Chicago and cofounder of the first juvenile court clinic in 1909, published many of these studies of delinquents. At that time there seemed to be a prevailing view that something organic was at the root of the adolescents' antisocial behavior, although Healy, a neurologist, was himself more concerned about environmental factors that were being overlooked. Healy in effect served as a counterbalance to the views of others, such as Lombroso, who believed that criminal tendencies were derived mainly from heredity. Thus in the study of juvenile delinquency a second major debate or theme in the study of childhood psychopathology began to take shape, namely, the relative roles of organic factors and environment. These two factors were seen initially mostly as an either–or proposition (the nature–nurture controversy) rather than as two interacting factors. Protagonists for both sides of the equation were often forceful in their views. In psychology too, at that time, Arnold Gesell (1952) at Yale, for example, was primarily a maturationist who largely ignored the environment, while John B. Watson (see Kessen, 1965) was essentially a behaviorist who largely ignored biological factors.

Psychoanalysis

Meanwhile a third major theme in the history of the study of childhood psychopathology began to emerge in 1909 when Sigmund Freud published his account of the psychopathology and treatment of Little Hans (Freud, 1909). The basic concepts of psychoanalysis, especially the concepts of an unconscious functioning of the mind and psychosexual phases of development, became a rich source of "explanation" of almost every symptom and behavior (as well as a popular hope for a universal cure for all psychological disorders).

While psychoanalysis as a method of research and as a form of treatment has changed little in its fundamental aspects since Freud first devised the method of free association, psychoanalysis as a theory has undergone a number of changes, from the early topographic model through to the structural model, ego psychology, object relations theory, and, more recently, self theories. Nevertheless, in spite of these changes, certain basic concepts, including psychic determinism, a dynamic unconscious, sexual and aggressive drive development, psychic conflicts, mechanisms of defense, and transference, have remained more or less intact. These concepts and the findings from which they were derived provided useful clinical explanations for a wide range of psychopathology in infants, children, and adolescents. Indeed, almost every psychiatric symptom was explained in part by various combinations of these basic concepts. Thus such symptoms as infant feeding and sleep difficulties, failure to thrive, bedwetting, encopresis, separation anxiety, learning and reading difficulties, phobias, compulsions, conversion symptoms, depression, and psychoses were understood, at least in part, in psychodynamic terms through the 1930s, 1940s, and 1950s.

Biological Research

A change then occurred: Scientific research began to focus increasingly on the biological processes involved in these disorders. Quite dramatically, almost every symptom and disorder now could be understood, again at least in part, in biological terms. Some examples of this change in our understanding will be described later. This blossoming of biological research, particularly during the past 10 years, soon overtook the virtual standstill in psychoanalytic research, and led to a more comprehensive biopsychosocial understanding of major psychiatric disorders in children and adolescents. The psychoanalytic constructs mentioned earlier nevertheless continue to play a useful role, as will be seen shortly.

Developmental Perspectives

Freud's psychoanalytic theory is a developmental theory, and as such it also provided a powerful impetus for a developmental point of view, which became an important fifth theme in the study of childhood psychopathology. One example of how this developmental perspective influenced our views of psychopathology in children can be seen in the continuing historical overview of our viewpoints on mental retardation.

Mental Retardation

Attitudes toward the mentally retarded have varied dramatically throughout recorded history; the mentally retarded have been held in contempt, believed to be demonic, and regarded with adoration (Rosen, Clark, & Kivitz, 1976). The distinction between emotional problems and mental retardation first was made during the eighteenth century in the writings of Locke (Doll, 1962). It was not until the turn of the nineteenth century, however, that a more humane and modern era in the field was ushered in by the work of a French psychiatrist, Itard, who was successful in educating the "Wild Boy of Aveyron" through a system of sensory input and allied habit training. Toward the middle of the nineteenth century (Seguin, 1866), who was inspired by Itard, continued to foster a progressive influence through the establishment of schools and residence centers for the humane care of "idiots and other feebleminded persons." This trend continued throughout the nineteenth century as the American Association of Mental Deficiency was founded (1876) and major attempts were made at educating and improving the lives of the mentally retarded. However, at the end of the nineteenth century the Parisian school of psychiatry and neurology focused its efforts on etiological factors and the identification of a common cerebral defect. This defect theory accounted for a tragic shift in attitudes toward the mentally retarded population. The approach was largely limited to education, and institutionalization of even the mildly retarded was encouraged for the protection of society. Sexual segregation and forced sterilization were commonly recommended (Zigler & Hodapp, 1985). This trend was supported by the popularity of the Binet test of intelligence along with the emphasis on inherited factors, which focused on the defects of a person. Unfortunately, American psychiatry at that time was so fascinated by the psychoanalytic treatment of the neuroses that it tended to neglect the area of mental retardation, since mentally retarded individuals were not seen as appropriate candidates for psychoanalysis.

The current trend is one of reinvolvement in the care and treatment of the mentally retarded. Parent and other advocacy groups brought pressure to bear to ensure the mentally retarded the opportunity to live in the least restrictive environments and have access to education services as mandated by federal law (PL 94-142). Research in developmental psychology meanwhile continued to investigate the sequential stage development of various retarded populations (Weisz & Zigler, 1979), and the implications of a developmental viewpoint for treatment and education began to take shape. Mentally retarded individuals were now seen to develop along the same developmental continuum as nonretarded individuals, albeit at slower rates. Further, mentally retarded children, it was found, could be educated to perform most common tasks adequately. One can readily see evidence of the popular effects of this research in the emotionally charged debates over such issues as educational mainstreaming and deinstitutionalization for community placement of the retarded person.

Based on this newer scientific understanding, a more enlightened attitude regarding the care and treatment of the mentally retarded person began to prevail. When given appropriate social and psychological supports, the majority of mentally retarded individuals were found not to develop psychiatric symptoms. At the same time, the common history of more frequent failure experiences and increased dependency in this population was likely to affect the conflicts, development, and self-esteem of the retarded individual. Mental retardation, nevertheless, was no longer synonymous with psychopathology. It is noteworthy that in DSM-III, and more recently DSM-III-R (American Psychiatric Association, 1980, 1987), mental retardation is considered a developmental disorder. Future trends will depend in large measure on the willingness of mental health professionals to continue their advocacy for this underserved population.

Thus while earlier viewpoints of mental retardation focused almost exclusively on the search for a specific defect in the child, the more recent developmental viewpoint has persuaded many clinicians of the validity of two important concepts: First, no matter what the organic condition (and more than 200 syndromes in which mental retardation is an outcome have been described), all retarded children follow a sequence of emotional and intellectual development that is identical to that followed by normal children, albeit at a slower rate and with a limited end point. Second, retarded children react in the same ways as normal children do to environmental encounters. True, retarded children experience an inordinate amount of failure, rejection, and deprivation. However, the mentally retarded child's *reactions* to these experiences are no different *in kind* from the reaction of a normal child who experiences an undue amount of failure, rejection, and deprivation. Thus many of the behavioral patterns seen in retarded children are now viewed as a result of this *normal reaction*, and are not an intrinsic part of the retardation. The importance of this change in viewpoint is that it radically changes our approach to the retarded child, who is now seen as having the same needs and therefore requiring and deserving the same treatments, in principle, that normal children receive.

Multiple Interactions

Subsequently, a sixth theme in childhood psychopathology emerged in which *all* the previously mentioned themes were viewed as useful contributory theories or models that individually might explain some behaviors, some symptoms, and some syndromes better than any one of the other existing theories, but which had the caveat that no single theory was sufficient to explain all behavior. The idea was that until we had a comprehensive theory we would have to utilize many different theories.

Subsequently, attempts were made to formulate an interactive model for the multiple theories. One such model was the goodness-of-fit framework proposed by Stella Chess, Alexander Thomas, and Herbert Birch (1956) in their New York Longitudinal Study of temperament in children. Temperament was first assessed through the evaluation of nine categories of behavior. Three common temperament groups were found: the "easy" child (40%), the "slow-to-warm-up" child (20%), and the child with a "difficult" temperament (10%). Each of these patterns was then examined in the context of the child's family, giving rise to many different final expressions, depending on whether there was a goodness of fit or a poorness of fit.

An overview of these historical phases in the study of childhood psychopathology reveals different degrees of emphasis at any given time on each of these six major themes: descriptive, environmental, psychoanalytic, biological, developmental, and interactional. Some of the different emphases can be clearly seen in our changing views on the psychopathology of particular disorders.

EXAMPLES OF CHANGING VIEWPOINTS

Infantile Autism

Our view of infantile autism has undergone several changes since Kanner's original description in 1943 of 11 cases of what he called early infantile autism. Kanner stressed the biological roots of the disorder, but also noted, mistakenly, as it happened, a class difference among the parents. Subsequently, psychoanalysts such as Bettelheim blamed "refrigerator mothers" for the condition, causing much guilt and further suffering among parents of autistic children. Then, beginning perhaps in the 1960s, it became clear through research that the type of parenting the child received did *not* account for the condition, although parents surely react to an autistic child, often with depression and social isolation. Today, most of the research findings point to neurobiological factors as being of primary etiological importance in infantile autism. Unfortunately, numerous anatomical and biochemical studies have not revealed any consistent ultimate cause or causes for the disorder (Rutter, 1984). Linguistic and social deficits are current areas of intense investigation.

Depression in Children

Another condition that clearly shows the shifts in emphasis in our understanding of childhood psychopathology is depression in children. Until the 1960s psychoanalysts, whose views prevailed at that time, posited that according to psychoanalytic theory (i.e., the development of the superego as a necessary condition for the occurrence of depression) depression in childhood was impossible. Rochlin (1959) stated the psychoanalysts' position unequivocally: "Classical depression, a superego phenomenon, as we psychoanalysts understand the disorder, does not occur in childhood" (p. 299). This view began to change in the 1960s and 1970s when the ideas that children *did* suffer from major depressive disorders and that childhood depression was *isomorphic* with adult depression began to prevail. This change in viewpoints culminated in the use of the same DSM-III (1980) major depressive disorder criteria for both children and adults. Numerous biological markers found in adults were then studied in children, confirming more or less this shift in our view of the psychopathology of depression in children and adolescents. Children were found to have test results that on the whole (sleep architecture was an exception) were in the same direction as those found in adults.

Having established this isomorphic viewpoint, clinicians then began to look for differences rather than similarities between depression in children and depression in adults. Thus a current approach in our view on depression in children is to look more closely at the consequences of developmental differences between children and adults who are depressed. Some of these developmental differences are reflected in DSM-III-R.

Attention Deficit Hyperactivity Disorder

The interactional approach is well illustrated in studies on attention deficit hyperactivity disorder (ADHD). In 1908, Tredgold coined the term *minimal brain damage*, one of a succession of many terms to label children who appear to be impulsive, inattentive, and hyperactive. However, in spite of numerous studies, no specific brain lesion for all children with ADHD has ever been reliably documented. Similarly, a wide range of etiological factors, including genetic factors, perinatal insult, infections, lead poisoning, head injury, metabolic disorders, neurotransmitter disorders, and dietetic and psychosocial factors, have at one time or another been implicated in the cause of ADHD. Since the disorder now appears to have a complex etiology, the prevailing view again tends to a more complex interactional model of pathogenesis. This interactional model has also served as a basis for the multimodal treatment approach that is now recommended for children with the disorder.

Violence in Children and Adolescents

Early views on the psychopathology of aggressive behavior in children and adolescents included Lombroso's presumed (but unproved) theory of genetic transmission, psychoanalytic theories such as the superego lacunae concept (Johnson & Szurek, 1952), sociological theories including role models (Shaw & McKay, 1942), social frustration (Merton, 1957), and a deprivation model describing a core of minority delinquents from socioeconomically deprived backgrounds (Wolfgang, Figlio, & Cellin, 1972). More recently, attention has been paid to neurobiological factors, including norepinephrine (Alpert, Cohen, Shaywitz, & Piccirillo, 1981) and 5-hydroxytryptamine (Valzelli, 1974) metabolism, hyporesponsive autonomic activity (Mednick & Christiansen, 1977), and elevated testosterone levels (Mattsson, Schalling, Oliwens, Löw, & Svensson, 1980).

Gradually, a belief has emerged that what we are dealing with in many instances of aggressive and violent behavior in children and adolescents is a symptom that represents a final common pathway brought about by the confluence of multiple psychosocial vulnerabilities including neurological deficits, psychosis, and severe physical abuse (both witnessed and suffered) (Lewis, Shenok, Pincus, & Glazer, 1979; Lewis, 1981). Thus a contemporary view of violent children is that the aggressive behavior is frequently caused by the interaction of multiple etiological factors, symptoms, and diagnoses, and that there is rarely a simple "cause" for the violence.

DISCUSSION

One further historical note worth mentioning is the oscillation between each of the viewpoints just outlined and illustrated; one example is the debate that apparently still continues between maturationists and developmentalists. Gesell, of course, was an early ardent proponent of the maturational point of view. Freud, Erikson, and others are obvious examples of early proponents of the developmental point of view. More recently, a maturational approach has reappeared in the form of a new concept called discontinuities. The leading example here is Kagan, who noted, for example, an enhancement of memory between 8 and 12 months of age and a shift from a perceptual mode to a symbolic–linguistic mode at about 17 months (Kagan, 1979). Kagan hypothesized that this shift was essentially a *discontinuity* that occurred almost entirely on the basis of CNS maturation. One consequence of this maturational viewpoint revisited was the suggestion that not *all* the experiences of the average infant with his or her parents necessarily have a long-lasting or cumulative effect, since new maturational phenomena might add to the plasticity of the infant and in effect supersede previous behaviors and experiences. Kagan in fact suggested that problems seen during the first year or so of life may linger for 2 or 3 years but may then diminish and eventually disappear. At the same time, Hunt (1979) has noted: "A major share of early losses can be made up if the development-fostering quality of experience improves, and a great deal of early gain can be lost if the quality of experience depreciates" (p. 136).

Nevertheless, the concept of a complex, interactional model is now widely employed in most research being undertaken in a wide variety of conditions, including obsessive-compulsive disorder, phobic disorder, panic disorder, pervasive developmental disorders, personality disorders, and Tourette's syndrome. The components of the interactions suggested by this research include psychodynamic, genetic, organic, neurochemical, cognitive, developmental, and socioenvironmental interactions. This current viewpoint is admittedly more complex than previously held "single" viewpoints, but it is probably more accurate. It remains to be seen precisely how these multiple factors interact to produce psychopathology in children and adolescents.

REFERENCES

Alpert, J.E., Cohen, D.J., Shaymitz, B.A., & Piccirillo, M. (1981). Neurochemical and behavioral organization: Disorder of attention, activity, and aggression. In D.O. Lewis (Ed.), *Vulnerabilities to delinquency*. New York: Spectrum.

American Psychiatric Association. (1980). *Diagnostic and statistical manual of mental disorders* (3rd ed.). Washington, DC: Author.

American Psychiatric Association. (1987). *Diagnostic and statistical manual of mental disorders* (3rd ed., rev.). Washington, DC: Author.

Doll, E.E. (1962). A historical survey of research and management of mental retardation in the United States. In E.P. Trapp & P. Himelstein (Eds.), *Readings on the exceptional child*. New York: Appleton-Century-Crofts.

Freud, S. (1909). Analysis of a phobia in a five-year-old boy. In J. Strachey (Ed. and Trans.), *The standard edition of the complete psychological works of Sigmund Freud* (Vol. 10, pp. 3–152). London: Hogarth Press, 1955.

Gesell, A. (1952). Arnold Gesell. In E.G. Boring, H.S. Langfeld, H. Werner, and R.M. Yerkes (Eds.), *History of psychology in autobiography* (Vol. 4). Worcester, MA: Clark University Press.

Glaser, K. (1967). Masked depression in children and adolescents. *American Journal of Psychotherapy, 11*, 565.

Goddard, H. (1912). *The Kallikak family*. New York: Macmillan.

Hunt, J. McV. (1979). Psychological development: Early experience. In L.W. Porter & M.R. Rosenzweig (Eds.), *Annual review of psychology* (Vol. 30). Palo Alto: Annual Review.

Johnson, A.M., & Szurek, S.A. (1952). The genesis of antisocial acting out in children and adults. *Psychoanalytic Quarterly, 21*, 323.

Kagan, J. (1979). The form of early development. *Archives of General Psychiatry, 36*, 1047–1054.

Kanner, L. (1943). Autistic disturbances of affective contact. *Nervous Children, 2*, 217–250.

Kessen, W. (1965). *The child*. New York: Wiley.

Lewis, D.O. (Ed.). (1981). *Vulnerabilities to delinquency*. New York: Spectrum.

Lewis, D.O., Shanok, S.S., Pincus, J.H., & Glazer, O.H. (1979). Violent juvenile delinquents: Psychiatric, neurological, psychological and abuse factors. *Journal of the American Academy of Child Psychiatry*, *18*, 307–319.

Mattsson, A., Schalling, D., Oliwens, D., Löw, H., & Svensson, J. (1980). Plasma testosterone, aggressive behavior, and personality dimensions in young male delinquents. *Journal of the American Academy of Child Psychiatry*, *19*, 476–491.

Mednick, S.A., & Christiansen, K.O. (Eds.). (1977). *Biosocial bases of criminal behavior*. New York: Gardner.

Merton, R.K. (1957). *Social theory and social structure*. New York: Free Press.

Rochlin, C. (1959). The loss complex: A contribution to the etiology of depression. *Journal of the American Psychoanalytic Association*, *7*, 299–316.

Rosen, M., Clark, G., and Kivitz, M. (1976). *The history of mental retardation* (Vol. 1). Baltimore: University Park Press.

Rutter, M. (1984). Cognitive deficits in the pathogenesis of autism. *Journal of Child Psychology and Psychiatry*, *24*, 513.

Sears, R.R. (1975). *Your ancients revisited: A history of child development*. Chicago: University of Chicago Press.

Seguin, E. (1866). *Idiocy: Its treatment by the physiological method*. New York: Teachers College, Columbia University.

Shaw, R.C., & McKay, H.D. (1942). *Juvenile delinquency and urban areas*. Chicago: University of Chicago Press.

Toolan, J.M. (1962). Depression in children and adolescents. *American Journal of Orthopsychiatry*, *32*, 404.

Valzelli, L. (1974). 5-hydroxytryptamine in aggressiveness. In E. Costa, G. Gessa, & M. Sanderl (Eds.), *Advances in biochemical psychopharmacology*. New York: Raven.

Weisz, J.R., & Zigler, E. (1979). Cognitive development in retarded and nonretarded persons: Piagetian tests of the similar-sequence hypothesis. *Psychological Bulletin*, *86*, 831–851.

Wolfgang, M.E., Figlio, R.M., & Cellin, T. (1972). *Delinquency in a birth cohort*. Chicago: University of Chicago Press.

Zigler, E., & Hodapp, R.M. (1985). Mental retardation. In J.O. Cavenar (Ed.), *Psychiatry* (Vol. 2). Philadelphia: Lippincott.

CHAPTER 2

A Nosological Approach to Assessing Childhood Psychiatric Disorders

PAUL V. TRAD

In spite of the fact that child psychiatric clinics throughout the United States and Europe see large numbers of children for a wide array of psychiatric, behavioral, and developmental conditions, research regarding this population is itself in its infancy. The fact that research into childhood disorders has only recently begun to yield useful information may be explainable in part by the difficulties inherent in evaluating members of this extremely heterogeneous cohort.

A child who may be demonstrating a psychiatric disturbance must be evaluated in terms of two basic parameters. The first is the child's *developmental level*. Is there a discrepancy between the child's behavior and his or her age, intelligence, or social status? Second, the *adaptive*, or *functional*, level of the child must be evaluated. In other words, does the problematic behavior interfere seriously with physical, mental, academic, or social functioning?

One of the problems that the clinician faces in evaluating and classifying a given child is the child's lack of expertise in fully and clearly expressing his or her feelings. Alternatively, when parents or teachers are relied upon, as they almost universally are, there is a risk of underestimating the severity of the disturbance (Weissman et al., 1986).

Another consideration to make on the way to obtaining an accurate diagnostic picture is whether the reason for referral lies with the child or with the parents. It may also be that the child's problem stems from the family's interactional dynamics and structure—considerations that we shall soon take up. When disorders suggest situation specificity, or are situation specific, it is necessary to collect information from several relevant sources, and to approach the disorder in interactional terms to account for interpersonal interactions and social contexts (Sullivan, 1956).

Since the mother or caregiver is usually the source of referral, the clinician must be on guard against developing a bias. It may be easy in many cases to overidentify with the child, blaming the parents for more than their share of the problem. Bias in the other direction must be guarded against as well. The assumption that an evaluation based on a brief office visit with the child is more valid than information given by the mother is often unjustified. The diagnostic procedures are made even more difficult by the fact that, in using current nosology, for example, the DSM-III-R (American Psychiatric Association, 1987), there is considerable room for overlap among currently recognized disorders.

In order to make these evaluations, it is crucially important to be able to interview not only the child but also the parents, teachers, and any others who may have valuable information. Skills in behavior observation are also a requisite, as is the ability to rule out other conditions that may be generating the same set of symptoms.

A second dimension that presents difficulties but that must nevertheless be taken into account comprises the *developmental changes* associated with normal maturation (Trad, 1986, 1987). Since the determination of continuities and discontinuities in the quality of adaptation from birth to adulthood is of fundamental importance to the field of developmental psychology, perhaps the most noticeable gap in the literature to date is the paucity of longitudinal studies.

When evaluating a child, it is essential to attend to the developmental context, since an understanding of the age-appropriate range of normal behaviors provides a mean of assessing the degree to which a given disturbance (or disturbances) has interfered with normal development. Additionally, the different phases of development, exemplified by the Piagetian system of cognitive development, are accompanied by different challenges and vulnerabilities that must be adjusted for.

Another component of the mind-set necessary for comprehensive psychiatric evaluation of children is the realization that, since childhood behaviors are embedded in the overall context of maturation and development, emotional problems must be viewed as exaggerations or deficiencies of behavior patterns seen in every child (Plenk & Hinchey, 1985). Symptoms in children cannot be regarded as a set of adjectives that will combine to describe a discrete psychologic state. Instead, childhood symptoms are more accurately viewed as existing, to one degree or another, along the entire behavioral continuum available to every child. Thus screening for psychopathology in childhood is largely a matter of assessing the behavioral manifestations along the dimensions of intensity, frequency, and duration, as well as the number of other abnormal behaviors, attitudes toward the problem, the extent of restriction of social activities, and the effects on others of the child's behavior.

Also important in diagnostic formulation is an examination of prior circumstances, precipitants, and contingencies in order to determine the significance of the behavior under scrutiny. The term *prior circumstances* refers to long-standing conditions that are helpful in determining the likelihood of certain behaviors. Precipitants are the events or circumstances that seem to initiate a problem, and contingencies are the expected responses to a specific behavior. Attention to these three surrounding factors can help in understanding the function and meaning of certain behaviors (Richman, 1985). Epidemiology regarding the nature and prevalence of psychiatric disorders must also be considered in diagnosis (Cox & Rutter, 1985), and, finally, a differential diagnosis must be performed before a course of treatment is formulated.

This discussion presents an overview of the tools and perspective needed in order to diagnose accurately the pathological texture of childhood behaviors. In addition to understanding the current status of DSM-III-R nosology for childhood, this will require knowledge about the effects of family variables, as well as the ability to conduct child and parent interviews, with expertise in the administration of standardized tests.

FACTORS INVOLVED IN MAKING THE DIFFERENTIAL DIAGNOSIS

Once the diagnostic procedure is under way, a range of discoveries is possible. If a significant problem exists, it may be a single stressful habit, such as temper tantrums. On the other hand, the problem may be a learning disorder or some other more pervasive condition, causing disturbances along a number of other behavioral axes. For example, children with autism must be differentiated from those who are mentally retarded or otherwise biologically impaired and from others who may be largely fearful and withdrawn; hyperactive and impulsive children must be separated from those who have problems with habit training or who display aggressive behavior. The foregoing example demonstrates the need for moment-to-moment awareness of the developmental context in which the child is embedded.

While the assessment procedure, consisting of family evaluation, child interview, observations and testing, and parent and/or teacher interview, should be directed at establishing the persistence and severity of the problem and the degree to which social functioning is impaired, it is important to guard against simply assembling a list of labels. The complete assessment goes beyond this stage, providing a picture of the child that is complete enough to allow closure when gaps occur.

One of the benefits derived from achieving a complete assessment is the discovery of the child's strengths as well as his or her weaknesses. This provides the opportunity to incorporate helpful attributes into the treatment schedule, a technique that will not only better equip the child to succeed but also be likely to put parents at their ease, making them feel that their child is not seen wholly as being dysfunctional.

CONTRIBUTIONS TO NOSOLOGY FROM FAMILY EVALUATIONS

Family Type

In addition to knowledge about the developmental context, the clinician will benefit from a clear understanding about the child's familial context. There are as yet few known direct correlations between family background and the development of abnormal behavior; however, family variables doubtless play a significant role in increasing or decreasing the risk for onset of some childhood disorders.

Parental marital status—specifically, separated, divorced, or remarried—has been noted innumerable times in the background of children with psychopathology. Brady, Bray, and Zeeb (1986) performed an excellent study with 703 children who were seen in a clinic. Looking for interactions between family type and age and sex of child, these investigators used the Conners Parent Questionnaire and found that the most severe problems occurred in children from separated families. Additionally, it was found that conduct problems and hyperactive behavior occurred more often in children from remarried families than in children from either divorced or separated families.

Boys in this study and in others (Guidubaldi, Perry, & Cleminshaw, 1984) appeared to suffer greater overall disturbance than girls as a result of family instability. Therefore, in terms of overall assessment, it is useful to know that boys tend to experience more difficulty in adjusting to a disordered family life than girls, and that the behavioral disturbance of a child from a separated or remarried home may tend to be more severe and to warrant more intensive assessment and care than that of a child from an intact or divorced home. While it should be kept in mind that these are gross generalizations very vulnerable to contradictions, these relationships nonetheless provide the clinician with a general framework he or she can use to test various hypotheses during the course of assessment and therapy.

Effect of Maternal Depression on Child Behavior

A study by Fergusson, Horwood, and Shannon (1984) casts additional light on the work of Brady and coworkers. The investigators looked for interrelations between the effects of stressful life events on the mother and the child. Specifically, Fergusson and colleagues studied the role of maternal mood and the effect of stressful life events and behavior problems in a cohort of 1265 children. These children were examined at birth, 4 months, and annually up to 5 years of age.

After excluding effects from a number of other family and social characteristics (e.g., family size and type; maternal educational level, age, and ethnicity; family living standards), Fergusson and coworkers found that correlations between family life events and maternal reports of child-rearing problems were largely attributable to the mediating effects of maternal depression.

As the authors point out, this result might have been produced by a mechanism in which the children of depressed mothers react to the mother's negative mood by developing more and more behavior problems. However, the result could just as well be explained by another mechanism in which the depressive condition changes the way in which the mother perceives her child's behavior. Due to the fact that the study was based on maternal reporting, it was not possible to isolate which mechanism was operative.

However, regardless of the particular mechanism, the role of parental mood as a mediator in children's behavior provides the clinician with an important diagnostic clue. For example, if in a given case the child's problematic behavior is difficult to substantiate, it may be advisable to consider maternal depression as the factor underlying referral of the child. Regardless of whether the child truly has a behavioral problem or whether the mother's perception is faulty, treatment of the maternal depression will likely benefit both mother and child.

Parental Role in the Etiology of Psychosis

Another area in which parents may play a strong mediational role in the pathologic development of their children is psychosis. One variable of concern is that children with a psychotic parent or parents are less likely to be exposed to persons who are cognitively more mature than they. Without this exposure, development is bound to be adversely affected.

Chandler (1978) has stressed the pathogenic effect of impaired cognitive development by focusing on the role of parental egocentric thinking in the genesis of childhood psychiatric disorders. Chandler noted that egocentric thinking was common in a population of mothers with histories of serious psychiatric disorders. Therefore, a test was devised to measure the degree of egocentric thinking among their offspring and the deficits attributable to the deficit. It was found that these children were slower to relinquish their own egocentric assumptions than were control children, and Chandler noted that these egocentric errors were comparable to those observed in seriously emotionally disturbed children.

Thus there may be a pathological relationship between parental egocentric thinking and child development in which the children are less likely to differentiate between themselves and their parents. Therefore, they are less motivated to establish a separate existence. In cases of suspected childhood psychosis, the clinician may be well advised to look for signs of parental egocentrism. It is clear that the investigation of family antecedents (genetic and social) widens the context for the assessment of psychopathology during the childhood years.

DSM-III-R AND MULTIAXIAL EVALUATIONS

In psychiatric assessment, many phenomena are difficult to describe in a manner devoid of personal, internal formulations. Thus Dr. Jaspers (1963) developed a technique for describing accurately nonobjective occurrences. This technique is called phenomenology, and it is similar in format to listings in the DSM-III-R.

When noting the occurrence of psychopathologic phenomena, observers need to differentiate clearly among those they observe directly, those that are derived from patient history, and those that are described by the patient. In recording, the clinician uses *sign* to denote his or her own observations and *symptom* to denote a patient's verbal indications. The psychiatric interview is the vehicle for collecting signs and symptoms, and these combine to constitute the mental status examination, which is used as a diagnostic tool.

A multiaxial evaluation requires assessment of each case on several *axes*, or through different types of information. There is a limited number of axes—five in the DSM-III-R multiaxial classification—ensuring maximal clinical utility. Axes I, II, and III make up the official diagnostic assessment. Use of the DSM-III-R multiaxial system ensures that attention is given to certain types of disorders, to aspects of the environment, and to areas of functioning that might be overlooked if the focus were on assessing a single presenting problem.

Each person is evaluated on each of these axes:

Axis I   Clinical Syndromes and V Codes
Axis II   Developmental Disorders and Personality Disorders

Axis III Physical Disorders and Conditions

Axis IV Severity of Psychosocial Stressors

Axis V   Global Assessment of Functioning

Axes I and II: Clinical Syndromes and V Codes

Axes I and II make up the entire classification of mental disorders plus V Codes. The Axis I–Axis II distinction highlights the need to consider disorders involving the development of cognitive, social, and motor skills when evaluating children.

Developmental disorders and personality disorders, listed on Axis II, usually present during childhood or adolescence and continue without either becoming more profound or going into remission through adult life. Axis I disorders are not usually characterized by these histories. It is not uncommon for a disorder to be on both Axis I and Axis II.

In some cases there may not be a disorder on Axis I; rather, treatment is for a disorder limited to Axis II, and a clinician would note this as follows: "Axis I: No diagnosis or condition on Axis I, or one of the conditions not attributable to a mental disorder." In instances where a disorder is noted on Axis I when there is no evidence of an Axis II disorder, the clinician would note the following: "Axis II: No diagnosis on Axis II."

When more than one diagnosis is given, the one that effected initial evaluation or clinical admission usually is regarded as the principal diagnosis, whether it is an Axis I or II diagnosis. If the principal diagnosis is on Axis II, the clinician should note *principal diagnosis*. If there are disorders on both Axis I and Axis II, the principal diagnosis is assumed to be on Axis I unless the Axis II diagnosis is followed by the qualifying phrase *principal diagnosis*.

To describe the current condition, *multiple diagnoses* should be made on both Axis I and II as indicated. When there are multiple diagnoses made on either Axis I or Axis II, they are listed within each axis in order of focus of attention or treatment. It is common, for example, to have multiple diagnoses of specific developmental disorders within Axis II. Specific personality traits or the habitual use of particular defense mechanisms can be indicated on Axis II, both when no personality disorder exists and to supplement a personality disorder diagnosis when personality traits are noted.

In some instances where there is not enough information to make a firm diagnosis, the clinician may wish to write *provisional* after the diagnosis, to indicate that a significant diagnostic uncertainty exists.

Diagnostic categories that are pertinent for children are listed in these sections. One section is called "Disorders Usually First Evident in Infancy, Childhood, and Adolescence." Other diagnostic categories that can be used for children are listed in the adult diagnoses section. This system permits a bidirectional crossover for children and adults. The following table lists all the diagnostic categories that may be evident in infancy, childhood, or adolescence. The main point of listing all of both child and adult diagnostic categories under one heading is to represent the degree of continuity between categories.

Disorders That May Be Evident in Infancy, Childhood, or Adolescence (DSM-III-R)

AXIS I

Adjustment Disorder. May begin at any age.

Anorexia Nervosa. Age of onset usually early to late adolescence, although it can range from prepuberty to early thirties (rare).

Attention-Deficit Hyperactivity Disorder. Onset before age of 7.

Autistic Disorder. Onset during infancy or childhood (if childhood, after 36 months).

Avoidant Disorder of Childhood or Adolescence. Age of onset at least 2½ years.

Body Dysmorphic Disorder. Most common age of onset is from adolescence through third decade.

Bulimia Nervosa. Usually begins in adolescence or early adult life.

Chronic Motor or Vocal Tic Disorder. Onset before the age of 21.

Cluttering. Usual onset is after 7 years.

Conduct Disorder. Usually prepubertal, particularly of solitary aggressive type.

Conversion Disorder. Usual age at onset is in adolescence or early adulthood, but symptoms may appear for first time during middle age, even in later decades.

Cyclothymia. Usually begins in adolescence or early adult life.

Depersonalization Disorder. Most often begins in adolescence.

Dyssomnias

> *Hypersomnia Disorders*: Hypersomnia related to another mental disorder; hypersomnia related to a known organic factor; primary hypersomnia. All can begin at any age.

> *Insomnia Disorders*: Insomnia related to another mental disorder; insomnia related to a known organic factor; primary insomnia.

> *Sleep–Wake Schedule Disorder*: Can begin at any age.

Dysthymia. Usually begins in childhood, adolescence, or early adult life.

Elective Mutism. Usually before 5 years.

Functional Encopresis. Primary functional encopresis begins by 4 years. Secondary functional encopresis occurs between 4 and 7 years.

Functional Enuresis. Primary functional enuresis begins by age 5. Secondary functional enuresis occurs between 5 and 8 years.

Gender Identity Disorder of Childhood. Majority of boys with this disorder begin to develop it before the fourth birthday. With females, onset is early, but exaggerated insistence on male activities and attire not apparent until late childhood or adolescence.

Gender Identity Disorder of Adolescence or Adulthood, Nontranssexual Type (GIDAANT). Occurs after person has reached puberty.

Hypochondrias. Can begin at any age; most common age of onset is between 20 and 30 years.

Identity Disorder. Onset during late adolescence, young adulthood, or even middle age.

Impulse Control Disorders Not Elsewhere Classified

    Intermittent Explosive Disorder: May begin at any stage of life.

    Kleptomania: Age of onset as early as childhood.

    Pathological Gambling: In males, usually begins during adolescence; in females, usually beings later in life.

    Pyromania: Age of onset usually in childhood.

    Trichotillomania: Age of onset usually in childhood.

Major Depressive Episode. Average onset is in late twenties but may begin at any age, even infancy.

Manic Episode. Mean age at onset is early twenties.

Mental Retardation. Onset before the age of 18 years.

Multiple Personality Disorder. Age of onset is almost invariably in childhood.

Oppositional Defiant Disorder. May appear in early childhood. Typically begins at 8 years and not usually later than early childhood.

Overanxious Disorder. No information on the age of onset.

Paraphilias

    Exhibitionism: Usually occurs before age 18.

    Fetishism: Usually begins by adolescence, although the fetish may have been endowed with special significance in childhood.

    Frotteurism: Usually begins by adolescence.

    Pedophilia: Usually begins in adolescence, although may begin at middle age.

    Sexual Dysfunction: Most common age of onset is early adulthood.

    Sexual Masochism: Likely to be present in childhood.

    Sexual Sadism: Likely to be present in childhood.

    Transvestite Fetishism: Begins with cross-dressing in childhood or early adolescence.

    Voyeurism: Usually has onset before the age of 15.

Parasomnias

    Dream Anxiety Disorder: Can start before age 10.

    Sleep Terror Disorder: Usually begins between the ages of 4 and 12 years.

    Sleep Walking Disorder: Usually begins between the ages of 6 and 12 years.

Pica. Age of onset usually 12 to 24 months; may begin earlier.

Psychogenic Amnesia. Most often observed in adolescence.

Psychogenic Fugue. Age of onset is variable.

Reactive Attachment Disorder of Infancy or Early Childhood. Age of onset before 5 years.

Rumination Disorder of Infancy. Usually appears between 3 and 12 months. In children with mental retardation, occasionally begins later.

Schizophrenia. Age of onset is usually during adolescence or early adulthood. May begin in middle or late adult life.

Schizophreniform Disorder. Age of onset similar to that of schizophrenia.

Separation Anxiety Disorder. Onset before age 18.

Somatization Disorder. Symptoms begin in teen years.

Somatization Pain Disorder. Can occur at any stage of life, from childhood to old age.

Stereotype/Habit Disorder. Usually first seen in childhood and may intensify in adolescence.

Stuttering. Typically begins between 2 and 7 years (peak onset around 5 years).

Tourette's Disorder. Onset before the age of 21.

Transient Tic Disorder. Onset before the age of 21.

Transsexualism. Usually full syndrome has onset by late adolescence or early adult life; in some cases, this disorder has a later onset.

Other diagnostic categories that are often appropriate for children and adolescents are the following:

Organic mental syndromes, for example, intoxication, organic hallucinosis
Organic mental disorder, for example, psychoactive substance use disorders

AXIS II
Developmental Disorders

Developmental Arithmetic Disorder: Usually apparent by 8 years old and not after 10 years.

Developmental Articulation Disorder: If severe, onset at 3 years; if less severe, onset at 6 years.

Developmental Coordination Disorder: Usually occurs when child first attempts such tasks as running, holding knife or fork, and/or buttoning clothes.

Developmental Expressive Language Disorder: If severe, onset at before 3 years; if less severe, may not occur until early adolescence

Developmental Expressive Writing Disorder: Usually apparent by age 7 in severe cases; 10 years if less severe.

Developmental Reading Disorder: Usually apparent by 7 years. If severe, onset at around 6 years; if less severe, onset at around 9 years.

Developmental Receptive Language Disorder: Typically occurs before 4 years. If severe, occurs at 2 years; if mild, may not be evident until child is 7 years or older when language becomes more complex.

V Codes are conditions that are a focus of attention or treatment but are not attributable to any of the mental disorders noted earlier.

V Codes

    Academic problem

    Borderline intellectual functioning

    Childhood or adolescent antisocial behavior

    Malingering

    Noncompliance with medical treatment

    Occupational problem

    Other interpersonal problem

    Other specified family circumstances

    Parent–child problem

    Phase of life problem or other life circumstance problem

    Uncomplicated bereavement

Personality *traits* are enduring patterns of perceiving, relating to, and thinking about the environment and oneself, and are exhibited in a wide range of important social and personal contexts. It is only when personality traits are inflexible and maladaptive and cause either significant functional impairment or subjective distress that they constitute *Personality Disorders*.

                                       (*DSM-III-R*, p. 335)

Personality disorder categories may be applied to children or adolescents in those instances in which the particular traits appear to be stable. However, one exception to this rule is antisocial personality disorder. (The diagnosis of Conduct Disorder should be made if the person is under 18 years of age.)

Personality Disorders

    Antisocial Personality Disorder

    Avoidant Personality Disorder

    Borderline Personality Disorder

    Dependent Personality Disorder

    Histrionic Personality Disorder

    Narcissistic Personality Disorder

    Obsessive-Compulsive Personality Disorder

    Paranoid Personality Disorder

    Passive-Aggressive Personality Disorder

    Schizoid Personality Disorder

    Schizotypal Personality Disorder

It is vital that the clinician not view the child as a presentation of symptoms that neatly add up to equal a definitive diagnostic label. Not only does such an approach deny the continuous change occurring in children; it also ignores the extensive overlap of symptoms among different disorders.

For example, a child may be referred for treatment because of depressed and irritable mood, symptoms found in many disorders, ranging from major depression to conduct disorder. Perhaps preliminary assessment indicates to the clinician that the field of possible diagnoses is restricted to, say, major depression, schizophrenia, gender identity disorder of adolescence and adulthood, nontranssexual type, and separation anxiety disorder.

A look into the possibility that the child is suffering from symptoms related to major depression may bear out a strong correlation between the child's symptoms and DSM-III-R criteria for diagnosing the disorder. Perhaps the clinician investigated thoroughly and decides, almost for certain, that what the child suffers from is, indeed, major depression. To approach a more positive diagnosis, the clinician must then perform a differential diagnosis. In the case where major depression is suspected, the differential diagnosis entails examination of the possibility that symptoms are really indicative of any of the following disorders: organic mood syndrome with depression; schizophrenia, catatonic type; schizoaffective disorder; dementia with depression; pseudodementia; psychological reaction to functional impairment associated with a physical illness; manic episode or unequivocal hypomanic episode; and dysthymia.

In the event that the suspected disorder is schizophrenia, the clinician must perform a differential diagnosis against organic mental disorder, mood disorder (depressive disorder NOS, or bipolar disorder NOS, or mood disorder with psychotic features), schizoaffective disorder, psychotic disorder NOS, schizophreniform disorder, delusional disorder, autistic disorder, pervasive developmental disorder NOS, obsessive-compulsive disorder, hypochondriasis, factitious disorder with psychological symptoms, mental retardation, beliefs or experiences of members of religious or other cultural groups, and personality disorders.

Clearly, the clinician who attempts to label a disorder based solely on the addition of clear symptoms will be prone to error. Approach should be made from a wide perspective, and narrowed according not only to symptoms but also to both the developmental significance of the symptoms and the possible other causes of the symptoms' presentation.

Axis III: Physical Disorders and Conditions

On Axis III, the clinician can note any current physical disorder or condition that may be relevant to understanding or managing a case. In some instances the physical condition is etiologically significant while in others it is not, but is still relevant to overall case management. In some cases the clinician may elect to note significant associated physical findings, such as soft neurologic signs. Multiple diagnoses are permitted.

Axis IV: Severity of Psychosocial Stressors

The Severity of Psychosocial Stressors Scale is a scale used to code the overall severity of a psychosocial stressor or multiple psychosocial stressors that confronted the child in the year preceding the current evaluation and may have played a role in any of the following:

1. Development of a new mental disorder
2. Recurrence of a prior mental disorder
3. Exacerbation of an already existing mental disorder

Although stressors often play a causative role in disorder, they might also be a consequence of a person's psychopathology.

Rating the severity of the stressor is based on the clinician's estimate of the stress that an average person, in similar circumstances and with similar sociocultural values, would endure as a result of a particular psychosocial stressor(s). This judgment entails consideration of the following: how much change is caused in the person's life due to the stressor; to what degree the occurrence is wanted and is under the person's control; and what the number of stressors is.

Specific psychosocial stressors are then further specified as either predominantly acute events (duration of shorter than 6 months), for example, acute psychotic decompensation of a bipolar parent, or predominantly enduring circumstances (duration of longer than 6 months), for example, paranoid-type schizophrenia in either of the parents.

Axis V: Global Assessment of Functioning

Axis V permits the clinician to present an overall judgment of a person's psychological, social, and occupational functioning using the Global Assessment of Functioning Scale (GAF scale), which asesses mental health or illness.

Ratings on the GAF scale need to be made for two time periods:

1. *Current*—the level of functioning at the time of the evaluation
2. *Past year*—the highest level of functioning that lasted for at least a few months during the past year. For children and adolescents, this should include at least a month during the school year

Ratings of current functioning generally reveal the current need for treatment. Ratings of highest level of functioning during the past year often have prognostic significance, as a person usually returns to his or her prior level of functioning after an illness.

DEVELOPMENTAL PSYCHIATRIC NOSOLOGY

Thus far, examples of the diagnostic clues inherent in the developmental and family contexts have been described. The need remains to discuss testing and observation techniques. However, it is first necessary to outline briefly the state of childhood diagnostic nosology. A comprehension of the current type of symptom systematization and its present level of sophistication will provide the clinician with the perspective needed to differentiate between firm diagnoses and those that may be more tentative.

Investigations into childhood psychopathology have most recently approached aberrant conditions being predominantly associated with one of two broad-band dimensions of behavior, the externalizing and internalizing dimensions. Externalizing symptoms are characterized by undercontrolled, aggressive behavior, while internalizing symptoms exist along a continuum of being overcontrolled, withdrawn, and anxious. This two-factor model of behavioral disorders is the basis of DSM-III-R nosology.

Fischer, Rolf, Hasafi, and Cousins (1984) performed a study whose results are typical of the information being derived from the DSM-III-R factor-analytic approach. These investigators followed 541 preschool children who were receiving either day or home care, evaluating them first as preschoolers and later when the children were 9 to 15 years of age. Like many other investigators (e.g., Kellman, Branch, Agrawal, & Ensminger, 1975; Kohn, 1977), Fischer and colleagues found there was continuity in internalizing and externalizing behaviors across the period from preschool to 7 years later.

The behavior that appeared to be most stable across time was angry–defiant behavior, suggesting that externalizing symptoms may be more predictive of later psychopathology. However, this result was in opposition to that of Kellam and colleagues, who found the withdrawn behaviors to be more stable than the externalizing symptoms. Additionally, unlike Fischer and colleagues Kohn found that early shy behavior was more predictive of later negative outcome.

Rescorla (1986) has attempted to explain these mixed results by noting that many preschool children demonstrate both internalizing and externalizing symptoms. In order to shed further light on the validity and usefulness of the broad-band factor-analytic system of nosology, Rescorla studied retrospectively the case records of 274 children 3 to 5 years old who had been evaluated and treated prior to the advent of DSM-III (APA, 1980).

The diagnostic categories used by the clinic prior to publication of DSM-III were severe atypical development (analogous to DSM-III childhood onset PDD); reactive disorder; and "other," which included children with language delay, hyperkinetic syndrome, or minimal brain dysfunction in the absence of neurologic disorder.

Thirty-four percent of the 274 children were classified as atypical to some degree. In opposition to the distinction of DSM-III, however, the majority of children in both atypical groups showed deviant development prior to 30 months. Thus the DSM-III method of distinguishing between different types of PDD in terms of age of onset was not validated. Significantly, this conceptualization has been eradicated in DSM-III-R, which recognizes autism as the only subcategory of PDDs.

Apart from demonstrating the considerable heterogeneity of symptoms in the child population and the applicability of more than one system of classification, the study by Rescorla demonstrated a close interrelationship between aggressive–destructive behavior and feelings of anxiety, sadness, and emotional insecurity. Thus the DSM-III-R demarcation between acting-out problems, such as conduct or oppositional disorder, and internalizing syndromes, such as anxiety disorders, may not be accurate.

Another finding that might lead to nosological changes was the very strong association between aggressive–destructive, acting-out behavior and problems of impulse control and attention. Forty percent of all girls and 45% of the boys scored high on both factors. This may indicate that, contrary to DSM-III-R nosology, impulsivity–hyperactivity is not distinct from conduct disorder. Instead, they may be two factors associated with the same disorder, as suggested by Quay (1979).

DIAGNOSTIC PROCEDURES

With the awareness that current nosology of childhood psychiatric disorders is still very much in flux, the diagnostic formulation can be integrated by combining information from the psychiatric history and family and parental evaluation with the signs and symptoms obtained from observation and testing (Akiskal, 1986). Plenk and Hinchey (1985) recommend that a complete evaluation should consist of standardized testing, behavioral observation and rating, a developmental history, and play interviews.

In their general structure and attention to detail, the evaluations performed by Plenk and Hinchey in their clinic provide an excellent model for discussion. Parent–child interactions are first observed in the waiting room, where such parameters as involvement with either parent, independence of play, propriety of verbal interchange, activity level of the child, and the ability of the parent to supervise the child are noted. The child is observed closely when the parent is invited into the inner office to give the developmental history. Variables such as comfort with separation are evaluated.

The developmental history should cover the child's physical and mental background, characteristics of infancy, attainment of motor milestones, self-help skills, and maturity of relationships with parents, peers, and siblings. It can also be advantageous to inquire as to what the parent likes best about the child, in order to set the stage for improved future rapport among all parties.

The test battery, consisting of a variety of developmental, intelligence, perceptual, academic achievement, projective, or social competence tests, can be administered following the developmental history. Parents are invited to observe testing through a one-way mirror in order to allay apprehension and allow them to appreciate fully the difficulties being encountered by the child.

In order to establish good rapport, thereby ensuring maximum motivation of the child, the examiner should adopt a positive, perhaps even playful attitude. Observation of the child begins as soon as the examiner enters the room. Seeking cooperation from the child by such ploys as asking him or her to help pick up toys allows the examiner to observe the child's reaction to such variables as limit setting, behavior toward strangers, eye contact, spontaneous outreach, dependence on adult direction, fine motor coordination, and so on.

Cognitive functioning can be assessed in the verbal child by the Stanford-Binet or the WISC-R (or WPPSI). Throughout testing, the examiner should be alert not only to the accuracy of responses but also the way in which the child responds. As is true for cognitive functioning, perceptual–motor capacity can be assessed by a variety of measurement tools. The child's motor performance can be assessed to some degree within the Stanford-Binet.

Finally, social–emotional functioning can be assessed by combining the rating scales from the parents with the behavioral observations. Projective tools, such as the Draw-A-Person and Draw-A-Family tests, can provide additional data pertaining to self-image and family relationships, as well as providing information about visual–motor functioning.

CONCLUSION

Because detection and analysis of psychiatric disorders can be an extremely difficult task within the heterogeneous childhood population, the clinician must learn to govern his or her own behavior in a way that maximizes results. Perhaps the single most rewarding behavior on the part of the clinician is the establishment of trust through empathic inquiry. Expending the energy to assure both the child and the parents of good intentions will make the tasks of diagnosis and treatment far easier and more effective. Measured expressions of concern and subtle emphasis on the child's strong points will quickly bring the family closer together and engender feelings of trust toward the therapist.

Once feelings of mutual trust have been established, it is vital to take the time to perform a complete assessment of the child's capabilities. The child's strengths should be woven into the assessment, to make it sufficiently broad to allow closure when inevitable gaps in the diagnostic continuum occur.

The developmental psychotherapist has the opportunity in many cases to preempt the development of a lifetime of disordered, unfulfilling behavior. While this is a large responsibility, its rewards are great and can merit the large expenditure of time and energy required to bring about a good result.

REFERENCES

Akiskal, H.S. (1986). Diagnosis in psychiatry and the mental status examination. In G. Winokur & P. Clayton (Eds.), *The mental basis of psychiatry*. Philadelphia: Saunders.

American Psychiatric Association. (1980). *Diagnostic and statistical manual of mental disorders* (3rd ed.). Washington, DC: Author.

American Psychiatric Association. (1987). *Diagnostic and statistical manual of mental disorders* (3rd ed., rev.). Washington, DC: Author.

Brady, C.P., Bray, J.H., & Zeeb, L. (1986). Behavior problems of clinic children: Relation to parental marital status, age and sex of child. *American Journal of Orthopsychiatry*, 56(3), 399–412.

Chandler, M.J. (1978). Role taking, referential communication, and egocentric intrusions in mother–child interactions of children vulnerable to risk of parental psychosis. In E.J. Anthony, C. Koupernik, & C. Chiland (Eds.), *The Child in His Family*, 4, 347–357.

Cox, A., & Rutter, M. (1985). Diagnostic appraisal and interviewing. In M. Rutter & L. Hersov (Eds.), *Child and adolescent psychiatry: Modern approaches*. Oxford: Blackwell.

Fergusson, D.M., Horwood, L.J., & Shannon, F. T. (1984). Relationship of family life events, maternal depression, and child-rearing problems. *Pediatrics, 7316*, 773–776.

Fischer, M., Rolf, J.E., Hasazi, J.E., & Cummings, L. (1984). Follow-up of a preschool epidemiological sample: Cross-age continuities and predictions of later adjustment with internalizing and externalizing dimensions of behavior. *Child Development, 55*, 137–150.

Guidubaldi, J., Perry, J.D., & Cleminshaw, H.K. (1984). The legacy of parental divorce: A nationwide study of family status and selected mediating variables on children's academic and social competencies. In B.B. Lahey & A. E. Kazdin (Eds.), *Advances in Clinical Child Psychology, 7*.

Jaspers, K. (1963). *General psychopathology* (J. Hoenig, Trans.). Manchester: Manchester University Press.

Kellman, S.G., Branch, J.D., Agrawal, K.C., & Ensminger, M.E. (1975). *Mental health and going to school*. Chicago: University of Chicago Press.

Kohn, M. (1977). *Social competence, symptoms and underachievement in childhood: A longitudinal perspective*. Washington, DC: Winston.

Plenk, A.M., & Hinchey, F.S. (1985). Clinical assessment of maladjusted preschool children. *Child Welfare League of America, 64*(2), 127–134.

Quay, H.C. (1979). Classification. In H.C. Quay & J.S. Werry (Eds.), *Psychopathological disorders of childhood*. New York: Wiley.

Rescorla, L.A. (1986). Preschool psychiatric disorders: Diagnostic classification and symptom patterns. *Journal of the Academy of Child Psychiatry, 25*(2), 162–169.

Richman, N. (1985). Disorder in pre-school children. In M. Rutter & L. Hersov (Eds.), *Child and adolescent psychiatry: Modern approaches*. Oxford: Blackwell.

Rutter, M. (1981). Stress, coping, and development: Some issues and some questions. *Journal of Child Psychology and Psychiatry, 22*, 323–356.

Sullivan, H.S. (1956). *Clinical studies in psychiatry*. New York: Norton.

Trad, P. (1986). *Infant depression paradigms and paradoxes*. New York: Springer-Verlag.

Trad, P. (1987). *Infant and childhood depression: Developmental factors*. New York: Wiley.

Vaughn, P.L., Boorse, M.A., & Jakobi, S.S. (1978). Mental health at preschool level: A preventive approach with a high-risk population. In E.J. Anthony, C. Koupernik, & C. Chiland (Eds.), *The Child and His Family, 4*, 597–618.

Weissman, M.W., Wickramaratne, P., Warner, V., John, K., Prusoff, B.A., Merikangas, K.R., & Gammond, G.D. (1987). Assessing psychiatric disorders in children. *Archives of General Psychiatry, 44*, 747–753.

CHAPTER 3

Reliability in Diagnostic Interviewing

ANTHONY COSTELLO

WHY RELIABILITY IN INTERVIEWING IS IMPORTANT

The essence of the scientific method is that a finding can be repeated by another investigator using the same techniques. If the observation cannot be replicated, then whatever the interest of the finding, no one can be confident that the observation was not made in error, or that it did not represent a chance association of variables that the experimenter had been unable to control. The principle applies as firmly to the less-well-defined techniques of clinical psychiatry as it does to the laboratory (if the former are to have any scientific status at all); hence the overriding importance of reliability. In using a measure that is reliable, we expect that it will consistently represent the status of the individual in whatever characteristic the instrument purports to measure. In other words, we have a concept of a "true" score, or category for the individual, which the instrument should identify correctly whenever it is used. If the true score is stable, then the measure should also be stable over time. Validity is closely related, for validity is based on the ability to predict anything other than the test performance itself. Without good reliability, validity will obviously be limited (Lord & Novick, 1968), though an instrument may have good reliability and still have little validity. It should be noted that reliability is not only a property of the instrument or method but is also affected by the population on which the method is tested. If the discrimination is an easy one, then reliability will be higher than if the discrimination is difficult. Reliability studies on mixtures of cases and controls should give high reliability, but in representative community samples, where more marginal cases may be found, reliability may well be lower.

Poor reliability can arise from many sources. The assumption usually made is that when observers disagree they do so because personal biases have affected their observations. Behavioral scientists have addressed the problem of reliability whenever they could by relying on techniques which they hope are objective and which introduce as little experimenter variance as possible. Examples are the many applications of direct observation in behavioral therapy, or the use of self-report inventories in diagnosis. Both give a structure to clinical procedures that reduces the variance contributed by the clinician. Of course, these methods may introduce other biases, but it is hoped that the bias will be more consistent than that introduced by the clinician, and potentially easier to identify, so that corrections can be made in analysis.

Another aspect of objective methods of assessment that is often overlooked in psychiatric assessment is the need to devise methods that are readily replicable. Some techniques place great emphasis on specialized training. Admittedly, it is unlikely that no training will ever be necessary, but the more elaborate training procedures paradoxically carry the danger of concealing those aspects of technique that are important. If a technique can only be learned by extensive personal training, it is possible that the need for such a pattern of training arises from a failure to specify with sufficient care the procedures that are used. If the procedures are not adequately specified, it is much easier for drift in the standard of measurement to occur over time. This problem should not be confused with the need for continued supervision, and continued tests of the stability of the procedure. Even with as straightforward a procedure as direct observation, drift in standards can develop if continued reliability checks are not maintained (Reid, 1970). It seems highly probable that such changes will happen even more frequently in such complex procedures as diagnostic interviewing, though the point has not been tested. The situation is complex, for in direct observation, if observers know who is the co-observer against which their own records will be checked, they are more likely to agree with that observer than with another whose observations are covert (Romanczyk, Kent, Diament, & O'Leary, 1973). In psychiatry this would argue that diagnoses are more likely to conform to the idiosyncratic standards of an "authority" if a senior is used as the standard of accurate diagnosis.

These methodological considerations, applied to psychiatric diagnosis, have prompted the development of structured and semistructured interviews that can be used to determine psychiatric diagnosis. Such interviews provide a standardized method for eliciting information, sometimes from more than one informant, and usually provide standardized procedures for reducing this information and evaluating it so that a diagnosis can be made. Often the complete procedure, including information gathering and information reduction, has been tested by comparing diagnoses made independently on the same individuals, and this test has been described as a test of "reliability." A moment's thought should convince the reader that to test agreement on diagnosis is to test many different aspects of the interview and diagnostic procedure at the same time, and it is not surprising that results have been mixed. The aims of this chapter are to analyze the many different aspects of standardized interviews that may be responsible for disagreement and to develop some suggestions for future study.

THE BACKGROUND—RELIABILITY IN CLINICAL PRACTICE

There have been many demonstrations of the poor agreement that is found between different diagnosticians making psychiatric diagnoses with conventional clinical procedures. It is important to note the reasons for such low reliability. One obvious source of disagreement is that different clinicians interviewing the same patient may obtain different information. One may rely more on spontaneous complaints by the patient, another on systematic questioning. More systematic review of possible symptoms by direct questioning has been shown to elicit more information (Cox, Rutter, & Holbrook, 1981), but many clinicians fear that this style of questioning will upset the patient, or create pressures to offer spurious information, despite the fact that no such tendencies can be demonstrated (Cox, Holbrook, & Rutter, 1981; Cox, Hopkinson, & Rutter, 1981; Cox, Rutter, & Holbrook, 1981).

Another source of disagreement on diagnosis is particularly likely for child psychiatric disorders, when it is often the case that to make an adequate diagnosis information must be sought from more than one informant. Parents, children, and teachers usually disagree on the nature and extent of a child's problem (Edelbrock Costello, Dulcan, Kales, & Conover, 1985; Herjanic, 1982; Reich, Herjanic, Welner, & Gandhy, 1982; Rutter, Tizard, & Whitmore, 1970), but there is little agreement in the scientific literature on how to interpret this disagreement, or on whose information should be given the most weight. Therefore, it is not surprising that clinicians are similarly perplexed and vary greatly in their practice in this regard.

Differing interpretations of diagnostic criteria may also give rise to disagreement. A further problem in clinical practice is that diagnostic systems have changed radically over a short time. A practicing clinician over the last decade may well have used at different times ICD 8, ICD 9, the GAP classification, DSM-II (APA, 1968), DSM-III (APA, 1980), and most recently may have started to explore the use of DSM-III-R (APA, 1987). Many of the earlier systems offered few criteria for a diagnosis. Even the most recent systems, despite an attempt to provide consistent criteria for diagnosis, rely on the clinician's subjective interpretation of such terms as *frequent* or *severe*. Though it can be argued that a diagnostic system for clinical use would become too inflexible if such terms were operationally defined, the failure to provide rigorous operational definitions is bound to generate diagnostic disagreements. Moreover, only the most enthusiastic nosologist is likely to maintain a good working knowledge of current diagnoses and their criteria, as so many alternative systems come and go. And at least in everyday practice there is likely to be some contamination of current nosologies from earlier classifications.

Another inevitable consequence of elaborating the diagnostic system itself is that, with more choices of diagnoses available, the probability of selecting a particular diagnosis falls, as does the chance of agreement between independent clinicians. This is one explanation of the disconcerting finding that clinicians making diagnoses from case history vignettes showed no better agreement using DSM-III, despite the introduction of clear diagnostic criteria, than when they used DSM-II (Mezzich, Mezzich, & Coffman, 1985).

Poor agreement on diagnosis between clinicians poses some difficult problems for the investigator devising new diagnostic procedures, since the reliability of clinical diagnosis is too low to make it useful as a standard against which to calibrate a new instrument. The dubious analogy of a monetary "gold standard" has been used to describe the mythical perfect criterion against which diagnostic procedures could be calibrated. The solution commonly adopted has been to use agreement between two independent, experienced clinicians as a reference point, negotiating agreement by discussion if their independent decisions differ. There have, however, been few if any demonstrations that agreement between two such pairs of experts working independently is superior to that between individual clinicians, and until this has been shown the procedure must be viewed with caution, particularly since it has not been shown that experience necessarily improves diagnostic agreement.

The default replacement for the gold standard proposed by R. L. Spitzer, which he picturesquely called the lead standard, is to obtain information from as many sources as possible, including follow-up data and response to treatment, and to have this information evaluated by experienced clinicians. Diagnosis based on such a wide range of information is likely to be more stable, particularly if explicit rules for the reduction of all this information are available. However, if outcome and response to treatment are conspicuously variable, as for example in the case of prepubertal depression (Puig-Antich et al., 1987), this solution may not offer any help. In the absence of convincing standards against which to measure validity, the field has tended to concentrate on reliability as a criterion to select a good measure, despite the convincing argument that this is a necessary but only intermediate step in evaluation.

THE ASSESSMENT OF RELIABILITY

Various strategies have been used to assess diagnostic reliability, and all have their limitations. *Interrater reliability* is sometimes offered as evidence of reliability. In such studies one interviewer conducts the interview, which is either observed directly or videotaped so that others can record and rate the information obtained. Such a design tests the adequacy of the recording system of the interview, and any subsequent procedures used to make a diagnosis, but does not test the consistency with which information is obtained. Since recording should not present problems if the instrument is well designed, very high interrater reliability should be expected unless the reliability of a diagnosis that depends on the rater's judgment is used as the criterion of agreement. Whenever possible it is preferable to evaluate agreement item by item, or by using a simple measure such as a specific symptom score, in which judgments by the rater or recorder are not involved. *Test–retest reliability* can be evaluated by using the same interviewer on both occasions, or by using a different interviewer for each interview. The single-interviewer design introduces the possibility that agreement between the first and second interview may be inflated by the interviewer's recollections of the first interview, which consciously or subconsciously may affect the responses recorded in the second interview. Both designs confound the reliability of the process with change that may occur with time, but if a very short test–retest interval is used the respondent may be remembering his or her responses to the first interview. A short test–retest interval design at least gives a reasonable upper limit to the estimate of reliability, and same-day interviewing with even so complex an interview as the Interview Schedule for Children (Kovacs, Feinberg, Crouse-Novak, & Paulaskas, 1984) is feasible (Last, personal communication). From a nosological standpoint we should be more interested in phenomena that can be elicited reliably over a longer time interval, since symptoms so ephemeral that they do not persist for 1 to 2 weeks can have little relevance to the concept of psychiatric diagnosis, though they may be of considerable interest as state-related phenomena. Unfortunately, it appears that children are likely to report fewer symptoms on reinterview, particularly of abnormal emotions rather than behavior, and that this tendency is most marked with younger children (Edelbrock et al., 1985). This limitation, which to some extent is found with diagnostic interviews of adults as well (Robins, 1985), may be so restrictive that differences between instruments cannot be evaluated by the test–retest design. But this has not yet been demonstrated convincingly.

THE MEASUREMENT OF RELIABILITY

Several statistical measures have been used to assess reliability, and though there are many relevant theoretical considerations, the choice of statistics is often determined by convention, since this facilitates comparisons. As always, the choice of statistics is much wider when the product of the instrument is a continuously distributed measure, with an approximation to a normal distribution. Though product-moment correlations are most commonly reported, it is of course possible for the correlation between observers to be high, but for one systematically to report higher values on a scale than the other. This may be overcome by calculating the reliability coefficient by means of analysis of variance (the intraclass correlation coefficient) so that systematic as well as random error will lower the coefficient (Shrout & Fleiss, 1979; Winer, 1971). The method is not without problems. For a review of the occasional difficulties of interpretation, see Lahey, Downey, and Saal (1983).

There is less agreement on the correct statistic to express agreement on categorical data. The simplest index, the percentage of agreement (i.e., the percentage of patients for which both diagnosticians agree), has several shortcomings. The most problematic for the case of psychiatric diagnosis is that, when a positive diagnosis is rarely made, agreement that the diagnosis was not made is going to be very high. This can be dealt with in several ways. One obvious solution is to use the percentage of agreements of those occasions when either diagnostician made the diagnosis, but then much of the ability of the procedure to discriminate between those that have and those that do not have the diagnosis is ignored, and quite small differences have an inflated effect on the index.

A more satisfactory procedure is to devise a correction for chance agreement. The most widely used statistic that embodies this correction is kappa (Cohen, 1960, 1968). This corrects for agreement by chance, which is calculated on the assumption that if chance agreement is operating each diagnostician is making diagnoses at random from the selection available. Although this assumption obviously does not correspond to reality, since diagnosticians inevitably favor one or more diagnoses at the expense of others, any other estimate of the judge's behavior involves even more problematic assumptions, and ignores the fact that judges may be influenced by the sample they diagnose even if agreement is poor, so that calculations made on the marginal frequencies of the agreement matrix reflect the sample as well as the diagnostic judges' behavior. An apparent problem with kappa is that if the base rate of a diagnosis is low it is hard to achieve a reasonable value; the sensitivity and specificity of the procedure used for reaching a diagnosis also affect the value of kappa.

A coefficient in many ways more desirable, since the assumptions on which it is based are more conservative, is the random error [RE] coefficient of agreement (Maxwell, 1977). This assumes that for many cases two diagnosticians agree confidently that a diagnosis can or cannot be made, and that there is a smaller proportion for which both are uncertain, and in the diagnosis of these cases chance factors may be operating. RE represents the sum of the proportions of cases for which agreement is based on a confident judgment that a diagnosis is present, and those in which it is absent. Numerically it varies between -1 and $+1$. Though it is in many ways a more useful statistic than kappa, it has not found wide favor. Janes (1979) argues that if the proportion of cases in nonagreement cells of the agreement matrix are quite unequal, the distribution of cases of chance agreement may be skewed, when the estimate of chance cases by calculating RE would be untrustworthy. Another contender, Yule's Y, suggested by Spitznagel and Helzer (1985), has proved equally unpopular. Though it is relatively independent of base rate, at times it has surprising values that do not seem to reflect the extent of agreement or disagreement found. Shrout, Spitzer, and Fleiss (1987) point out that the conditions under which Y is equivalent to kappa are so restrictive that they will rarely apply, and if they do not apply, then Y is not a true reliability coefficient.

THE DISADVANTAGES OF INTERNAL RELIABILITY AS AN ESTIMATE FOR STRUCTURED DIAGNOSTIC INTERVIEWS

The problems of test–retest designs are familiar in other fields of assessment, notably cognitive testing. Though the solution of alternative forms may be used when it is not the case that items within an instrument are correlated (Nunnally, 1978), it is probably not a feasible solution for psychiatric diagnostic instruments. This is the case since the criteria are so restrictive that if alternative items were devised, either they would be mere paraphrases of the original or they could only be achieved by reducing the number of criteria explored in each form, which would do rough justice to the concept of diagnostic syndromes. A similar limitation applies to the measures of internal consistency that have been used to estimate the reliability of some psychological measures. The split-half strategy, in which items from a test are divided into two parts and correlated (the Kuder-Richardson formula [Kuder & Richardson, 1937]), and other more sophisticated procedures for assessing the internal homogeneity of a measure have little application to measures that derive diagnoses by using a nosology based on multiple criteria. Only if the concept evaluated can be treated as a continuously varying dimension or set of dimensions can such procedures be used. Some diagnostic instruments have been used to generate symptom scores (e.g., the K-Sads [Chambers et al., 1985] or the DISC [Costello, Edelbrock, Dulcan, Kalas, & Klaric, 1984]), and for these scores such a procedure would be applicable. Since the scales are usually based on ad hoc assemblages of items that have not been derived empirically, it would not be surprising if internal consistency were only moderate. But this is a necessary constraint if the primary function of the instrument is to elicit the data needed to satisfy the criteria of a diagnostic system that itself is only loosely based on formal empirical investigation. Good internal reliability is usually only obtained if preliminary factor analysis is used in the selection of items to ensure homogeneity.

INTEROBSERVER AGREEMENT

Another limited aspect of performance that is sometimes described as reliability is the demonstration that two independent observers of the same interview can agree on the data that are recorded. This measure, usually presented as a product-moment correlation, or as a kappa statistic in the case of categorical responses (Cohen, 1960), reflects the care with which response categories have been defined, the ability of the questions to generate unambiguous responses, and the training of the observers. Good interobserver agreement is clearly needed before reasonably high measures of more demanding aspects of reliability can be obtained, and it is necessary in order to demonstrate that the instrument has the potential for the replication of findings. By itself it is not a sufficient indication that the instrument is reliable.

Not surprisingly, given the nature of the decisions that have to be made by the recorder, interobserver agreement is typically somewhat lower for semistructured interviews in which responses by the informant are typically rated on a scale that assesses severity than for highly structured interviews that usually only demand 2- or 3-point response recording (yes–no, or yes–maybe–no). Examples for those instruments for which data are available are given in Table 3.1.

TEST–RETEST RELIABILITY

Since psychiatric diagnoses are supposed to be moderately persistent conditions that continue for some time even when treatment has been initiated, and without treatment may last for at least several months, it should be expected that an interview when repeated after several hours, days, or even weeks should generate the same diagnosis.

TABLE 3.1.   Interrater Reliability

	DICA	K-SADS	CAS	ISC	DISC (CHILD)
Range	80–90%	.86 (parent)	.44	.5	.94
		.89 (child)	to .82	to 1.0	to 1.0
Average	85%	—	.74	.91	.98
Median	—	—	.70	.87	.99

As a procedure, the test–retest strategy is fraught with problems. If the child (or parent) is not given some explanation of the rationale for repeating exactly what has already been completed, then the interviewer's sanity is likely to be suspect. If an explanation is given before the first interview, as ethical considerations would advise, then the knowledge that the questions will be repeated at a later date may motivate for improved recall. If the explanation is delayed until the second interview, then it may not be feasible to arrange the very short test–retest intervals that are needed to make valid comparisons of different interviewers. Moreover, even a delayed explanation may give the subject some opportunity to rehearse recall of the original interview. These objections argue for inflation of reliability, but it is equally possible that subjects will be poorly motivated to undergo a second comprehensive interview, and will use whatever strategies shorten the second interview, a hypothesis that is consistent with some of the findings.

Another issue to be treated with care, particularly if long test–retest intervals are employed, is the time window of the interview. Many diagnostic instruments focus on a specific or general time frame, such as the events of the last year, or of the last 6 months. With longer intervals between first and second interviews, consistent responses can only be expected if the behavior is unusually stable. If an instrument distinguishes between the recent and distant past, so that so-called "lifetime" diagnoses can be made, then this difficulty may be overcome, though it should be expected that retrospective recall is not going to agree perfectly with a contemporaneous report. Only the epidemiological version of the K-SADS (Orvaschel, Puig-Antich, Chambers, Tabrizi, & Johnson, 1982) has attempted to make this distinction, and the evidence of long-term reliability for the instrument, though encouraging, is based on a somewhat biased sample of subjects who were mostly depressed.

Test–retest reliability must have an upper bound limited by interobserver agreement. Within this limit the demonstration that the same answer is obtained on two successive occasions can be, first, a measure of the ability of the instrument to impose uniformity of practice, when a different interviewer gives the interview on each occasion. Second, it can be a measure of the stability of the underlying concept the instrument purports to measure. Since it is commonly the case that a different interviewer gives the interview on each occasion, the two are often confounded. So far no published studies have compared test–retest data obtained using the same interviewer with test–retest data obtained using different interviewers. And, indeed, the majority of the available data come from the latter design. From same-day test–retest interview with the Interview Schedule for Children (ISC [Kovacs, 1984]) obtained by Last (1986, personal communication), we know that the variance contributed by well-trained interviewers using a semistructured interview can be very small, and much less than that found reinterviewing within a 48- to 72-hour interval with a very similar interview (Chambers et al., 1985).

One can argue, of course, that a child reinterviewed the same day may appear very consistent because the replies he or she gives on the second occasion are more influenced by recollections of the answers given in the first interview than by a reconsideration of how he or she actually felt or behaved. The point is an important one, but like many of the theoretically important considerations that underlie diagnostic interviewing, it has not been tested. It can also be argued that if test–retest reliability

TABLE 3.2.   Test–Retest Reliability (Kappa)

	DICA (CHILD)	K-SADS	CAS	ISC	DISC
Range	.76	.09	—	—	(P) .40
	to 1.0	to .89	—	—	to .86
					(C) .26
					to .77
Average	.88	.57	—	—	(P) .80
					(C) .69
Median	.83	.56	—	—	(P) .83
					(C) .74

is reduced over longer intervals, then the interview is not measuring constructs of any clinical interest. If the concept of psychiatric disorder has any significance, then disorders must have at least some short-term temporal stability.

Though it is true that some instruments show quite poor test–retest reliability over intervals as short as 7 to 21 days when younger children are interviewed (e.g., see the data on the Diagnostic Interview Schedule for Children [DISC] in Edelbrock et al., 1985), neither the instrument nor the diagnostic concepts can be readily dismissed. In this particular case the validity of both instruments and the underlying concepts of DSM-III child psychiatric disorder are good when discriminant validity is tested (Costello, Edelbrock, & Costello, 1985), and the test–retest reliability is adequate for older children and good for the parent account (Edelbrock et al., 1985). This introduces a further variable that must be taken into account when assessing the performance of an interview. The age of the child may make a profound difference. This may be because some interviews are not suitably worded for a particular age group, though it should be noted that even when readability is taken into account in instrument construction (Costello et al., 1984) this problem is not overcome. It seems equally plausible that some concepts entrenched in our definitions of psychiatric disorders, such as a persistent mood state largely independent of the immediate circumstances, may not be cognitively appropriate for younger children. Until more psychometric data are available on several of the diagnostic interviews for children, the point remains speculative. A summary of the test–retest data available so far is presented in Table 3.2.

It should be noted that, since the methodology is slightly different and the samples in each study are of different size and composition, these comparisons can only be taken as an indication of what is currently possible, and do not necessarily demonstrate that one or another interview is superior. Choice of an interview should be based on many factors, of which reliability is only one. And, as has been noted earlier, reliability achieved for one population may not be achieved on another even when the same interview method is used.

THE CONCEALED COMPONENTS OF RELIABILITY

From what has already been written, it should be evident that the term *reliability* has been used in a variety of ways, and that all of these are important in assessing the usefulness of an instrument. This chapter does not attempt to address the equally important and even more elusive issue of validity—the evidence that an instrument measures what it purports to measure. Probably in the end the validity of psychiatric diagnostic instruments, like that of intelligence tests, will have to depend on the demonstration of practical predictive utility. It is well to remember though that there are other aspects of test performance related to reliability that should be evaluated. For example, it is common in clinical practice for a clinician to have idiosyncratic tendencies in making certain diagnoses. One clinician may be readier than another, for example, to diagnose depression, while another places greater emphasis than most on conduct disorder. Such biases may easily become part of an institutional culture, and a sturdy diagnostic instrument should be immune to such predispositions. Similarly, it is possible that an instrument may be more sensitive to nonspecific psychiatric symptomatology, so that diagnoses tend to congregate in a few individuals in the population studied, who receive several diagnoses.

If the agreement matrix is visualized as a three-dimensional array, with individuals on one axis, independent diagnosticians on the second, and diagnoses on the third, then reliability can be seen as maximizing the number of empty columns when this matrix is viewed from the diagnosis-by-individuals plane (see Fig. 3.1). If diagnostic preferences are to be overruled, then when the matrix is viewed from the judge-by-diagnosis plane, the spread over the columns should be similar for each judge. Finally, the sensitivity of the instrument to specific diagnoses rather than nonspecific psychiatric distress can be evaluated by examining the distribution in the columns when viewed from the judge-by-individuals plane, when again the desired distribution is a more even one across all columns. The specificity, sensitivity, and efficiency

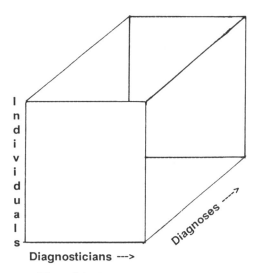

Figure 3.1. A complete agreement matrix.

of the instrument as a way of making diagnoses or measuring disorder must also be considered.

FUTURE DEVELOPMENTS

From the material reviewed it is evident that there is much basic work still to be done. Not only is there an urgent need for more adequate and uniform psychometric data on the existing instruments, but there may well be some fundamental issues to be explored before the science of diagnostic interviewing can be advanced. We need to be able to separate the test–retest variance due to the child's changing self-report from that introduced by a change of interviewer. We need to know whether the poor reliability of reporting by younger children is influenced by the style of interviewing, and if so, what style of interviewing maximizes reliability. We need to know what psychological principle, if any, lies behind the great discrepancies between reliability on the report of feelings and on reports of conduct problems. Though there has been much speculation on these and other aspects of the performance of diagnostic interviews for children, what is needed now is some patient exploration of these and related methodological issues. Without such work it is only too probable that the field will be influenced more by fashion than by informed judgment.

REFERENCES

American Psychiatric Association (1968). *Diagnostic and statistical manual of mental disorders* (2nd ed.). Washington, DC: Author.

American Psychiatric Association (1980). *Diagnostic and statistical manual of mental disorders* (3rd ed.). Washington, DC: Author.

American Psychiatric Association (1987). *Diagnostic and statistical manual of mental disorders* (3rd ed., rev.). Washington, DC: Author.

Chambers, W.J., Puig-Antich, J., Hirsch, M., Paez, P., Ambrozini, P., Tabrizi, M.A., & Johnson, R. (1985). The assessment of affective disorders in children and adolescents by semi-structured interview. *Archives of General Psychiatry, 42,* 696–702.

Cohen, J. (1960). A coefficient of agreement for nominal scales. *Educational & Psychological Measurement, 20,* 37–46.

Cohen, J. (1968). Weighted kappa: Nominal scale agreement with provision for scaled disagreement or partial credit. *Psychological Bulletin, 70,* 213–220.

Costello, A.J., Edelbrock, C., Dulcan, M.K., Kalas, R., & Klaric, S.A. (1984). Final Report to NIMH on the Diagnostic Interview Schedule for Children.

Costello, E.J., Edelbrock, C., & Costello, A.J. (1985). Validity of the NIMH Diagnostic Interview Schedule for Children: A comparison between psychiatric and pediatric referrals. *Journal of Abnormal Child Psychology, 13,* 579–595.

Cox, A., Holbrook, D., & Rutter, M. (1981). Psychiatric interviewing techniques. VI. Experimental study: Eliciting feelings. *British Journal of Psychiatry, 139,* 144–152.

Cox, A., Hopkinson, K., & Rutter, M. (1981). Psychiatric interviewing techniques II.

Naturalistic study: Eliciting factual information. *British Journal of Psychiatry*, *138*, 283–291.

Cox, A. Rutter, M., & Holbrook, D. (1981). Psychiatric interviewing techniques V. Experimental study: eliciting factual information. *British Journal of Psychiatry*, *139*, 29–37.

Edelbrock, C., Costello, A.J., Dulcan, M.K., Kalas, R.L., & Conover, N.C. (1985). Age differences in the reliability of the psychiatric interview of the child. *Child Development*, *56*, 265–275.

Herjanic, B., & Reich, W. (1982). Development of a structured psychiatric interview for children: Agreement between child and parent on individual symptoms. *Journal of Abnormal Child Psychology*, *10*, 307–324.

Janes, C.L. (1979). Agreement measurement and the judgment process. *Journal of Nervous & Mental Disease*, *167*, 343–347.

Kovacs, M., Feinberg, T.L., Crouse-Novak, M.A., & Paulaskas, S.L. (1984). Depressive disorders in childhood. *Archives of General Psychiatry*, *41*, 229–237.

Kuder, G.F., & Richardson, M.W. (1937). The theory of the estimation of test reliability. *Psychometrika*, *2*, 151–160.

Lahey, M.A., Downey, R.G., & Saal, F.E. (1983). Intraclass correlations: There's more there than meets the eye. *Psychological Bulletin*, *93*, 586–595.

Lord, F.M., & Novick, M.R. (1968). *Statistical theories of mental test scores*. Reading, MA: Addison-Wesley.

Maxwell, A. E. (1977). Coefficients of agreement between observers and their interpretation. *British Journal of Psychiatry*, *130*, 79–83.

Mezzich, A.C., Mezzich, J.E., & Coffman, G. A. (1985). Reliability of DSM-III vs. DSM-II in child psychopathology. *Journal of the American Academy of Child Psychiatry*, *24*, 273–280.

Nunnally, J. (1978). *Psychometric theory* (2nd ed.). New York: McGraw-Hill.

Orvaschel, H., Puig-Antich, J., Chambers, W. Tabrizi, M.A., & Johnson, R. (1982). Retrospective assessment of prepubertal major depression with the Kiddie-SADS-E. *Journal of the American Academy of Child Psychiatry*, *21*, 392–397.

Puig-Antich, J., Perel, J.M., Lupatkin, W., Chambers, W.J., Tabrizi, M.A., King, J., Goetz, R., Davies, M., & Stiller, R.L. (1987). *Imipramine in prepubertal major depressive disorders*. Unpublished manuscript.

Reich, W., Herjanic, W., Welner, Z., & Gandhy, P. (1982). Development of a structured psychiatric interview for children: Agreement on diagnosis comparing child and parent interviews. *Journal of Abnormal Child Psychology*, *10*, 325–336.

Reid, J.B. (1970). Reliability assessment of observation data: A possible methodological problem. *Child Development*, *41*, 1143–1150.

Robins, L.N. (1985). Epidemiology: Reflections on testing the validity of psychiatric interviews. *Archives of General Psychiatry*, *42*, 918–924.

Romanczyk, R.G., Kent, R.N., Diament, C., & O'Leary, K.D. (1973). Measuring the reliability of observational data: A reactive process. *Journal of Applied Behavior Analysis*, *6*, 175–184.

Rutter, M., Tizard, J., & Whitmore, K. (1970). *Education, health and behaviour*. London: Longman.

Shrout, P.E., & Fleiss, J.L. (1979). Intraclass correlations: Uses in assessing rater reliability. *Psychological Bulletin*, *86*, 420–428.

Shrout, P.E., Spitzer, R.L., & Fleiss, J.L. (1987). Quantification of agreement in psychiatric diagnosis revisited. *Archives of General Psychiatry*, *44*, 172–177.

Spitznagel, E.L., & Helzer, J.E. (1985). A proposed solution to the base rate problem in the kappa statistic. *Archives of General Psychiatry*, *42*, 725–728.

Winer, B.J. (1971). *Statistical principles in experimental design* (2nd ed.). New York: McGraw-Hill.

CHAPTER 4

Validating Diagnostic Categories

DONALD K. ROUTH

To me, validity simply means truth. Therefore, within the field of child psycho-pathology, validating a diagnostic category means investigating whether inferences based on it are correct or incorrect. The diagnostic category should convey some clinically important information about a child's condition beyond what was known before the category was assigned. What this new information might be depends on the particular diagnostic construct and how much solid scientific information there is about it, but typically clinicians are most concerned about: (1) the prognosis of the condition (its natural history and outcome in the absence of any particular intervention); (2) its etiology (known antecedents or causes); and (3) its response to various possible treatments. So validating diagnostic categories boils down, at least in part, to hypothesis testing about their implications for prognosis, etiology, and treatment.

The categories cannot be any more valid than the state of our knowledge of child psychopathology at the moment. In a recent *Annual Review of Psychology* chapter, my associates and I (Quay, Routh, & Shapiro, 1987) tried to convey the view just presented at some length, with examples from a number of different types of child psychopathology. This chapter, written about a year subsequent to the preparation of the one by Quay and colleagues, provides some elaborations of it based on further reflection, and some updating in terms of the more recent literature of child psy-chopathology. It also focuses to a greater extent than did Quay and colleagues on the history of my own research evaluating the validity of the syndrome labeled by DSM-III (American Psychiatric Association, 1980) as attention deficit disorder with hyperactivity, and DSM-III-R (APA, 1987) or attention deficit hyperactivity dis-order.

The field of mental testing has been responsible for a number of conceptual and empirical advances, and some confusion, about the notion of "validity" over the last several decades. The earlier *Standards for Educational and Psychological Tests* (American Psychological Association, 1974) managed to convey the idea that there were different "types" of validity, namely, criterion-related validity (concurrent and predictive), content validity, and construct validity. This has subsequently been referred to as the trinitarian view of validity (Landy, 1986). These "types" of validity are undoubtedly familiar to the reader. In assessing criterion-related validity, one must first establish a kind of gold standard or well-accepted criterion measure of the particular category or dimension to be assessed. Thus in validating his new measure of intelligence, Alfred Binet took as the criterion teachers' judgments of children's academic aptitude. In validating the original scales of the Minnesota Multiphasic Personality Inventory, Hathaway and McKinley took as their criteria the diagnostic categories applied to patients by psychiatrists. The idea of content validity, in contrast, is basically one of systematically sampling from a domain or universe of skills or behaviors. It is most obviously applicable to academic achievement testing. If one wants to know how well a person can spell, a spelling list could in principle be made up by taking every nth word from a dictionary. The results of the test then could presumably be generalized back to the entire set of words in the dictionary. The idea of construct validity (Cronbach & Meehl, 1955) is more complicated (and nebulous) than those of criterion-related or content validity. Originally, construct validation was supposed to be applicable only to those situations where there was no obvious criterion or universe of content. A measure was to be validated by the correspondence between its empirical relationships to other variables and the corresponding relationships specified by the investigator's theory (or nomological net, as it was called). Thus a measure could be invalidated not only by the absence of theoretically predicted relationships with other variables but by the presence of theoretically unpredicted ones. In other words, the validity of the measure stood or fell with the validity of the theory of which it was a part. Bechtoldt (1959) long ago complained that Cronbach and Meehl seemed to be trying to set up a separate philosophy of science for the psychometric part of the field. (I think Bechtoldt's complaint was well justified.)

The newest edition of the *Standards for Educational and Psychological Testing* (Novick, 1985) appears to endorse a unified view of validity in which all validity is essentially equated with construct validity. Landry (1986) makes this view even more explicit. In other words, in the current view it is impossible to validate a test, a set of observations, or a diagnostic category without some kind of theory or hypothesis as to how the variable is related to other measures, categories, or processes. The previous other "types" of validity simply become types of *evidence* for or against validity. Therefore, the evidence that may be applicable to the question of validity is no longer limited to "criterion" or "content" relationships but depends only on one's ingenuity in setting up research designs to test hypotheses. In other words, validity means truth.

Another influential approach to evaluating validity has been that of Campbell and Fiske (1959). The scheme they prescribed was to set up a multitrait, multimethod matrix in which each of several traits (e.g., intelligence, aggressiveness, and anxiety) was to be assessed by each of several methods (e.g., self-report, teacher, and peer ratings). *Convergent validity* refers to the agreement of assessments of the same trait by different methods—in this example it would hold if peer and teacher ratings agreed highly as to which children were more aggressive. *Discriminant validity* refers to the lack of relationship of supposedly independent traits when measured by the same method—here, it might refer to an absence of positive or negative halo effects in which peers (or teachers) rate certain positive or negative children favorably or unfavorably on all traits. The multitrait, multimethod matrix has proven to be an excellent scheme for systematically ordering the presentation of data from different sources. However, it is hard to find a set of actual clinical data that meets their somewhat arbitrary assumptions. For one thing, it now seems unrealistic to assume one would get *exactly* the same information from various sources about the same clinical phenomenon. For example, some colleagues and I are currently involved in a study of children's reactions to injections with and without their mothers present (Routh et al., 1987). We videotape the children and carry out detailed coding of their behaviors, such as crying, screaming, flailing, and others. Physiological recordings of changes in heart rate and respiration are made. After the injection, the children who are old enough to do so are also asked to rate how scared they were (or how much pain they had) during the shot. In a crude sense, the behavioral, physiological, and self-report measures are attempting to capture aspects of the same phenomenon of distress and coping, yet I would be very surprised if they all correlated perfectly. Theorists of anxiety such as Lang (e.g., Lang, Levin, Miller, & Kozak, 1983) would agree that there are several rather separate aspects of such reactions. A second point against taking a multitrait, multimethod approach too literally is that phenomena of clinical interest are often not as independent as the model assumes. To take a physical example, suppose the characteristics being measured are height and weight. These convey meaningful separate information yet are highly correlated. Should we therefore regard their correlation when measured (e.g., in grams and centimeters) as unwanted "method" variance? No, of course not. The point is, the assumptions about what correlations are to be expected in a multitrait, multimethod matrix should not be taken as given as laid down by the general Campbell and Fiske (1959) model but should be the subject of careful theoretical reasoning in each substantive area of research.

AN EXAMPLE: THE QUESTION OF A SYNDROME
OF HYPERACTIVITY

The preceding comments are necessarily rather general. It might help the reader to gain a clearer understanding of my views on validating diagnostic categories if I go through some of the history of how I came to them. As a graduate student and as a psychology intern, I was deeply impressed with the clinical phenomenon of hyperactivity in children. For example, as an intern at the University of Oklahoma Health Sciences Center, I was once asked to evaluate a school-age child who was not able to sit still for testing until I sat behind him with one knee up against the back of his chair. He would look briefly at each Rorschach inkblot card, give a simple response (usually "a bat," or "a bug"), and then sail the card off into the air. After completing this testing session with him, I foolishly allowed him to go out into the open courtyard next to the examining room. He raced around the yard, spied a large tree, and before he could be stopped had climbed high into its branches. In this case, his impulsivity was on my side, however. He soon tired of being in the tree and came down without being coaxed to do so. It was a relief to deliver him safely back into the care of his parents.

When I was on my first job out of graduate school, I worked part of my time in the University of Iowa Child Development Clinic, in the Department of Pediatrics. We saw many hyperactive children there, and the most common diagnosis they received was that of minimal cerebral dysfunction. They were generally put on Ritalin by the pediatricians, with the dosage being titrated upward until maximum benefit seemed to be obtained, or side effects became a problem. At that time we believed that the behavior problems would tend to fade by adolescence, and so informed the child and parents. It certainly seemed to me to be a successful example of the medical model in action, since the diagnostic category seemed to convey specific information about etiology, prognosis, and treatment.

However, my own scientific training would not let me feel secure with that seemingly rather satisfactory state of affairs. The rationale for the particular symptoms that went into the diagnosis was rather unclear. The most interesting document I came across in trying to understand this rationale was Clements's (1966) monograph on minimal brain dysfunction. It reviewed the massive available literature on the topic and listed 99 possible symptoms of MBD that had been suggested by various authors. The one at the top of the list was hyperactivity. Other symptoms prominently featured included short attention span, impulsivity, specific learning problems, neurological soft signs such as poor motor skills, and so on. I immediately planned a study of the interrelationship of the major symptoms on Clements's list in children seen at our Child Development Clinic. My assumptions at that time about validating diagnostic categories were (I now admit) rather simplistic. The first assumption I made was that all symptoms ought to "go together" in the sense of being correlated with each other. The study (Routh & Roberts, 1972) showed not only that the intercorrelations were disappointingly low, but also that, after one took the precaution of partialing out age and IQ from the correlation matrix, there was little common variance left among the symptoms. Our article was published under the title "Minimal Brain Dysfunction: Failure to Find Evidence for a Behavioral Syndrome."

Actually, there was something quite interesting in the data of that study that we did not detect. Loney and her associates (Langhorne, Loney, Paternite, & Bechtoldt, 1976) later factor-analyzed our correlation matrix and were able to demonstrate "source" factors there. They replicated and extended these findings with a larger sample and better defined measures. It seems that each "source" of information, that is, the parents, the teacher, the physician, sees certain children as having the most severe behavioral problems, but the sources do not agree very well as to which children these are. It is just what Campbell and Fiske (1959) were referring to when they spoke of "method variance" or a lack of discriminant validity.

I went on also to try to develop better measures of what appeared to be the core symptoms of a hypothesized hyperactivity syndrome, specifically hyperactivity and attention deficit. We set up a standardized playroom in a pediatric clinic at the University of North Carolina where we could observe how much a child moved around, crossing between different quadrants of the room, and how often the child shifted attention from one toy to another. We also adapted a standardized clinical interview developed by Werry (1968) and his associates into a parent activity questionnaire. In a study of 140 normal children aged 3 to 9 years (Routh, Schroeder, & O'Tuama, 1974), we were able to demonstrate that there was a decrease of activity with age, whether activity was measured by quadrant entries in the playroom or by parent ratings. (The attentional measure did not work out so well, however.) We were also able to demonstrate that both the playroom activity measure and the parent ratings significantly discriminated children referred for the evaluation of hyperactivity from nonclinic controls matched for age (Routh & Schroeder, 1976). In a longitudinal study, Milich, Loney, and Roberts (1986) later confirmed our cross-sectional age changes in activity. One interesting facet of our research, however, was the lack of correlation of different measures of activity or of hyperactivity. Even though both our playroom activity measures and parent ratings of activity were correlated with age and with clinical hyperactivity, the two measures were not correlated with each other. In fact, the parent activity measure could be factor-analyzed into seven independent dimensions. Barkley and Ullman (1975) developed a more detailed set of measures, all putatively a part of the hyperactivity syndrome, and found few correlations among them.

These kinds of findings confront one with an important validity issue. If one has good measures of symptom A and of symptom B and they are not correlated with each other, either the diagnostic category supposedly consisting of A and B does not exist, or the notion of covariation as a requirement of a diagnostic category is flawed. I have now come to believe that the covariation requirement should be relaxed. Symptoms do not necessarily have to be correlated to be part of a diagnostic category. All that is necessary is that the symptoms be reliably measurable and (especially) that they relate to (1) prognosis, (2) etiology, or (3) response to treatment.

Let me provide a couple of examples of legitimate diagnostic categories that have some symptoms uncorrelated with each other. One is Down's syndrome. This condition, which is uniformly associated with mental retardation of increasing severity as the individual grows older, received strong confirmation as a meaningful diagnostic category when it was discovered to be associated with extra chromosomal material usually appearing as trisomy 21 (three number 21 chromosomes in the karyotype instead of the usual two). Gibson's work (e.g., Gibson, Pozsonyi, & Zarfas, 1964) has shown that the physical stigmata of Down's syndrome are quite variable from one individual to another and are often uncorrelated with each other within a Down's syndrome population. Another perhaps more psychopathologically relevant example is schizophrenia. Meehl (1973) has pointed out that many symptoms of the schizophrenia spectrum are uncorrelated with each other in affected individuals, even though in a mixed group of persons they are statistically associated with schizophrenia. What I want to say is that in my present concept of hyperactivity it is not necessary for the behavioral symptoms such as overactivity, short attention span, or impulsivity to be correlated with each other, or even for two valid measures of hyperactivity to be correlated, so long as they are statistically associated with the presence of the syndrome, and relate to prognosis, etiology, or response to treatment.

Let us therefore move on to discuss the prognosis of hyperactivity (or attention deficit disorder with hyperactivity). It is certainly clear that our previous ideas about hyperactivity disappearing at age 12 or so were incorrect. Recent longitudinal studies, for example, that of Weiss and Hechtman (1986), have confirmed that, although the core symptoms may decrease somewhat with age, adults who were formerly hyperactive children continue to manifest many of the same behavioral characteristics that set them apart as children, and their educational, vocational, and interpersonal histories are somewhat adversely affected by their residual psychopathology. The main research issue with respect to the prognosis of hyperactivity is whether it can be separated from that of other "externalizing" disorders, such as unsocialized aggressive conduct disorder. Existing research data suggest that most hyperactive children have conduct disorder, and, conversely, most conduct-disordered children are also hyperactive. In a group of children including many with both problems, Milich and Loney (1979) were able to show that it was aggression rather than hyperactivity that predicted a poor social outcome. In fact, they actually found aggression to be a better predictor of future hyperactivity than was present hyperactivity. Hyperactivity seemed to predict only future academic difficulties (of course, the question here would be whether academic problems themselves would not be a better predictor of future ones than hyperactivity would). Future research needs to examine whether there is a different prognosis for "pure" conduct disorder than for mixed hyperactive–conduct-disordered children. In order to do this kind of research, it is crucial that diagnostic measures for the assessment of both ADD and conduct disorder be purged of items that fail to discriminate between the two related conditions. Loney and Milich's (1982) development of separate teacher rating scales for Inattention–Overactivity on the one hand and Aggression on the other is a step in the right direction in this respect. At this point, the question about the differential prognosis of ADD is unresolved. The jury is still out.

What about the etiology of hyperactivity? In a sense, we know less about this topic than we thought we knew a few years ago. For example, one used to be able to cite an expanding number of papers by Morrison and Stewart (e.g., 1973) among others about the familial nature of hyperactivity and the predictive value of knowing whether an adopted child had biological relatives with a history of hyperactivity. Stewart, for one, seems to have changed his mind about the interpretation of these studies and now thinks it is conduct problems rather than hyperactivity that are familial. One can raise the same general question about most other studies of etiological factors. For a second example, in Nichols and Chen's (1981) prospective longitudinal studies of pregnant women and their offspring, was maternal smoking really linked to hyperactivity or only to its correlates, such as learning disabilities or conduct problems?

Last, what about the specificity of treatment? It continues to be true that the efficacy of stimulant medication for improving hyperactive children's behavior is the best documented finding in child psychopharmacology. The drugs decrease activity, increase on-task behavior, temporarily improve performance on arithmetic and certain other academic tasks, decelerate various disruptive behaviors that are irritating to peers, and improve the quality of adult–child interaction. Yet reports come from England that there is so little demand for Ritalin that pharmacies have stopped carrying it. How can both of these sets of statements be true?

One problem is that stimulant drug effects are short lived. Other than certain rebound phenomena (e.g., Porrino et al., 1983), stimulant drugs seem to have their behavioral effects only for about 4 hours. In Weiss and Hechtman's (1986) long-term study, the formerly hyperactive adults generally described their memories of stimulant drug effects a little more favorably than those of neuroleptic medications, yet they did not feel drugs were the most helpful to their long-term well-being. (In fact, they usually singled out as most helpful to them some adult, whether a parent, teacher, or principal, who continued to "believe" in them despite their difficulties.)

Second, and more important from a theoretical point of view, is that stimulant drugs seem to have approximately the same effect on behaviorally normal, healthy children that they have on hyperactive ones (Rapoport et al., 1978).

To me, the most intriguing current question concerning stimulant drugs is how one can predict favorable or unfavorable response to them. In Barkley's (1977) widely cited review, and subsequently, it is generally stated that about 75% are favorable responders. How can we determine ahead of time who these responders are, and will the discovery of predictors of this help us define the nature of ADD with more specificity?

SOME BETTER VALIDATED DIAGNOSTIC CATEGORIES

The reader may find it annoying to be provided with guidelines for validating diagnostic categories and then to read so much about hyperactivity—surely a prime example of a diagnostic category that has up to this point resisted validation. (I have certainly found it frustrating to continue to do research on this particular issue, and, in fact, in recent years seem to have "delegated" continuing work on it to more persistent colleagues such as Russell Barkley, Jan Loney, and Richard Milich.) Let me therefore spend the remainder of the chapter listing some examples of categories that *do* have some established validity.

Mental Retardation and Intelligence

Concepts of mental retardation emerged long before the scientific era in child psychopathology. Common clinical experience demonstrates that certain children, often ones who are odd looking (with small or grossly large heads, hemiparalysis, or malformed facial features), are slow to develop intellectually and fail to become fully mentally competent as adults. The development of formal intelligence tests (and measures of "adaptive behavior") came along much later and made it possible to identify milder degrees of mental handicap in children with normal physical appearance whose retardation may be evident only in relation to the intellectual demands of school. Perhaps this is a paradigm for the relationship between categories and dimensions (which are sometimes seen as incompatible, alternative diagnostic constructs). Historically, the category seems to appear first, based on clinical observation. The dimension comes along later, based on more refined scientific evidence; it does not replace the category and, in fact, may have a hard fight for general acceptance. In this example, we could note that, although concepts of mental retardation are universal, IQ tests are still illegal in California for use in educational placement decisions and have been rejected on similar grounds in large areas of the world: for example, the Soviet Union and mainland China.

Is the concept of mental retardation "valid"? I would certainly say that it is, if only on the basis that this category conveys some definite information about prognosis. Children who are observed to be retarded in their mental development usually keep having difficulty in school. They will likely never develop Piagetian formal operational thought. Their vocational options will therefore probably not include positions where higher educational attainment or high levels of logical reasoning are required. Intelligence tests share in being "validated" by some of this same prognostic utility. The test scores of individuals tend to be relatively stable over long periods of time. The major exception to this statement has been infant test scores, which generally showed little prognostic value. This limitation may be decreased or eliminated with the emergence of new infant assessment technology from the laboratories of developmental psychologists (e.g., Bornstein & Sigman, 1986).

One important development in the psychometric assessment of intelligence is the use of a profile of abilities rather than a single IQ score. With the publication of the newest edition of the Stanford-Binet (Thorndike, Hagen, & Sattler, 1986), which also uses a profile of scores, there is not a single individual IQ test in common use that provides a single score. The forecast of academic performance these days typically uses different combinations of predictors for different outcomes. Thus for example in selecting a prospective engineering student, one would give a heavier weight to the quantitative score of the Scholastic Aptitude Test, while in selecting a journalism student one would give more weight to the verbal SAT score. Similarly, prediction of vocational success involves the use of differential weights for various aptitude measures, depending on the occupation (Schmidt & Hunter, 1981). Eventually, the clinical use of these profiles may be the impetus for developing new, more differentiated concepts of children's limitations in particular intellectual domains. This would be an advantage in stating a child's intellectual prognosis more precisely.

Mental retardation as a category conveys very little specific information about etiology. It has been stated that there are more than 300 separate etiological factors in mental retardation, with new ones being discovered all the time (e.g., a larger and larger catalog of inborn errors of metabolism and chromosomal anomalies). However, no one of these etiological factors explains much of the overall variance in mental retardation. It is still true that most affected persons are only mildly retarded, seem biologically normal, and fit only into the ambiguous etiological category of cultural–familial retardation (i.e., their difficulty is presumably attributable to some combination of polygenetic heredity and life experiences). The use of intelligence test information allows one to be a little more specific about etiology in that persons with IQs under 50 are far more likely than those with scores from 50 to 70 to have some identifiable biological difficulties related to their retardation.

Unfortunately, different profiles of intellectual abilities do not seem to correspond very well to particular etiological factors.

There is, in general, no known treatment for mental retardation once it becomes well established. This is not a counsel of despair, because much can be done to "normalize" the lives of mentally retarded children and adults, but the main thrust of work aimed at producing normal mental development must be preventive. Preventive work generally depends upon firm scientific knowledge about causes, or at least about risk factors. An often-told success story in the prevention of mental retardation is that of the low phenylalanine diet for infants identified as having PKU. On the cultural–familial end of the etiological spectrum, I would cite the development day-care program of Ramey and his associates (e.g., Ramey & Haskins, 1981) as a somewhat successful effort to prevent mental retardation. In principle, children with different profiles of academic skills might require different remedial educational strategies. However, this approach has not yet been developed very far in the special education of the mentally retarded.

Conduct Disorder and Aggression

The second example of a valid category of child psychopathology I would like to give is that of conduct disorder (unsocialized aggressive conduct disorder, as it is termed in DSM-III, or solitary, aggressive type, as it is termed in DSM-III-R). As in the case of mental retardation, the firmest evidence for the validity of the conduct disorder category concerns prognosis. Robins's (1966) classic 30-year follow-up study showed that a significant proportion of child psychiatric patients identified as showing antisocial behavior as a presenting complaint became adult sociopaths (equivalent to DSM-III and DSM-III-R antisocial personality disorder), as compared to child patients with other presenting complaints or neighborhood control subjects. Once more it is possible to identify a dimension of aggressiveness roughly corresponding to the category of conduct disorder. Here, for example, one can cite the peer-rated measures of aggression developed for 8-year-old children by Eron and his colleagues. In their latest follow-up studies, when these youngsters had grown into adults 30 years old, it was found that childhood-peer-rated aggression predicted adult MMPI aggression scores, trouble with the law, spouse abuse, and other such variables. Aggression had predictive value over a 22-year period even after IQ was controlled statistically (Huesmann, Eron, Lefkowitz, & Walder, 1984). Among the most sophisticated approaches to the measurement of childhood aggressive behavior at present is that of Patterson (1986), who combines child self-reports and parent, teacher, and peer ratings with direct observation of family interaction in the home. Patterson believes that the use of these diverse sources in measuring aggressive behavior should maximize the predictive value of these measures (as well as their values as outcome measures in treatment studies).

Knowledge about etiological factors in conduct disorder and aggression has not yet reached a high level of consensus. If one simply looks at the individuals in prisons or other correctional facilities in the United States, it is clear that far more males than females are incarcerated, that adolescents and young adults are the largest age group, and that lower SES and members of disadvantaged racial minorities are greatly overrepresented. Unfortunately, none of these demographic facts is very easy to interpret. First of all, many persons in prison do not fit into any category of psychopathology, although those with antisocial personality disorder (with a history of childhood conduct disorder) are common. Conversely, many children with conduct disorder fail to become involved with the law. Most scholars discount the importance of SES and race in themselves as artifactual and focus on other correlated variables such as the presence of an antisocial parent in the home (or in the child's biological background) or of models for aggressive or antisocial behavior in the family, neighborhood, or school. Rigorous experimental studies demonstrating the effects of aggressive models (live or televised) on children's behavior abound, but the explanatory value of these in relation to actual conduct disorder is disputed. Male children as a group are clearly more aggressive in their behavior than females (Maccoby & Jacklin, 1974), yet the extent to which this is due to biological as opposed to social factors is unclear. In conclusion, the diagnostic category of conduct disorder in children cannot yet be stated to be validated by the etiological information it conveys.

The treatment of conduct disorders is notoriously difficult. The most rigorously studied treatments so far are behavioral ones, some of which have taken place in family settings (Patterson, 1974), some in group homes (Fixsen, Phillips, & Wolf, 1973), and some in schools (reviewed by Routh, 1979). The effect of positive reinforcement, time out for misbehavior, and other behavioral variables on various aggressive behaviors can be considered to be well established but nonspecific to those behaviors. There is also the problem that behavioral researchers are still often scornful of the utility of diagnostic categories or "the medical model," and so they do not document the diagnostic status of children in their studies—even studies that are otherwise very rigorous. The long-term efficacy of behavioral treatments in decreasing conduct disorder has not yet been adequately studied. In short, knowledge about differential response to treatment cannot be considered to validate conduct disorders as a diagnostic category.

Tourette's Syndrome

Although Tourette's syndrome is not a common type of child psychopathology (certainly not as common as mental retardation or conduct disorder), it may be worth discussing here as a category that seems to be validated not only by knowledge about prognosis but also by knowledge about its etiology and response to treatment. Tourette's syndrome, defined by multiple tics including vocal ones, has as its most dramatic symptom (in adolescents and adults) coprolalia, or the use of obscence language, as part of the tic. It has a somewhat intermittent course, which may be lifelong (Shapiro, Shapiro, Brunn, & Sweet, 1978).

The general etiology of Tourette's syndrome is not known, but what is interesting as a phenomenon of child psychopathology is that the full-blown disorder has been shown to emerge as a side effect to stimulant medication (Golden, 1974). This may even be clinically important because such a large proportion of Tourette's patients have been found to meet criteria for attention deficit disorder (Comings & Comings, 1984). Therefore, the presence of tics, especially vocal ones, has come to be viewed as a contraindication of the prescription of stimulant medication to a hyperactive child. Stimulant medication can be viewed as a significant iatrogenic factor in Tourette's syndrome even if it is not typically the main cause of the syndrome. I consider this discovery to provide one type of evidence for the validity of this diagnostic category.

However, it was a treatment discovery that probably did the most to move Tourette's syndrome from its status as an obscure curiosity to its present greater prominence as a diagnostic category. The drug haloperidol (Haldol) was found to have the effect of reducing the tics in Tourette's patients. One always must be a bit cautious in regarding a treatment effect as "validation" of a diagnostic category. For example, Kendell (1982) commented that headaches, bruises, rheumatic fever, and rheumatoid arthritis all respond to aspirin, and yet we do not therefore regard these disorders as having anything fundamental in common. Haloperidol, the drug that has an effect on tics in Tourette's syndrome, is one of a broad category of neuroleptic or antipsychotic drugs, yet most other drugs of this general type do not cause the antitic effect. Also, the effects of the drug on the frequency of tics in Tourette's syndrome seem to be relatively specific ones and not due to any general sedation or other inhibitory effects. So the haloperidol effect may be seen as one kind of information validating Tourette's syndrome as a diagnostic category.

Beyond Hypotheses about Prognosis, Etiology, and Treatment

This chapter began by equating "validity" with truth, and the validation of diagnostic categories with testing hypotheses about child psychopathology. Although hypotheses about prognosis, etiology, and treatment are of high interest to clinicians, they are hardly the only hypotheses of interest. Theories and research concerning child psychopathology will obviously range far beyond these issues and should not be limited to them.

One important aspect of child psychopathology, for example, is the fact that it occurs in immature, developing organisms. Therefore, a natural set of questions and hypotheses concerns the relationships between child psychopathology and development.

In my own research on hyperactivity, already discussed, one of the main hypotheses of interest concerned the relationship of hyperactivity to normal child development. The hypothesis was basically that the hyperactive child resembled a younger normal child in activity level and attention span. In a series of studies of normal children (e.g., Routh et al., 1974; Routh, Walton, & Padan-Belkin, 1978), my associates and I tried to investigate the development of activity level in children, indexed by quadrant entries in a standardized playroom. Indeed, we were able to find some support for the expectation that activity level would increase, from about age 10 months to a peak in toddlers 18 months old, and (under certain experimental conditions) decline thereafter, with an especially reliable decline during the late preschool years. Children referred for the evaluation of hyperactivity were indeed found to resemble somewhat younger normal children in terms of their number of quadrant entries in the playroom (Routh & Schroeder, 1976). As already stated, Milich and colleagues (1986) confirmed some of our cross-sectional age differences by his observation of longitudinal age changes in children's activity level. Eaton and Enns (1986) have tried to build a case for changes in activity level as a life span developmental phenomenon. Thinking about activity level in these terms causes one to wish to investigate the biological and social mechanisms underlying age changes in activity level and how these might be related to the phenomenon of hyperactivity, and also the mechanisms by which stimulant drugs reduce children's activity (e.g., Porrino et al., 1983).

In another area of research, there has always been great interest on the part of researchers in studying mental retardation in relation to normal mental development. One of the criteria used by Binet in constructing his mental scale was that each item must demonstrate an increase in the percentage of children passing it with age. For each item one could therefore construct a developmental curve from the age when no child could pass it through intermediate ages up to the age at which all children could pass the item. Many years later, Inhelder (1968) studied the performance of adult mentally retarded individuals on Piagetian tasks. She found that mildly retarded individuals performed at a concrete operational level, like normal children of elementary school age. More severely retarded individuals performed at a preoperational or even a sensorimotor level on the Piagetian tasks. In longitudinal research reviewed by Woodward (1963), retarded individuals passed the Piagetian developmental milestones in the same general sequence as normal infants and children, but of course at a much later age and at a slower pace.

Child psychologists working within an information-processing theoretical framework have also been interested in the relationship between normal development and mental retardation in terms of strategic behaviors. In a memory task, for example, normal older children will show a bowed serial position curve, remembering both the first and the last items presented better than the middle items (the so-called primacy and recency effects). The primacy effect (better recall of the early items) is generally considered to be due to the use of rehearsal or other cognitive strategies. Indeed, younger children do not show such a primacy effect unless they are taught to rehearse items, and then they do show it. Mentally retarded children perform on such memory tasks like younger normal children, that is, showing no primacy effect. Like the young children, the retarded can be taught to rehearse, and when they do, it increases primacy and normalizes their performance. Therefore, the "deficit" shown by the retarded on such memory tasks represents not an absolute incapacity, but only a failure on their part spontaneously to devise strategies for optimum task performance. Using a computer analogy, these retarded children have not a "hardware" but a "software" problem. It is of considerable interest theoretically to know this, and to an extent it contributes to the construct validity of the diagnostic category of mental retardation.

CHOOSING BETWEEN ALTERNATIVE DEFINITIONS

Even the best accepted categories in child psychopathology have somewhat different specific definitions in DSM-III, DSM-III-R, ICD-9, or the literature. Kendell (1982), in discussing the choice of diagnostic criteria for research, advises the use of several definitions simultaneously to see which one produces the best results. If a hunter is trying to hit a target and is not sure of its precise location, a shotgun would be a better choice of weapon than a rifle. Another good reason for using formal diagnostic criteria in subject selection is to produce better comparability between studies by different investigators.

Barkley (1982), in trying to provide better guidelines for the assessment of hyperactivity, pointed out that most researchers do not use *any* operational criteria beyond their own unsupported clinical judgment that their subjects are hyperactive. The single operational measure in most common use, the Conners Teacher Rating Scale, has recently been criticized for its lack of discriminant validity; it reportedly is more likely to pick out children with conduct disorder than those who are purely hyperactive (Ullman, Sleator, & Sprague, 1985).

Zigler, Balla, and Hodapp (1984) have argued that the official definition of mental retardation should be changed from being based on IQ and adaptive behavior measures to being defined by IQ alone. This would correspond to what many diagnosticians actually do now, that is, ignore measures of adaptive behavior even if available (Adams, 1973). Beyond this, it would undoubtedly define a population of individuals with greater stability over time, since IQ scores have greater long-term reliability (and greater internal consistency) than do measures of adaptive behavior (Sparrow, Balla, & Cicchetti, 1984). The problem with such a change, it seems to me, would come in the area of evaluating treatment rather than in the area of prognosis. Treatments of retarded individuals are usually aimed not at changing IQ scores but at changing adaptive behavior: for example, teaching self-help, communication, academic, vocational, or interpersonal skills. If an adult individual with an IQ of 65 is earning a living in competitive employment and is happily married, what clinical (or scientific) purpose is served by labeling the person mentally retarded? This may be too high a price to pay for mere stability and internal consistency in the definition of retardation.

Conduct disorder is inherently defined by social criteria, and so the recent trend toward assessing it to a greater extent by ratings of other people (i.e., parents, teachers, peers) rather than depending exclusively on self-report or behavioral observation seems praiseworthy. As already noted, peer measures of aggression (like measures of peer rejection in general) have extremely high stability over time (Cowen, Pederson, Babigian, Izzo, & Trost, 1973; Huesmann et al., 1984).

INVALIDATING DIAGNOSTIC CATEGORIES

According to the philosophy of science espoused by Karl Popper (1962) and his followers, scientific theories shoud be falsifiable, and progress occurs through efforts to disconfirm hypotheses rather than to confirm them. The picture that has been painted in this chapter of a valid diagnostic category is mainly one that predicts something about future outcomes, provides information about etiology, or is responsive to specific treatment(s). If a theory made stronger statements, such as that *all* cases of X have a particular outcome, it could be disconfirmed by a single negative case. However, few theoretical statements about diagnostic categories in child psychopathology are so rash. Most would be in probabilistic terms, and the counterargument, that X is *not* predictive of some particular outcome, amounts to accepting the null hypothesis. Present theories are thus difficult to disconfirm, and to that extent rather unsatisfactory.

CONCLUSION

It has been argued here that validating diagnostic categories amounts to testing scientific hypotheses about children to whom these categories apply. At this rather early stage in the progress of child psychopathology, most of the hypotheses have to do with prognosis, and to a lesser extent etiology and response to treatment. The strongest evidence that could be adduced for the validity of child diagnostic categories was thus seen in ones like mental retardation and conduct disorder, because these disorders have been shown to have high stability over time.

In the future it is hoped that more explicit theories can be be developed about categories and dimensions of child psychopathology, ones that are both strongly grounded in empirical research findings and subject to disconfirmation by contrary facts.

REFERENCES

Adams, J. (1973). Adaptive behavior and measured intelligence in the classification of mental retardation. *American Journal of Mental Deficiency, 78*, 77–81.

American Psychiatric Association (1980). *Diagnostic and statistical manual of mental disorders* (3rd ed.). Washington, DC: Author.

American Psychiatric Association (1987). *Diagnostic and statistical manual of mental disorders* (3rd ed., rev.). Washington, DC: Author.

American Psychological Association (1974). *Standards for educational and psychological tests.* Washington, DC: Author.

Barkley, R.A. (1977). A review of stimulant drug research with hyperactive children. *Journal of Child Psychology and Psychiatry, 18*, 137–165.

Barkley, R. (1982). Guidelines for defining hyperactivity in children (Attention Deficit Disorder with Hyperactivity). In B.B. Lahey & A.E. Kazdin (Eds.), *Advances in clinical child psychology* (Vol. 5). New York: Plenum.

Barkley, R.A., & Ullman, D.G. (1975). A comparison of objective measures of activity level and distractibility in hyperactive and nonhyperactive children. *Journal of Abnormal Child Psychology, 4*, 327–348.

Bechtoldt, H.P. (1959). Construct validity: A critique. *American Psychologist, 14,* 619–629.

Bornstein, M.H., & Sigman, M.D. (1986). Continuity in mental development from infancy. *Child Development, 57,* 251–274.

Campbell, D.T., & Fiske, D.W. (1959). Convergent and discriminant validation by the multitrait–multimethod matrix. *Psychological Bulletin, 56,* 81–105.

Clements, S. (1966). *Minimal brain dysfunction in children.* Washington, DC: U. S. Government Printing Office. (NINDB Monograph No. 3.)

Comings, D.E., & Comings, B.G. (1984). Tourette syndrome and attention deficit disorder with hyperactivity: Are they genetically related? *Journal of the American Academy of Child Psychiatry, 23,* 138–146.

Cowen, E.L., Pederson, A., Babigian, H., Izzo, L.D., & Trost, M.A. (1973). Long-term follow-up of early detected vulnerable children. *Journal of Consulting & Clinical Psychology, 41,* 438–446.

Cronbach, L.J., & Meehl, P.E. (1955). Construct validity in psychological tests. *Psychological Bulletin, 52,* 281–300.

Eaton, W.O. & Enns, L.R. (1986). Sex differences in human motor activity level. *Psychological Bulletin, 100* 19–28.

Fixsen, D.L., Phillips, E.L., & Wolf, M.M. (1973). Achievement Place: Experiments in self-government with pre-delinquents. *Journal of Applied Behavior Analysis, 6,* 31–47.

Gibson, D.L., Pozsonyi, J., & Zarfas, D.E. (1964). Dimensions of mongolism: II. The interaction of clinical indices. *American Journal of Mental Deficiency, 68,* 503–510.

Golden, G.S. (1974). Gilles de la Tourette's syndrome following methylphenidate administration. *Developmental Medicine & Child Neurology, 16,* 76–78.

Huesmann, L.R., Eron, L.D., Lefkowitz, M.M., & Walder, L.O. (1984). The stability of aggression over time and generations. *Developmental Psychology, 20,* 1120–1134.

Inhelder, B. (1968). *The diagnosis of reasoning in the mentally retarded* (W.B. Stephens, Trans.). New York: John Day.

Kendell, R.E. (1982). The choice of diagnostic criteria for biological research. *Archives of General Psychiatry, 39,* 1334–1339.

Landy, F. (1986). Stamp collecting versus science: Validation as hypothesis testing. *American Psychologist, 41,* 1183–1192.

Lang, P.J., Levin, D.N., Miller, G., & Kozak, M.J. (1983). Fear behavior, fear imagery, and the psychophysiology of emotion: The problem of affective response integration. *Journal of Abnormal Psychology, 92,* 276–306.

Langhorne, J.E., Loney, J., Paternite, C., & Bechtoldt, H.P. (1976). Childhood hyperkinesis: A return to the source. *Journal of Abnormal Psychology, 85,* 201–209.

Loney, J., & Milich, R. (1982). Hyperactivity, inattention, and aggression in clinical practice. In M. Wolraich & D.K. Routh (Eds.), *Advances in developmental and behavioral pediatrics* (Vol. 3). Greenwich, CT: JAI.

Maccoby, E.E., & Jacklin, C.N. (1974). *The psychology of sex differences.* Stanford, CA: Stanford University Press.

Meehl, P.E. (1973). Maxcov-hitmax: A taxonomic search method for loose genetic syndromes. In P. E. Meehl (Ed.), *Psychodiagnosis: Selected papers.* New York: Norton.

Milich, R., & Loney, J. (1979). The role of hyperactive and aggressive symptomatology in predicting adolescent outcome among hyperactive children. *Journal of Pediatric Psychology*, *4*, 93–112.

Milich, R., Loney, J., & Roberts, M.A. (1986). Playroom observations of activity level and sustained attention: Two-year stability. *Journal of Consulting & Clinical Psychology*, *54*, 272–274.

Morrison, J.R., & Stewart, M.A. (1973). The psychiatric status of the legal families of adopted families of hyperactive children. *Archives of General Psychiatry*, *28*, 888–891.

Nichols, P., & Chen, T.-C. (1981). *Minimal brain dysfunction: A prospective study*. Hillsdale, NJ: Erlbaum.

Novick, M.R. (1985). *Standards for educational and psychological testing*. Washington, DC: American Educational Research Association, American Psychological Association, and National Council on Measurement in Education.

Patterson, G.R. (1974). Interventions for boys with conduct problems: Multiple settings, treatments, and criteria. *Journal of Consulting & Clinical Psychology*, *42*, 471–481.

Patterson, G.R. (1986). Performance models for antisocial boys. *American Psychologist*, *41*, 432–444.

Popper, K.R. (1962). *Conjectures and refutations: The growth of scientific knowledge*. New York: Basic.

Porrino, L.J., Rapoport, J.L., Behar, D., Sceery, W., Ismond, D.R., & Bunney, W.E., Jr. (1983). A naturalist assessment of the motor activity of hyperactive boys. *Archives of General Psychiatry*, *40*, 681–687.

Quay, H.C., Routh, D.K., & Shapiro, S.K. (1987). Psychopathology of childhood: From description to validation. In M.R. Rosenzweig & L.W. Porter (Eds.), *Annual Review of Psychology* (Vol. 38). Palo Alto, CA: Annual Reviews, Inc.

Ramey, C.T., & Haskins, R. (1981). The modification of intelligence through early experience. *Intelligence*, *5*, 5–19.

Rapoport, J.I., Buchsbaum, M. S., Zahn, T.P., Weingartner, H., Ludlow, C., & Mikkelsen, E.J. (1978). Dextroamphetamine: Cognitive and behavioral effects in normal prepubertal boys. *Science*, *199*, 560–563.

Robins, L.N. (1966). *Deviant children grown up*. Baltimore: Williams & Wilkins.

Routh, D.K. (1979). Activity, attention, and aggression in learning disabled children. *Journal of Clinical Child Psychology*, *8*, 183–187.

Routh, D.K., Gonzalez, J., Saab, P., Armstrong, F.D., Guerra, E., Shifman, L., & Fawcett, N. (1987, August). *The effects of mother presence on children's reactions to medical stress: Subjective and physiological aspects*. Presented at the meeting of the American Psychological Association, New York.

Routh, D.K., & Roberts, R.D. (1972). Minimal brain dysfunction in children: Failure to find evidence for a behavioral syndrome. *Psychological Reports*, *31*, 307–314.

Routh, D.K., & Schroeder, C.S. (1976). Standardized playroom measures as indices of hyperactivity. *Journal of Abnormal Child Psychology*, *4*, 199–207.

Routh, D.K., Schroeder, C.S., & O'Tuama, L.A. (1974). Development of activity level in children. *Developmental Psychology*, *10*, 163–168.

Routh, D.K., Walton, M.D., & Padan-Belkin, E. (1978). Development of activity level in children revisited: Effects of mother presence. *Developmental Psychology*, *14*, 571–581.

Schmidt, F.L., & Hunter, J.E. (1981). Employment testing: Old theories and new research findings. *American Psychologist, 36,* 1128–1137.

Shapiro, A.K., Shapiro, E.S., Brunn, R.D., & Sweet, R.D. (1978). *Gilles de la Tourette syndrome.* New York: Raven.

Sparrow, S.S., Balla, D., & Cicchetti, D.V. (1984). *Vineland Adaptive Behavior Scales: Manual.* Circle Pines, MI: American Guidance Service.

Thorndike, R.L., Hagen, E.P., & Sattler, J.M. (1986). *The Stanford-Binet Intelligence Scale: Fourth Edition. Guide for administering and scoring.* Chicago: Riverside.

Ullman, R.K., Sleator, E.K., & Sprague, R.L. (1985). A change of mind: The Conners Abbreviated Rating Scales reconsidered. *Journal of Abnormal Child Psychology, 13,* 553–565.

Weiss, G., & Hechtman, L.T. (1986). *Hyperactive children grown up: Empirical findings and theoretical considerations.* New York: Guilford.

Werry, J.S. (1968). Developmental hyperactivity. *Pediatric Clinics of North America, 15,* 581–599.

Woodward, M. (1963). The application of Piaget's theory to research in mental deficiency. In N.R. Ellis (Ed.), *Handbook of mental deficiency.* New York: McGraw-Hill.

Zigler, E., Balla, D., & Hodapp, R. (1984). On the definition and classification of mental retardation. *American Journal of Mental Deficiency, 89,* 215–230.

PART 2

Specific Diagnoses

CHAPTER 5

Mental Retardation

ALAN A. BAUMEISTER AND ALFRED A. BAUMEISTER

DEFINITION

The notion that people are "created equal" is firmly rooted in American historical and political traditions. But, examined from biological and behavioral perspectives, it is clear not only that in many health-related aspects people are unequal, but also that individual differences are profound, manifold, and enduring. Variability is inherent in nature, human and otherwise.

A major feature of human variability is the extent to which effective adjustments to changing environmental exigencies are moderated by intelligent behavior. The concept of intelligence has been and continues to be the subject of considerable and sometime acrimonious debate in the professional literature, in the legal arena, and in the popular press. Nevertheless, the construct of intelligence is and always has been central to the definition of mental retardation.

Mental retardation represents an enormous constellation of symptoms, etiologies, and outcomes, requiring diverse interventions. In some instances mental retardation can be attributed to observed or inferred biological perturbation. But in most cases, the source is more socially complex, and disability, in turn, must be related to prevailing attitudes and values. In the broadest sense, then, mental retardation is a culturally defined disorder. In any event, we are dealing here with perhaps the most heterogeneous of human morbidities; generalizations can only be proffered in the largest sense. Each of the specific conditions or causes, numbering more than 350, must be considered separately with respect to prevention, treatment, and prognosis.

Mental retardation, by most definitions, currently and historically, presents two fundamental general features: It is primarily a behavioral concept and is defined relative to standards for different ages, cultures, and situations. Over the years, specific definitions of mental retardation have taken varied forms, depending on existing scientific information as well as on prevailing attitudes and values. Moreover, different aspects have been emphasized from culture to culture. Also, consider the various disciplines concerned with mental retardation. Each approaches the problem with particular concepts, methods, and assumptions. So general definitions that drive policy decisions, that generate service systems, and that provide the conceptual basis for individual interventions frequently represent compromises. But in so doing we are often left with a certain vagueness and looseness accompanied by conceptual contradictions that may produce a Procrustean model of mental retardation and lead to internal definitional contradictions (Baumeister & Muma, 1975).

A detailed account of the various definitions of mental retardation and how these have evolved is not possible here. We shall identify the major consensus definitions and briefly attend to some alternative considerations that have diagnostic and policy implications. It is important, though, to emphasize that definition of mental retardation is much more than an idle academic exercise, because millions of people are directly and indirectly affected by classification of disability. A rational and equitable system of service delivery depends on valid classification. Science, too, requires a specific and veridical terminology for definitional purposes.

Early definitions and classification systems of mental retardation tended to focus on relatively severe types, especially those that presented obvious neurological disturbance. But even then attention was directed to social adaptation as a criterion (e.g., Jervis, 1952; Tredgold, 1908). However, evolving social values, accelerated sophistication in the behavioral and medical sciences, and increasing reliance on technology for successful adaptation have led to emphasis on multifaceted criteria. Over time greater focus came to be placed on mild mental retardation, criteria for which are reflected primarily in behavioral and social variables. This is a concept of mental retardation heavily laden with significant socioeconomic implications.

Probably the first to suggest all-inclusive criteria for defining and classifying mental retardation was Doll (1941). We mention Doll because the conditions he proposed are thoroughly embedded in the public view of mental retardation. His definition included six criteria: (1) social incompetence; (2) mental incompetence; (3) developmental deficiency; (4) of constitutional origin; (5) persistence into adulthood; and (6) essentially incurable. Some of the primary features of Doll's 1941 definition are contained in current formal systems, such as that proposed by the American Association of Mental Deficiency (AAMD) and the American Psychiatric Association. There are, of course, some differences, particularly in the area of "incurability." Moreover, it is clear that Doll confused diagnosis with prognosis, although the fact is that most children diagnosed as mentally retarded will become adults with mental retardation. In practice, Doll's definition probably is still commonly accepted, particularly in the form of publicly held beliefs, beliefs that are reflected in treatment practices, policies, and resource allocation.

The American Association on Mental Deficiency Terminology and Classification

The AAMD, for many years, has proposed systems of definition, terminology, and classification. The first such effort produced a manual in 1921. Various editions appeared until a comprehensive new version, basically the current one, was published in 1959. That system, too, was revised and fine-tuned in 1973 and 1977, eventuating in the present system of classification and terminology (Grossman, 1983).

According to the current definition promulgated by the AAMD (Grossman, 1983), three criteria are employed for making diagnoses and for classification: (1)

subaverage general intellectual functioning; (2) existing concurrently with deficits in adaptive behavior; and (3) exhibited during the developmental period. A major purpose guiding the formulation of this system was to produce "world-wide use of a common nosology with definitional criteria" (p. 3). Although certainly influential, the AAMD system has not entirely achieved this goal, even in the United States, either in the sense of acceptance of the basic definitional elements or in terms of their specific description (Frankenberger, 1984; Huberty, Koller, & Tenbrink, 1980; Lowitzer, Utley, & Baumeister, 1987; Patrick & Reschly, 1982; Utley, Lowitzer, & Baumeister, 1987). The factors weighing against universal acceptance of the AAMD definition include: (1) rapid changes in eligibility criteria for services; (2) fiscal implications; (3) civil rights litigation; (4) professional preferences; (5) agency disagreements; and (6) interest group influence.

The criterion of subaverage general intelligence refers to an IQ of approximately 70, obtained on a standardized general intelligence test, usually the Stanford-Binet or one of the Wechsler variants. However, the latest AAMD manual indicates that the upper limit of 70 is but a guideline and that, depending on setting factors, clinical considerations, and the particular instrument, the cutting level might be extended to 75.

In the earlier 1977 version the IQ cutting level was lowered from 1 standard deviation to 2 standard deviations below the mean, or from an IQ of about 85 to one of about 70. This was a definitional change of major consequence because many people who previously qualified for available services were no longer technically eligible. While there are some very compelling reasons for making the IQ cutoff more stringent, an alteration of this magnitude met with resistance, frustration, confusion, and disagreement. In fact, some states continue to rely on the older system or to identify a "borderline" category of people in need of services. Obviously public policy implications were as profoundly affected as clinical issues, because the change of a single standard deviation greatly decreased mental retardation prevalence, as estimated within a statistical model. Because of what appeared to be an absolute IQ criterion, the 1983 version is somewhat more flexible, in that, based on clinical judgments, some people may be diagnosed as retarded even with IQs well above the cutoff.

The second principal element of the AAMD definition describes impairments in adaptive behavior—that is, limitations in the effectiveness with and the extent to which an individual demonstrates social adaptation and personal independence typical for his or her age group and cultural setting. During infancy and early childhood, adaptive behavior includes such characteristics as sensorimotor function, communication, and self-help skills. In later childhood and early adolescence greater emphasis is placed on academic skills. Because academic performance can be measured with high reliability and because academic achievement is so obviously salient as adaptive behavior during the school period, it weighs heavily in the diagnostic process in later childhood and early adolescence. The fact that academic skills are so clearly important and so readily measured may account for the relatively high prevalence of mental retardation during school years. Before and after, measures of adaptive behavior are not so clear-cut or universally accepted, nor is failure to adjust so clearly evident.

From a clinical point of view the concept of adaptive behavior is rather nebulous and does not lend itself to easy assessment (except in the case of academic skills), especially in marginal cases. Of course, there are many adaptive behavior scales in the literature (Meyers, Nihira, & Zetlin, 1979). Some of these, such as the AAMD Adaptive Behavior Scale and the Vineland Maturity Scale, have been rather rigorously standardized in terms of their psychometric properties, among both institutional and public school samples. These two instruments are the most widely employed in formal evaluation, although there are many others available.

Serious questions have been raised about the relative importance of intelligence and adaptive behavior in the diagnosis and classification process. On the one hand, critics of the IQ remind us that this is a single component score that may have little validity outside the closed and self-contained system of the school, that the IQ is a culturally laden concept that places certain ethnic, minority, and racial groups at differential risk for false diagnosis and mislabeling, that the IQ is programmatically unclear as an indicator for intervention strategies, that infant and later measures of intelligence do not correlate well, and that the concept of general intelligence is based on a fixed-capacity, inborn, and unitary theory of adaptation. These are hardly new arguments, but they have enormous policy, educational, and clinical significance and implication; as a recent example, in California a federal court has prevented placement of minority pupils in special classes on the basis of standard IQ tests.

But, on the other hand, serious criticisms can also be levied at adaptive behavior as a basis upon which to diagnose and classify. The standardized adaptive behavior scales are extremely limited in their content and range, they are typically based on informants' imprecise and unreliable perceptions of an individual's capabilities, and they are developed within a person-oriented defect model of adaptation. This last criticism becomes all the more salient as one considers that different environments define competence differently, and that requirements for adaptations must be evaluated against the demands set by a particular context. Because adaptive behavior scales tend to be constructed from a conventional psychometric perspective, they focus on individual behavior without systematic consideration of variable environmental constraints and demands. The argument can and occasionally has been made that environments are defective, not children.

If our taxonomy of adaptive behavior is inadequate, a taxonomy of environments is nonexistent. Although there may be some standard features of adaptive behaviors that cut across environments, these are events that are also likely to be tapped by tests of intelligence. In fact, despite the apparent bivariate nature of the AAMD definition, scores from intelligence tests and standard adaptive behavior scales correlate significantly. The point is that, not only are intelligence and adaptive behavioral measures nonorthogonal, but neither may be sensitive to specific but important environmental constraints.

In all likelihood, recent federal court orders notwithstanding, more professional and programmatic credibility currently is attached to standardized intelligence scores than to adaptive behavior measures. A study by Adams (1973) showed that, despite tacit professional and administrative reliance on both aspects of behavior for making differential diagnoses, in practice most clinicians rely on the IQ for the final determination.

For this and for other practical as well as theoretical reasons, Zigler and his colleagues have argued that the IQ should be the only formal basis for evaluation of mental retardation (e.g., Zigler, Balla, & Hodapp, 1984). Adaptive behavior measures might provide an adjunctive measure of information concerning education intervention, but the primary diagnosis in their view ought to be based on IQ (see Clausen, 1977, for a similar conclusion). It should be added that the vast research literature, cutting across many disciplines, relies much more heavily on IQ scores than on any other index in describing samples of subject.

The third criterion, an age distinction, is that mental retardation should be manifested in the developmental period, which, depending on where one happens to be reading in the manual, is the period between conception and the eighteenth or twenty-first birthday. Developmental deficits are regarded as slow, arrested, or incomplete development owing to brain injury, degenerative central nervous system effects, or psychological factors. There is a certain arbitrariness to the age criterion, in that development is a continuous process in which different physical and behavioral functions progress at different rates, mature at different times, and may, in fact, change at different rates depending on social variables. Moreover, mental retardation is a behavioral concept and, from that perspective, it makes little difference whether a person receives brain trauma the day before or the day after the eighteenth birthday. Even though these conditions would take different diagnostic labels, the required treatment would obviously be little influenced by the labels. However, accessibility to services might be drastically affected.

Once the diagnosis of mental retardation is made, then the procedure typically is to determine level of retardation. Level of retardation is as much a social as a biological or a psychometric test. Obviously, mentally retarded people comprise a very heterogeneous group in which some are totally dependent while others can function quite independently.

In addition, mentally retarded individuals vary greatly with respect to causation, prognosis, behavioral manifestations, physical handicaps, and stigmata. A generally accepted rule of thumb is that about 25% of the retarded population exhibits some type of biomedical etiology, while the majority appear to have no clear-cut neurological involvement and no evident biological sign. These considerations constitute part of the rationale for the two classification systems development by the AAMD, one based entirely on measured intelligence and the other on medical taxonomy.

Classification Based on Measured Intelligence

Assuming that an individual is diagnosed as mentally retarded, then the functional classification is based on IQ as follows:

Mild	50–55 to about 70
Moderate	35–40 to 50–55
Severe	20–25 to 35–40

Profound	below 20–24
Unspecified	

This is not an entirely new system in that most of these terms have been used in previous editions of the AAMD manual. The bands, defining the boundaries, reflect the fact that IQ is subject to error of measurement and that clinical judgment may be required to classify an individual appropriately. The "unspecified" category is included to permit professional latitude in classification when circumstances prohibit valid or complete assessment, especially when unusual features are presented.

Whether this particular classification has any great functional or clinical value is of some debate. Obviously, the purpose of classification, such as school placement, will greatly affect the particular system applied. Certainly from an administrative point of view the wide, but not universal, acceptance of the AAMD terminology suggests that it has utility from a planning perspective. The educational classification system, not developed by AAMD, has traditionally roughly corresponded to the AAMD system, except that a different terminology based on educability has historically been employed. Even then, however, a much more complete educational and behavioral assessment is required to design and implement educational programs, as reflected in the Individual Educational Plan (IEP).

Nevertheless, the AAMD classification system has been widely employed for epidemiological analyses as well as for programmatic and policy purposes. Most of the data we have concerning the distribution of mental retardation, with analysis of accompanying resources, are based on the level of retardation conception. In the broader sense the functional classification system has some face and predictive validity and may be useful for population description.

Medical Classification

The medical classification system of AAMD was revised in the 1983 manual to make it as compatible as possible with the World Health Organization International Classification of Diseases (ICD-9, 1978) and the *Diagnostic and Statistical Manual of Mental Disorders* of the American Psychiatric Association (1980). Earlier efforts by these organizations were similarly motivated in order to achieve consistency. But, owing to a number of factors, primarily having to do with the missions of the three organizations, there still remain differences. Obviously, the WHO and the APA have a much broader mandate and, therefore, had to cover many more topics, yet within an internally consistent framework. In this sense, the AAMD medical classification system is more complete because of its greater specificity regarding etiology. On the other hand, the ICD-9 system has wider application. Because ICD-9 is a comprehensive system for classifying medical conditions, the Health Care Finance Administration (HCFA, 1985) issued a regulation requiring use of ICD-9 for Medicaid reimbursement. In turn, this ruling has had an effect on medical classification systems employed in some states with respect to primary disability, and will undoubtedly affect others (Lowitzer et al., 1987).

By way of summary, the AAMD Medical Etiological Classification is organized into 10 categories. We describe each in a later section dealing with clinical features. The major categories are as follows:

1. Infections and intoxications—both maternal and child infections and intoxications occurring prenatally or postnatally

2. Trauma or physical agent—those cases in which brain damage has resulted from trauma, mechanical, or physical causes

3. Metabolism or nutrition—metabolic, nutritional, endocrine, or growth disorders that produce deviant mental development

4. Gross brain disease in the postnatal period—neoplasms and degenerative disease, and cerebral–cranial disorders of unknown or uncertain etiology coded here

5. Unknown prenatal influences—etiology not certain, but the condition exists at or prior to birth

6. Chromosomal anomalies—those conditions producing mental retardation that involve numerical and/or structural chromosomal aberrations

7. Other conditions originating in the perinatal period—prematurity, low birth weight, fetal malnutrition, or growth retardation

8. Mental retardation following psychiatric disorder—important to mental retardation that follows a psychiatric disorder such as psychosis, with no evidence of cerebral pathology

9. Environmental influences—perhaps the largest category because it includes cases where there is evidence of deprivation but no significant neural pathology; poverty would be a contributing factor

10. Other conditions—a catchall category including ill-defined or unknown conditions and sensory defects

American Psychiatric Association (DSM-III)

The definition of mental retardation set forth by the American Psychiatric Association in the *Diagnostic and Statistical Manual of Mental Disorders* (APA, 1980) was deliberately prepared to be consistent with that proposed by the American Association on Mental Deficiency. Again, the essential features are: (1) significantly subaverage general intellectual function; (2) that results in or coexists with impairments in adaptive behavior; and (3) is evident before the age of 18.

Given that standard intelligence tests involve some error of measurement, the IQ cutoff is considered to be a band from 75 to 65. This also allows for flexibility in the exercise of professional clinical judgment for diagnosis of mental retardation.

The same consideration applies to the evaluation of adaptive behavior criteria, which, in the DSM definition, refers to the individual's capacity to meet standards of independence and socialization consistent with expectations for age and cultural groups. While there are standardized scales available for assessment of general adaptation, none is considered sufficient to evaluate the individual independent of clinical judgment. These considerations are essentially identical to those noted with respect to the AAMD definition.

There are some differences, though, in terminology that may seem slight enough, but in principle could be significant. The DSM-III definition, by employing the phrase "resulting in," suggests that subaverage intelligence *causes* the deficit in adaptive behavior. The AAMD does not distinguish causality from association because of the assumption that in most instances direction of causality cannot be determined. Perhaps this is in large measure a semantic distinction, but it is hard to ignore the clinical or even commonsense experience that maladaptive behavior, such as excessive noncompliance, juvenile delinquency, and school truancy, can produce subaverage IQs.

Another, less meaningful, distinction is that the APA uses the term *impairments* in adaptive behavior, while the AAMD definition is limited to *deficits*. This wording difference, however, may have social implications in that *deficits* may imply a more structural basis.

With regard to classification, the subtypes identified by the two systems are virtually the same. The difference lies in the more flexible IQ cutoff points, or ranges, identified by AAMD. In identifying level of retardation, the coding system developed by AAMD was modified to make it consistent with DSM-III.

School Classification

A somewhat different system of classification is typically employed in school settings. Although the IQ score remains an important feature, the educational approach tends to focus on severity, particularly with respect to learning ability. Educational classification, just like those in medicine, behavior analysis, and sociology, has changed and evolved over time. But basically three categories have been commonly utilized: (1) educable mentally retarded (EMR); (2) trainable mentally retarded (TMR); and (3) severely and profoundly mentally retarded (SMR and PMR). The IQ cutoffs are 50–55 to 70–75, 25–35 to 50–55, and below 25–35, respectively. The particular ranges in each category will vary somewhat with school districts. Functionally, the three groups differ with respect to the type of educational expectations placed on them and the relative emphasis on academic and self-help skills.

HISTORICAL BACKGROUND

A number of accounts of the history of the field of mental retardation have appeared in the literature over the past three decades. In some instances these reviews focus on a relatively specific problem issue or topic such as eugenics (e.g., Smith, 1985), institutions (e.g., Baumeister & Butterfield, 1970), classification (Blanton, 1975), economics (Braddock, 1986), or special education (Semmel, Gottlieb, & Robinson, 1979). Others have taken a more comprehensive and long-range view. Perhaps the first extensive and influential treatment of the history of mental retardation was prepared by Kanner (1964); in it he carefully traced scientific, social, and clinical developments. Undoubtedly the most thorough, scholarly, and integrative history of the field of mental retardation is the one recently published by Scheerenberger (1983).

Most early discussions of mental retardation appear in religious or literary contexts. To the extent that the subject was addressed in a scientific sense, reference was to neurological and emotional disorders. Viewed against today's perspective, the treatment accorded the mentally retarded has historically been rather dismal, although there have been some very notable periods and places of enlightenment and exception.

Certainly, treatment of the mentally retarded has been erratic and cyclic. It is only in fairly recent times that mental retardation services and research have been elevated to the level of a national priority. Important recent advances have been made in the scientific realm at the same time that services have enormously expanded and improved. Much of this activity can be traced to political and social events of the early 1960s, during which time the federal government entered the field in a major way, in providing resources, in setting the conditions for sustained moral and legal commitment to the treatment and care of the retarded, and in direct support of a major research effort.

Scientific advances, both in biomedical and behavioral realms, are too numerous and complicated to cover here. But with increased understanding of genetic and neurological factors, together with a burgeoning technology, many medical interventions are now available that can dramatically and drastically alter the outcome of the course of some disorders such as PKU and kernicterus. At the same time behavioral interventions can also significantly alter the patterns of deviant and impoverished behavior. Prenatal screening, surgical techniques, behavior modification, early intervention, and drugs have all affected rate and severity of mental retardation.

Prevention

Yet, there is another, darker side to this recent history that needs to be appreciated. A great deal of mental retardation, based on what we currently know, could be prevented or ameliorated if public health and education programs were vigorously pursued and amply funded. Some years ago the President's Committee on Mental Retardation established as a national goal the reduction by 50% in incidence of mental retardation by the year 2000. A number of commentators (e.g., Baumeister, 1981; Clarke & Clarke, 1977; Zigler, 1978) have all concluded that this national goal will not be attained. The reasons are complex—partly scientific, social, political, and economic. The knowledge is available, but the resolve is not. Prevention has, in fact, received more rhetoric than action.

There is still another lesson to be learned from recent history. Despite dramatic advances in basic science, in the vast majority of cases we do not know the cause of mental retardation. Various studies of those severely affected show that diagnosis is possible in fewer than one-third (Milunsky, 1983), and in those instances where diagnosis has been made, it is in error in almost 50% of the cases (Baumeister & MacLean, 1979). These are the severely affected, and for patients whose mental retardation is mild, uncertainty about precise causes is even greater. Causes are subtle, multivariate, and interactive and not yet fully appreciated. As one examines classification systems with a view toward identifying those cases of retardation due to acquired causes, it becomes painfully obvious that opportunities for treatment and cure are not well understood and are extremely unlikely.

So while recent scientific history reveals an enormous enlargement of our knowledge base about some of the causes and effects of mental retardation, relative to the size and complexity of the problem we have but irritated the surface. On reflection, it is not really astonishing that we have such a long distance to go, because, while mental retardation is by definition treated more or less as a unitary problem, with different degrees of severity, in clinical practice we deal with hundreds of different causes, with manifold manifestations. Most of these are not interchangeable in the sense that knowledge gained from one is directly applicable to another. The problem of mental retardation is far too heterogeneous to be solved in a simple stroke or two. The problem is medically and socially complex; the solutions can be no less so.

Prevention, it may be argued, while not high on any but a verbal agenda, may be more scientifically, economically, and socially feasible than case-by-case treatment. The issue hinges on how one regards "cause." The traditional disease model regards cause in a proximal sense in that the link between event and outcome is clear and direct. In a preventive health model, cause may be thought of as more distal in that living conditions, environmental factors, personal stress, and community pressures may be implicated as precursors to the more immediate cause. Space does not permit extended discussion here of this issue, but Baumeister (1988) has expressed the hope and implications of prevention in terms of an elaborated "new morbidity" model. Here, again, the theory is advanced that mental retardation, particularly mild expression, is but one manifestation of a constellation of biological and environmental factors that combine to place certain children at risk for disabilities.

Civil Rights

The recent history of mental retardation has also emphasized the civil rights of retarded persons. Expressions of these conceptual developments are to be found in professional practices, legislation, but most dramatically in judicial determinations. Value issues that have been addressed include: (1) normalization; (2) mainstreaming; (3) right to treatment; and (4) social integration. One of the best known and most influential events of the recent past is the class action suit known as *Wyatt vs. Stickney*, a highly publicized judicial breakthrough that established what have come to be known as minimum constitutional standards for adequate habilitation for the mentally retarded.

In ruling for plaintiffs' rights to habilitation, Judge Johnson observed that retarded people in institutions have "the right to habilitation including medical treatment, education, and care, suited to their needs, regardless of age, degrees of retardation, or handicapped condition" (Poling & Breuning, 1982, p. 396).

This lawsuit set into action a major civil rights initiative for the mentally retarded. In addition, it implicitly involved some conceptual scientific and social issues that had been and still are under debate. For instance, in asserting that every resident has a right to treatment, Judge Johnson implicitly assumed that all can profit from educational or clinical interventions, at least to some extent. While not going as far as some others who followed, Johnson also, by virtue of the standards he imposed, clearly accelerated the deinstitutionalization movement. A variety of federal laws have been enacted that bolster the case for treatment and habilitation of the retarded. Congress has been and continues to be very active in this respect. For instance, last year the basic provisions of PL 94-142 were extended downward to include all children under 3 at risk for developmental disabilities. While PL 94-142 has been widely adopted, the final chapter has yet to be written concerning programmatic and cost effectiveness. Mainstreaming is an issue yet far from resolution.

In short, the recent history of mental retardation reveals some important and profound changes in scientific understanding of mental retardation. But there remains a great deal to be done because progress follows a wavelike rather than a linear course. As we invent new approaches to treatment, more serious and difficult ethical and value decisions will undoubtedly emerge and will inevitably be confronted.

CLINICAL PICTURE

Beyond the characteristics identified in connection with definition and classification and beyond specific clinical types (more than 350), there is no standard typology that can describe mentally retarded people as a diagnostic group. Occasionally, the reader will find in the literature case studies or histories that are intended to be illustrative of a particular behavior manifestation, clinical type, or treatment possibility. Mental retardation is a syndrome with myriad clinical features resulting from numerous etiologies. Obviously, not only does such variability have significant implications for diagnosis and classification, but it is essential to understand this variability when designing intervention strategies. Moreover, mental retardation is frequently accompanied by other handicapping conditions that may be more immediately clinically significant than the mental retardation.

In an effort to convey the clinical picture in a summary way, we shall follow the AAMD etiological classification system, briefly illustrating each of the major categories.

Infections and Intoxication

Prenatal Infection

Infectious diseases may be transmitted from the mother to the fetus through the placenta. Infectious agents that have been associated with mental retardation include cytomegalovirus, the rubella virus, the bacterium responsible for syphilis, and a protozoan parasite that causes toxoplasmosis.

CYTOMEGALIC INCLUSION DISEASE.   Cytomegalic inclusion disease is caused by infection with the herpes virus cytomegalovirus. Cytomegalovirus can be transmitted from mother to fetus via placental blood pathways. The consequences to the fetus can be severe and include encephalitis (inflammation of the brain), meningitis (inflammation of the meninges), and necrosis of brain tissue, especially in the periventricular region. Microcephaly, seizures, and mental retardation are common findings among infants who survive the disease.

CONGENITAL RUBELLA.   The clinical manifestations of congenital rubella include visual and hearing problems, heart defects, and mental retardation. Type and severity of symptoms depend greatly on the gestational age at the time of infection. Infections occurring during the first 2 months of age are fatal in about 50% of the cases. Among the survivors about 20% display some form of abnormality. Pathological effects on brain development include reduced proliferation of brain cells, encephalitis, and necrosis. Although there is no specific treatment for congenital rubella, the development of a rubella vaccine makes it a preventable disease. Yet there is still a problem because not all girls receive the vaccine.

CONGENITAL SYPHILIS.   A woman who is infected with the syphilis bacterium prior to or during pregnancy may transmit the bacterium to the fetus. In congenital neurosyphilis the organism attacks the infant's brain, causing inflammation and necrosis of neural tissue. Clinical manifestations include mental retardation, blindness, deafness, convulsions, hydrocephalus, and paralysis. With the advent of antibiotics, incidence of syphilis declined dramatically, though recent years have witnessed a rise in its incidence (Ingall & Norins, 1976). In fact, we currently appear to be undergoing another epidemic of syphilis.

CONGENITAL TOXOPLASMOSIS.   Prenatal infection with toxoplasmosis protozoan may result in stillbirth, abortion, or multiple abnormalities, especially of the nervous system and eyes. Sequelae are most severe when infection occurs during the first trimester. The invading organism attacks the blood vessels of the brain, causing inflammation and the formation of granulomas. Neurological symptoms of congenital toxoplasmosis may include mental retardation, paralysis, and convulsions.

Postnatal Cerebral Infection

Mental retardation may also be caused by infectious diseases occurring postnatally. In most of these cases, damage to the nervous system is associated with encephalitis or meningitis. Encephalitis is typically associated with viral infections, whereas bacterial infections are usually responsible for meningitis. Three categories of encephalitis are recognized: (1) viral encephalitis, in which a virus directly attacks the nervous system; (2) postvaccinal encephalitis, which may occur following vaccination against smallpox or rabies; and (3) postinfectious encephalitis, which occurs after an infectious disease such as measles, mumps, smallpox, pertussis, or influenza. Possible etiologic factors in addition to a direct action of the virus include production of a toxin by the virus and development of an allergic reaction (Merritt, 1973). The symptoms of encephalitis and meningitis are similar and may include headache, fever, lethargy, delirium, movement disorders, convulsions, and coma. Neurological sequelae, including mental retardation, occur in approximately 10 to 25% of the cases, depending on the nature of the infectious organism and the age of the child at the time of infection.

Intoxication

It is now well established that exposure to toxic substances during pregnancy can produce severe abnormalities in the developing fetus. We now are fully aware that prenatal exposure to a wide range of environmental pollutants may cause mental retardation. Lead, for example, has long been known to be teratogenic. Exposure to high levels of lead during pregnancy has been associated with miscarriage, stillbirths, preterm deliveries, retarded growth and development, microcephaly, and a variety of neurological symptoms including seizures and mental retardation (Schroeder, 1987).

Another problem that has come to light in recent years is that consumption of alcohol during pregnancy can have severe deleterious effects on the developing fetus. Fetal alcohol syndrome (FAS) is characterized by growth retardation, facial abnormalities, microcephaly, motor dysfunction, and mental retardation. Estimates of the incidence of FAS in the general population are 1 to 2 per 1000 live births, although among some groups, especially native Americans, incidence is much higher. Among children born to alcoholic mothers approximately 25 per 1000 display the syndrome. The percentage of births with subtle abnormalities attributable to alcohol consumption may be greatly underestimated. Susceptibility to the teratogenic influences of alcohol appears to be dependent on a number of factors, including dose, duration of exposure, and gestational timing. At present it has not been possible to establish a threshold below which alcohol consumption during pregnancy is safe.

It has also been reported that smoking during pregnancy may have harmful effects of the fetus. Infants born to women who smoked during pregnancy have shorter gestational periods and weigh less at birth than those born to nonsmokers. In addition, there is evidence that smoking during pregnancy may damage the nervous system. Infants born to women who smoked during pregnancy exhibit behavioral abnormalities shortly after birth. Maternal smoking has also been linked to long-term cognitive and behavioral deficits in children. However, it should be noted that numerous methodological problems render interpretation of these studies difficult. Specific conclusions about the behavioral sequelae of maternal smoking during pregnancy on intellectual function in the offspring cannot now be made.

Mental retardation associated with toxemias of pregnancy is also classified under "Intoxication." *Toxemia of pregnancy* is a term used to describe a disorder occurring during late pregnancy that is characterized by a sudden rise in blood pressure, edema, and excretion of large amounts of protein in the urine. In severe cases convulsions followed by coma may occur. Toxemia of pregnancy in the absence of convulsions is called preeclampsia. When convulsions are present the condition is called eclampsia. The unborn child is at risk for mental retardation due to prematurity or anoxia.

Fetal Neurotoxicity

This also results from maternal–fetal Rh incompatibility. Rh factors are proteins on the surface of red blood cells. These proteins are inherited as a dominant trait.

When an Rh-negative mother has an Rh-positive fetus, and there is sufficient mixing of maternal and fetal blood as is common during birth, the mother's immune system may form antibodies against the Rh factors. In subsequent pregnancies in which the fetus is again Rh positive, the mother's antibodies cross the placenta and destroy fetal red blood cells. Hemoglobin released from blood cells is converted to bilirubin, which is deposited in the fetal brain, producing mental retardation and motor impairment. The development of Rh incompatibility disease can be prevented by treating the mother with Rh immunoglobulin shortly after delivery. Rh immunoglobulin prevents the mother's immune system from manufacturing antibodies against the Rh factors by destroying the infant red blood cells.

Trauma or Physical Agent

This is a large and varied category intended to include mental retardation owing to brain injury resulting from numerous types of trauma, including physical agents. The common estimate is that about 8 to 10% of the mentally retarded in the mild and moderate categories have suffered brain trauma of this sort. Obviously, the more severe and extensive the damage to the brain the greater the physical and behavioral effects are likely to be. Consequently, those in the severe and profound groups are apt to be included in this particular category.

Prenatal Injury

Although prenatal injury is typically regarded as a rare source of mental retardation, as we examine the enormous range of factors that can produce prenatal insult, more prenatal damage is caused by trauma than is commonly assumed, including overexposure to irradiation, hypoxia, and drugs. There is clear overlap here with other categories such as intoxications, for example, maternal PKU. Abnormal phenylalanine metabolities may contain a teratogen that can cause brain damage prenatally.

Mechanical Birth Injuries

Again, the results may be similar to brain damage arising from other sources. Although signs of brain damage may appear early, the long-term consequences are difficult to anticipate and when they do occur, they take a variety of forms.

Perinatal Problems

These may be somewhat more common, especially asphyxia. Such conditions are almost always reflected in seriously low Apgar scores.

Postnatal Injury

Childhood accidents represent a serious health problem, and many of them could be prevented. Child abuse is another condition that sometimes gives rise to health problems. Clinical manifestations may be highly variable varying from mild behavior deviations to clear physical signs such as microcephaly.

Postnatal Exposure to Toxic Agents

Postnatal exposure to a wide variety of toxic agents can produce injury to the nervous system. A significant postnatal cause of neurological dysfunction in children has been lead intoxication. Frank lead poisoning in children most frequently results from ingestion of lead-based paint. Although manufacture of lead-based paint is now prohibited, lead is still present on the walls of many older low-income dwellings. Inadequate maintenance resulting in flaking of paint from the walls and the propensity of young children for pica are important factors in lead poisoning. Acute ingestion of high levels of lead produces severe pathological changes in the brain and neurological symptoms that include drowsiness, stupor, ataxia, paralysis, convulsions, and coma. Among children with a history of severe lead encephalopathy mental retardation is a common finding. In recent years there has been growing concern that exposure either prenatally or postnatally to lead at levels below those that produce frank encephalopathy may cause subtle neurological symptoms, such as mild cognitive impairments and disordered behavior. Despite considerable research (e.g., Schroeder, 1987), we feel that the evidence bearing on this latter point is inconclusive at the present time.

Metabolism or Nutrition

This category includes disorders due to inherited errors of metabolism, dysfunction of endocrine glands, or dietary imbalances. A large number of conditions are subsumed under this category.

Errors of Metabolism

Numerous syndromes in which mental retardation is a feature are caused by an inherited impairment of metabolism in specific biosynthetic pathways. These disorders, which usually have an autosomal recessive mode of inheritance, are classified as inborn errors of metabolism. Autosomal recessive inborn errors of metabolism associated with MR can be divided into three groups of disorders: (1) aminoacidurias; (2) errors of carbohydrate metabolism; and (3) errors of lipid metabolism.

In the aminoacidurias, large amounts of amino acids or related compounds are excreted in the urine. A well-known example of an inborn error of amino acid metabolism is phenylketonuria (PKU). The metabolic basis of PKU is an inherited deficiency of phenylalanine hydroxylase, the enzyme responsible for catalyzing the conversion of phenylalanine to tyrosine. Clinical manifestations of this enzyme defect include reduced pigmentation of the skin, eyes, and hair, delayed motor development, seizures, and severe to profound mental retardation. The biochemical consequences of a deficiency of phenylalanine hydroxylase include an accumulation of phenylalanine and its metabolite, phenylpyruvic acid, and a reduction of tyrosine and its byproducts. The former consequences appear to be of greatest etiological significance with regard to the neurological disorder since this disorder can be prevented by placing the child on a low phenylalanine diet. Toxicity due to phenylalanine or its metabolites appears to be greatest during early postnatal years when the brain is still developing, because the low phenylalanine diet may be discontinued when the child reaches school age without major deleterious effects. However, when female patients later decide to become pregnant it is advisable to reinstate the low phenylalanine diet to prevent high maternal levels of phenylalanine from damaging the fetus. In fact, recent studies suggest that maternal PKU rates are so high as to offset completely the reduced incidence of mental retardation due to dietary management within one generation.

Maple syrup urine disease is another example of an aminoaciduria having an autosomal recessive mode of inheritance. The metabolic error in this disease is a block in the pathway responsible for decarboxylation of branched-chain amino acids. The presence of high concentrations of these amino acids in urine gives these patients an odor characteristic of maple syrup. Clinical symptoms are usually present within the first week after birth and include poor feeding, vomiting, lethargy, and convulsions. If untreated, death usually occurs within the first month of life. The primary pathologic change in the brain appears to be a deficiency of myelin synthesis. Patients respond favorably when placed on diets low in branched-chain amino acids at an early age. As is not the case for phenylketonuria, however, there is no indication that dietary restrictions may be eliminated once the child has matured sufficiently.

Another group of recessive disorders result from errors in carbohydrate metabolism. For example, in galactosemia there is a deficiency of an enzyme that converts galactose to glucose. Clinical manifestations are failure to thrive, vomiting and diarrhea, signs of liver abnormalities such as jaundice, convulsions, cataracts, and mental retardation. The mechanism by which this enzyme defect produces mental retardation is not known, though a deficiency of serotonin has been implicated. Dietary restriction of galactose begun early in life may be an effective treatment.

Another group of autosomal recessive disorders are those that result from a derangement of lipid metabolism. Two such diseases are Tay-Sachs and Niemann-Pick diseases, both of which occur most frequently among persons of Jewish ancestry. Both disorders are attributed to enzyme deficiencies, which lead to accumulation of lipids in the brain. There is no effective treatment for either of these disorders and both are ultimately fatal, usually by the third year of age.

Errors of metabolism associated with mental retardation may also be caused by genes carried on the X sex chromosome. A good example of such a disorder is the Lesch-Nyhan syndrome (Baumeister & Frye, 1985). The Lesch-Nyhan syndrome occurs almost exclusively in males, a pattern consistent with a recessive X-linked mode of inheritance. The metabolic basis of the Lesch-Nyhan syndrome is a deficiency of an enzyme (hypoxanthine-guanine phosphoribosyltransferase) that plays an important role in purine biosynthesis. Clinical manifestations of this enzyme defect include choreoathetosis, mental retardation, and severe self-injurious behavior. Recent evidence suggests that the self-injurious behavior exhibited by these patients may be related to a deficiency of brain dopamine (Breese et al., 1984; Breese, Baumeister, Napier, Frey, & Mueller, 1985).

Dysfunction of Endocrine Glands

The most common endocrine disorder associated with mental retardation is hypothyroidism, an underproduction of thyroid hormones. When severe hypothyroidism occurs prenatally or during early childhood it may produce a syndrome called cretinism, with abnormalities in both mental and physical development. Skeletal growth is retarded and there is a thickening of subcutaneous tissues. Dwarfism, moderate obesity, enlargement of the lips and tongue, and a protruding abdomen are common. Permanent mental retardation due to a disruption in physical development may also occur. The severity of symptoms depends on the timing, duration, and degree of thyroid insufficiency. The disorder can usually be completely prevented by treatment with thyroid hormone if begun early enough.

Nutritional Disorders

Nutritional disorders are probably more common than is typically acknowledged. Part of the diagnostic and treatment problem is that the clinical picture may present only subtle signs of deviation. Sometimes diets not only are calorically inadequate but also may be related to aberrant eating customs and to other disease processes.

Gross Brain Disease (Postnatal)

The category of postnatal gross brain disease includes several neurocutaneous diseases, that is, diseases affecting both the nervous system and the skin. Neurofibromatosis is inherited as an autosomal dominant trait with variable expression. This disease is characterized by patches of cutaneous pigmentation and the presence of multiple benign tumors of the skin and nervous system. The incidence of neurofibromatosis in the general population is about 1 in 2000, but mental retardation is present in about 10% of the cases. The only "treatment" for neurofibromatosis is surgical removal of the tumors. Removal of tumors is not advised unless they are causing some serious problem because of the possibility that they will become malignant.

Another neurocutaneous disease with a dominant mechanism of inheritance is tuberous sclerosis. The clinical manifestation of tuberous sclerosis is characterized by a triad of symptoms: (1) epilepsy; (2) tumors of the sweat glands of the face; and (3) mental retardation, usually severe. The epilepsy and mental retardation are due to the presence of multiple tumors in the brain. There is no specific treatment for the underlying pathology in tuberous sclerosis. Control of seizures and early environmental stimulation to minimize mental retardation are indicated. Estimates of the incidence of tuberous sclerosis in the general population vary from 1 in 150,000 to 1 in 300,000—rare, in any event.

A third example of a gross brain disease that also has a dominant genetic mechanism is the Sturge-Weber syndrome. A prominent symptom of this syndrome is a vascular nevus on one side of the face, which is often called a port wine stain because of its reddish-purple color. Other characteristics of Sturge-Weber syndrome include epilepsy, paralysis, and mental retardation. The underlying neuropathology is an extensive angioma and accompanying calcification in one cerebral hemisphere. The only treatment for this disorder is surgical removal of the affected brain tissue, the effectiveness of which is not certain.

Unknown Prenatal Influence

Craniostenosis

Craniostenosis is the premature closure of one or more skull bones. At birth the bones that form the skull are separated to allow continued growth and expansion of the brain. Normally, complete closure of the skull bones does not occur until early adulthood. If the skull bones fuse too early, the growing brain becomes compressed and intracranial pressure increases. Increased intracranial pressure produces compensatory enlargement of regions of the head where the skull bones have not fused. In addition to deformation of the skull, intracranial pressure may produce visual problems, anosmia, and deafness due to nerve damage. Mental retardation may also result.

Microcephaly

The term *microcephaly* refers to an abnormally small brain. Two etiological categories of microcephaly are recognized: (1) true or primary microcephaly, which is thought to result from a genetic failure of brain development; and (2) secondary microcephaly, which results from a wide variety of environmental influences such as intrauterine infections, anoxia, prenatal irradiation, and teratogenic exposure. Primary microcephaly presents characteristic abnormalities that include a progressive narrowing of the head from the base to the top, a forehead that slants sharply backward, furrowing of the scalp due to reduced surface area of the top of the head, and facial features that are of normal size but appear large because of the reduced size of the head. Clinical features of secondary microcephaly are variable. A variety of architectural abnormalities of the cerebrum have been noted in microcephaly, including agyra, micropolygyra, and absence of lamination of the cortex. Mental retardation is usually present in severe microcephaly.

Hydrocephaly

The term *hydrocephaly* refers to an abnormally high volume of cerebral spinal fluid (CSF) in the cranium due to: (1) an overproduction of CSF; (2) an obstruction that interferes with the normal flow of CSF; or (3) impairment of reabsorption of CSF into the blood. Hydrocephaly may be classified as communicating or noncommunicating. In noncommunicating hydrocephaly there is an obstruction that prevents the flow of CSF from the ventricles to the subarachnoid space. Communicating hydrocephaly results from an impairment in either the synthesis or the absorption of CSF or to an obstruction located within the subarachnoid space. Increased volume of CSF increases pressure within the ventricles. As a result the ventricles expand and compress surrounding brain tissue against the skull, causing damage to the cerebral hemispheres. In young children increased intracranial pressure may cause the sutures to separate, leading to gross enlargement of the head. Neurological sequelae are variable, depending on the extent and nature of the underlying pathology and the age of onset.

Anencephaly

The term *anencephaly* refers to congenital malformation of the brain that is characterized by absence of the cerebrum. It is one of the most common major congenital disorders of the brain, occurring in between 0.5 and 4 per 1000 births, depending on geographical region. Anencephaly is attributed to a failure of the anterior neuropore to close during early development, though the etiological factors responsible for the abnormal development are not known.

Chromosomal Anomalies

Mental retardation is often associated with abnormalities in the number or structure of chromosomes. Among disorders caused by chromosomal abnormalities the most common is Down's syndrome. Three distinct chromosomal abnormalities have been associated with Down's syndrome. The most common is the presence of an extra chromosome 21 resulting from nondysfunction during meiosis. In the second type of abnormality, which accounts for approximately 4% of the cases of Down's syndrome, material from chromosome 21 is translocated to another chromosome, usually number 14. In the third form, called mosaicism, some cells contain the extra chromosome but others are normal. This latter abnormality results from nondysfunction during mitotic division occurring shortly after formation of the zygote. Down's syndrome occurs in about 1 in 650 live births, the risk increasing dramatically as maternal age increases. Down's syndrome is associated with a variety of physical abnormalities such as the presence of epicanthal folds, congenital heart defects, short stature, microcephaly, unusually shaped ears, a flattening of the back of the head, furrowing of the tongue, and stubby fingers and toes. The brains of persons with Down's syndrome tend to be reduced in size and display a simplified convolutional pattern. Microscopic abnormalities include a reduction in the number and density of neurons, abnormalities in dendritic spines, and the presence of neuritic plaques and neurofibrillary tangles. These last two abnormalities are characteristic of Alzheimer's syndrome, suggesting some commonality in the pathogenesis of these neurological disorders (Coyle, Oster-Granite, & Gearhart, 1986).

Mental retardation has also been linked to abnormalities of the X sex chromosome. A new syndrome with mental retardation as a feature has recently been described among males in which there is a narrowing near the end of the long arm of the X chromosome. In some cases part of the distal end of the chromosome actually breaks off. For this reason the syndrome is called fragile-X syndrome. The incidence of fragile-X syndrome is not known, though there has been speculation that, among the diagnosable causes of mental retardation, its incidence may be second only to that of Down's syndrome (Abuelo, 1983).

Other Conditions Originating in the Perinatal Period

The primary attribute for inclusion in this category is prematurity or low birth weight. The risk for infant mortality is extremely high for low-birth-weight infants and, not surprisingly, the risk is directly related to birth weight. Baumeister and Kupstas (in press) have reported that the literature shows a forty-fold risk of infant mortality owing to prematurity. Mortality rates are a common index of the health of a population. As mortality increases, so does morbidity. Low-birth-weight infants are at extreme risk for many problems, collectively called the "new morbidity," including mental retardation.

It is very difficult to identify which premature infant is at risk for mental retardation. In fact, the best indices are not biological or medical, but behavioral and social. Various studies have shown that a powerful predictor of morbidity, including mental retardation, is maternal education level. Socioeconomic factors weigh heavily in the outcome.

Following Psychiatric Disorder

When there is no evidence of cerebral pathology, but when an individual has experienced psychosis or other psychiatric disorder, then this category is applicable. In fact, if the conditions exist concomitantly then another category should be applied. It is doubtful whether this particular category includes many individuals.

Environmental Influences

This category includes the largest subgroups of mentally retarded persons, particularly those whose retardation is mild or borderline. Here there is no evidence of significant organicity, but rather indications of adverse environmental contributing factors.

By far the most common designation is *psychosocial disadvantage*: the current term. Over the years there have been a variety of descriptive labels applied to this large group of people, the labels changing more as a function of social pressure than from a deepening of professional understanding. One earlier designation that is still frequently employed is *cultural–familial*.

In any case, the basic criterion, aside from the absence of organic disease, is subnormal intelligence in one or both parents and in one or more siblings. The causes of mental retardation are complex, multivariate, and interactive. Clearly, the intention is to implicate familial tendencies.

But it is here also that poverty is seen to play a critical role. Actually, poverty itself is better regarded as a moderating variable that sets conditions for increased risk of different types of morbidity, including mental retardation. Baumeister (1988) and Baumeister and Kupstas (in press) have described conditions that give rise to the new morbidity: those events that are the outcome (including mental retardation, learning disabilities, emotional disturbance, growth failure, accidents, and so on), and those circumstances that intervene to set the conditions.

Risk factors do not operate independently but rather interact in such a way as to produce a range of causality, both in absolute and relative terms. Psychosocial and biological risks may be multiplicative rather than additive.

One of the most consistent relationships in our literature is that between socioeconomic status and intelligence. Correlations between these two general factors range from .40 to .62 in every modern industrial society. Incidence of mental retardation appears to be at least six times greater in the lowest as compared with the highest SES level.

Why is poverty associated with mental retardation? What is the direction of causality? What are the implications for prevention? An examination of the literature suggests that there are at least five different conceptual systems that aim toward explanation of retarded education and development within low-income groups (Laosa, 1984). Each produces a different perception as to the nature and cause of ethnic inequality:

1. The genetic or, better, polygenic model
2. The cultural deficit or pathology model—the "culture of poverty" notion; the idea of social disadvantage owing to behavioral defects
3. The institutional deficiency model—basically one that blames schools for perpetrating incompatibilities
4. The structure characteristic model—minorities are denied access to more desirable social and occupational roles
5. The developmental, socioculture model—no society or subculture is superior to the other, so behavior must be understood in its own terms (i.e., within the values, systems, and institutions that comprise a particular culture)

We suggest that the relatively high risk of the new morbidity, including mental retardation, among poor people and those in lower SES groups, is best characterized by an interactional process in which certain children are behaviorally and biologically vulnerable to environmental and social variations predisposing them to an array of disabling conditions. The connection between poverty and mental retardation is not direct, but is mediated by a host of proximal and distal variables. The truth is that our knowledge of the precise nature of these correlations, causes, and effects is imperfect. But we do know enough about some of these conditions to intervene preventively in ways that improve quality of life and are cost-effective.

Poverty is not good for children. And here, in summary, are some of these considerations, not all of which are entirely new (e.g., Birch & Gussow, 1970). The environments in which economically disadvantaged children develop are less conducive to good physical, mental, and behavioral development than the environment of children not disadvantaged. These differences are deep rooted, fundamental, enduring, and intergenerational, a fact that has not received sufficient respect. Similar to their offspring, mothers of disadvantaged children are not so well nourished, they are smaller, and they receive less nurturing care. When of childbearing age, they have children younger (frequently as teenagers), more rapidly, more often, and they continue to bear them to an older age. When such a mother is pregnant her general health will be poorer than that of a woman who is better off, and her fetus faces greater risk of infection, intoxication, and trauma. Prenatal and general health care is less accessible to her. She is more likely to deliver her child under substandard conditions. Children of such mothers, on the average, are smaller for gestational age, are more likely to be premature, die more readily and suddenly, are sicker in infancy, suffer a greater rate of accidents, and run a greater risk of neglect than children born into better circumstances. If they survive the first few weeks of life, their mortality thereafter is excessively high; their illnesses more frequent, more persistent, and more severe. Development is negatively influenced by the mother's health, age, income level, education, and habits. During school years, children's nutrition may be inadequate, they miss school more frequently, their housing is frequently substandard, family income is low, and family disorganization is high. They will present a higher rate of learning problems, behavior disturbances, allergies, and speech difficulties (Freeman, 1985).

Disadvantage, whether economic, educational, or biologic, occurs through time, each generation passing on to the next the unfortunate and cumulative consequences of its own experience, as in a circle, with no clear beginning and no clear end. Neither the much-rehearsed cultural deficit nor the vulnerable genetic inheritance theory is adequate to explain the development of different forms of social competence, economic inequality, and biological vulnerability.

ASSOCIATED FEATURES

Mental retardation is often accompanied by other forms of handicap or disability, such as movement disorder, physical defects, and emotional disturbance. In some instances, the associated disability has a particularly high frequency among individuals who present a specific etiology. Heart defects in Down's syndrome, dwarfism in hypothyroidism, and cataracts in galactosemia are representative of such disease–defect associations. In other instances the pathological aspects, such as seizures and cerebral palsy, may cut across a number of conditions. The risks of epilepsy and cerebral palsy vary greatly depending on the primary problem.

Psychopathology

An examination of the research and clinical literature reveals a current and long-standing concern with the connection between personality and affective disorders and mental retardation. A generally accepted conclusion is that disorders of psychopathology are much more frequently observed among persons identified as mentally retarded than among nonretarded persons; the range is from 2.5 to 10 times as common (Thompson, 1988). Among some groups prevalence rates are extremely high (Reid, 1985). These would be considered psychiatric problems in the more traditional sense. When we examine specific behavior disorders at a functional and more specific level, then we may conclude that retarded persons are at considerable risk. These reactions include such behavior disorders as excessive stereotyped movements, rage reactions, pica, aggression, and extreme noncompliance, personality, and affective disorders. These disorders are related to general functional level and are much more common among those with IQs below 50, those for whom the risk of brain damage is greatly increased. Likewise, Kopp (1983) has pointed to a large number of distinctly genetic and/or exogenous biological risk factors for mental retardation that are also associated with emotional problems.

There is no doubt that mentally retarded people, for a variety of reasons, are at significant risk for psychiatric, affective, and behavior disorders. These include childhood psychoses, attention deficits, functional behavior problems, neurosis, and various forms of conduct disorders. In many instances the treatment, such as pharmacological intervention, is indicated as it would be for anyone presenting the disorder. In other instances, the mental retardation itself may be a limiting factor in treatment, such as in the instance of conventional psychotherapy. In addition, setting factors as well as more pervasive family disorganization must be taken into account.

Epilepsy

Seziure disorders are especially common among mentally retarded people, with the risk increasing as a function of degree of CNS involvement. Certain mental retardation etiologies almost always carry convulsions as a presenting problem. In other diseases the risk of epilepsy is not particularly elevated. But we should note that even among mildly retarded people there appears to be increased incidence of seizure disorder. It has been reported that frequency of seizures among mentally retarded people with evidence of organicity is about 20%, whereas among mildly retarded individuals the rate may be about 5% (Corbett, Harris, & Robinson, 1975).

Usually, the connection between epilepsy and mental retardation occurs in early childhood or infancy. This fact, too, suggests an underlying common central nervous system involvement. But this is not always the case, and various seizure disorders can occur later, as with the general population.

Inevitably, the question is raised as to what leads to what. That is, does the mental retardation (or putative cause) also produce convulsive disorders, or do the seizures result in diminished intellectual function? Probably both circumstances occur. Status epilepticus does appear to cause impaired intellectual functioning in some cases. It should also be noted that there is a link between behavior disorders and epilepsy, especially the temporal lobe variant.

The literature on epilepsy is enormous and complicated. We can only offer a generalization by saying that mentally retarded people are at increased risk for all of the various types of seizures, that a lesion often produces both disorders, that there appears to be a familial pattern, in most cases the disorder is found in childhood, and drug control, especially of the grand mal seizures, is very effective.

Cerebral Palsy

Cerebral palsy is a generally descriptive term for a cluster of movement and postural disorders. The range of involvement is considerable. Mental retardation is associated with cerebral palsy, but certainly not inevitably. Mental retardation of perinatal origin is most frequently found in connection with cerebral palsy (Hagberg & Hagberg, 1985), but can occur in both the prenatal and postnatal periods as well.

There are basically four categories, with a number of subvariations, of cerebral palsy: (1) spastic—the most common variant, involving muscular rigidity and restriction in range; (2) dyskinetic—restricted motion with uncontrolled and sometimes, jerky movements, usually athetosis or choreoathetosis; (3) ataxic—characterized by standing and walking difficulties due to poor balance; and (4) a mixture of the first three. Retarded people are found in all these categories, but predominantly in the spastic form.

Unfortunately, the behavioral problems of mental retardation are often compounded when cerebral palsy is involved. For instance, speech abnormalities are commonly found in cerebral palsied patients. Other deficits include visual, auditory, and perceptual deficiencies. Clearly, too, assessment of competence is compromised because of deficiencies in language and motor abilities, abilities required by most standard instruments. There are, however, specialized testing procedures available.

Other Features

Of course, there are a great many other impairments and processes that put mentally retarded people into special risk. It is an unfortunate (and seemingly unfair) state of nature that problems tend to be linked to each other. One might assume that one major disability is enough, but the fact is that each one creates a special vulnerability for another.

COURSE AND PROGNOSIS

As we have noted previously, mental retardation has multiple causes and diverse behavioral, cognitive, and medical manifestations. As such, few generalizations regarding course and prognosis can be made. However, one generalization that seems to have wide acceptance is that mental retardation caused by organic brain disease has relatively poor prognosis compared to mental retardation caused by environmental factors. In the former case intellectual deficits may appear at an earlier age, they tend to be more severe, they are less amenable to behavioral interventions, and they are more likely to be chronic and progressive. Nevertheless, because of the enormous variability of etiologies and deficits displayed, and because in most cases etiology cannot be specified, such generalizations are of little value in trying to predict outcome in individual cases. In fact, certain organic conditions, as we have already observed, can now be treated very effectively.

IMPAIRMENT

The DSM-III defines impairment in terms of deficits in two particular classes of adaptive behavior: social and occupational functioning. Because mental retardation, by definition, involves deficits in adaptive behavior, impairments of social and occupational functioning are probable. The extent to which an individual displays such impairment, however, depends greatly on the magnitude of the intellectual deficit as well as existence of associated features, such as psychopathology.

COMPLICATIONS

Complications in DSM terminology refers to secondary conditions that result from mental retardation. The major complications of mental retardation are social isolation and dependency on others.

EPIDEMIOLOGY

Obviously in order to conduct a comprehensive inquiry into the epidemiology of mental retardation, we shall require a standard definition of that condition. However, there is not a universally accepted set of specific criteria from state to state, among disciplines, or over time—for reasons noted earlier. As an example, since 1977 prevalence of learning disability has continued to displace that of mental retardation.

Although there have been a number of surveys in the United States and Europe of mentally retarded people (Richardson & Koller, 1985), most general estimates of either incidence or prevalence are derived from a statistical or inferential model. Assuming a normal distribution for IQ scores (which is not an entirely good assumption), we could readily determine how many individuals will fall below 70 points, or any cutoff, for that matter. These estimates, then, would at least be subject to empirical verification. At the same time we understand that many factors, such as age, sex, geography, method of ascertainment, social class, and ethnic group membership, will lead to variations in prevalence estimates.

Often, too, we tend to confuse prevalence and incidence. *Prevalence* refers to the number of cases at a particular point in time, while *incidence* describes those diagnosed within a time frame. As a general rule mental retardation incidence will be higher than prevalence because some cases diagnosed as mentally retarded at one point may not be so designated at another. Thus, for example, incidence is particularly high during the school period and drops markedly before and after. But prevalence can also increase without a concomitant increase in incidence. For example, the number of Down's syndrome babies has declined in some localities, but because these individuals are living longer, prevalence may now increase.

In general, and despite survey variations, the prevalence estimate of mental retardation has been assumed to be about 3%. However, recent developments, both statistical and political, have led others to suggest that the "true" prevalence is about 1%. Incidence, that is, those who were ever labeled retarded, is probably closer to 3%. In any case, there has been no large-scale descriptive epidemiological study conducted in the United States, and the best we have, for the population as a whole, are rough estimates of incidence and prevalence. Broad national policy is dependent on these coarse and variable figures.

When the condition of mental retardation is examined in terms of more specific components, then incidence and prevalence data may be more trustworthy and useful. For example, we know how many people reside in institutions and we can describe this group in fairly good detail. The same applies to public school enrollments. Then, too, there are certain types or subclasses about which we can make more definitive epidemological statements. For example, we have relatively good information regarding prevalence of Down's syndrome and other genetic disorders.

There is another consideration that should be addressed in the context of the epidemiology of mental retardation. As noted earlier, overall estimates of incidence and prevalence are typically derived from statistical models with assumed mathematical properties—that is, a normal distribution. But we also noted that IQ is not normally distributed, a fact that is not surprising and one that can be readily ascertained. The observed distribution is actually bimodal in that at the lower end there is a great excess of cases beyond what would be predicted from the statistical model. This skewing may be called the "bump of pathology." Assaults upon the nervous system, genetic errors, accidents, diseases, and unfavorable living conditions are but a few factors that tend to have directional effects; that is, a lesion to the brain is much more likely to depress than to raise the IQ.

Quite beyond the problem of establishing reliable and valid epidemiological data, skewness of IQs also brings into focus certain conceptual issues that have long been debated but that have never been satisfactorily resolved. There are those who argue for a two-class distinction—brain injured versus cultural–familial (e.g., Zigler, 1978). Classification based on this distinction can have profound theoretical, programmatic, and policy implications because in one case a disease process is implicated, whereas the other represents the inevitable outcome of polygenic variation (Baumeister, 1984, 1987).

FAMILIAL PATTERN

It is well established that mental retardation tends to occur more frequently among relatives of a mentally retarded proband than it does among the general population. Of course, this fact alone does not necessarily imply a genetic basis for mental retardation, because relatives tend to share a common environmental as well as a common genetic heritage. Without a doubt, adverse environmental conditions contribute to the familial pattern observed in mental retardation, especially in cases classified as psychosocial. Nevertheless, there are numerous instances of mental retardation, particularly in the severe and profound ranges, which clearly have a genetic basis.

Mental retardation can be caused by inheritance of dominant or recessive genes. Syndromes caused by dominant genes are relatively rare because of the high probability that carriers of the gene will display the syndrome. To the extent that a syndrome severely limits reproductive potential, genetic transmission of the trait is precluded. However, not all dominant genes are manifested phenotypically (incomplete penetrance). In addition, the nature and severity of symptoms associated with a dominantly inherited disorder may be quite variable (variable expression). These characteristics (i.e., incomplete penetrance and variable expression) serve to reduce selection pressure against dominant genes that may have severe deleterious effects in some individuals. Several dominant gene disorders associated with mental retardation are known, such as neurofibromatosis, tuberous sclerosis, and Sturge-Weber syndrome.

Recessive genes associated with mental retardation are more common and more consistent in their manifestation than are dominant genes. This is because in the heterozygous state there is little selection pressure against deleterious recessive genes. However, when both parents are heterozygous there is a one-in-four chance that offspring will inherit the recessive gene from each parent and consequently display the disorder. Several disorders that have mental retardation as a feature are caused by inheritance of two recessive genes. In most of these syndromes the recessive genes exert their deleterious effects by impairing metabolism in specific biosynthetic pathways. As detailed earlier, such disorders are classified inborn errors of metabolism.

Genes that cause mental retardation may occur on the autosomes or sex chromosomes. Traits that are coded by genes on the sex chromosomes occur with different frequencies in males and females. Recessive X-linked traits occur more frequently in males because males have only one X chromosome and consequently there is no allele to oppose the expression of recessive genes carried on that chromosome. X-linked disorders such as the Lesch-Nyhan syndrome and fragile-X syndrome may account, in part, for the greater rate of mental retardation among males.

DIFFERENTIAL DIAGNOSIS

The DSM-III distinguishes among several disorders of childhood that have symptoms overlapping those that define mental retardation. Mental retardation is distinguished from pervasive developmental disorders primarily on the basis that the latter is characterized by extreme qualitative departures from normal developmental patterns (e.g., in infantile autism), whereas in mental retardation development is delayed but is otherwise characteristic of patterns that are normal for an earlier age. Mental retardation is also distinguished from specific developmental disorders. The latter involve a delay in a particular area of development such as language, with other areas of development being unaffected. In mental retardation the development delay is more pervasive, affecting many different areas at once.

CLINICAL MANAGEMENT: RESEARCH FINDINGS

Treatment of the mentally retarded is a multifaceted endeavor involving experts in fields as diverse as medicine, psychology, and education. Because of the enormity of the problems that attend mental retardation, a detailed discussion of treatment is well beyond the scope of this chapter. Instead we shall briefly discuss approaches to dealing with the behavioral deficiencies and excesses exhibited by the mentally retarded.

Pharmacological Therapy

Medications are used frequently in the treatment of mentally retarded persons, especially those who reside in institutions (Aman & Singh, 1983). Approximately 50 to 70% of the institutionalized mentally retarded receive some form of psychoactive medication. The most common uses of psychoactive medication in this group are to control seizures and to suppress aberrant behavior. The types of aberrant behavior that have been treated pharmacologically include hyperactivity, aggression, stereotypy, and self-injury. The drugs used most frequently for behavioral control are neuroleptics; 40 to 50% of the institutionalized mentally retarded receive neuroleptic medication. Other less frequently used drugs include stimulants (2 to 3%), antidepressants (4%), and anxiolytics (8 to 13%). Despite the high frequency with which drugs are used in the mentally retarded there is very little evidence to support the efficacy of this approach to behavioral management. There is some weak evidence that neuroleptics sometimes suppress stereotyped and self-injurious behavior, but beyond this there is little evidence that psychoactive drugs are useful for controlling aberrant behavior. Moreover, it is clear that some of these drugs have undesirable side effects. For example, between 20 and 30% of mentally retarded persons treated with neuroleptics display a side effect (called tardive dyskinesia) of the medication that is characterized by a variety of involuntary movements of the face, tongue, trunk, and limbs (Kalachnik, 1984). Other questions about possible adverse side effects of psychoactive medication, such as their effect on cognitive function, remain unanswered. Notwithstanding the preceding discussion, the pharmacological approach has the potential to contribute significantly to efforts to treat the mentally retarded. However, more methodologically sound studies of the efficacy and side effects of psychoactive drugs in the mentally retarded are clearly needed. In addition, a more sound theoretical basis needs to be employed for the selection of pharmacological therapies than has been used in the past. Additional basic and clinical research is needed to determine the neural mechanisms that underlie particular forms of abnormal behavior. Drugs can then be selected for experimental trials based on their ability to alter selectively the substrates that mediate the target behavior. This approach is yielding promising results in efforts to understand and control self-injurious behavior through pharmacological means (Baumeister & Frye, 1985; Baumeister, Frye, & Schroeder, 1985; Breese et al., 1984; Breese et al., 1985; Goldstein, Anderson, Reuben, & Dancis, 1985).

Behavioral Therapy

Clearly, the most widely used method for eliminating unwanted behavior and for instilling new adaptive forms of behavior in the mentally retarded involves the application of a variety of procedures based on the principles of learning, an approach that is well known as behavior modification. One of the hallmarks of behavior modification is the conceptualization of mental retardation in terms of observed behavior, without regard to etiology or to underlying neurological dysfunction. The influence of this approach is apparent in the inclusion of the criterion that deficits in adaptive behavior be present before a diagnosis of mental retardation is made. Viewing mental retardation as a problem primarily of behavioral deficiencies, the behavior modifier seeks to incorporate new skills into the retarded person's repertoire through the contingent application of appetitive stimuli. Complex skills (e.g., learning how to dress) are broken down into their component parts and are gradually shaped through the reinforcement of successive approximations to the desired behavioral end point.

On the other hand, the behavior modifier attempts to suppress maladaptive behavior through extinction or through punishment. In the former procedure it is assumed the undesirable behavior is being reinforced by some stimulus such as attention from caretakers. Under such circumstances, it may be possible to extinguish the behavior by noncontingently withdrawing the reinforcement. If such efforts are unsuccessful punishment may be tried. A variety of punishment procedures have been developed for use with the mentally retarded, including time out, overcorrection, and contingent application of electric shock. Generally, the behavior modifier tries the least aversive procedure first and proceeds to more aversive procedures only if the preceding attempt to suppress the behavior is unsuccessful. Extremely aversive procedures, such as contingent electric shock, are generally reserved for the most severe forms of aberrant behavior, such as life-threatening self-injury. Although behavior modification justifiably remains the treatment of choice with the mentally retarded, its efficacy has often been greatly exaggerated; the gains achieved through this approach, especially with those who are severely impaired, are often modest at best.

Psychotherapy

Psychotherapy may be distinguished from behavior modification on the basis of differing assumptions about the nature of mental retardation, the specific problems addressed, and the methods used. A basic distinction is that behavior modification is focused on attainment of technical skills, whereas psychotherapy attempts to achieve certain psychological goals, such as self-understanding and self-confidence or elimination of emotional disorder. The latter approach includes such methods as art and music therapy, individual and group therapy, and counseling. Although the methods employed may differ greatly, there may be considerable overlap in the results obtained. Thus the music therapy, in addition to instilling a sense of mastery and self-confidence, may develop fine-motor or social skills, whereas acquisition of skills through behavior modification may enhance self-esteem. Nevertheless, the extent to which psychotherapy is a useful treatment for the mentally retarded cannot be assessed at this time because research into the efficacy of such procedures has traditionally been of low quality.

Special Education

Clinical management of the mentally retarded defies quick and ready prescriptions, primarily because of the enormous heterogeneity among this population, the significant lack of knowledge about many of the causes of disability, how the effects are mediated, and, finally, the paucity of resources. Choices must inevitably be made as to socially responsible utilization of what resources exist. Yet decisions as to how to treat mentally retarded people are daily events in the lives of literally thousands of people, in turn necessitating many compromises.

Although the term *clinical management* does not typically include special education, we offer a brief general discussion here because: (1) free and appropriate education is now mandated by federal law for all retarded children; (2) special education, in its various forms, is by far the most universally relied-on form of intervention; and (3) recent legislation has greatly altered the concept of education, from traditional school experiences, to focus on basic self-help skills, health aspects, and social adaptation.

Of the various laws that pertain to the education of mentally retarded children, the best known, most far-reaching, and most hotly discussed is Public Law 94-142, the Education for All Handicapped Act. It must be noted, however, that the major policy initiatives contained in this law are not based on research findings, but rather derive from shifting public and professional views and values concerning the disabled. Essential features of the act include the following: (1) Every child regardless of handicap is entitled to free and appropriate public education; (2) designation of a child must be based on nondiscriminatory, culture-fair assessments; (3) every pupil must have a regularly updated individualized education program (IEP) that is specifically pertinent to the child's special needs, along with documentation of those needs and the programs designed to intervene; (4) special-needs children must be included, unless otherwise clearly contraindicated in the child's best interests, in the regular school setting along with nonretarded children, a "least restrictive" concept; (5) the law requires "due process" in classification and school placement, essentially meaning that parents have access to school records, guaranteed impartial placement hearings, and opportunity for independent evaluation; and (6) parents may participate in the planning and decision-making process and challenge recommendations.

In short, Public Law 94-142 represents one of the most fundamental and far-reaching educational policy decisions and intervention measures ever enacted affecting mentally retarded children. In principle, at least, a number of well-established educational concepts were dramatically altered. Perhaps the most fundamental of these are: (1) the practice of separate and homogeneous grouping in favor of individualized programming in more "normalized" settings; and (2) the assertion of rights of severely and profoundly retarded children to receive free and appropriate education, whereas previously these individuals were often excluded from public school.

Whether this law is as revolutionary as it is often touted to be remains to be seen. There is evidence that some changes have been more cosmetic than substantive.

The ultimate criterion hinges on outcome or criterion measures that have yet to be addressed, or even agreed upon.

A more recent law, Part H of the Education of the Handicapped Act, provides federal funding to states for further development of comprehensive, coordinated interdisciplinary and interagency programs for early intervention. This new law, just being implemented, will extend handicapped services to preschool children as well as those who are of school age. In fact, these programs will serve, once implemented, many young children who are "at risk" for mental retardation.

DSM-III-R

The most recent edition of the *Diagnostic and Statistical Manual of Mental Disorders* (DSM-III-R) has recently been released (APA, 1987). The essential aspects of the description, definition, and discussion of mental retardation remain much the same as in the previous edition of the manual. There are a few changes, along with some updating of information.

Again the threefold criterion system is applied to definition: (1) subaverage general intellectual function; (2) significant deficits in adaptive behavior; and (3) onset before age of 18. Perhaps the most obvious alteration concerns the relation between low intelligence and deficits in adaptive behavior. Whereas in the earlier version, as we have noted, low intelligence can "result" in deficits or impairments in adaptive behavior, the latest APA position is that one "accompanies" the other. Causality is no longer a definitional issue. This change brings the APA definition into virtual identity with the AAMD definition of mental retardation.

As before, there is recognition that clinical judgment is important to classification in that hard and fast IQ criteria are not desirable. Furthermore, with young children clinical judgment substitutes for IQ estimates because conventional tests do not yield numerical IQ values. Indeed there is a clear indication that informed clinical judgment of adaptive behavior is at least as vital to diagnosis as scores of standard scales of adaptive behavior. There is also an effort to distinguish between mental retardation and other behavior delays such as reading or language. The distinction is made in terms of generality of the deficits. That is, the more "general" or pervasive the delays, the more appropriate the designation *mental retardation.*

Otherwise, the revised manual provides a general discussion of such issues as course, complications, prevalence of etiological factors, family patterns, prevalence, and so on. All of this material is very similar to that in the earlier version of the manual and in the diagnosis and treatment of the individual case, too general to be of much assistance.

REFERENCES

Abuelo, D.N. (1983). Genetic disorders. In J.L. Matson & J.A. Mulick (Eds.), *Handbook of mental retardation.* New York: Pergamon.

Adams, J. (1973). Adaptive behavior and measured intelligence in the classification of mental retardation. *American Journal of Mental Deficiency, 78,* 77–81.

Aman, M.G., & Singh, N.N. (1983). Pharmacological intervention. In J.L. Matson & J.A. Mulick (Eds.), *Handbook of mental retardation.* New York: Pergamon.

American Psychiatric Association (1980). *Diagnostic and statistical manual of mental disorders* (3rd ed.). Washington, DC: Author.

American Psychiatric Association (1987). *Diagnostic and statistical manual of mental disorders* (3rd ed., rev.). Washington, DC: Author.

Baumeister, A.A. (1981). Mental retardation policy and research: The unfulfilled promise. *American Journal of Mental Deficiency, 85,* 449–456.

Baumeister, A.A. (1984). Some conceptual and methodological issues on the study of cognitive progresses. In P. Brooks, R. Sperber, & C. McCauley (Eds.), *Learning and cognition in the mentally retarded.* Hillsdale, NJ: Erlbaum.

Baumeister, A.A. (1987). Mental retardation: Some conceptions and dilemmas. *American Psychologist, 42,* 796–800.

Baumeister, A.A. (1988). Effective planning strategies to prevent mental retardation among socially disadvantaged populations. In *National conference on state planning for the prevention of mental retardation and related developmental disabilities.* U.S. Department of Health and Human Services. Washington, DC: U.S. Government Printing Office.

Baumeister, A.A., & Butterfield, E. (1970). *Residential facilities for the mentally retarded.* Chicago: Aldine.

Baumeister, A.A., & Frye, G.D. (1985). The biochemical basis of the behavioral disorder in the Lesch-Nyhan syndrome. *Neuroscience & Biobehavioral Reviews, 9,* 169–178.

Baumeister, A.A., Frye, G.D., & Schroeder, S.R. (1985). Neurochemical correlates of self-injurious behavior. In J.A. Mulick & B.L. Mallory (Eds.), *Transitions in mental retardation: Advocacy, technology, and science.* Norwood, NJ: Ablex.

Baumeister, A.A., & Kupstas, F. (in press). *The new morbidity: Implications for prevention and amelioration.* In A.B.D. Clarke (Ed.), *Combating mental handicap—A multidisciplinary approach.* London: Taylor & Francis.

Baumeister, A.A., & MacLean, W.E., Jr. (1979). Brain damage and mental retardation. In N.R. Ellis (Ed.), *Handbook of mental deficiency: Psychological theory and research.* Hillsdale, NJ: Erlbaum.

Baumeister, A.A., & Muma, J.R. (1975). On defining mental retardation. *Journal of Special Education, 9,* 294–306.

Birch, H., & Gussow, G.O. (1970). *Disadvantaged children.* New York: Grune & Stratton.

Blanton, R.L. (1975). Historical perspectives on classification of mental retardation. In N. Hobbs (Ed.), *Issues in the classification of children* (Vol. I). San Francisco: Jossey-Bass.

Braddock, D. (1986). From Roosevelt to Reagan: Federal spending for mental retardation and development disabilities. *American Journal of Mental Deficiency, 90,* 479–489.

Breese, G.R., Baumeister, A., Napier, T.C., Frey, G.D., & Mueller, R.A. (1985). Evidence that D-1 receptors contribute to the supersensitive behavioral responses induced by L-dihydroxyphenylalinine in rats treated neonatally with 6-hydroxydopamine. *Journal of Pharmacology & Experimental Therapeutics, 235,* 287–295.

Breese, G.R., Baumeister, A.A., McCown, T.J., Emerick, S.G., Frye, G.D., Crotty, K., & Mueller, R.A. (1984). Behavioral differences between neonatal and adult 6-hydroxydopamine agonists: Relevance to neurological symptoms in clinical syndromes with reduced brain dopamine. *Journal of Pharmacology & Experimental Therapeutics*, *231*, 343–354.

Clarke, A.D.B., & Clarke, A.M. (1977). Prospects for prevention and amelioration of mental retardation: A guested editorial. *American Journal of Mental Deficiency*, *81*, 523–533.

Clausen, J.A. (1977). Quo vadis, AAMD? *Journal of Special Education*, *6*, 51–60.

Corbett, J.A., Harris, R., & Robinson, R.G. (1975). Epilepsy. In J. Wortis (Ed.), *Mental retardation and developmental disabilities* (Vol. 8). New York: Brunner/Mazel.

Coyle, J.T., Oster-Granite, M.J., & Gearhart, J.D. (1986). The neurobiologic consequences of Down syndrome. *Brain Research Bulletin*, *16*, 773–787.

Doll, E.A. (1941). The essentials of an inclusive concept of mental deficiency. *American Journal of Mental Deficiency*, *46*, 214–219.

Frankenberger, W. (1984). A survey of state guidelines for identification of mental retardation. *Mental Retardation*, *22*, 17–20.

Freeman, J.M. (Ed.). (1985). *Prenatal and perinatal factors associated with brain disorders*. Washington, DC: U.S. Department of Health and Human Services.

Goldstein, M., Anderson, L.T., Reuben, R., & Dancis, J. (1985). *Lancet*, *1*, 338.

Grossman, J.H. (Ed.). (1983). *Classification in mental retardation*. Washington, DC: American Association on Mental Deficiency.

Hagberg, B., & Hagberg, G. (1985). Neuropaediatric aspects of prevalence, aetiology, prevention and diagnosis. In A.M. Clarke, A.D.B. Clarke, & M. Berg (Eds.), *Mental deficiency: The changing outlook*. New York: Free Press.

Huberty, T.J., Koller, J.R., & Tenbrink, T.D. (1980). Adaptive behavior in the definition of the mentally retarded. *Exceptional Children*, *46*, 256–264.

Ingall, D., & Norins, L. (1976). Syphilis. In J.S. Remington & J.O. Klein (Eds.), *Infectious diseases of the fetus and newborn infant*. Philadelphia: Saunders.

Jervis, G.A. (1952). Medical aspects of mental deficiency. *American Journal of Mental Deficiency*, *57*, 175–188.

Kalachnik, J.E. (1984). Tardive dyskinesia and the mentally retarded: A review. *Advances in Mental Retardation and Developmental Disabilities*, *2*, 329–356.

Kanner, L. (1964). *A history of the care and study of the mentally retarded*. Springfield, IL: Thomas.

Kopp, C. (1983). Risk factors in development. In P. H. Mussen (Ed.), *Handbook of child psychology* (4th ed.). New York: Wiley.

Laosa, L.M. (1984). Social policies toward children of diverse ethnic, racial, and language groups in the United States. In H.W. Stevenson & A.E. Siegel (Eds.), *Child development research and social policy*. Chicago: University of Chicago Press.

Lowitzer, A.C., Utley, C.A., & Baumeister, A.A. (1987). AAMD's 1983 *Classification in mental retardation* as utilized by state mental retardation/developmental disability agencies. *Mental Retardation*, *25*, 287–291.

Meyers, C.E., Nihira, K., & Zetlin, A. (1979). The measurement of adaptive behavior. In N.R. Ellis (Ed.), *Handbook of mental deficiency: Psychological theory and research*. Hillsdale, NJ: Erlbaum.

Merritt, H.H. (1973). *A textbook of neurology*. Philadelphia: Lea & Febiger.

Milunsky, A. (1983). Genetic aspects of mental retardation: From prevention to cure. In F.J. Menolascino, R. Norman, & J.A. Stark (Eds.), *Curative aspects of mental retardation: Biomedical and behavioral advances*. Baltimore: Brooks.

Patrick, J.L., & Reschly, D.J. (1982). Relationships of state educational criteria and demographic variables to school-system prevalance of mental retardation. *American Journal of Mental Deficiency, 86,* 351–360.

Poling, A., & Breuning, S.E. (1982). Overview of mental retardation. In S.E. Breuning & A.D. Poling (Eds.), *Drugs and mental retardation.* Springfield, IL: Thomas.

Reid, A.H. (1985). Psychiatric disorders. In A.M. Clark, A.D.B. Clarke, & J.M. Berg (Eds.), *Mental deficiency: The changing outlook* (4th ed.). New York: Free Press.

Richardson, S.A., & Koller, H. (1985). Epidemiology. In A.M. Clarke, A.D.B. Clarke, & J.M. Berg (Eds.), *Mental deficiency: The changing outlook.* New York: Free Press.

Scheerenberger, R.C. (1983). *A history of mental retardation.* Baltimore: Brooks.

Schroeder, S.L. (1987). *Toxic substances and mental retardation: Neurobehavioral toxicology and teratology.* Washington, DC: American Association on Mental Deficiency.

Semmel, M.I., Gottlieb, J., & Robinson, N. (1979). Mainstreaming: Perspectives on educating handicapped children in the public schools. In D.C. Berlinger (Ed.), *Review of research in education.* Washington, DC: American Educational Association.

Smith, J.D. (1985). *Minds made feeble: The myth and legacy of the Kallikaks.* Rockville, MD: Aspen.

Thompson, T. (1988). Prevention and treatment of behavior disorders of children and youth with retardation and autism. In. J.A. Stark, F.J. Menolascino, M.H. Albarelli, and V.C. Gray (Eds.), *Mental retardation and mental health: Classification, diagnosis, treatment, services* (pp. 98–105). New York: Springer-Verlag.

Utley, C.A., Lowitzer, A.C., & Baumeister, A.A. (1987). A comparison of the AAMD's definition, eligibility criteria, and classification schemes with state departments of education guidelines. *Education & Training in Mental Retardation, 22,* 35–43.

World Health Organization. (1978). *International classification of diseases* (9th ed.). Geneva: Author.

Wyatt v. Stickney (1972). Civil Action No. 3195-N, U.S. District Court, Middle District of Alabama, North Division.

Zigler, E. (1978). Dealing with retardation. *Science, 196,* 1192–1194.

Zigler, E., Balla, D., & Hodapp, R. (1984). On the definition and classification of mental retardation. *American Journal of Mental Deficiency, 89,* 215–230.

CHAPTER 6

Attention Deficit Disorders

MINA K. DULCAN

DEFINITION

The third edition of the *Diagnostic and Statistical Manual of Mental Disorders* (DSM-III) (American Psychiatric Association, 1980) defined the essential features of attention deficit disorder (ADD) as developmentally inappropriate inattention and impulsivity. Two subtypes of the active disorder were specified: ADD with hyperactivity (ADD/H) and ADD without hyperactivity (ADD/WO). It remains controversial whether these are in fact two forms of a single disorder or two distinct disorders (Carlson, 1986). In addition, ADD, residual type (ADD/R), included "individuals once diagnosed as having ADD/H in which hyperactivity is no longer present, but other signs of the disorder persist" (p. 41).

ADD with Hyperactivity

In addition to attentional difficulties and impulsivity, hyperactivity inappropriate for the child's mental and chronological age must be reported by adults who know the child well, such as parents and teachers. These behaviors may or may not be observed by the clinician or when the child is in a new or a one-to-one situation. DSM-III recommended that when parents and teachers disagree "primary consideration should be given to the teacher reports because of greater familiarity with age-appropriate norms" (p. 43). A specific number of symptoms was required in each of three categories: inattention, impulsivity, and hyperactivity.

Required onset was before the age of 7, with a duration of at least 6 months. The clinician must determine that the symptoms are not due to schizophrenia, affective disorder, or severe or profound mental retardation.

ADD without Hyperactivity

The criteria were the same as for ADD/H, except there were never signs of hyperactivity. In practice, there are many children who have mild hyperactivity, or meet only one of the hyperactivity criteria. DSM-III did not indicate how these children should be diagnosed.

ADD, Residual Type

To be given this diagnosis, the patient must once have met the criteria for ADD/ H. Hyperactivity is no longer present, but attentional deficits and impulsivity persist. The individual must experience impairment in social or occupational functioning as a result of the symptoms. The symptoms must not be due to schizotypal or borderline personality disorder, or any of the exclusionary diagnoses listed for ADD/H.

In this chapter the term *hyperactivity* is used to describe older studies that predate DSM-III and more recent studies that did not use DSM-III criteria. When the subtype is specified, it is used here.

HISTORICAL BACKGROUND

In the more than 80 years since Still (1902) described children with symptoms of overactivity and poor impulse control, the evaluation and treatment of hyperactive children have been plagued with myths and controversy (Henker & Whalen, 1980). Many of the early studies referred to children who were retarded or neurologically impaired. Reports in the 1920s noted hyperactivity, antisocial behavior, and emotional instability as sequelae of childhood encephalitis or head trauma (Rutter, 1982). In the 1940s, it was believed that, since these behaviors occurred in children who had obvious brain damage, all such children must have some degree of brain damage (Rutter, 1982). Despite the lack of evidence for this assumption, terms such as *minimal brain damage*, *minimal brain dysfunction* (Wender, 1971), *minimal cerebral dysfunction*, and *minor cerebral dysfunction* came into use for children who were hyperactive and had neurological "soft signs" or learning disabilities. Despite the lack of evidence for this assumption (Rutter, 1977, 1982), it has been difficult to eliminate these concepts.

In the 1930s, Bradley (1937) fortuitously discovered that benzedrine (dl-amphetamine) had positive effects on a mixed group of child patients in a psychiatric hospital. In the subsequent three decades, treatment with dextroamphetamine (Dexedrine) and then methylphenidate (Ritalin) became increasingly common for a disparate group of "hyperactive" children.

Unfortunately, several notions that were later demonstrated to be incorrect were widely promulgated. In the 1950s and 1960s it was accepted that hyperactivity vanished at puberty (Brown & Borden, 1986) and that the so-called paradoxical effect of stimulants reversed in adolescence (Wender, 1971). Until it was realized in the 1970s that adolescents and even some adults continued to be symptomatic (Brown & Borden, 1986), and that stimulants work in exactly the same way in hyperactive adolescents (Varley, 1983, 1985), and, in fact, in normal children, adolescents, and adults (Rapoport, 1983; Rapoport et al., 1978; Rapoport et al., 1980; Weingartner et al., 1980; Zahn, Rapoport, & Thompson, 1980) that they do in hyperactive children, many patients were unnecessarily deprived of effective drug treatment. "Positive response" to stimulants was once considered pathognomonic of hyperactivity. This is no longer believed to be the case (Ferguson & Rapoport, 1983; Rapoport, 1983; Taylor, 1983).

DSM-II (APA, 1968) used the diagnosis hyperkinetic reaction of childhood (or adolescence), characterized by overactivity, restlessness, distractibility, and short attention span. Other diagnostic terms that have been used to describe children with some features of ADD include: hyperkinetic syndrome of childhood (ICD-9), hyperkinetic impulse disorder, and hyperactive child syndrome.

Public outcry in the lay press in the 1970s that stimulants were being inappropriately used to drug normal children into submission spurred a wave of better designed studies to define a syndrome and to measure the efficacy of medication, in which the rating scales developed by Conners (1973) were critical tools.

Research on motor activity led to disappointment, as mechanical measures were found to correlate poorly with each other and with behavioral ratings (McMahon, 1984).

Hypotheses regarding both consistent overarousal and consistent underarousal in hyperactive children have not been unambiguously supported by research data (McMahon, 1984). Proposed alternatives included an inability to modulate arousal in response to environmental demands (Rosenthal & Allen, 1978) or heterogeneity among hyperactive children in habitual arousal levels (Sroufe, 1975).

The work of Douglas and her group at McGill University focused on deficits in attention, rather than on the measurement of activity level. Her presidential address to the Canadian Psychological Association, titled "Stop, Look and Listen: The Problem of Sustained Attention and Impulse Control in Hyperactive and Normal Children" (Douglas, 1972), changed the direction of research in hyperactivity, and led to the new name of ADD. While research on attention as it relates to diagnosis, impairment, and treatment has been productive, current frustration with inconsistency among different measures of attention and among hyperactive children has led to an increased interest in motivation (Glow & Glow, 1979). It has recently been suggested that abnormalities in youngsters with ADD/H may be caused by an elevated reward threshold (Haenlein & Caul, 1987).

In the late 1970s, Campbell (1975) and Barkley (Barkley & Cunningham, 1979) emphasized the problems in compliance and in social relationships that make hyperactive children so difficult for parents and teachers to manage. Barkley's 1981 book, *Hyperactive Children: A Handbook for Diagnosis and Treatment*, guided a generation of clinicians.

The landmark study by Meichenbaum and Goodman (1971) suggested that a specific psychological treatment, cognitive training, could address the primary deficit in impulsive children, leading the way for others to develop models of cognitive behavior modification (Kendall & Braswell, 1985).

One of the most controversial areas has been whether hyperactivity or MBD or ADD represents a syndrome at all (Barkley, 1982; Ross & Ross, 1982; Rutter, 1983). The water has been muddied by differing diagnostic practices and schemata in different countries (especially Great Britain vs. the United States) (Thorley, 1984a) and by the use of rating scales that do not distinguish between aggressive and hyperactive children (Loney, 1987). The weight of current opinion is that ADD does constitute at least one syndrome, although it frequently co-occurs with oppositional disorder (OD) and conduct disorder (CD) and with learning disabilities (Ross & Ross, 1982).

CLINICAL PICTURE

Ross and Ross (1982) provide detailed descriptions. Briefly, in the classroom, children with ADD have difficulty staying with tasks and have difficulty organizing and completing work. Classroom and playroom observations find them frequently off task. Written work is often sloppy and is characterized by impulsive, careless errors that are a result of not following directions or guessing without considering all of the alternatives. Children often seem not to be listening to adult instructions. Group situations and those that require sustained attention are the most difficult.

Attentional problems at home are shown by failure to follow through on parental requests (in contrast to the *refusal* to comply, characteristic of OD), and relative inability for age to stick to activities, including play (APA, 1980).

Youngsters with ADD/H also show hyperactivity, which is seen in excessive running and climbing, especially in young children. Adults describe them as always on the go, "running like a motor," or having difficulty sitting still. Older children and adolescents may be extremely fidgety and restless. The excess motor activity tends to be inappropriate for the situation, poorly organized, and not consistent with the goals of the environment.

It is typical of the disorder for symptoms to vary from time to time and between situations. It is controversial whether situational and pervasive hyperactivity differ in severity only, in other ways, or at all (Cohen & Minde, 1983; Lambert, Sandoval, & Sassone, 1978; Rutter, 1983). In one U.S. study of carefully diagnosed ADD/H children, direct observation and activity measures did not distinguish between those rated hyperactive by teachers only and those rated hyperactive by both parents and teachers (Rapoport, Donnelly, Zametkin, & Carrougher, 1986).

In reviewing the literature that describes the features of ADD, it is important to distinguish between hyperactivity studies (which often include children with coexisting CD, OD, or learning disabilities) and more recent studies of ADD, ADD/H, ADD/WO, and ADD/R. Subject characteristics also vary according to the method of recruitment, for example, psychiatric clinics, pediatricians' offices, teacher identification, or school screening.

Douglas (1983) identified the following as primary deficits in ADD: (1) lack of investment, organization, and maintenance of attention and effort in completing tasks; (2) inability to inhibit impulsive responding; (3) lack of modulation of arousal levels to meet the demands of the situation; and (4) unusually strong inclination to seek immediate reinforcement.

Hyperactive children have been found to differ from controls in tests of sustained attention and effortful search but do not show consistently increased distractibility or impaired selective attention (Aman & Turbott, 1986). Performance can be improved to normal or near normal levels by having the examiner present during the test, testing individually rather than in groups, making tasks more interesting, delivering auditory stimuli through earphones, letting the child pace the task, frequently repeating instructions, using contingent rewards or response costs, and/or administering stimulant medication (Barkley, in press; Douglas, 1983; Draeger, Prior, & Sanson, 1986). Noncontingent schedules of rewards may actually impair performance (Douglas & Parry, 1983). Often, the deficit seems to be more in motivation than in attentional capacity per se (Glow & Glow, 1979).

In laboratory tests, children with ADD/H have difficulty inhibiting impulsive responding (O'Dougherty, Nuechterlein, & Drew, 1984) and typically choose more immediate rewards, rather than delaying to obtain a large prize (Rapport, Tucker, DuPaul, Merlo, & Stoner, 1986).

Using a monitor of truncal movement in a naturalistic setting, boys with ADD/H demonstrate higher levels of motor activity than controls, regardless of the time of day, including during sleep and on weekends, although the differences are most pronounced during structured school activities (Porrino et al., 1983). Even more important, hyperactive children do not regulate their activity in accord with situational demands (Routh, 1978).

Barkley (1981a) believes that noncompliance, or failure of rule-governed behavior, is the key deficit in hyperactive children. Under conditions of delayed or no re-inforcement, they do not comply with verbal instructions as well as normal children the same age. In addition, their ability to generate and/or follow social and problem-solving rules is impaired (Barkely, in press).

ADD can be observed even in some preschool children who, in an unstructured situation, do not show excess total gross motor activity but do shift activities more often and engage in less sustained play. During structured tasks they are more restless and fidgety, more often out of seat and off task, and less able to delay reward (Campbell, 1985).

For ADD/WO, DSM-III stated that "all of the features are the same as those of ADD/H except for the absence of hyperactivity; the associated features and impairment are generally milder" (p. 44). Some investigators find, however, rather different patterns of behavior. Both groups have learning problems and peer difficulties, although children with ADD/H are more likely to be aggressive and behaviorally impulsive. Children with ADD/WO are perceived as forgetful, sluggish, drowsy, and apathetic and tend to be anxious, shy, and socially withdrawn (Carlson, 1986; Lahey et al., 1987; Lahey, Schaughency, Hynd, Carlson, & Nieves, 1987).

ASSOCIATED FEATURES

DSM-III listed "obstinacy, stubbornness, negativism, bossiness, bullying, increased mood lability, low frustration tolerance, temper outbursts, low self-esteem, and lack of response to discipline" (p. 42). Many of these features, however, are more closely associated with OD or CD than with ADD (Loney, Kramer, & Milich, 1981).

Compared to normal controls, children with ADD have been reported to have lower self-esteem (Kelly, Cohen, & Atkinson, 1986), more depressive symptoms, and more external attributions (Borden, Brown, Jenkins, & Clingerman, 1987).

In social situations, both adults and other children find the behavior of children with ADD intrusive, irritating, and objectionable. Unless OD or CD is also present, the problems seem to be due to impulsivity and lack of ability to observe themselves and others, rather than intentional misbehavior. In classrooms, they are more talkative than normal children and more likely to initiate social interactions. Their actions tend to be intense, out of synchrony with the situational context, and insensitive to social expectations and interpersonal nuances, despite normal performance on tests of social knowledge or perspective-taking skills (Pelham & Bender, 1982; Whalen & Henker, 1985). Hyperactive children may have deficits in vicarious social learning (Whalen & Henker, 1985).

Hyperactive girls are referred less often for hyperactivity and aggressive behavior disorders and more often for learning difficulties and speech disorders. They are more fearful, more likely to be enuretic, and more likely to be rejected by peers (Berry, Shaywitz, & Shaywitz, 1985; Kashani, Chapel, Ellis, & Shekim, 1979).

Despite parental reports of restless sleep in ADD children, polysomnography discloses no differences from controls except decreased REM activity (Greenhill, Puig-Antich, Goetz, Hanlon, & Davies, 1983).

Investigators have recently focused on children who are both hyperactive and aggressive. In classroom observation studies, both hyperactive (H) and hyperactive/aggressive (H/A) boys are more frequently off task than children who are aggressive only (A) or normal controls. The H/A boys also engage in rule-violating behavior while off task. By all measures, A and H/A boys engage in significantly more peer-directed aggression than H boys. Differences in the patterns and motivation of the aggression remain to be studied. H/A boys are more likely to be verbally or physically aggressive toward and less compliant with adults than are H boys. This results in teachers directing more negative attention to H/A boys than to either H or A boys. H/A and A boys also engage in more nonaggressive antisocial behaviors than H boys (Milich & Pelham, 1986).

Associations between hyperactivity and soft signs, minor physical anomalies, and EEG abnormalities are weak, and many normal children and children with other psychiatric disorders have them (Ferguson & Rapoport, 1983; Rutter, 1982; Shaffer, O'Connor, Shafer, & Prupis, 1983). DSM-III estimated that 5% of cases of ADD are associated with diagnosable neurological disorder, which should be coded on Axis III.

Compared to normal controls, hyperactives are more likely to have had poor coordination, delay in bowel control, delay in talking, and speech problems (Hartsough & Lambert, 1985).

Mothers of preschoolers with ADD/H report discipline problems, temper tantrums, inability to play alone, and difficulties getting along with peers and siblings (Campbell, 1985). In free play, mothers of hyperactive preschoolers are more likely to suggest alternative activities, to make statements aimed at slowing their children down and helping them to regain control, and to give reprimands (Campbell, Breaux, Ewing, Szumowski, & Pierce, 1986).

BIOLOGICAL ASPECTS

Predisposing Factors

The following historical items significantly discriminate between hyperactives and controls: poor maternal health during pregnancy, toxemia or eclampsia, first pregnancy, maternal age less than 20, postmaturity (but not prematurity), longer duration of labor, and health problems during infancy (Hartsough & Lambert, 1985). Prenatal factors account for only a small portion of the variance, however, and interact in complex ways with environmental factors. They also seem more likely to be related to nonspecific psychopathology, not just ADD, and they are not particularly helpful in making diagnoses or predictions in individual cases (Ferguson & Rapoport, 1983).

There are suggestions that maternal alcohol use and smoking contribute to hyperactivity and/or attentional problems (Denson, Nanson, & McWatters, 1975; Shaywitz, Cohen, & Shaywitz, 1980; Steinhausen & Spohr, 1986; Streissguth et al., 1984).

Malnutrition in the first year of life (Galler, Ramsey, Solimano, & Lowell, 1983) and subclinical chronic lead poisoning (Gittelman & Eskenazi, 1983; Ross & Ross, 1982) have been implicated. There is an increased risk of ADD in children with phenylketonuria (even with diet restriction) (Realmuto et al., 1986) or glucose-6-phosphate dehydrogenase (G6PD) deficiency (Meijer, 1984).

Pathophysiology

Gualtieri and colleagues (Evans, Gualtieri, & Hicks, 1986; Gualtieri, Hicks, & Mayo, 1983) suggest that the core problem in ADD is excessive variability in both rate and magnitude of change in arousal level and reactivity. Various dimensions of arousal are less well synchronized, parameters of response are widely set, and oscillations are extreme and unpredictable. As a result, ADD children do not regulate their activity, either in goal or amount, in response to situational demands. In this model, stimulants are seen as acting by canalizing, or reducing variability in, arousal and reactivity.

Despite a variety of theories and investigations, the evidence for a single neurochemical abnormality in ADD is ambiguous. The majority of studies have found no or inconsistent biochemical differences between ADD children and controls. Likely candidates for neurotransmitter system abnormalities include dopamine, norepinephrine, and serotonin, as well as a number of other more recently identified neurotransmitters (Shaywitz, Shaywitz, Cohen, & Young, 1983). More likely than simple excess or deficiency is imbalance in receptor sensitivity or between several neurotransmitter systems (Zametkin & Rapoport, 1986).

Current theories favor the frontal lobe as the anatomic site of abnormality in ADD. The proposed mechanism is delayed or abnormal maturation. This is derived from four sources:

1. Extrapolation from the behavior of patients with documented frontal lobe damage (Evans et al., 1986; Mattes, 1980)
2. Studies of cerebral blood flow, using xenon inhalation and computerized tomography, indicating hypoperfusion in this region, compared to normal sibling controls (Lou, Henriksen, & Bruhn, 1984)
3. Differences from controls shown by adults diagnosed ADD/H or ADD/R in glucose metabolism in the anterior frontal and posterior medial orbital regions on PET scan during an auditory attention task (Zametkin, 1986)
4. Deficits in ADD children on neuropsychological tests presumed to measure frontal lobe inhibitory control (Chelune, Ferguson, Koon, & Dickey, 1986). (These differences have not been found consistently, however, and may be more closely related to CD than ADD [Schaughency, Lahey, Hynd, Stone, & Piacentini, 1987].)

COURSE AND PROGNOSIS

In many cases, signs of ADD are apparent very early. Parents of hyperactives are more likely to report difficulty establishing routines even during infancy (Hartsough & Lambert, 1985). Parent-referred children identified as hyperactive at age 3 demonstrate a mixture of problems in attention, impulse control, noncompliance, and aggression (Campbell, Breaux, Ewing, & Szumowski, 1986). They show developmental progress but continuing overactivity and impulsivity at age 4. At age 6, at least 30% of the boys meet DSM-III criteria for ADD, while girls are more likely to "outgrow" their problems (Campbell, 1985; Campbell, Ewing, Breaux, & Szumowski, 1986). Persistent hyperactivity and aggression at age 6 are predicted by the occurrence at age 3 of lower social class, greater family stress, higher maternal ratings of child aggression and hyperactivity, observed negative and directive maternal behavior and negative and noncompliant child behavior, and laboratory measures of inattention and overactivity (Campbell et al., 1986).

From 50 to 80% of hyperactive children continue to show symptoms of hyperactivity, impulsivity, and/or inattention in adolescence, frequently also with poor academic performance, depression, low self-esteem, and poor peer relationships. The incidence of antisocial behaviors varies from 10 to 50%, according to the source of the sample and the original percentage with aggressive behavior. Age at time of reevaluation influences findings (Brown & Borden, 1986; Cantwell, 1986; Weiss, 1985b).

In the cohort followed by August, Stewart, and Holmes (1983), antisocial behavior was found only in the group with CD as well as hyperactivity initially.

The most extensive controlled prospective study of hyperactive children followed into adulthood, done at Montreal Children's Hospital, now has 15-year follow-up data (Weiss, Hechtman, Milroy, & Perlman, 1985). Educational achievement continued to be limited, and 66% of subjects complained of at least one symptom (restlessness, poor concentration, impulsivity, explosiveness). Compared to controls, hyperactives reported more physical aggression and suicide attempts. Forty-four percent were observed to be restless or fidgety. They scored lower on a global measure of functioning, and were more often diagnosed as antisocial personality disorder. Drug and alcohol abuse were *not* more common (Hechtman & Weiss, 1986).

A more recent clinical sample of boys diagnosed hyperactive followed into adolescence showed persistence of the full syndrome of ADD/H in one-third. Interestingly, only 5% were found to have ADD/R, and an equal number had hyperactivity with impulsivity or with inattention, a group that is not described in DSM-III or DSM-III-R. Despite efforts to eliminate children with concurrent CD from the original sample, 27% were diagnosed CD at follow-up (although the Conners rating scales used in subject selection may have inadvertently led to inclusion of youth with CD). Nearly all of the CD was found in youth with a continuing diagnosis of ADD/H. Findings for substance abuse were similar. Rates of these problems were significantly higher in early adolescence than in the late teens and early twenties, demonstrating improvement with age (Gittelman, Mannuzza, Shenker, & Bonagura, 1985). A smaller sample of hyperactive girls followed into adolescence did not show significant gender-related differences (Mannuzza & Gittelman, 1984).

Studies of outcome suffer from a variety of methodological difficulties, including the changing conceptualization of the disorder, variability in diagnostic methods and selection criteria, nonrepresentative samples, inadequate control groups, overly brief follow-up periods, lack of attention to medication status, and high rates of attrition (Brown & Borden, 1986; Cantwell, 1985; Thorley, 1984b; Wallander & Hubert, 1985).

Consistent predictors of poor prognosis include aggression, low IQ, poor mother–child relationship, brain damage, low socioeconomic status, and poor family environment (Paternite & Loney, 1980; Weiss, 1985a; Whalen & Henker, 1980). Adult-directed oppositional and aggressive behavior may be a much more powerful negative prognostic sign than peer-directed aggression (Johnston & Pelham, 1986).

IMPAIRMENT

Academic Performance

At the time of diagnosis, virtually all youngsters with ADD show cognitive, achievement, and/or school performance deficits to some degree. One cohort of hyperactive boys (without CD) has been shown to have significantly lower IQ scores than their siblings, but equivalent achievement scores, when corrected for IQ (Halperin & Gittelman, 1982). Far more hyperactive youngsters than controls score significantly lower on tests of academic achievement than predicted from their IQ. Hyperactives tend to lag more severely and in more subjects (Cantwell & Satterfield, 1978; Lambert & Sandoval, 1980). The Montreal group found that only 20% of their hyperactive adolescents made a satisfactory academic adjustment (Weiss, Minde, Werry, Douglas, & Nemeth, 1971).

Children with ADD/WO are at higher risk for repeating a grade at school than those with ADD/H (Edelbrock, Costello, & Kessler, 1984).

Peer Relations and Social Function

Hyperactive children have a bossy, uncooperative, aggressive, and bothersome interpersonal style (Pelham & Bender, 1982) and are viewed by their peers as deviant and problematic (Whalen & Henker, 1985). Immature, negative, attention-seeking behaviors as well as unpredictability, attempts to dominate peers, and temper outbursts lead to rapid identification and rejection by peers (Ross & Ross, 1982). Hyperactives receive more active rejection and less positive attention from peers than do controls (Carlson, Lahey, Frame, Walker, & Hynd, in press; Milich & Landau, 1982; Pelham & Bender, 1982). Children with ADD/WO tend to be neglected rather than actively rejected (Carlson et al., in press).

COMPLICATIONS

Depending on the sample, definitions, and diagnostic methodology used, from 40 to 75% of hyperactive children in clinic populations also have CD (Lahey, Piacentini et al., in press). Youngsters with both disorders tend to have an earlier age of onset, be referred at a younger age, exhibit a greater total number of antisocial behaviors, display more physical aggression, and engage in more serious delinquency, and are more likely to have the "versatile" pattern of antisocial behavior associated with a poor prognosis than those with CD alone (Offord, Sullivan, Allen, & Abrams, 1979; Walker, Lahey, Hynd, & Frame, in press).

Hyperactive children are significantly more likely to be reported by their parents to be accident prone than normals (Hartsough & Lambert, 1985) or psychiatric clinic controls (Gayton, Bailey, Wagner, & Hardesty, 1986). Data suggest an increased risk for accidental poisoning (Stewart, Thach, & Freidin, 1970) and for car accidents (Weiss, Hechtman, Perlman, Hopkins, & Werner, 1979).

The problem behaviors of hyperactive children lead, through a reciprocal feedback system, to negative attitudes and behavior toward them from parents and teachers, resulting in increasing dysfunction in the child (Barkley, 1981a, 1981b; Milich & Landau, 1982; Whalen & Henker, 1985). Mothers of hyperactive children report their own levels of stress to be high (Mash & Johnston, 1983).

EPIDEMIOLOGY

The epidemiology of hyperactivity has been controversial. In a disorder that represents one end of a continuum, the cutoff point for diagnosis is to some extent artificial. Prevalence also varies according to the type and number of informants, cultural expectations (Shapiro & Garfinkel, 1986), and whether pervasive symptoms, clinical diagnosis and functional impairment, teacher identification, or only scores on screening tests are used.

Between 14 and 20% of preschool and kindergarten boys and approximately a third as many girls can be considered hyperactive (Campbell, 1985).

Two well-designed studies of elementary school populations (Bosco & Robin, 1980; Sandoval, Lambert, & Sassone, 1980) found that approximately 3% of students had ever been diagnosed by a physician as hyperactive. An additional 5 to 7% had scores equal to the hyperactives on rating scales but had never been identified or treated. Boys outnumber girls by from four to one to eight to one.

FAMILY PATTERNS

Early studies that demonstrated family genetic and/or environmental transmission of hyperactivity and a linkage between hyperactivity and antisocial disorders suffered from methodologic flaws (Ross & Ross, 1982) and contained unspecified proportions of children who were aggressive in addition to being hyperactive or even *instead of* being hyperactive (Loney & Milich, 1982).

More recently, August and Stewart (1983) found that hyperactive children with a parental history of antisocial personality, hysteria, or alcohol and/or drug abuse had a high frequency of CD in themselves and in siblings, while hyperactive children and their siblings who did not have a parent with an antisocial spectrum disorder had little evidence of CD. These children had more learning and academic difficulties, as did their siblings, who also tended to have attentional problems.

Twin studies, which are limited by very small numbers, suggest that monozygotic twins have a higher concordance rate for hyperactivity than dizygotic twins (Heffron, Martin, & Welsh, 1984).

Biederman and colleagues (Biederman, Munir, & Knee, 1986; Biederman, Munir, Knee et al., 1986) conducted a family study using blind structured interviews of probands and first-degree relatives of carefully diagnosed clinically referred boys with ADD and matched normal controls. Sixty-four percent of the ADD patients also had a diagnosis of OD or CD. Relatives of ADD patients both with and without CD or OD had a higher rate of ADD than relatives of controls. Relatives of children with ADD *and* CD or OD had a significantly higher rate of CD, OD, and antisocial personality disorder than those with ADD *without* CD or OD, which equaled relatives of controls.

ADD patients were also significantly more likely to have major depressive disorder (MDD) than controls, as were their relatives, compared to control relatives. Probands with both ADD and MDD did not have a higher prevalence of MDD in relatives than probands without MDD or normal controls.

Another study (Lahey, Piacentini, et al., in press) found that parents of children with ADD/H but *without* CD did not have an increased incidence of psychopathology compared to clinic controls, although questions were not asked about childhood ADD or ADD/R. Fathers of children with *both* ADD/H and CD were markedly more likely to have a history of aggression, arrest, and imprisonment, even when compared to fathers of children with CD alone. The finding of significantly lower SES for the ADD/H plus CD group is a potentially complicating factor.

Although the direction of causality is unclear, there is an increased incidence of depression in mothers and marital discord between parents of hyperactive children (Barkley, 1981a).

DIFFERENTIAL DIAGNOSIS

A discussion of the clinical issues in evaluation of children and adolescents suspected to have attention deficits is beyond the scope of this chapter, but may be found in Barkley (1981a). ADD must first be distinguished from normal, age-appropriate overactivity. At all developmental levels, information from multiple sources is vital (Campbell, Szumowski, Ewing, Gluck, & Breaux, 1982; Gittelman & Mannuzza, 1985). Clinical interviews and standardized rating scales provide complementary data (Lahey, McBurnett et al., 1987; Shekim et al., 1986). Laboratory tests of learning and attention are valuable adjuncts, when available (Pelham, 1982; Swanson, 1985).

Other Psychiatric Disorders

According to DSM-III, patients may have diagnoses *in addition to* ADD, although the presumed ADD symptoms must not be "due to" schizophrenia, affective disorder, or severe or profound mental retardation. Children in clinical settings are more likely to have several disorders, due to referral bias.

If there is a late onset or brief duration of symptoms, one should suspect an adjustment disorder in reaction to a stressor such as family crisis or disorganization, child abuse or neglect, inappropriate school placement, or teacher–child or parent–child conflict.

After years of controversy, it is now clear that CD can be distinguished from hyperactivity by parent interview, teacher ratings, and associated features (Lahey, Piacentini, et al., in press; Loney & Milich, 1982; McGee, Williams, & Silva, 1984; Taylor, Everitt et al., 1986; Taylor, Schachar, Thorley, & Wieselberg, 1986), although as many as two-thirds of hyperactive children in clinical settings also have conduct problems. Noncompliance with rules is common to ADD, OD, and CD, although the presumed intent differs.

Children with pervasive developmental disorders may show hyperactivity, in-attention, and impulsivity, but a PDD diagnosis preempts a diagnosis of ADD (APA, 1980).

Schizophrenia or mood disorders, such as agitated depression or mania, may be associated with overactivity and decreased concentration, but the episodic nature of the disturbance and the presence of other signs and symptoms should make the distinction relatively easy. Mania may, however, take uncharacteristic forms in prepubertal children, and children with presumed hyperactivity, especially those with a family history of bipolar affective disorder, may later develop full-blown mania, with or without precipitation by methylphenidate (Dvoredsky & Stewart, 1981; Koehler-Troy, Strober, & Malenbaum, 1986).

Children who are fidgety and seem preoccupied may have an anxiety disorder rather than or in addition to ADD. A diagnosis of anxiety disorder requires verbalization of worries and/or fears, which is not present in pure ADD. Anxious children usually improve with increased experience in a situation, while ADD children worsen. The overlap is greatest between anxiety disorders and ADD without hyperactivity (Carlson, 1986).

Mental retardation can be mistaken for ADD, but ADD can be diagnosed in retarded youngsters if symptoms are excessive for the child's mental age. A recent study found that a substantial proportion of children described as hyperactive by teachers but not parents were found to have mental retardation or learning disabilities rather than ADD (Landman & McCrindle, 1986).

Much of the older literature has confused the distinction between ADD (or MBD) and learning disabilities. The DSM-III definitions of specific developmental disorders are not particularly helpful here. When learning disabilities are defined as delays in specific skills demonstrated on psychoeducational testing such as dyslexia, dyscalculia, agraphia, or spelling disorder, a proportion of children with ADD are found to have specific learning disabilities also (Barkley, 1982).

Drug Effects

The use of phenobarbital as an anticonvulsant is commonly associated with the development of hyperactivity, which may be only partially reversible (Wolf & Forsythe, 1978).

Theophylline (used in the treatment of asthma) has been demonstrated to increase impulsivity, distractibility, and irritability and decrease ability to finish a task (Rachelefsky et al., 1986).

Abuse of amphetamines may lead to apparent hyperactivity.

Medical Disorders

Hyperthyroidism may superficially resemble hyperactivity.

Patients with Tourette's syndrome (TS) often demonstrate overactivity, impulsivity, and distractibility. It is controversial whether these are part of TS or due to a coexisting ADD, and whether ADD and TS are genetically related (Comings & Comings, 1984; Pauls et al., 1986; Young, Leven, Knott, Leckman, & Cohen, 1985).

CLINICAL MANAGEMENT: RESEARCH FINDINGS

A comprehensive review of the clinical aspects of the treatment of ADD may be found in Dulcan (1986).

Pharmacotherapy

See Dulcan (1986, 1988) for a detailed discussion of the therapeutic and side effects of medications used to treat ADD.

The stimulant drugs methylphenidate (Ritalin), dextroamphetamine (Dexedrine), and magnesium pemoline (Cylert) are the most commonly used. On global measures, parents, teachers, and clinicians rate 75% of hyperactive children "improved" on stimulant medication, as opposed to 40% on placebo. Twenty-five percent are judged "no change" or "worse" (Barkley, 1981a). On closer inspection, however, the situation is not so simple, due to the dissociation of magnitude and direction of stimulant effects on various behavioral, cognitive, cardiovascular, neuroendocrine, and electrophysiological measures (Gualtieri et al., 1983). When used in appropriate doses, methylphenidate, dextroamphetamine, and, to a somewhat lesser extent, sustained-release methylphenidate and pemoline (Dulcan, 1986; Pelham et al., in press) decrease motor activity, vocalization, noise, classroom disruption, distractibility, off-task behavior, intensity of behavior, impulsivity, defiance (Taylor et al., 1987), and negative social behavior (Whalen et al., 1987) and improve sustained attention, compliance, and handwriting in the short term in the majority of hyperactive youngsters (Dulcan, 1986; Henker, Astor-Dubin, & Varni, 1986). Gains in both learning and academic productivity can be demonstrated, if the tasks and the measures are correctly chosen (Pelham, 1983, 1985; Pelham, Bender, Caddell, Booth, & Moorer, 1985; Pelham & Murphy, 1986). Gains in achievement testing may require educational remediation as well as medication (Winsberg, Maitinsky, Kupietz, & Richardson, 1986). Aggression has been reduced in some children in some studies, but not in others. Stimulant-produced increase in compliance in hyperactive children can result in changes in the behavior of mothers and teachers toward them (Barkley, 1981b; Whalen, Henker, Fink, & Dotemoto, 1979). A pilot study found methylphenidate improved school grades in children with ADD/WO (Famularo & Fenton, 1987).

Studies of long-term stimulant effects have been disappointing, especially with regard to academic achievement, but this can be attributed to flaws in the studies, including problems in the medication regimens such as dosages too high, too low, or timed poorly, medication discontinued too soon, or no measures of compliance, which is known to be poor (Brown, Borden, & Clingerman, 1985a; Firestone, 1982; Kauffman, Smith-Wright, Reese, Simpson, & Jones, 1981). Other deficits or problems such as specific learning disabilities, academic deficits, conduct problems, social skills deficits, and family pathology were not addressed. Methodologic defects include heterogeneous samples, inappropriate control groups, insensitive outcome measures, and lack of attention to individual response variation (Gadow & Swanson, 1985; Pelham, 1985; Pelham & Murphy, 1986).

Stimulant responsiveness in an individual youngster with ADD/H is difficult to predict (Barkley, 1976; Halperin, Gittelman, Katz, & Struve, 1986; Loney, 1986; Taylor, 1983). Positive placebo response to stimulants in children with ADD is as high as 18% (Ullmann & Sleator, 1986).

Other drugs that have some demonstrated efficacy in the treatment of ADD that can be used if response to stimulants is poor or if tics (Denckla, Bemporad, &

MacKay, 1976; Lowe, Cohen, Detlor, Kremenetzer, & Shaywitz, 1982) or other side effects preclude their use, including the tricyclics imipramine (Pliszka, 1987; Rancurello, 1985; Rapoport, Quinn, Bradbard, Riddle, & Brooks, 1974) and desipramine (Biederman, Gastfriend, & Jellinek, 1986; Garfinkel, Wender, Sloman, & O'Neill, 1983; Gastfriend, Biederman, & Jellinek, 1984) and the alpha-adrenergic agonist clonidine (Hunt, Minderaa, & Cohen, 1985).

Combinations of drugs are not advised (Dulcan, 1986; Grob & Coyle, 1986).

Behavior Therapy

Behavior modification is able to address symptoms that stimulants do not, but the cooperation of parents and teachers is required. Parents find behavior management training more difficult to sustain than pharmacotherapy (Firestone, Kelly, Goodman, & Davey, 1981), but some parents may prefer behavioral to medical treatment (Thurston, 1981). Programs differ in their duration and intensity, and not all behavior therapy studies have positive results. Interestingly, classroom operant programs may have beneficial effects on students not specifically targeted (Loney, Weissenburger, Woolson, & Lichty, 1979).

Behavioral interventions with hyperactive children are effective in the short term in improving behavior, social skills, and academic performance if specifically targeted (Mash & Dalby, 1979). Programs may be conducted directly with children and adolescents, or through teachers (Ayllon & Rosenbaum, 1977) or parents (Dubey, O'Leary, & Kaufman, 1983). While a relatively brief operant program at home and school decreased aggression in hyperactive children to the level of controls, it did not substantially reduce inattention, activity, or impulsivity (Abikoff & Gittelman, 1984). Unmedicated ADD children do not respond to a general classroom program of attention and reward for positive behavior alone, but require the addition of a response cost system (Pelham & Murphy, 1986). Hyperactive children often require both instruction to remedy deficits in social or academic skills and contingency management to induce them to use the skills (Pelham & Bender, 1982). In addition, interventions need to be continued for months or years to produce permanent behavior changes (Pelham & Bender, 1982).

Limitations in existing studies include small numbers of subjects, poorly specified subject populations, brief duration of treatment, limited generalization and maintenance of treatment effects, and virtually nonexistent follow-up evaluations leading to no knowledge of long-term effects (Mash & Dalby, 1979).

Cognitive Behavior Modification (CBM) or Problem-Solving Therapy

This treatment, which may be administered individually or in a group, combines behavior modification techniques such as contingency management (Douglas, 1980) and modeling with teaching cognitive strategies such as stepwise problem solving and self-monitoring (Meichenbaum & Goodman, 1971). It was developed in an attempt to improve the generalization and durability of behavior modification techniques and to improve long-term outcome over stimulant medication. It is theoretically appealing, because it directly addresses presumed deficits in control of impulsivity and in problem solving and provides a structure for work with children who otherwise gain little benefit from psychotherapy.

Early studies showed improvement on measures of cognitive impulsivity and social behavior (Douglas, 1980; Douglas, Parry, Marton, & Garson, 1976; Hinshaw, Henker, & Whalen, 1984b; Yellin, Kendall, & Greenberg, 1981) and additive effects with stimulants (Hinshaw et al., 1984a; Horn, Chatoor, & Conners, 1983), and a model was developed to teach aggressive, impulsive, and hyperactive children self-control and problem-solving strategies (Kendall & Braswell, 1985). Subsequent results in hyperactive children have been somewhat disappointing, and have not demonstrated that CBM is able to improve results over stimulant medication alone (Abikoff, 1985; Abikoff & Gittelman, 1985b; Brown, Wynne, & Medenis, 1985). Possible reasons are inappropriate patient selection, variation in individual response that is obscured in group data, lack of attention to generalization, omission of behavioral contingencies from the training, lack of individualization of the training in response to actual deficits, and insufficiently intensive and extensive training.

CBM has had the most success when used in a summer day program (Kirby & Grimley, 1986), where it was integrated into all of the activities, specific attention was given to generalization to academic and social situations, and in-school booster sessions were conducted. Unfortunately, this study did not look at interactive effects with medication.

A recent study using cognitive therapy with nonmedicated hospitalized children with conduct problems, some of whom also had ADD, showed improvement at 1-month and 1-year follow-up, although most children were still not in the normal range on behavior measures (Kazdin, Esveldt-Dawson, French, & Unis, 1987).

Academic Therapy

Stimulation reduction techniques are popular in classrooms, despite lack of empirical support. In general, teaching techniques and curricular adaptations that would be helpful to youngsters with ADD have received little attention (Ross & Ross, 1982; Sprague, 1983).

Other Treatment Methods

Reviews of the methodologically adequate studies show that at most 5% of hyperactive children may show behavioral or cognitive improvement on the so-called Kaiser-Permanente diet, but these changes are not as dramatic as those induced by stimulants (Barkley, 1981a; Varley, 1984; Wender, 1986). No one has been able to predict which children will respond, although preschoolers are more likely to respond than older children.

Controlled studies have been unable to demonstrate consistently that ingestion of sugar has an effect on the behavior or cognitive performance of normal or hyperactive children, even those identified by their parents as sugar responsive (Milich, Wolraich, & Lindgren, 1986).

The efficacy of biofeedback techniques, separate from relaxation training and contingency management, remains to be demonstrated (Ross & Ross, 1982).

Combinations of Treatments

For most ADD youngsters, neither stimulant medication nor behavior therapy alone is sufficient to normalize behavior and academic performance, and there are non-responders to each intervention (Pelham & Murphy, 1986). Behavior modification has been shown to be additive in effect to methylphenidate for many ADD children (Pelham & Bender, 1982; Pelham, Milich, & Walker, 1986; Pelham, Schnedler, Bologna, & Contreras, 1980). Although with a sufficiently intensive and structured behavioral program it is possible to nearly normalize the behavior of children with ADD while in the treatment setting, 30 to 60% will improve further with the addition of low-dose methylphenidate (Pelham & Murphy, 1986). Similarly, behavior therapy has been demonstrated to add to the efficacy of methylphenidate, yielding ratings equal to normal peers, with methylphenidate alone superior to behavior therapy alone (Gittelman et al., 1980). Studies with less intensive interventions have not found behavior modification to add significantly to pharmacotherapy (Firestone et al., 1981; Wolraich, Drummond, Salomon, O'Brien, & Sivage, 1978).

Due to the multiple deficits in youngsters with ADD and the limitations of existing treatments, multimodality treatment programs have been advocated (Pelham & Murphy, 1986; Satterfield, Satterfield, & Cantwell, 1981). Unfortunately, these are often difficult to implement and to evaluate systematically (Brown, Borden, & Clingerman, 1985b). One longitudinal study combining methylphenidate and in-dividual, group, parent, family, and/or educational therapy based on individualized evaluation and treatment planning found at follow-up in adolescence a reduction in delinquency over boys treated with medication alone (Satterfield, Satterfield, & Schell, 1987). Unfortunately, methodologic deficiencies limit the usefulness of this study other than as a guide to future work.

DSM-III-R

ADD criterion items in the three categories in DSM-III proved to be difficult to operationalize in practice. In DSM-III-R (APA, 1987) there is a single category of attention deficit hyperactivity disorder (ADHD), under the subclass of disruptive behavior disorders. The inclusion criteria form a single list of 14 items chosen to improve discrimination from oppositional defiant disorder and conduct disorder. The threshold of 8 symptoms for a diagnosis of ADHD was determined by field trial. Required onset is before the age of 9, with a minimum duration of 6 months. Pervasive developmental disorder is an exclusionary diagnosis.

The diagnosis of ADD/WO has been eliminated, because it was rarely made in the field trial. In response to protest over this decision, a new category, undifferentiated attention deficit disorder, was created, which does not have signs of impulsiveness and hyperactivity. There are no criteria specified for this diagnosis. Unfortunately, since some children and adolescents called ADD/WO will meet criteria for ADHD, and others will be classified in the undifferentiated ADD category, this is likely to worsen, rather than reduce, the confusion.

ADD/R will no longer be specifically listed, since each DSM-III diagnosis is presumed to have a residual state.

In contrast, the tenth revision of the *International Classification of Diseases* (World Health Organization, 1987), which permits only one diagnosis per axis, uses the overall term *hyperkinetic disorder* for a group of disorders including simple disturbance of activity and attention, hyperkinetic conduct disorder, and hyperkinetic disorder, not otherwise specified.

RESEARCH ISSUES IN DIAGNOSIS

There is currently little consensus among researchers on the criteria or methods to diagnose ADD or on the validity of various subtypes. DSM-III-R has not improved the situation significantly. There is general agreement that the following dimensions are important in studying the externalizing or disruptive disorders: inattention, overactivity, impulsivity, covert antisocial acts, verbal and physical aggression (toward peers and toward adults), and oppositional behaviors. Unfortunately, opinions are diverse on the way to measure these dimensions and how to group them into categories. Even the desirability of categories has been questioned (Achenbach & Edelbrock, 1978).

Standardized assessment measures vary in the amount of time and professional expertise they require, and their purpose, which may include screening, diagnosis, sample characterization, and measurement of treatment effect. Some are used just for ADD, and others are more general.

There is variable agreement among different types of measures in the same setting (Atkins, Pelham, & Licht, 1985; Lahey, McBurnett, et al., 1987; Schachar, Sandberg, & Rutter, 1986). In general, questionnaires tend to have more test–retest stability than observational measures but lower interrater reliability (Rutter, 1983). This may be due in part to the global impressions solicited by questionnaires that favor highly salient but relatively infrequent behaviors (Collins, Whalen, & Henker, 1980). Loudness and inappropriateness of behaviors tend to increase salience and frequency ratings (Mintz & Collins, 1985). There are also differences between settings, which may relate to real differences in behavior in different contexts.

Examples include:

Rating Scales (see Conners & Barkley, 1985; Edelbrock & Rancurello, 1985)

    Parent

        Conners Parent Symptom Questionnaire (Goyette, Conners, & Ulrich, 1978)

        MOMS (Mother's Measure for Subgrouping) (Loney, 1987)

        Child Behavior Checklist and Profile (Achenbach & Edelbrock, 1983)

        Home Situations Questionnaire (Barkley & Edelbrock, in press)

Yale Children's Inventory (Shaywitz, Schnell, Shaywitz, & Towle, 1986)

Teacher

Conners Teacher Rating Scale (Conners, 1969; Goyette et al., 1978)

IOWA Conners (Loney & Milich, 1982)

SNAP (DSM-III criteria) (Atkins et al., 1985)

Child Behavior Checklist and Profile (Achenbach & Edelbrock, 1986)

CAP (Child Attention Problems) (Edelbrock, 1986)

ACTeRS (ADD-H: Comprehensive Teacher Rating Scale) (Ullmann, Sleator, & Sprague, 1984, 1985b)

School Situations Questionnaire (Barkley & Edelbrock, in press)

Self-Report

ADD-H Adolescent Self-Report Scale (Conners & Wells, 1985)

Self-Evaluation (Teenager's) Self-Report (Gittelman, 1985)

Interviews (see also Orvaschel, 1985)

Structured (see Chapter 23)

DICA (Herjanic, 1981)

DISC (Costello, Edelbrock, & Costello, 1985)

Semistructured

KSADS (Schedule for Affective Disorders & Schizophrenia for School-Age Children) (Chambers et al., 1985)

PACS (Parental Account of Children's Symptoms) (Taylor, Schachar, Thorley, & Weiselberg, 1986)

Observational Scales

Classroom

Classroom Observation Code (Abikoff & Gittelman, 1985a)

During testing

Hillside Behavior Rating Scale (Gittelman & Klein, 1985)

Standard playroom (Milich, Loney, & Roberts, 1986; Roberts, Ray, & Roberts, 1984; Routh, 1978)

Playground or other unstructured activity (Abikoff, Martin, & Gittelman, 1985; Whalen et al., 1987)

Laboratory Measures of Activity (Conners & Kronsberg, 1985)

Computerized Measures of Cognitive Function (Conners, 1985; Swanson, 1985)

Tests of Academic Performance (Gadow & Swanson, 1985; Pelham, 1985)

Standard Psychological Tests (e.g., WISC-R)

Sociometrics (Carlson et al., in press)

(See also Reatig, 1985)

Rating scales developed by Conners have come to be the most widely used in research and clinical practice. The Conners Parent Symptom Questionnaire (CPSQ) (Goyette et al., 1978) does not correlate well with activity or attention measured by behavior observations but it does correlate with measures of child noncompliance, academic problems, and response to medication (Barkley, 1981a). The 10-item Hyperkinesis Index contained in both the CPSQ and the Conners Teacher Rating Scale (CTRS) (Conners, 1969; Goyette et al., 1978) has been used extensively (Conners, 1973). It is sensitive to differences between active drug and placebo (Goyette et al., 1978) but is problematic when used for diagnosis or subject selection in hyperactivity research. It is not sensitive to inattention without hyperactivity (Ullmann, Sleator, & Sprague, 1985a), and is overly sensitive to conduct problems (Ullmann et al., 1985a; Loney & Milich, 1982). Many items correlate with both hyperactivity and aggression. Samples selected by using the conventional cutoff score of 15 will have excessive numbers of boys who are *both* aggressive and hyperactive. Even worse, boys who are only aggressive are selected as often as boys who are only hyperactive (Loney & Milich, 1982; Ullmann et al., 1985a). Also, defiance toward the teacher increases the likelihood of being rated as hyperactive or inattentive (Schachar et al., 1986). In addition, the score tends to decrease from first to second administration, which may be a practice effect (Werry & Sprague, 1974; Zentall & Zentall, 1986) or a statistical regression effect (Milich, Roberts, Loney, & Caputo, 1980).

The single worst problem in interpreting past research on hyperactivity or ADD is the contamination of samples with unspecified amounts of CD (for reviews see Hinshaw, 1987; Loney, 1987). "We do not have a literature about childhood hyperactivity as such; instead, we have a literature about childhood externalizing behavior problems (hyperactivity *and* aggression) that we *call* a literature about childhood hyperactivity" (Loney & Milich, 1982, p. 143).

Loney and Milich (1982) developed a new teacher rating scale called the IOWA (*I*nattention and *O*veractivity *w*ith *A*ggression) Conners using individual items from the CTRS that loaded on *either* a hyperactivity factor or an aggression factor (which included negative affect and defiant interpersonal behavior), but not both. Norms have been determined (Pelham, Milich, & Murphy, 1986).

Edelbrock (1986) has developed an extensively normed short rating scale called the CAP (Child Attention Problems) from the Teacher CBCL (Achenbach & Edelbrock, 1986) with Inattentive and Overactive factors.

FUTURE DIRECTIONS

Future work will be improved with more homogeneous and better described samples, paying particular attention to IQ, learning disabilities, presence of aggressive and nonaggressive conduct problems, presence or absence of hyperactivity, situational versus pervasive symptoms, description of the source of the sample and the methods of recruitment and selection, and standardized diagnostic and evaluation instruments, so that samples can be compared and collaborative studies conducted. Descriptive studies should compare youngsters with ADHD with other psychiatric patients as well as normal controls.

Promising directions for treatment research include the effects of stimulants on sociability (Hinshaw & McHale, in press; Milich & Landau, 1982; Whalen et al., 1987), conduct problems (Taylor et al., 1987), aggression, and learning (Pelham, 1985; Weiss, 1985b). Drugs other than stimulants require more systematic evaluation. Combinations of treatment modalities should be studied in an effort to improve generalization and long-term efficacy, with attention paid to order effects and individual variation.

REFERENCES

Abikoff, H. (1985). Efficacy of cognitive training interventions in hyperactive children: A critical review. *Clinical Psychology Review*, *5*, 479–512.

Abikoff, H., & Gittelman, R. (1984). Does behavior therapy normalize the classroom behavior of hyperactive children? *Archives of General Psychiatry*, *41*, 449–454.

Abikoff, H., & Gittelman, R. (1985a). Classroom Observation Code: A modification of the Stony Brook Code. *Psychopharmacology Bulletin*, *21*, 901–909.

Abikoff, H., & Gittelman, R. (1985b). Hyperactive children treated with stimulants: Is cognitive training a useful adjunct? *Archives of General Psychiatry*, *42*, 953–961.

Abikoff, H., Martin, D., & Gittelman, R. (1985). Social Interaction Observation Code. *Psychopharmacology Bulletin*, *21*, 869–873.

Achenbach, T.M., & Edelbrock, C.A. (1978). The classification of child psychopathology: A review and analysis of empirical efforts. *Psychological Bulletin*, *85*, 1275–1301.

Achenbach, T.M., & Edelbrock, C.S. (1983). *Manual for the Revised Child Behavior Checklist and Profile*. Burlington, VT: University Associates in Psychiatry.

Achenbach, T.M., & Edelbrock, C. (1986). *Manual for the Teacher's Report Form and Teacher Version of the Child Behavior Profile*. Burlington, VT: University of Vermont Department of Psychiatry.

Aman, M.G., & Turbott, S.H. (1986). Incidental learning, distraction, and sustained attention in hyperactive and control subjects. *Journal of Abnormal Child Psychology*, *14*, 441–455.

American Psychiatric Association (1968). *Diagnostic and statistical manual of mental disorders* (2nd ed.). Washington, DC: Author.

American Psychiatric Association (1980). *Diagnostic and statistical manual of mental disorders* (3rd ed.). Washington, DC: Author.

American Psychiatric Association (1987). *Diagnostic and statistical manual of mental disorders* (3rd ed., rev.). Washington, DC: Author.

Atkins, M.S., Pelham, W.E., & Licht, M.H. (1985). A comparison of objective classroom measures and teacher ratings of attention deficit disorder. *Journal of Abnormal Child Psychology*, *13*, 155–167.

August, G.J., & Stewart, M.A. (1983). Familial subtypes of childhood hyperactivity. *Journal of Nervous & Mental Disease, 171*, 362–368.

August, G.J., Stewart, M.A., & Holmes, C.S. (1983). A four-year follow-up of hyperactive boys with and without conduct disorder. *British Journal of Psychiatry, 143*, 192–198.

Ayllon, T., & Rosenbaum, M.S. (1977). The behavioral treatment of disruption and hyperactivity in school settings. In B. B. Lahey & A. E. Kazdin (Eds.), *Advances in clinical child psychology* (Vol. 1). New York: Plenum.

Barkley, R.A. (1976). Predicting the response of hyperkinetic children to stimulant drugs: A review. *Journal of Abnormal Child Psychology, 4*, 327–348.

Barkley, R.A. (1981a). *Hyperactive children: A handbook for diagnosis and treatment*. New York: Guilford.

Barkley, R.A. (1981b). The use of psychopharmacology to study reciprocal influences in parent–child interaction. *Journal of Abnormal Child Psychology, 9*, 303–310.

Barkley, R.A. (1982). Guidelines for defining hyperactivity in children (attention deficit disorder with hyperactivity). In B.B. Lahey & A.E. Kazdin (Eds.), *Advances in clinical child psychology*. New York: Plenum.

Barkley, R.A. (in press). Do as we say, not as we do: The problem of stimulus control and rule-governed behavior in attention deficit disorder with hyperactivity. In J. Swanson & L. Bloomingdale (Eds.), *Attention deficit disorders IV: Emerging trends in the treatment of attention and behavior problems in children* (Monograph). *Journal of Child Psychology and Psychiatry*.

Barkley, R.A., & Cunningham, C. (1979). The effects of Ritalin on the mother–child interactions of hyperactive children. *Archives of General Psychiatry, 36*, 201–208.

Barkley, R.A., & Edelbrock, C. (in press). Assessing situational variation in children's problem behaviors: The Home and School Situations Questionnaires. In R. Prinz (Ed.), *Advances in behavioral assessment of children and families*. Greenwich, CT: JAI.

Berry, C.A., Shaywitz, S.E., & Shaywitz, B.A. (1985). Girls with attention deficit disorder: A silent minority? A report on behavioral and cognitive characteristics. *Pediatrics, 76*, 801–809.

Biederman, J., Gastfriend, D.R., & Jellinek, M.S. (1986). Desipramine in the treatment of children with attention deficit disorder. *Journal of Clinical Psychopharmacology, 6*, 359–363.

Biederman, J., Munir, K., & Knee, D. (1986). Attention deficit disorder with and without conduct and oppositional disorder: A controlled family study. *Journal of the American Academy of Child and Adolescent Psychiatry, 26*, 724–727.

Biederman, J., Munir, K., Knee, D., Habelow, W., Armentano, M., Autor, S., Hoge, S. K., & Waternaux, C. (1986). A family study of patients with attention deficit disorder and normal controls. *Journal of Psychiatric Research, 20*, 263–274.

Borden, K.A., Brown, R.T., Jenkins, P., & Clingerman, S.R. (1987). Achievement attributions and depressive symptoms in attention deficit disordered and normal children. *Journal of School Psychology, 25*, 399–404.

Bosco, J.J., & Robin, S.S. (1980). Hyperkinesis: Prevalence and treatment. In C.K. Whalen & B. Henker (Eds.), *Hyperactive children: The social ecology of identification and treatment*. New York: Academic.

Bradley, C. (1937). The behavior of children receiving benzedrine. *American Journal of Psychiatry, 94*, 577–585.

Brown, R.T., & Borden, K.A. (1986). Hyperactivity at adolescence: Some misconceptions and new directions. *Journal of Clinical Child Psychology, 15*, 194–209.

Brown, R.T., Borden, K.A., & Clingerman, S.R. (1985a). Adherence to methylphenidate therapy in a pediatric population: A preliminary investigation. *Psychopharmacology Bulletin, 21*, 28–35.

Brown, R. T., Borden, K. A., & Clingerman, S. R. (1985b). Pharmacotherapy in ADD adolescents with special attention to multimodality treatments. *Psychopharmacology Bulletin, 21*, 192–211.

Brown, R.T., Wynne, M.E., & Medenis, R. (1985). Methylphenidate and cognitive therapy: A comparison of treatment approaches with hyperactive boys. *Journal of Abnormal Child Psychology, 13*, 69–87.

Campbell, S. (1975). Mother–child interaction: A comparison of hyperactive, learning disabled, and normal boys. *Developmental Psychology, 45*, 51–57.

Campbell, S.B. (1985). Hyperactivity in preschoolers: Correlates and prognostic implications. *Clinical Psychology Review, 5*, 405–428.

Campbell, S.B., Breaux, A.M., Ewing, L.J., & Szumowski, E.K. (1986). Correlates and predictors of hyperactivity and aggression: A longitudinal study of parent-referred problem preschoolers. *Journal of Abnormal Child Psychology, 14*, 217–234.

Campbell, S.B., Breaux, A.M., Ewing, L.J., Szumowski, E.K., & Pierce, E.W. (1986). Parent-identified problem preschoolers: Mother–child interaction during play at intake and 1-year follow-up. *Journal of Abnormal Child Psychology, 14*, 425–440.

Campbell, S.B., Ewing, L.J., Breaux, A.M., & Szumowski, E.K. (1986). Parent-referred problem three-year-olds: Follow-up at school entry. *Journal of Child Psychology & Psychiatry, 27*, 473–488.

Campbell, S.B., Szumowski, E.K., Ewing, L.J., Gluck, D.S., & Breaux, A.M. (1982). A multidimensional assessment of parent-identified behavior problem toddlers. *Journal of Abnormal Child Psychology, 10*, 569–592.

Cantwell, D.P. (1985). Pharmacotherapy of ADD in adolescents: What do we know, where should we go, how should we do it? *Psychopharmacology Bulletin, 21*, 251–257.

Cantwell, D.P. (1986). Attention deficit disorder in adolescents. *Clinical Psychology Review, 6*, 237–247.

Cantwell, D.P., & Satterfield, J.H. (1978). The prevalence of academic underachievement in hyperactive children. *Journal of Pediatric Psychology, 3*, 168–171.

Carlson, C.L. (1986). Attention deficit disorder without hyperactivity: A review of preliminary experimental evidence. In B.B. Lahey & A.E. Kazdin (Eds.), *Advances in clinical child psychology* (Vol. 9). New York: Plenum.

Carlson, C.L., Lahey, B.B., Frame, C.L., Walker, J., & Hynd, G.W. (in press). Sociometric status of clinic-referred children with attention deficit disorders with and without hyperactivity. *Journal of Abnormal Child Psychology.*

Chambers, W.J., Puig-Antich, J., Hirsch, M., Paez, P., Ambrosini, P.J., Tabrizi, M.A., & Davies, M. (1985). The assessment of affective disorders in children and adolescents by semistructured interview. *Archives of General Psychiatry, 42*, 696–702.

Chelune, G.J., Ferguson, W., Koon, R., & Dickey, T.O. (1986). Frontal lobe disinhibition in attention deficit disorder. *Child Psychiatry & Human Development, 16*, 221–234.

Cohen, N.J., & Minde, K. (1983). The "hyperactive syndrome" in kindergarten children: Comparison of children with pervasive and situational symptoms. *Journal of Child Psychology & Psychiatry, 24*, 443–455.

Collins, B.E., Whalen, C.K., & Henker, B. (1980). Ecological and pharmacological influences on behaviors in the classroom: The hyperkinetic behavioral syndrome. In S. Salzinger, J. Antrobus, & J. Glick (Eds.), *The ecosystem of the "sick" child*. New York: Academic.

Comings, D.E., & Comings, B.G. (1984). Tourette's syndrome and attention deficit disorder with hyperactivity: Are they genetically related? *Journal of the American Academy of Child Psychiatry, 23*, 138–146.

Conners, C.K. (1969). A teacher rating scale for use in drug studies with children. *American Journal of Psychiatry, 126*, 152–156, 884–888.

Conners, C.K. (1973). Rating scales for use in drug studies with children. *Psychopharmacology Bulletin* (Special Issue—Pharmacology of Children), 35–42.

Conners, C.K. (1985). The computerized continuous performance test. *Psychopharmacology Bulletin, 21*, 891–892.

Conners, C.K., & Barkley, R.A. (1985). Rating scales and checklists for psychopharmacology. *Psychopharmacology Bulletin, 21*, 809–815.

Conners, C.K., & Kronsberg, S. (1985). Measuring activity level in children. *Psychopharmacology Bulletin, 21*, 893–897.

Conners, C.K., & Wells, K.C. (1985). ADD-H Adolescent Self-Report Scale. *Psychopharmacology Bulletin, 21*, 921–922.

Costello, E.J., Edelbrock, C.S., & Costello, A.J. (1985). Validity of the NIMH Diagnostic Interview Schedule for Children: A comparison between psychiatric and pediatric referrals. *Journal of Abnormal Child Psychology, 13*, 579–595.

Denckla, M.B., Bemporad, J.R., & MacKay, M.C. (1976). Tics following methylphenidate administration: A report of 20 cases. *Journal of the American Medical Association, 235*, 1349–1351.

Denson, R., Nanson, J.L., & McWatters, M.A. (1975). Hyperkinesis and maternal smoking. *Canadian Psychiatric Association Journal, 20*, 183–187.

Douglas, V.I. (1972). Stop, look and listen: The problem of sustained attention and impulse control in hyperactive and normal children. *Canadian Journal of Behavioral Science, 4*, 259–281.

Douglas, V.I. (1980). Treatment and training approaches to hyperactivity: Establishing internal or external control. In C.K. Whalen & B. Henker (Eds.), *Hyperactive children: The social ecology of identification and treatment*. New York: Academic.

Douglas, V.I. (1983). Attentional and cognitive problems. In M. Rutter (Ed.), *Developmental neuropsychiatry*. New York; Guilford.

Douglas, V.I., & Parry, P.A. (1983). Effects of reward on delayed reaction time task performance of hyperactive children. *Journal of Abnormal Child Psychology, 11*, 313–326.

Douglas, V.I., Parry, P.A., Marton, P., & Garson, C. (1976). Assessment of a cognitive training program for hyperactive children. *Journal of Abnormal Child Psychology, 4*, 389–410.

Draeger, S., Prior. M., & Sanson, A. (1986). Visual and auditory attention performance in hyperactive children: Competence or compliance. *Journal of Abnormal Child Psychology, 14*, 411–424.

Dubey, D. R., O'Leary, S.G., & Kaufman, K.F. (1983). Training parents of hyperactive children in child management: A comparative outcome study. *Journal of Abnormal Child Psychology, 11*, 229–246.

Dulcan, M.K. (1986). Comprehensive treatment of children and adolescents with attention deficit disorders: The state of the art. *Clinical Psychology Review*, *6*, 539–569.

Dulcan, M.K. (1988). Treatment of children and adolescents. In J.A. Talbott, R.E. Hales, & S.C. Yudofsky (Eds.), *The American Psychiatric Press textbook of psychiatry*. Washington, DC: American Psychiatric Press.

Dvoredsky, A.E., & Stewart, M.A. (1981). Hyperactivity followed by manic-depressive disorder: Two case reports. *Journal of Clinical Psychiatry*, *42*, 212–214.

Edelbrock, C. (1986). *Child Attention Problems Rating Scale*. Unpublished manuscript.

Edelbrock, C., Costello, A.J., & Kessler, M.D. (1984). Empirical corroboration of attention deficit disorder. *Journal of the American Academy of Child Psychiatry*, *23*, 285–290.

Edelbrock, C., & Rancurello, M.D. (1985). Childhood hyperactivity: An overview of rating scales and their applications. *Clinical Psychology Review*, *5*, 429–445.

Evans, R.W., Gualtieri, C.T., & Hicks, R.E. (1986). A neuropathic substrate for stimulant drug effects in hyperactive children. *Clinical Neuropharmacology*, *9*, 264–281.

Famularo, R., & Fenton, T. (1987). The effect of methylphenidate on school grades in children with attention deficit disorder without hyperactivity: A preliminary report. *Journal of Clinical Psychiatry*, *48*, 112–114.

Ferguson, H.B., & Rapoport, J.L. (1983). Nosological issues and biological validation. In M. Rutter (Ed.), *Developmental neuropsychiatry*. New York: Guilford.

Firestone, P. (1982). Factors associated with children's adherence to stimulant medication. *American Journal of Orthopsychiatry*, *52*, 447–457.

Firestone, P., Kelly, M.J., Goodman, T.J., & Davey, J. (1981). Differential effects of parent training and stimulant medication with hyperactives: A progress report. *Journal of the American Academy of Child Psychiatry*, *20*, 135–147.

Gadow, K.D., & Swanson, H.L. (1985). Assessing drug effects on academic performance. *Psychopharmacology Bulletin*, *21*, 877–886.

Galler, J.R., Ramsey, F., Solimano, G., & Lowell, W.E. (1983). The influence of early malnutrition on subsequent behavioral development: II. Classroom behavior. *Journal of the American Academy of Child Psychiatry*, *22*, 16–22.

Garfinkel, B.D., Wender, P.H., Sloman, L., & O'Neill, I. (1983). Tricyclic anti-depressant and methylphenidate treatment of attention deficit disorder in children. *Journal of the American Academy of Child Psychiatry*, *22*, 343–348.

Gastfriend, D.J., Biederman, J., & Jellinek, M. (1984). Desipramine in the treatment of adolescents with attention deficit disorder. *American Journal of Psychiatry*, *141*, 906–908.

Gayton, W.F., Bailey, C., Wagner, A., & Hardesty, V.A. (1986). Relationship between childhood hyperactivity and accident proneness. *Perceptual & Motor Skills*, *63*, 801–802.

Gittelman, R. (1985). Self-evaluation (teenager's) self-report. *Psychopharmacology Bulletin*, *21*, 925–926.

Gittelman, R., Abikoff, H., Pollack, E., Klein, D.F., Katz, S., & Mattes, J. (1980). A controlled trial of behavior modification and methylphenidate in hyperactive children. In C.K. Whalen & B. Henker (Eds.), *Hyperactive children: The social ecology of identification and treatment*. New York: Academic.

Gittelman, R., & Eskenazi, B. (1983). Lead and hyperactivity revisited: An investigation of nondisadvantaged children. *Archives of General Psychiatry*, *40*, 827–833.

Gittelman, R., & Klein, D. (1985). Hillside Behavior Rating Scale (behavior during testing). *Psychopharmacology Bulletin*, *21*, 898–899.

Gittelman, R., & Mannuzza, S. (1985). Diagnosing ADD-H in adolescents. *Psychopharmacology Bulletin*, *21*, 237–242.

Gittelman, R., Mannuzza, S., Shenker, R., & Bonagura, N. (1985). Hyperactive boys almost grown up. I: Psychiatric status. *Archives of General Psychiatry*, *42*, 937–947.

Glow, P.H., & Glow, R.A. (1979). Hyperkinetic impulse disorder: A developmental defect of motivation. *Genetic Psychology Monographs*, *100*, 159–231.

Goyette, C.H., Conners, C.K., & Ulrich, R.F. (1978). Normative data on revised Conners Parent and Teacher Rating Scales. *Journal of Abnormal Child Psychology*, *6*, 221–236.

Greenhill, L., Puig-Antich, J., Goetz, R., Hanlon, C., & Davies, M. (1983). Sleep architecture and REM sleep measures in prepubertal children with attention deficit disorder with hyperactivity. *Sleep*, *6*, 91–101.

Grob, C.S., & Coyle, J.T. (1986). Suspected adverse methylphenidate-imipramine interactions in children. *Developmental & Behavioral Pediatrics*, *7*, 265–267.

Gualtieri, C.T., Hicks, R.E., & Mayo, J.P. (1983). Hyperactivity and homeostasis. *Journal of the American Academy of Child Psychiatry*, *22*, 382–384.

Haenlein, M., & Caul, W.F. (1987). Attention deficit disorder with hyperactivity: A specific hypothesis of reward dysfunction. *Journal of the American Academy of Child Psychiatry*, *26*, 356–362.

Halperin, J.M., & Gittelman, R. (1982). Do hyperactive children and their siblings differ in IQ and academic achievement? *Psychiatry Research*, *6*, 253–258.

Halperin, J.M., Gittelman, R., Katz, S., & Struve, F.A. (1986). Relationship between stimulant effect, electroencephalogram, and clinical neurological findings in hyperactive children. *Journal of the American Academy of Child Psychiatry*, *25*, 820–825.

Hartsough, C.S., & Lambert, N.M. (1985). Medical factors in hyperactive and normal children: Prenatal, developmental, and health history findings. *American Journal of Orthopsychiatry*, *55*, 190–201.

Hechtman, L., & Weiss, G. (1986). Controlled prospective 15-year follow-up of hyperactives as adults: Non-medical drug and alcohol use and antisocial behavior. *Canadian Journal of Psychiatry*, *31*, 557–567.

Heffron, W.A., Martin, C.A., & Welsh, R.J. (1984). Attention deficit disorder in three pairs of monozygotic twins: A case report. *Journal of the American Academy of Child Psychiatry*, *23*, 299–301.

Henker, B., Astor-Dubin, L., & Varni, J.W. (1986). Psychostimulant medication and perceived intensity in hyperactive children. *Journal of Abnormal Child Psychology*, *14*, 105–114.

Henker, B., & Whalen, C.K. (1980). The changing faces of hyperactivity: Retrospect and prospect. In C.K. Whalen & B. Henker (Eds.), *Hyperactive children: The social ecology of identification and treatment*. New York: Academic.

Herjanic, B., & Reich, W. (1982). Development of a structured psychiatric interview for children: Agreement between child and parent on individual symptoms. *Journal of Abnormal Child Psychology*, *10*, 307–324.

Hinshaw, S.P. (1987). On the distinction between attentional deficits/hyperactivity and conduct problems/aggression in child psychopathlogy. *Psychological Bulletin*, *101*, 443–463.

Hinshaw, S.P., Henker, B., & Whalen, C.K. (1984a). Cognitive–behavioral and pharmacologic interventions for hyperactive boys: Comparative and combined effects. *Journal of Consulting & Clinical Psychology*, *52*, 739–749.

Hinshaw, S.P., Henker, B., & Whalen, C.K. (1984b). Self-control in hyperactive boys in anger-inducing situations: Effects of cognitive–behavioral training and methylphenidate. *Journal of Abnormal Child Psychology, 52,* 739–749.

Hinshaw, S.P., & McHale, J.P. (in press). Stimulant medication and the social interactions of hyperactive children: Effects and implications. In D. Gilbert & J. Conley (Eds.), *Personality, social skills and psychopathology: An individual differences approach.* New York: Plenum.

Horn, W.F., Chatoor, I., & Conners, C.J. (1983). Additive effects of dexedrine and self-control training. *Behavior Modification, 7,* 383–402.

Hunt, R.D., Minderaa, R.B., & Cohen, D.J. (1985). Clonidine benefits children with attention deficit disorder and hyperactivity: Report of a double-blind placebo-crossover therapeutic trial. *Journal of the American Academy of Child Psychiatry, 24,* 617–629.

Johnston, C., & Pelham, W.E. (1986). Teacher ratings predict peer ratings of aggression at 3-year follow-up in boys with attention deficit disorder with hyperactivity. *Journal of Consulting & Clinical Psychology, 54,* 571–572.

Kashani, J., Chapel, J.L., Ellis, J., & Shekim, W.O. (1979). Hyperactive girls. *Journal of Operational Psychiatry, 10,* 145–148.

Kauffman, R.E., Smith-Wright, D., Reese, C.A., Simpson, R., & Jones, F. (1981). Medication compliance in hyperactive children. *Pediatric Pharmacology, 1,* 231–237.

Kazdin, A.E., Esveldt-Dawson, K., French, N.H., & Unis, A.S. (1987). Problem-solving skills training and relationship therapy in the treatment of antisocial child behavior. *Journal of Consulting & Clinical Psychology, 55,* 76–85.

Kelly, P.C., Cohen, M.L., & Atkinson, A.W. (1986). Self-esteem of children treated medically for attention deficit disorder. *Developmental Medicine & Child Neurology, 28,* Supplement, 46.

Kendall, P.C., & Braswell, L. (1985). *Cognitive–behavioral therapy for impulsive children.* New York: Guilford.

Kirby, E.A., & Grimley, L.K. (1986). *Understanding and treating attention deficit disorder.* New York: Pergamon.

Koehler-Troy, C., Strober, M., & Malenbaum, R. (1986). Methylphenidate-induced mania in a prepubertal child. *Journal of Clinical Psychiatry, 47,* 566–567.

Lahey, B.B., McBurnett, K., Piacentini, J.C., Hartdagen, S., Walker, J., & Hynd, G.W. (1987). *Agreement of parent and teacher rating scales with comprehensive clinical assessments of attention deficit disorder with hyperactivity.* Unpublished manuscript.

Lahey, B.B., Pelham, W.E., Schaughency, E.A., Atkins, M.S., Murphy, H.A., Hynd, G.W., Russo, M., Hartdagen, S., & Lorys-Vernon, A. (1988). Dimensions and types of attention deficit disorder/hyperactivity in children: A factor cluster analytic approach. *Journal of the American Academy of Child and Adolescent Psychiatry, 27,* 330–335.

Lahey, B.B., Piacentini, J.C., McBurnett, K., Stone, P., Hartdagen, S., & Hynd, G. (in press). Psychopathology and antisocial behavior in the parents of children with conduct disorder and hyperactivity. *Journal of the American Academy of Child Psychiatry.*

Lahey, B.B., Schaughency, E.A., Hynd, G.W., Carlson, C.L., & Nieves, N. (1987). Attention deficit disorder with and without hyperactivity: Comparison of behavioral characteristics of clinic referred children. *Journal of the American Academy of Child and Adolescent Psychiatry, 26,* 718–723.

Lambert, N.M., & Sandoval, J. (1980). The prevalence of learning disabilities in a sample of children considered hyperactive. *Journal of Abnormal Child Psychology, 8,* 33–50.

Lambert, N.M., Sandoval, J., & Sassone, D. (1978). Prevalence of hyperactivity in elementary school children as a function of social system definers. *American Journal of Orthopsychiatry*, *48*, 446–463.

Landman, G.B., & McCrindle, B. (1986). Pediatric management of nonpervasively "hyperactive" children. *Clinical Pediatrics*, *25*, 600–604.

Loney, J. (1986). Predicting stimulant drug response among hyperactive children. *Psychiatric Annals*, *16*, 16–18.

Loney, J. (1987). Hyperactivity and aggression in the diagnosis of attention deficit disorder. In B.B. Lahey & A.E. Kazdin (Eds.), *Advances in clinical child psychology* (Vol. 10). New York: Plenum.

Loney, J., Kramer, J., & Milich, R. (1981). The hyperkinetic child grows up: Predictors of symptoms, delinquency, and achievement at follow-up. In J. Gadow & J. Loney (Eds.), *Psychosocial aspects of drug treatment for hyperactivity*. Boulder, CO: Westview.

Loney, J., & Milich, R. (1982). Hyperactivity, inattention, and aggression in clinical practice. In M. Wolraich & D.K. Routh (Eds.), *Advances in developmental and behavioral pediatrics* (Vol. 3). Greenwich, CT: JAI.

Loney, J., Weissenburger, F.E., Woolson, R.F., & Lichty, E.C. (1979). Comparing psychological and pharmacological treatments for hyperactive boys and their classmates. *Journal of Abnormal Child Psychology*, *7*, 133–143.

Lou, H.C., Henriksen, L., & Bruhn, P. (1984). Focal cerebral hypoperfusion in children with dysphasia and/or attention deficit disorder. *Archives of Neurology*, *41*, 825–829.

Lowe, T.L., Cohen, D.J., Detlor, J., Kremenetzer, M.W., & Shaywitz, B.A. (1982). Stimulant medications precipitate Tourette syndrome. *Journal of the American Medical Association*, *247*, 1168–1169.

Mannuzza, S., & Gittelman, R. (1984). The adolescent outcome of hyperactive girls. *Psychiatry Research*, *13*, 19–29.

Mash, E.J., & Dalby, J.T. (1979). Behavioral interventions in hyperactivity. In R.L. Trites (Ed.), *Hyperactivity in children: Etiology, measurement and treatment implications*. Baltimore: University Park Press.

Mash, E.J., & Johnston, C. (1983). Parental perceptions of child behavior problems, parenting self-esteem, and mothers' reported stress in younger and older hyperactive and normal children. *Journal of Consulting & Clinical Psychology*, *51*, 86–99.

Mattes, J.A. (1980). The role of frontal lobe dysfunction in childhood hyperkinesis. *Comprehensive Psychiatry*, *21*, 358–368.

McGee, R., Williams, S., & Silva, P.A. (1984). Behavioral and developmental characteristics of aggressive, hyperactive and aggressive–hyperactive boys. *Journal of the American Academy of Child Psychiatry*, *23*, 270–279.

McMahon, R.C. (1984). Hyperactivity as dysfunction of activity, arousal, or attention: A study of research relating to DSM-III's attention deficit disorder. *Journal of Clinical Psychology*, *40*, 1300–1308.

Meichenbaum, D., & Goodman, J. (1971). Training impulsive children to talk to themselves: A means of developing self-control. *Journal of Abnormal Psychology*, *77*, 115–126.

Meijer, A. (1984). Psychiatric problems of children with glucose-6-phosphate dehydrogenase (G6PD) deficiency. *International Journal of Psychiatry in Medicine*, *14*, 207–214.

Milich, R., & Landau, S. (1982). Socialization and peer relations in hyperactive children. *Advances in Learning & Behavioral Disabilities*, *1*, 283–339.

Milich, R., Loney, J., & Roberts, M.A. (1986). Playroom observations of activity level and sustained attention: Two year stability. *Journal of Consulting & Clinical Psychology*, *54*, 272–274.

Milich, R., & Pelham, W.E. (1986). Differentiating valid subgroups of hyperactive and aggressive children. Presented in W.E. Pelham (Chair), *Subgrouping research in externalizing disorders of childhood: Toward an integration*. Symposium presented at the Annual Meeting of the American Psychological Association, Washington, DC.

Milich, R., Roberts, M.A., Loney, J., & Caputo, J. (1980). Differentiating practice effects and statistical regression on the Conners Hyperkinesis Index. *Journal of Abnormal Child Psychology*, *8*, 549–552.

Milich, R., Wolraich, M., & Lindgren, S. (1986). Sugar and hyperactivity: A critical review of empirical findings. *Clinical Psychology Review*, *6*, 493–513.

Mintz, L.I., & Collins, B.E. (1985). Qualitative influences on the perception of movement: An experimental study. *Journal of Abnormal Child Psychology*, *13*, 143–153.

O'Dougherty, M., Nuechterlein, K.H., & Drew, B. (1984). Hyperactive and hypoxic children: Signal detection, sustained attention, and behavior. *Journal of Abnormal Psychology*, *93*, 178–191.

Offord, D.R., Sullivan, K., Allen, N., & Abrams, N. (1979). Delinquency and hyperactivity. *Journal of Nervous & Mental Disease*, *167*, 734–741.

Orvaschel, H. (1985). Psychiatric interviews suitable for use in research with children and adolescents. *Psychopharmacology Bulletin*, *21*, 737–745.

Paternite, C.E., & Loney, J. (1980). Childhood hyperkinesis: Relationships between symptomatology and home environment. In C.K. Whalen & B. Henker (Eds.), *Hyperactive children*. New York: Academic.

Pauls, D.L., Hurst, C.R., Kruger, S.D., Leckman, J.F., Kidd, K.K., & Cohen, D.J. (1986). Gilles de la Tourette's syndrome and attention deficit disorder with hyperactivity: Evidence against a genetic relationship. *Archives of General Psychiatry*, *43*, 1177–1179.

Pelham, W.E. (1982). *Laboratory measures of attention in the diagnosis of hyperactivity/ attention deficit disorder*. Paper presented at the annual meeting of the American Psychological Association, Washington, DC.

Pelham, W.E. (1983). The effects of psychostimulants on academic achievement in hyperactive and learning-disabled children. *Thalamus*, *3*, 1–47.

Pelham, W.E. (1985). The effects of stimulant drugs on learning and achievement in hyperactive and learning disabled children. In J. K. Torgesen & B. Wong (Eds.), *Psychological and educational perspectives on learning disabilities*. New York: Academic.

Pelham, W.E., & Bender, M.E. (1982). Peer relationships in hyperactive children: Description and treatment. *Advances in Learning & Behavioral Disabilities*, *1*, 365–436.

Pelham, W.E., Bender, M.E., Caddell, J., Booth, S., & Moorer, S.H. (1985). Methylphenidate and children with attention deficit disorder: Dose effects on classroom academic and social behavior. *Archives of General Psychiatry*, *42*, 948–952.

Pelham, W.E., Milich, R., & Murphy, D.A. (1986). *Normative data on the IOWA Conners Teacher Rating Scale*. Unpublished manuscript.

Pelham, W.E., Milich, R., & Walker, J.L. (1986). Effects of continuous and partial reinforcement and methylphenidate on learning in children with attention deficit disorder. *Journal of Abnormal Psychology*, *95*, 319–325.

Pelham, W.E., & Murphy, H.A. (1986). Attention deficit and conduct disorders. In M. Herson (Ed.), *Pharmacological and behavioral treatment: An integrative approach.* New York: Wiley.

Pelham, W.E., Schnedler, R.W., Bologna, N.C., & Contreras, J.A. (1980). Behavioral and stimulant treatment of hyperactive children: A therapy study with methylphenidate probes in a within-subject design. *Journal of Applied Behavioral Analysis, 13,* 221–236.

Pelham, W.E., Sturges, J., Hoza, J., Schmidt, C., Bijlsma, J.J., Milich, R., & Moorer, S. (1987). The effects of sustained release 20 and 10 mg Ritalin b.i.d. on cognitive and social behavior in children with attention deficit disorder. *Pediatrics, 80,* 491–501.

Pliszka, S.R. (1987). Tricyclic antidepressants in the treatment of children with attention deficit disorder. *Journal of the American Academy of Child and Adolescent Psychiatry, 26,* 127–132.

Porrino, L.J., Rapoport, J.L., Behar, D., Sceery, W., Ismond, D.R., & Bunney, W.E. (1983). A naturalistic assessment of the motor activity of hyperactive boys: I. A comparison with normal controls. *Archives of General Psychiatry, 40,* 681–687.

Rachelefsky, G.S., Wo, J., Adelson, J., Mickey, M.R., Spector, S.L., Katz, R.M., Siegel, S.C., & Rohr, A.S. (1986). Behavior abnormalities and poor school performance due to oral theophylline use. *Pediatrics, 78,* 1133–1138.

Rancurello, M.D. (1985). Clinical applications of antidepressant drugs in childhood behavioral and emotional disorders. *Psychiatric Annuals, 15,* 88–100.

Rapoport, J.L. (1983). The use of drugs: Trends in research. In M. Rutter (Ed.), *Developmental neuropsychiatry.* New York: Guilford.

Rapoport, J., Buchsbaum, M., Weingartner, H., Zahn, T., Ludlow, C., Bartko, J., & Mikkelsen, E.J. (1980). Dextroamphetamine: Cognitive and behavioral effects in normal and hyperactive boys and normal adult males. *Archives of General Psychiatry, 37,* 933–943.

Rapoport, J., Buchsbaum, M., Zahn, T., Weingartner, H., Ludlow, L., & Mikkelsen, E. (1978). Dextroamphetamine: Behavioral and cognitive effects in normal prepubertal boys. *Science, 199,* 560–563.

Rapoport, J.L., Donnelly, M., Zametkin, A., & Carrougher, J. (1986). "Situational hyperactivity" in a U.S. clinical setting. *Journal of Child Psychology & Psychiatry, 27,* 639–646.

Rapoport, J.L., Quinn, P.O., Bradbard, G., Riddle, K.D., & Brooks, E. (1974). Imipramine and methylphenidate treatments of hyperactive boys: A double-blind comparison. *Archives of General Psychiatry, 30,* 789–793.

Rapport, M.D., Tucker, S.B., DuPaul, G.J., Merlo, M., & Stoner, G. (1986). Hyperactivity and frustration: The influence of control over and size of rewards in delaying gratification. *Journal of Abnormal Child Psychology, 14,* 191–204.

Realmuto, G.M., Garfinkel, B.D., Tuchman, M., Tsai, M.Y., Chang, P., Fisch, R.O., & Shapiro, S. (1986). Psychiatric diagnosis and behavioral characteristics of phenylketonuric children. *Journal of Nervous & Mental Disease, 174,* 536–540.

Reatig, N. (1985). Bibliography on rating and assessment instruments for attention deficit disorder. *Psychopharmacology Bulletin, 21,* 929–930.

Roberts, M.A., Ray, R.S., & Roberts, R.J. (1984). A playroom observation procedure for assessing hyperactive boys. *Journal of Pediatric Psychology, 9,* 177–192.

Rosenthal, R.H., & Allen, T.W. (1978). An examination of attention, arousal, and learning dysfunctions of hyperkinetic children. *Psychological Bulletin, 85,* 689–715.

Ross, D.M., & Ross, S.A. (1982). *Hyperactivity: Current issues, research, and theory* (2nd ed.). New York: Wiley-Interscience.

Routh, D.K. (1978). Developmental and social aspects of hyperactivity. In C. K. Whalen & B. Henker (Eds.), *Hyperactive children: The social ecology of identification and treatment.* New York: Academic.

Rutter, M. (1977). Brain damage syndromes in childhood: Concepts and findings. *Journal of Child Psychology & Psychiatry, 18,* 1–21.

Rutter, M. (1982). Syndromes attributed to "minimal brain dysfunction" in childhood. *American Journal of Psychiatry, 139,* 21–33.

Rutter, M. (1983). Behavioral studies: Questions and findings on the concept of a distinctive syndrome. In M. Rutter (Ed.), *Developmental neuropsychiatry.* New York: Guilford.

Sandoval, J., Lambert, N.M., & Sassone, D. (1980). The identification and labeling of hyperactivity in children: An interactive model. In C.K. Whalen & B. Henker (Eds.), *Hyperactive children.* New York: Academic.

Satterfield, J.H., Satterfield, B.T., & Cantwell, D.P. (1981). Three-year multimodality treatment study of 100 hyperactive boys. *Journal of Pediatrics, 98,* 650–655.

Satterfield, J.H., Satterfield, B.T., & Schell, A.M. (1987). Therapeutic interventions to prevent delinquency in hyperactive boys. *Journal of the American Academy of Child Psychiatry, 26,* 56–64.

Schachar, R., Sandberg, S., & Rutter, M. (1986). Agreement between teachers' ratings and observations of hyperactivity, inattentiveness, and defiance. *Journal of Abnormal Child Psychology, 14,* 331–345.

Schaughency, E.A., Lahey, B.B., Hynd, G.W., Stone, P.A., & Piacentini, J.C. (1987). *Neuropsychological test performance and the attention deficit disorders.* Unpublished manuscript.

Shaffer, D., O'Connor, P.A., Shafer, S.Q., & Prupis, S. (1983). Neurological "soft signs": Their origins and significance for behavior. In M. Rutter (Ed.), *Developmental neuro-psychiatry.* New York: Guilford.

Shapiro, B.A., & Garfinkel, B.D. (1986). The occurrence of behavior disorders in children: The interdependence of attention deficit disorder and conduct disorder. *Journal of the American Academy of Child Psychiatry, 25,* 809–819.

Shaywitz, S.E., Cohen, D.J., & Shaywitz, B.A. (1980). Behavior and learning difficulties in children of normal intelligence born to alcoholic mothers. *Journal of Pediatrics, 96,* 978–982.

Shaywitz, S.E., Schnell, C., Shaywitz, B.A., & Towle, V.R. (1986). Yale Children's Inventory (YCI): An instrument to assess children with attentional deficits and learning disabilities: I. Scale development and psychometric properties. *Journal of Abnormal Child Psychology, 14,* 347–364.

Shaywitz, S.E., Shaywitz, B.A., Cohen, D.J., & Young, J.G. (1983). Monoaminergic mechanisms in hyperactivity. In M. Rutter (Ed.), *Developmental neuropsychiatry.* New York: Guilford.

Shekim, W.O., Cantwell, D.P., Kashani, J., Beck, N., Martin, J., & Rosenberg, J. (1986). Dimensional and categorical approaches to the diagnosis of attention deficit disorder in children. *Journal of the American Academy of Child Psychiatry, 25,* 653–658.

Sprague, R.L. (1983). Behavior modification and educational techniques. In M. Rutter (Ed.), *Developmental neuropsychiatry.* New York: Guilford.

Sroufe, L.A. (1975). Drug treatment of children with behavior problems. In F. Horowitz (Ed.), *Review of child development research* (Vol. 4). Chicago: University of Chicago Press.

Steinhausen, H., & Spohr, H. (1986). Fetal alcohol syndrome. In B.B. Lahey & A.E. Kazdin (Eds.), *Advances in clinical child psychology* (Vol. 9). New York: Plenum.

Stewart, M.A., Thach, B.E., & Freidin, M. (1970). Accidental poisoning and the hyperactive child syndrome. *Diseases of the Nervous System, 31*, 403–407.

Still, G.F. (1902). Some abnormal psychical conditions in children. *Lancet, 1*, 1077–1082.

Streissguth, A.P., Martin, D.C., Barr, H.M., Sandman, B.M., Kirchner, G.L., & Darby, B.L. (1984). Intrauterine alcohol and nicotine exposure: Attention and reaction time in 4-year-old children. *Developmental Psychology, 20*, 533–541.

Swanson, J.M. (1985). Measures of cognitive functioning appropriate for use in pediatric psychopharmacological research studies. *Psychopharmacology Bulletin, 21*, 887–890.

Taylor, E. (1983). Drug response and diagnostic validation. In M. Rutter (Ed.), *Developmental neuropsychiatry*. New York: Guilford.

Taylor, E., Everitt, B., Thorley, G., Schachar, R., Rutter, M., & Wieselberg (1986). Conduct disorder and hyperactivity: II. A cluster analytic aproach to the identification of a behavioural syndrome. *British Journal of Psychiatry, 149*, 768–777.

Taylor, E., Schachar, R., Thorley, G., & Wieselberg (1986). Conduct disorder and hyperactivity: I. Separation of hyperactivity and antisocial conduct in British child psychiatric patients. *British Journal of Psychiatry, 149*, 760–767.

Taylor, E., Schachar, R., Thorley, G., Wieselberg, H.M., Everitt, B., & Rutter, M. (1987). Which boys respond to stimulant medication? A controlled trial of methylphenidate in boys with disruptive behavior. *Psychological Medicine, 17*, 121–143.

Thorley, G. (1984a). Hyperkinetic syndrome of childhood: Clinical characteristics. *British Journal of Psychiatry, 144*, 16–24.

Thorley, G. (1984b). Review of follow-up and follow-back studies of childhood hyperactivity. *Psychological Bulletin, 96*, 116–132.

Thurston, L.P. (1981). Comparison of the effects of parent training and of Ritalin in treating hyperactive children. In M. Gittelman (Ed.), *Strategic interventions for hyperactive children*. New York: M.E. Sharpe.

Ullmann, R.K., & Sleator, E.K. (1986). Responders, nonresponders and placebo responders among children with attention deficit disorder. *Clinical Pediatrics, 25*, 594–599.

Ullmann, R.K., Sleator, E.K., & Sprague, R.L. (1984). A new rating scale for diagnosis and monitoring of ADD children. *Psychopharmacology Bulletin, 20*, 160–164.

Ullmann, R.K., Sleator, E.K., & Sprague, R.L. (1985a). A change of mind: The Conners Abbreviated Rating Scales reconsidered. *Journal of Abnormal Child Psychology, 13*, 553–565.

Ullmann, R.K., Sleator, E.K., & Sprague, R.L. (1985b). Introduction to the use of ACTeRS. *Psychopharmacology Bulletin, 21*, 915–920.

Varley, C.K. (1983). Effects of methylphenidate in adolescents with attention deficit disorder. *Journal of the American Academy of Child Psychiatry, 22*, 349–350.

Varley, C.K. (1985). A review of studies of drug treatment efficacy for attention deficit disorder with hyperactivity in adolescents. *Psychopharmacology Bulletin, 21*, 216–221.

Walker, J.L., Lahey, B.B., Hynd, G.W., & Frame, C.L. (in press). Comparison of specific patterns of antisocial behavior in children with conduct disorder with or without coexisting hyperactivity. *Journal of Consulting & Clinical Psychology*.

Wallander, J.L., & Hubert, N.C. (1985). Long-term prognosis for children with attention deficit disorder with hyperactivity (ADD/H). In B.B. Lahey & A.E. Kazdin (Eds.), *Advances in clinical child psychology* (Vol. 8). New York: Plenum.

Weingartner, H., Ebert, M.H., Mikkelsen, E.J., Rapoport, J.L., Buchsbaum, M.S., Bunney, W.E., & Caine, E.D. (1980). Cognitive processes in normal and hyperactive children and their response to amphetamine treatment. *Journal of Abnormal Psychology*, *89*, 25–37.

Weiss, G. (1985a). Follow-up studies on outcome of hyperactive children. *Psychopharmacology Bulletin*, *21*, 169–177.

Weiss, G. (1985b). Hyperactivity: Overview and new directions. *Psychiatric Clinics of North America*, *8*, 737–753.

Weiss, G., Hechtman, L., Milroy, T., & Perlman, T. (1985). Psychiatric status of hyperactives as adults: A controlled prospective 15-year follow-up of 63 hyperactive children. *Journal of the American Academy of Child Psychiatry*, *24*, 211–220.

Weiss, G., Hechtman, L., Perlman, T., Hopkins, J., & Werner, A. (1979). Hyperactives as young adults: A controlled prospective ten-year follow-up of 75 children. *Archives of General Psychiatry*, *36*, 675–681.

Weiss, G., Minde, K., Werry, J.S., Douglas, V.I., & Nemeth, E. (1971). Studies on the hyperactive child, VIII: Five-year follow-up. *Archives of General Psychiatry*, *24*, 409–414.

Wender, E.H. (1986). The food additive-free diet in the treatment of behavior disorders: A review. *Journal of Developmental and Behavioral Pediatrics*, *7*, 35–42.

Wender, P.H. (1971). *Minimal brain dysfunction in children*. New York: Wiley-Interscience.

Werry, J.S., & Sprague, R.L. (1974). Methylphenidate in children: Effect of dosage. *Australian & New Zealand Journal of Psychiatry*, *8*, 9–19.

Whalen, C.K., & Henker, B. (1980). The social ecology of psychostimulant treatment: A model for conceptual and empirical analysis. In C.K. Whalen & B. Henker (Eds.), *Hyperactive children: The social ecology of identification and treatment*. New York: Academic.

Whalen, C.K., & Henker, B. (1985). The social worlds of hyperactive (ADDH) children. *Clinical Psychology Review*, *5*, 447–478.

Whalen, C.K., Henker, B., Finck, D., & Dotemoto, S. (1979). A social ecology of hyperactive boys: Medication effects in structured classroom environments. *Journal of Applied Behavioral Analysis*, *12*, 65–81.

Whalen, C.K., Henker, B., Swanson, J.M., Granger, D., Kliewer, W., & Spencer, J. (1987). Natural social behaviors in hyperactive children: Dose effects of methylphenidate. *Journal of Consulting & Clinical Psychology*, *55*, 187–193.

Winsberg, B., Maitinsky, S., Kupietz, S., & Richardson, E. (1986). *Effects of methylphenidate on academic achievement in hyperactive reading disabled children with attention deficit disorder*. Presented at the annual meeting of American Academy of Child and Adolescent Psychiatry, Los Angeles.

Wolf, S.M., & Forsythe, A. (1978). Behavior disturbance, phenobarbital, and febrile seizures. *Pediatrics*, *61*, 728–731.

Wolraich, M., Drummond, T., Salomon, M.K., O'Brien, M.L., & Sivage, C. (1978). Effects of methylphenidate alone and in combination with behavior modification procedures on the behavior and academic performance of hyperactive children. *Journal of Abnormal Child Psychology*, *6*, 149–161.

World Health Organization (1987). *International classification of diseases* (10th ed.), 1986 Draft of Chapter V: Mental, behavioral and developmental disorders. Geneva: Author.

Yellin, A.M., Kendall, P.C., & Greenberg, L.M. (1981). Cognitive–behavioral therapy and methylphenidate with hyperactive children: Preliminary comparisons. *Research Communications in Psychology, Psychiatry & Behavior*, *6*, 213–227.

Young, J.G., Leven, L.I., Knott, P.J., Leckman, J.F., & Cohen, D.J. (1985). Tourette's syndrome and tic disorders. In J.M. Wiener (Ed.), *Diagnosis and psychopharmacology of childhood and adolescent disorders*. New York: Wiley.

Zahn, T.P., Rapoport, J.L., & Thompson, C.L. (1980). Autonomic and behavioral effects of dextroamphetamine and placebo in normal and hyperactive prepubertal boys. *Journal of Abnormal Child Psychology*, *8*, 145–160.

Zametkin A.J. (1986). *Brain metabolism in hyperactive parents of hyperactive children*. Paper presented at the annual meeting of the American Academy of Child and Adolescent Psychiatry, Los Angeles.

Zametkin, A.J., & Rapoport, J.L. (1986). The pathophysiology of attention deficit disorder with hyperactivity: A review. In B.B. Lahey & A.E. Kazdin (Eds.), *Advances in clinical child psychology* (Vol. 9). New York: Plenum.

Zentall, S.S., & Zentall, T.R. (1986). Hyperactivity ratings: Statistical regression provides an insufficient explanation of practice effects. *Journal of Pediatric Psychology*, *11*, 393–396.

CHAPTER 7

Conduct and Oppositional Disorders

ALAN E. KAZDIN

Conduct and oppositional disorders encompass a range of disruptive, annoying, and occasionally even dangerous behaviors among children and adolescents. The behaviors are quite clear to those in contact with such children and of course to mental health practitioners. It is useful at the outset to distinguish in a preliminary way conduct and oppositional disorders. *Conduct disorder* has been recognized for some time as a specific type of dysfunction that includes a broad range of antisocial behaviors such as aggressive acts, theft, vandalism, fire setting, lying, truancy, and running away. Although these behaviors are diverse, their common characteristic is that they tend to violate major social rules and expectations. Many of the behaviors often reflect actions against the environment, including both persons and property.

Oppositional disorder reflects a category that has only been delineated relatively recently in psychiatric diagnosis (American Psychiatric Association, 1980). Generally, the behaviors are much less severe than those associated with conduct disorder. An oppositional child is stubborn, defies authority, and often has tantrums. The delineation of oppositional disorder is more controversial and tenuous because it is not clear that the dysfunction is different from the type of behavior that many nonreferred ("normal") children evince or has long-term implications for psychiatric dysfunction or adjustment.

It is useful to view oppositional disorder and conduct disorder as on a continuum. Oppositional disorder includes obnoxious and disruptive behavior but no pattern of clearly dangerous acts or major rule violation. More severe behaviors may be sufficient to be considered conduct disorder. There is another reason for viewing these disorders together. Some evidence suggests that noncompliance and oppositional behaviors are initial behaviors that occur in children who are likely to develop conduct disorder and to engage in more serious antisocial behavior (cf. Loeber & Schmaling, 1985a; Patterson, 1986). Thus oppositional disorder may be a precursor of more severe problems of conduct.

Completion of this chapter was facilitated by a Research Scientist Development Award (MH00353) and a grant (MH35408) from the National Institute of Mental Health.

For the present chapter, the primary emphasis is on conduct disorder. The reason is based on the extensive research on the diagnosis, assessment, and prognosis of conduct disorder. There are major questions regarding conduct disorder but these questions do not overshadow the agreement that there is a constellation of behaviors that reflect significant problems of conduct. Oppositional disorder has not been well studied and basic questions regarding the constellation are not resolved.

DEFINITION

The term *conduct disorder* is used to refer to instances when the children or adolescents evince a *pattern of antisocial behavior*, when there is *significant impairment* in everyday functioning at home or school, or when the behaviors are *regarded as unmanageable by significant others*. Thus the term *conduct disorder* is reserved here for antisocial behavior that is clinically significant and clearly beyond the realm of normal functioning.[1] Clinically severe antisocial behavior is likely to bring the youth into contact with various social agencies. Mental health services (clinics, hospitals) and the criminal justice system (police, courts) are the major sources of contact for youths whose behaviors are identified as severe. Within the educational system, special services, teachers, and classes are often provided to manage such children on a daily basis.

Many symptoms of conduct and oppositional disorders emerge in some form over the course of normal development. Fighting, lying, stealing, destruction of property, and noncompliance are relatively high at different points in childhood (Achenbach & Edelbrock, 1981; MacFarlane, Allen, & Honzik, 1954). For the most part, these behaviors diminish over time, do not interfere with everyday functioning, and do not predict untoward consequences in adulthood. There are several features of conduct disorder that make the behaviors clearly discrepant from what is seen in everyday life.

First, the behaviors such as fighting, temper tantrums, stealing, and others are relatively *frequent*. In some cases, the behaviors may be of a low frequency (e.g., fire setting), in which case *intensity* or *severity*, rather than frequency, is the central characteristic. Second, *repetitiveness* and *chronicity* of the behaviors are critical features. The behaviors are not likely to be isolated events or to occur within a brief period where some other influences or stressors (e.g., change in residence, divorce) are operative. Third, the *breadth of the behaviors* is central as well. Rather than an individual *symptom* or target behavior, there are usually several behaviors that occur together and form a *syndrome* or constellation of symptoms. Conduct disorder, as a syndrome, includes several core features such as fighting, engaging in temper tantrums, theft, truancy, destroying property, defying or threatening others, and running away, among others (see Quay, 1986a). Obviously, any individual

---

[1] The term *conduct disorder* here is used generically to delineate clinically severe levels of antisocial behavior and dysfunction. In the discussion of a specific psychiatric diagnosis, *Conduct Disorder* also refers to a constellation of behaviors. The uppercase letters will be used when the specific diagnostic category is delineated.

child is not likely to show all of the symptoms. The notion that they are all part of a syndrome merely indicates that they are likely to come in packages.

In the United States, the diagnosis of syndromes and disorders was advanced considerably with the appearance of the third edition of the *Diagnostic and Statistical Manual of Mental Disorders* (DSM-III) (American Psychiatric Association, 1980). The major diagnostic category within DSM-III for coding antisocial behavior in children and adolescents is Conduct Disorder. The essential feature is a "repetitive and persistent pattern of conduct in which either the basic rights of others or major age-appropriate societal norms or rules are violated" (APA, 1980, p. 45). In order for the diagnosis to be made, one or more problematic behaviors (e.g., fighting, stealing, running away) must be evident and have a duration of at least 6 months.

In the 1980 version of the DSM, four subtypes of the diagnostic category Conduct Disorder were delineated based on the type of antisocial behavior (aggressive or nonaggressive) and the presence or absence of social attachments (socialized or undersocialized). Children who meet the *aggressive* type violate the rights of others by physical violence (e.g., fighting, mugging, theft involving confrontation of the victim). Children who meet the *nonaggressive* type are characterized by the absence of physical violence as evident in such acts as running away, truancy, and persistent lying or stealing. *Undersocialized* types are characterized by a failure to establish affection, empathy, and relationships with others. *Socialized* types show evidence of attachment and relationships with others. In the use of this system, the most frequently diagnosed subtype has been undersocialized–aggressive type.

In the 1980 version of the DSM, the diagnostic category of oppositional disorder was delineated with the essential feature being "a pattern of disobedient, negativistic, and provocative opposition to authority figures" (APA, 1980, p. 63). The symptoms included violations of minor rules, temper tantrums, argumentativeness, provocative behavior, and stubbornness. The disorder clearly is different from Conduct Disorder. Oppositional disorder includes obviously bothersome behaviors but no major rule violation or dangerous acts. By the rules for invoking diagnostic criteria, children who meet criteria for oppositional disorder would not also meet the criteria for Conduct Disorder. Children who meet criteria for Conduct Disorder would be likely to meet the criteria for oppositional disorder but the latter diagnosis would not be given as well.

HISTORICAL BACKGROUND

Conduct Disorder has long been recognized in part because of the impact of constituent behaviors beyond the formal development of clinical child psychology and child psychiatry. Antisocial behaviors that comprise Conduct Disorder include aggressive behavior, theft, and vandalism and have been of interest as part of legal codes for children and adults. Within clinical work, the dysfunction has been identified readily as well. Conduct Disorder reflects externalizing behaviors that act against the environment and are more readily apparent diagnostically than internalizing disorders that reflect reactions directed inward (e.g., social withdrawal, depression).

Early studies of clinical disorders among children identified antisocial behaviors quite clearly. For example, one of the earliest studies that utilized statistical techniques to examine childhood disorders was completed by Hewett and Jenkins (1946). These investigators analyzed the case records of children ($N = 500$) referred to a child guidance clinic. They measured several different symptoms from the records to identify the joint occurrence of specific problems. On the basis of the pattern of intercorrelations, they identified three major behavioral syndromes: unsocialized aggressive, socialized delinquent, and overinhibited. The first two of these reflect antisocial behavior and have clear parallels in contemporary views of Conduct Disorder and its subtypes. In subsequent studies, the constellation of behaviors comprising Conduct Disorder, particularly in relation to an aggressive type, has been repeatedly demonstrated (see Quay, 1986b). In contrast, oppositional disorder has not been studied or identified in this fashion.

The significance of antisocial behavior has been made salient by longitudinal studies. In the 1950s, Glueck and Glueck (1950, 1959) examined characteristics of delinquent youths and attempted to identify child, parent, and family predictors of delinquency and recidivism. In the 1960s Robins (1966) completed the now-classic study that followed clinically referred youths 30 years later. The study demonstrated the long-term consequences of antisocial behavior as reflected in psychiatric symptoms, criminal behaviors, and physical and social adjustment problems. These findings were replicated with separate samples and with follow-up evaluations of different durations (see Robins, 1978, 1981). These studies made salient the severity and prognosis of antisocial behavior over the developmental spectrum.

CLINICAL PICTURE

Although the definition and diagnostic criteria convey the characteristics of conduct disorder, the clinical picture itself is often very complex. The complexity derives from the range of dysfunctions that the child may evince and family and parent factors that may be involved as well. Even though the behavioral problems that constitute conduct disorder are familiar, it is useful to illustrate the level of severity and the surrounding circumstances that characterize clinically severe levels of impairment.

CASE STUDY

Mitch is an 8-year-old boy who lives at home with his mother and one older and one younger brother. At home he constantly fought with his brothers. The intensity of the fighting exceeded the usual boundaries of sibling interactions. On one occasion, Mitch stabbed his younger brother in the chest and emergency treatment and a hospital stay were required. On another occasion, immediately preceding hospitalization, Mitch attacked a child in his class with a baseball bat. He hit the child twice, causing a broken arm. Apart from extremely aggressive acts at home and at school, he constantly defied authority and destroyed other children's property whenever he was angry. He argued frequently with his mother and would leave home for several hours at a time after an argument. On three occasions, he remained out overnight after arguments with his mother and could not be found by police. He stayed with friends on two occasions and stayed with his father (outside of the home) on the other occasion. Apart from his aggression and running away, he occasionally stole things from others. He stole purses from his teachers at school on two occasions within the year preceding his referral at the clinic. On each occasion, his mother found the purse in Mitch's closet and phoned the school to arrange for its return. Mitch denied that he had taken the purses.

Mitch was brought to the clinic because his mother felt she could no longer manage him and because his behavior seemed too dangerous for her and her other children. Also, he had recently been suspended from school for three days because of his last fight. Consequently he was at home more than usual and engaged in more frequent and extreme aggressive behavior with his mother. Mitch's mother brought him to a clinic to seek treatment. The psychiatric evaluation at the clinic revealed that Mitch had become significantly more aggressive at home and at school in the past few months. His fighting, threats to others, and destruction of property all had seemed to worsen. Both the mother and Mitch's siblings had been physically injured, and there was no consistent way to keep Mitch in the home at night. Based on the description of Mitch's recent behavior and in consultation with the mother, it was decided that Mitch should be hospitalized for a brief period to begin treatment and to help develop a program to integrate him back into school.

Several features of Mitch's home life and family are worth noting. Mitch lived with his mother. His mother and father were divorced three years earlier, when Mitch was five years old. Prior to the divorce, there had been considerable spouse and child abuse by the father. The father was a diagnosed alcoholic. When he came home inebriated, he often beat his wife and children. On more than one occasion, he awakened one of the boys to beat him for not doing a chore like taking out the trash or washing the dishes. The mother and children moved to a women's shelter. This was followed by legal separation and divorce. The mother and boys eventually moved back into their home. The father remained nearby but did not seek further contact with the children after the divorce.

Mitch's mother worked part-time at a dry cleaner and also was on public assistance. She was at home in the afternoon and evenings when her children returned from school. Occasionally, her mother would help babysit for the children when she had to go to work and the children were home from school. Mitch's mother has a history of major depressive disorder, although she has been out of treatment for 2 years with no further episodes.

At school, Mitch was in the third grade. His academic performance and grades were consistently low. He had been placed in a special class for emotionally disturbed children because of his disruptive annd aggressive behavior. Also, his high level of activity led to his being labeled hyperactive. His level of intelligence, when tested, fell within the low normal range (Full Scale IQ score of 92 on the Wechsler Intelligence Scale for Children—Revised [WISC-R]). However, his work led to barely C grades in academic subjects because he missed so much class time and had such difficulty completing his work.

General Comments

The case illustrates briefly the type and severity of problems that conduct disorder represents and underscores a few important points. First, the child engaged in rather severe behaviors. The problems were not merely failing to comply with his mother's requests, getting into arguments with siblings, and not completing school work. Each of these behaviors was evident but did not serve as the primary basis for seeking professional attention. Second, the mother felt that the child was out of control and no longer manageable. The school could not manage the child, either, and had suspended Mitch for fighting. Third, the mother's situation was difficult to manage. She was a single parent, on welfare, with two other children to maintain, and had a history of and was at risk for continued depression.

ASSOCIATED FEATURES

The central features of conduct and oppositional disorders are antisocial, aggressive, and defiant behaviors. There are several correlates or associated features as well. Among alternative symptoms that have been found among antisocial children, those related to *hyperactivity* have been the most frequently identified. These symptoms include excessive motor activity, restlessness, impulsiveness, and inattentiveness. In fact, the co-occurrence of hyperactivity and conduct disorder has made their diagnostic delineation and assessment a topic of considerable research.[2] Several other behaviors have been identified as problematic among antisocial youths, such as boisterousness, showing off, and blaming others (Quay, 1986a). Many of these appear to be relatively mild forms of obstreperous behavior in comparison to aggression, theft, vandalism, or other acts that cause damage to persons or property.

Children with conduct disorder are also likely to suffer from *academic deficiencies*, as reflected in achievement level, grades, and specific skill areas, especially reading (e.g., Ledingham & Schwartzman, 1984; Sturge, 1982). Such children are often seen by their teachers as uninterested in school, unenthusiastic toward academic pursuits, and careless in their work (Glueck & Glueck, 1950). They are more likely to be left behind in grades, to show lower achievement levels, and to end their schooling sooner than their peers matched in age, socioeconomic status, and other demographic variables (Bachman, Johnston, & O'Malley, 1978; Glueck & Glueck, 1968).

Poor interpersonal relations are likely to correlate with antisocial behavior. Children high in aggressiveness or other antisocial behaviors are rejected by their

---

[2] The combination of antisocial and hyperactive behavior in children has been recognized by the ICD-9 system of classification. A special diagnostic category is delineated as hyperkinetic conduct disorder, which includes hyperactivity and antisocial behavior that go together.

peers and show poor social skills (e.g., Behar & Stewart, 1982; Carlson, Lahey, & Neeper, 1984). Such youths have been found to be socially ineffective in their interactions with an array of adults (e.g., parents, teachers, community members). Specifically, antisocial youths are less likely to defer to adult authority, to show politeness, and to respond in ways that promote further positive interactions (Freedman, Rosenthal, Donahoe, Schlundt, & McFall, 1978; Gaffney & McFall, 1981).

The correlates of antisocial behavior involve not only overt behaviors but also a variety of *cognitive and attributional processes*. Antisocial youths have been found to be deficient in cognitive problem-solving skills that underlie social interaction (Dodge, 1985; Kendall & Braswell, 1985). For example, such youths are more likely than their peers to interpret gestures of others as hostile and are less able to identify solutions to interpersonal problem situations and to take the perspective of others.

COURSE AND PROGNOSIS

The course and prognosis of antisocial behavior have been studied relatively exten-sively, and several different features have been identified. To begin with, among childhood disorders, conduct disorder tends to be relatively stable over time (Beach & Laird, 1968; Robins, 1978). The stability departs from many other disorders that often are age specific and remit over the course of development. Thus when children evince consistent antisocial behavior such as aggressive acts toward others, it is unlikely that they will simply "grow out of it."

For the children who are diagnosed with conduct disorder and who are seen clinically for their antisocial behavior, the course and prognosis are relatively clear. Longitudinal studies have consistently shown that antisocial behavior identified in childhood or adolescence predicts a continued course of social dysfunction, problematic behavior, and poor school adjustment (e.g., Bachman et al., 1978; Gersten, Langner, Eisenberg, Simcha-Fagan, & McCarthy, 1976; Glueck & Glueck, 1968; Jessor & Jessor, 1977; McCord, McCord, & Zola, 1959). One of the most dramatic illustrations of the long-term prognosis of clinically referred children was the classic study by Robins (1966) who evaluated their status 30 years later. The results demonstrated that antisocial child behavior predicted multiple problems in adulthood. Youths who had been referred for their antisocial behavior, compared to youths with other clinical problems or matched normal controls, as adults suffered dysfunction in psychiatric symptoms, criminal behavior, physical health, and social adjustment. Several studies attest to the breadth of dysfunction of conduct-disordered children as they mature into adulthood. Table 7.1 highlights the characteristics that these children are likely to evince when they become adults.

Even though conduct disorder in childhood portends a number of other significant problems in adulthood, not all antisocial children suffer impairment as adults. Nevertheless, data suggest that a high percentage of children are likely to do so. Across several different samples, Robins (1978) noted that, among the most severely antisocial children, less than 50% become antisocial adults. Even though less than

TABLE 7.1.   Long-Term Prognosis for Conduct-Disordered Youths: Overview of Major Characteristics Likely to Be Evident in Adulthood

Area of Functioning	Characteristics in Adulthood
Psychiatric status	Greater psychiatric impairment including sociopathic personality, alcohol and drug abuse, and isolated symptoms (e.g., anxiety, somatic complaints); also, greater history of psychiatric hospitalization
Criminal behavior	Higher rates of driving while intoxicated, criminal behavior, arrest records, and conviction, and period of time spent in jail; greater seriousness of the criminal acts
Occupational adjustment	Less likely to be employed; shorter history of employment, lower status jobs, more frequent change of jobs, lower wages, and more frequent dependence on financial assistance (welfare); served less frequently and performed less well in the armed services
Educational attainment	Higher rates of dropping out of school, lower attainment among those who remain in school
Marital status	Higher rates of divorce, remarriage, and separation
Social participation	Less contact with relatives, friends, and neighbors; little participation in organizations such as church
Physical health	Higher mortality rate; higher rate of hospitalization for physical (as well as psychiatric) problems

Note. These characteristics are based on comparisons of clinically referred children identified for antisocial behavior relative to control clinical referrals or normal controls or from comparisons of delinquent and nondelinquent youths (see Bachman et al., 1978; Glueck & Glueck, 1950; Huesmann, Eron, Lefkowitz, & Walder, 1984; Robins, 1966, 1978; Wadsworth, 1979).

half of the children continue antisocial behavior into adulthood, the percentage is still quite high.

If diverse diagnoses are considered, rather than serious antisocial behavior alone, the picture of impairment in adulthood is much worse. Among children referred for antisocial behavior, 84% received a diagnosis of psychiatric disorder as adults (Robins, 1966). Although these diagnoses vary in degree of impairment (e.g., psychoses, neuroses), the data suggest that the majority of children with clinically referred antisocial behavior will suffer from a significant degree of impairment.

As noted above, not all antisocial youths become antisocial adults. Major factors that influence whether antisocial youths are likely to continue their behavior into adulthood include parent antisocial behavior, alcoholism, poor parental supervision of the child, harsh or inconsistent discipline practices, marital discord in the family, large family size, older siblings who are antisocial, and so on. The most significant predictors of long-term outcome are characteristics of the child's antisocial behavior. Early onset of antisocial behaviors, antisocial acts evident across multiple settings (e.g., home and school), and many and diverse antisocial behaviors (e.g., several vs. few, covert and overt acts) are the primary factors that predict untoward long-term consequences (Loeber & Dishion, 1983; Rutter & Giller, 1983).

IMPAIRMENT AND COMPLICATIONS

The impairment and complications associated with antisocial behavior stem from the pervasiveness of the dysfunction and its correlates and stability over time. In terms of the former, youths with conduct disorder are likely to show dysfunction in diverse areas of their lives. They are likely to be functioning poorly at home and at school, and within a given setting multiple problems are likely to be evident. For example, at school, antisocial youths are likely to be performing poorly in their academic tasks and to have few prosocial relationships with their peers. The core symptoms of the dysfunction appear to begin a sequence of events that support continued dysfunction. Thus failure to complete homework and possible truancy or lying are not likely to increase the attention of teachers to aid the student. Consequently, the initial dysfunctions at school are likely to portend further deterioration. Apart from the characteristics in a particular setting, the associated features convey the breadth of dysfunction in academic, cognitive, and interpersonal domains.

The poor prognosis of antisocial behavior leads to a variety of complications. The reason is that a large proportion of antisocial youths remain in continued contact with mental health and criminal justice systems well into adulthood. Over the course of childhood and adolescence, antisocial youths are likely to be exposed to various forms of psychiatric and psychological treatment, family social work, juvenile adjudication and incarceration, and special education programs. Indeed, in light of the poor prognosis and continued contact with various social agencies, antisocial behavior has been identified as one of the most costly mental disorders to society (Robins, 1981).

The poor prognosis for the individual is not the only source of complications. Antisocial behavior is stable over time not only *within individuals* but also *within families*. Antisocial behavior in childhood predicts similar behaviors in one's offspring (Huesmann et al., 1984; Robins, 1981). The continuity is evident across multiple generations. Grandchildren are more likely to show antisocial behaviors if their grandparents have a history of these behaviors (Glueck & Glueck, 1968). Thus the social consequences of antisocial behavior may be perpetuated.

It is evident that conduct disorder in children and adolescents leads to major impairment of the individual. A discussion of the nature and scope of the social problem neglects the personal tragedy that antisocial behavior reflects. There is, of course, the chronic maladjustment and unhappiness of those whose conduct is of clinically severe proportions. In addition, there are the many victims of acts of murder, rape, robbery, arson, drunk driving, and spouse or child abuse, which are carried out to a much greater extent by persons with a history of antisocial behavior than by other persons. Because of the many victims, antisocial behavior plays a role unlike that of many other psychiatric problems (e.g., psychoses) that receive center-stage attention in research on the mental disorders.

EPIDEMIOLOGY OF CONDUCT DISORDER

Prevalence

The prevalence of conduct disorder is difficult to estimate given very different definitions that have been used and variations in rates for children of different age, sex, socioeconomic class, and geographical locale. Estimates of the rate of conduct disorder among children have ranged from approximately 4 to 10% (Rutter, Cox, Tupling, Berger, & Yule, 1975; Rutter, Tizard, & Whitmore, 1970).

When rates are evaluated for specific behaviors that comprise conduct disorder, and youths themselves report on their activities, the prevalence rates are extraordinarily high. For example, among youths (ages 13 to 18) more than 50% admit to theft; 35% admit to assault; 45% admit to property destruction; and 60% admit to engaging in more than one type of antisocial behavior (such as aggressiveness, drug abuse, arson, vandalism) (see Feldman, Caplinger, & Wodarski, 1983; Williams & Gold, 1972). Even though it is difficult to pinpoint how many children might be defined as conduct disordered at a particular age, data consistently reveal that the problem is great by most definitions.

The extent of the problem is attested to further by the utilization of clinical services by youths with antisocial behavior and their families. The rates of referrals of conduct disorder to clinical services are relatively high. Estimates have indicated that referrals to outpatient clinics for aggressiveness, conduct problems, and antisocial behaviors encompass from one-third to one-half of all child and adolescent cases (Gilbert, 1957; Robins, 1981).

Sex and Age Variations

Conduct disorder in children and adolescents varies as a function of sex (Gilbert, 1957; Robins, 1966). The precise sex ratio is difficult to specify because of varying criteria and measures of conduct disorder among the available studies. Nevertheless, antisocial behavior appears to be at least three times more common among boys (Graham, 1979). The sex differences are not merely due to biases in the referral process for identifying boys more than girls as problematic. Assessment of antisocial behavior through self-report reveals that male juveniles report higher rates of these behaviors than do females (Empey, 1982; Hood & Sparks, 1970).

Sex differences also are apparent in the age of onset of dysfunction. Robins (1966) found that the median age of onset of dysfunction for children referred for antisocial behavior was in the range of 8 to 10 years. Most (57%) boys had an onset before age 10 (median = 7). For girls, onset of antisocial behavior was concentrated in the age range of 14 to 16 (median = 13). Characteristic symptom patterns were different as well. Theft was more frequent as a basis of referral among antisocial boys than among antisocial girls. For boys, aggression was also likely to be a presenting problem. For girls, antisocial behavior was much more likely to include sexual misbehavior.

FAMILY CHARACTERISTICS

The families of antisocial youths have been studied relatively extensively. Evidence has suggested that antisocial behavior clearly is transmitted across generations. Both adoption and twin studies have revealed that there are genetic and environmental influences that contribute to the appearance of conduct disorder. The simultaneous contribution of genetic and environmental factors can be illustrated by the studies that show that the occurrence of antisocial behavior in both the biological and adoptive parent increases the risk of antisocial behavior in the child (Mednick & Hutchings, 1978), although the influence of the biological parent appears to be much greater. A variety of specific factors have been found in the homes of antisocial youth (see Kazdin, 1987).

Psychopathology and Criminal Behavior

Parents of antisocial youths are more likely to suffer from various psychiatric disorders than parents of children in the general population (Rutter et al., 1970). Criminal behavior and alcoholism, particularly of the father, are two of the stronger and more consistently demonstrated parental characteristics of conduct-disordered youths (Robins, 1966; Rutter & Giller, 1983; West, 1982).

Interestingly, selected antisocial and associated behaviors are highly related between parent and child. For example, Robins (1978) reported the relationship between school truancy and dropping out of high school between parents and their children. If one (vs. neither) parent evinced either of these behaviors, the likelihood of the child showing the same behavior was greater. If both parents showed the behavior, the risk was greater still. This study shows that specific antisocial and maladaptive parental behaviors, through whatever mechanism, clearly are related across generations.

Most studies of parental dysfunction have focused on the parents of the antisocial child. Grandparents of antisocial children and adolescents, on both paternal and maternal sides, are more likely to show antisocial behavior (criminal behavior and alcoholism) compared to the grandparents of youths who are not antisocial (Glueck & Glueck, 1968). Longitudinal studies have shown that aggressive behavior is stable across generations within a family. More specific statements can be made. For example, a good predictor of how aggressive the child will be is the level of aggressiveness of the father when he was about the same age (Huesmann et al., 1984). In general, antisocial or aggressive children are likely to come from families with a history of antisocial behavior.

Parent–Child Interaction

Discipline Practices

Several features related to the interaction of parents with their children characterize families of conduct-disordered youths. Parent disciplinary practices and attitudes have been especially well studied. Parents of conduct-disordered youths tend to be harsh in their attitudes and disciplinary practices with their children (e.g., Farrington, 1978; Glueck & Glueck, 1968; McCord, McCord, & Howard, 1961; Nye, 1958). Studies have also shown the degree of child aggression in nonclinic populations is positively correlated with severity of punishment in the home (e.g., Sears, Maccoby, & Levin, 1957). Indeed, conduct-disordered youths are more likely than normals and clinical referrals without antisocial behavior to be victims of child abuse and to be in homes where spouse abuse is evident (Behar & Stewart, 1982; Lewis, Shanok, Pincus, & Glaser, 1979).

It is not only harsh punishment that characterizes families of antisocial youths. Studies have shown that more lax, erratic, and inconsistent discipline practices for a given parent and between the parents are related to conduct disorder. For example, severity of punishment on the part of the father and lax discipline on the part of the mother have been implicated in delinquent behavior (Glueck & Glueck, 1950; McCord et al., 1959). When parents are consistent in their discipline practices, even if they are punitive, children are less likely to be at risk for antisocial behavior (McCord et al., 1959).

Apart from punishment practices, research suggests that the other ways of controlling child behavior are problematic among parents of antisocial youths. Direct observation of families in the home has revealed that parents of antisocial children are more likely to give commands to their children, to reward deviant behavior directly through attention and compliance, and to ignore or provide aversive consequences for prosocial behavior (see Patterson, 1982). Fine-grained analyses of parent–child interaction suggest that antisocial behavior, particularly aggression, is systematically, albeit unwittingly, trained in the homes of antisocial children.

Supervision and Monitoring of the Child

Supervision of the child, as another aspect of parent–child contact, has been frequently implicated in conduct disorder (Glueck & Glueck, 1968; Goldstein, 1984; Robins, 1966). Parents of antisocial or delinquent children are less likely to monitor their children's whereabouts or to make arrangements for their care when they are temporarily away from the home. Other factors considered to reflect poor supervision and to constitute risk factors include not providing rules in the home stating where the children can go and when they must return home, allowing children to roam the streets, and permitting them to engage in many independent and unsupervised activities (Wilson, 1980).

Quality and Emotional Expressiveness

Features that reflect the quality of parent–child and family relationships also have been identified as risk factors. Parents of antisocial youths, compared with parents of normal youths, show less acceptance of their children, less warmth, affection, and emotional support, and report less attachment (Loeber & Dishion, 1984; McCord et al., 1959; West & Farrington, 1973). At the level of family relations, less supportive and more defensive communications among family members, less participation in activities as a family, and more clear dominance of one family member also distinguish families of antisocial youths (Alexander, 1973; Hanson, Henggeler, Haefele, & Rodick, 1984; West & Farrington, 1973).

Broken Homes and Marital Discord

Separation of one's parents during childhood ("broken homes") has been found to be related to antisocial child behavior and delinquency (Glueck & Glueck, 1968; McCord et al., 1959; Nye, 1958). Yet broken homes are related to psychiatric impairment across a variety of disorders in children, not just conduct disorder (Rutter et al., 1970). Also, the separation of the parents may be due to several factors, such as death, institutionalization, or marital discord. Research has consistently demonstrated that unhappy marital relationships, interpersonal conflict, and aggression characterize the parental relations of delinquent and antisocial children (see Hetherington & Martin, 1979; Rutter & Giller, 1983). Whether or not the parents are separated, it is the extent of discord that is associated with antisocial behavior and childhood dysfunction.

Birth Order and Family Size

Birth order is related to antisocial behavior. Antisocial behavior is more likely among middle children in comparison to only, firstborn, or youngest children (e.g., Glueck & Glueck, 1968; McCord et al., 1959; Nye, 1958; Wadsworth, 1979). In general, an extended period of time as the only or the youngest child before the sibling is born reduces risk for antisocial behavior (Wadsworth, 1979).

Antisocial youths are more likely to come from families of larger sizes (Glueck & Glueck, 1968; Nye, 1958; West, 1967). Family size obviously relates to findings of birth order of the children. Efforts to separate them have looked at birth spacing of offspring and family size. Children with older siblings are more likely to be delinquent, and the older the siblings (i.e., space in age between them), the greater the likelihood of antisocial behavior (Wadsworth, 1979). Interestingly, the risk is associated with the number of brothers rather than sisters in the family (Offord, 1982). If one of the brothers is antisocial, the others are at increased risk for antisocial behavior (Robins, West, & Herjanic, 1975).

Social Class

There is a preponderance of conduct disorder and delinquency from lower socioeconomic classes (West, 1982). However, interpretation of this finding is complicated because of the association of social class with family size, overcrowding, poor child supervision, and other variables known to relate to antisocial behavior. When these separate factors are controlled, social class shows little or no relation to antisocial behavior (Robins, 1978; Wadsworth, 1979). Yet in many instances, the impact of separate factors is not evaluated. Lower socioeconomic class, as a summary label or conglomerate variable that includes a number of class-related factors, at a global level characterizes families of antisocial youths.

General Comments

The present discussion does not exhaust the range of characteristics of parents and families of conduct-disordered youths. Other characteristics such as mental retardation of the parent, early marriage of the parents, lack of parent interest in the child's school performance, and lack of participation of the family in religious or recreational activities have been found as well (Glueck & Glueck, 1968; Wadsworth, 1979). Many of the factors discussed separately are interrelated and come in "packages." For example, family size, overcrowding, poor housing, poor parental supervision, parent criminality, and marital discord are likely to be related. Thus the long list of risk factors reflects different ways of identifying the same or at least overlapping factors. Identification of the unique contribution of any specific factor requires a careful effort to partial out other factors with which it may be associated.

Apart from their co-occurrence, individual risk factors may interact with each other. For example, large family size has been repeatedly shown to be a risk factor for conduct disorder and delinquency. However, the importance of family size as a predictor is moderated by (i.e., interacts with) income. If family income and living accommodations are adequate, family size is less likely to be a risk factor. Family size exerts a greater influence on risk in lower-family-income homes where over-crowding and other problems are likely to emerge (West, 1982). Apparently, families with adequate income can manage larger numbers of children and reduce the impact of any adverse influences associated with lower socioeconomic disadvantage.

DIFFERENTIAL DIAGNOSIS

Antisocial and Oppositional Behavior in Other Disorders

The diagnosis of conduct disorder is not entirely straightforward because characteristic behaviors may be evident in other diagnostic categories. Two diagnoses in particular are worth noting. The first is an adjustment disorder with disturbance of conduct. In the case of this disorder, the symptoms may be evident but they usually can be traced to the onset of a particular stressor or change (e.g., divorce, loss of a relative) in the environment. The onset of symptoms within 3 months of the stressor would constitute an adjustment disorder. Symptoms such as increased fighting, vandalism, or truancy would be expected to decrease over time as the impact of the stressor attenuates. If the pattern continues, the diagnosis could be altered to Conduct Disorder.

Symptoms of Conduct Disorder also would be evident in conditions not due to a particular disorder.[3] These conditions would include isolated acts rather than a pattern of antisocial behavior. Conflict between the parent and child would be the most common instance of one of these conditions. In such cases, the dysfunction is restricted in time and place and includes isolated symptoms rather than the more protracted syndrome.

Attention Deficit Disorder (ADD)

Perhaps the most salient issue regarding differential diagnosis pertains to the relationship of ADD to Conduct Disorder. The primary characteristics of ADD are persistent and excessive activity, distractibility, short attention span, and impulsivity (APA, 1980). In the 1980 version of DSM, two forms of ADD were acknowledged, with and without hyperactivity. In DSM-III-R, the disorder is referred to as Attention Deficit–Hyperactivity Disorder (ADHD). This reflects the experience that few ADD youths have been identified who do not show hyperactivity.[4]

Although this is not a core feature of the diagnosis, children with ADD often show aggressive behavior, negativism, and other characteristics of conduct or oppositional disorder. Similarly, children who are characterized as aggressive or oppositional often are regarded as hyperactive. Multivariate studies have shown that hyperactivity and aggression often emerge as separate factors (see Kazdin, 1987). Even so, children's scores on these factors (as evaluated from parent or teacher ratings) typically are correlated in the moderate range (r's $= .40$ to $.60$).

Current evidence suggests that many children who meet diagnostic criteria for Conduct Disorder may also meet criteria for ADD with hyperactivity (see Prinz, Connor, & Wilson, 1981; Stewart, DeBlois, Meardon, & Cummings, 1980). The disorders can be distinguished and are associated with different background characteristics and prognoses (Loney, Kramer, & Milich, 1981; Loney, Langhorne, & Paternite, 1978). On the other hand, there is overlap as well that is important to recognize in discussing either disorder. In DSM-III, children who meet criteria can receive both diagnoses. It is not likely that the presence of one disorder would necessarily be confused with another. The diagnostic issue is the need for careful assessment to evaluate whether the criteria for each disorder are met.

---

[3] Conditions not attributable to a specific mental disorder are referred to as V Codes in DSM-III. This coding system has been adopted from the Internal Classification of Diseases (WHO, 1979). Parent–child problems (e.g., child abuse) or isolated antisocial behaviors of the child (e.g., fighting with the parent) might be categorized as a V code.

[4] In DSM-III-R, there has been an acknowledgement that attention deficit disorder symptoms may occur without hyperactivity. This has been recognized in a special category called undifferentiated attention-deficit disorder. This latter category has been proposed to be distinct from ADHD, which has more data on its behavior as a diagnostic entity. Undifferentiated ADD has been proposed as a category that remains to be validated.

CLINICAL MANAGEMENT AND TREATMENT

Management of Referred Youths

Conduct-disordered children who are referred for treatment often pose several issues that need to be addressed immediately. The family may require special attention because of child abuse, clinical problems with nonreferred siblings, or psychopathology of the parent. These characteristics may not only present crises other than the difficulties associated with the referred child, but also place constraints on what can be attempted or accomplished in treatment.

Characteristics of the referred child of course also may raise special issues in managing the case. It is possible that the child's behavior is dangerous or the parents cannot manage or care for the child. In such cases the child may need to be removed from the home either on a temporary (e.g., brief psychiatric hospitalization) or permanent basis (e.g., placement into a foster home). In most instances, the child can be seen in outpatient treatment and remain at home.

Management of the case often requires involvement with other social agencies. For example, it is usually the case that severe problems at school are evident. A history of suspensions and special placements is common. Casework may be needed to integrate the child back into the school or to find an alternative placement at another school. The child may also have had some contact with the juvenile justice system. In such cases, contacts may need to be maintained with the court. Parents may have been ordered to seek and obtain treatment and the courts may need to be apprised of progress for further decision making about the placement of the child. In short, by the very nature of the clinical problem and the consequences that derive from the antisocial behaviors themselves, considerable effort is needed in managing the case. In extreme cases, the extensive efforts in managing the disposition of the case often supersede any efforts to provide treatment.

Treatment

Several treatments have been implemented for antisocial behavior, including diverse forms of individual and group therapy, behavior therapy, residential treatment, pharmacotherapy, psychosurgery, and a variety of innovative community-based treatments (Kazdin, 1985; McCord, 1982; O'Donnell, 1985; Shamsie, 1981). At present no treatment has been demonstrated to ameliorate conduct disorder and to controvert its poor prognosis. This conclusion is particularly unfortunate given the points, noted earlier, that antisocial behavior is one of the most frequent bases for clinical referrals and that the behaviors are quite stable over the course of development.

Several promising treatments have emerged, including parent-management training, problem-solving skills training, and functional family therapy. In parent-management training, parents are trained to alter their interactions and child-rearing practices with the child. In problem-solving skills training, interpersonal cognitive problem-solving skills are trained in the child. In functional family therapy, the communication and problem-solving skills of the family are altered and specific behaviors are developed in the family to support prosocial child behavior. Each of these techniques has evidence attesting to changes in antisocial youths (see Kazdin, 1985). The long-term effects of these treatments and their range of applicability to antisocial youths pose significant questions that remain to be addressed. In clinical lore, youths with a diagnosis of conduct disorder usually are regarded as poor candidates for treatment and not especially rewarding to deal with on a session-by-session basis. Part of the difficulty may be the fact that to date few treatments have been identified that can have even short-term impact on the problems.

REVISION OF DSM-III DIAGNOSTIC CRITERIA

Beginning in 1983, the diagnostic categories of DSM-III have been reevaluated to incorporate research findings on alternative disorders and experience in applying the specific diagnostic categories. In the revised DSM-III criteria (DSM-III-R, APA, 1987), a broad category was introduced and referred to as disruptive behavior disorders. This category includes Conduct Disorder, Oppositional Defiant Disorder, and Attention Deficit Hyperactivity Disorder. For Conduct Disorder, the diagnostic criteria have been better specified than in DSM-III. Table 7.2 presents the range of symptoms that are required for the diagnosis. The requirement of at least four symptoms for the diagnosis differs from the 1980 version where only one symptom was sufficient, if the duration and other criteria were met.

There has been a reconsideration of the fourfold classification for subtyping Conduct Disorder based on aggressive versus nonaggressive and socialized versus undersocialized dichotomies. In the DSM-III-R, there are two major subtypes of

---

TABLE 7.2.   DSM-III-R Criteria for Conduct Disorder

A disturbance of conduct lasting at least 6 months, during which at least three of the following have been present:
 1. Has stolen without confrontation of a victim on more than one occasion (including forgery)
 2. Has run away from home overnight at least twice while living in parental or parental surrogate home (or once without returning)
 3. Often lies (other than to avoid physical or sexual abuse)
 4. Has deliberately engaged in fire setting
 5. Is often truant from school (for older person, absent from work)
 6. Has broken into someone else's house, building, or car
 7. Has deliberately destroyed others' property (other than by fire setting)
 8. Has been physically cruel to animals
 9. Has forced someone into sexual activity with him or her
10. Has used a weapon in more than one fight
11. Often initiates physical fights
12. Has stolen with confrontation of a victim (e.g., mugging, purse snatching, extortion, armed robbery)
13. Has been physically cruel to people

Source: Reprinted with permission from the *Diagnostic and Statistical Manual of Mental Disorders*, Third Edition, Revised. Copyright 1987 American Psychiatric Association.

TABLE 7.3.   DSM-III-R Criteria for Oppositional Defiant Disorder

A disturbance of at least 6 months during which at least five of the following are present:
1. Often loses temper
2. Often argues with adults
3. Often actively defies or refuses adult requests or rules, for example, refuses to do chores at home
4. Often deliberately does things that annoy other people, for example, grabs other children's hats
5. Often blames others for his or her own mistakes
6. Is often touchy or easily annoyed by others
7. Is often angry and resentful
8. Is often spiteful or vindictive
9. Often swears or uses obscene language

Source: Reprinted with permission from the *Diagnostic and Statistical Manual of Mental Disorders*, Third Edition, Revised. Copyright 1987 American Psychiatric Association.

Conduct Disorder, referred to as group type and solitary aggressive type. In the group type, the conduct problems occur primarily as a group activity in the company of friends who have similar problems and to whom the individual is loyal. Physical aggression may be present. Children are included in the solitary aggressive type if they show physically or verbally aggressive behavior. The behavior usually is initiated by the individual rather than as part of group activity, and no attempt is made to conceal the behavior. The subtype notes that social isolation often may be evident.

A few points about these subtypes are noteworthy. First, the two subtypes better reflect research findings on patterns of antisocial behavior. As is evident in the discussion of multivariate approaches to diagnosis, aggressive and delinquent types have consistently emerged in research. Second, a problem with the DSM-III version was that aggressive or nonaggressive types were mutually exclusive when in fact many children show features of both. In the DSM-III-R, aggressive behavior might be evident in either the group or solitary aggressive types. Finally, in the 1980 version of the DSM, the majority of Conduct Disorder youths were subtyped as undersocialized–aggressive type. The revised version recognizes this pattern of behavior, which would now fall in the solitary aggressive type category, in which social isolation is often evident.

Oppositional disorder is also treated differently in the DSM-III-R. The criteria for the disorder, now referred to as oppositional defiant disorder, are presented in Table 7.3. The criteria elaborate a wider range of symptoms and include the term *defiant* in the label of the disorder better to reflect the characteristic pattern of responding. As in the DSM-III, there are no subtypes specified for this disorder.

OTHER APPROACHES TO DIAGNOSIS

Other approaches to diagnosis of conduct and oppositional disorders have engendered major advances and promise important contributions and warrant discussion in their own right. Conduct disorder as a distinct type of dysfunction has been recognized by alternative approaches, which have made special gains in focusing on various subtypes.

Multivariate Approaches

Clinically derived diagnosis as represented by DSM-III and DSM-III-R relies on clinical observation and abstractions from these observations to identify discrete constellations of behaviors or syndromes. The resulting diagnostic systems have been *categorical* or typological. Various disorders are regarded as present or absent. The task of diagnosis is to identify which symptoms are present, if any, and then to assign or rule out the presence of discrete disorders.

Multivariate approaches to diagnosis are fundamentally dimensional rather than categorical. Thus the approaches do not lead to the statement that a person has a particular disorder. Rather, one can describe the degree to which one or many characteristics are evident. Multivariate approaches depend on determining the correlations among several specific characteristics (symptoms, problems) and then summarizing them through quantitative techniques (see Blashfield, 1984). Typically, the process begins by having parents, teachers, or others complete a measure that includes a large number of items about the child's behavior. Data obtained from a large number of children are subjected to *factor analysis* to identify symptoms (items) that go together (correlate). Rating scales typically yield multiple factors. An individual child has a score on each of the different factors or dimensions. The scores for an individual on all of the factors constitute a profile or pattern. From evaluating profiles of many children, diagnostic categories or typologies can be devised through *cluster analysis*. The clusters serve as empirically derived diagnostic entities analogous to disorders derived from clinical methods.

Efforts to identify syndromes empirically have utilized a wide array of measures, raters, clinical samples, and methods of data analyses. Across a wide range of multivariate studies of childhood disorders, Quay (1986b) has identified six factors that emerged consistently. The factors include conduct disorder, socialized aggression, attention problems, motor activity, anxious–depressed withdrawal, and schizoid–unresponsive. Table 7.4 provides the two factors that reflect conduct disorder and the six frequently associated characteristics of each. The characteristics of these

TABLE 7.4.   Conduct-Disorder-Related Dimensions from Multivariate Analyses and Six Frequently Associated Characteristics of Each

Conduct Disorder	Socialized Aggression
Fighting, hitting	Has "bad" companions
Disobedient, defiant	Absent from home
Temper tantrums	Truant from school
Destructiveness	Steals in company of peers
Impertinent, impudent	Loyal to delinquent friends
Uncooperative, resistant	Belongs to gang

Source: Adapted from Quay (1986b).

factors (rather than the names of the factors) reflect aggressive and delinquent subtypes. Cluster analyses to identify a typology of childhood disorders have been less frequently used than factor analyses. Even so, some consistencies have emerged here as well. Studies using cluster analyses with normal, inpatient, and outpatient samples of children (ages 4 to 17) have identified clusters reflecting aggression and/ or delinquent types of behaviors (e.g., Edelbrock & Achenbach, 1980; Lessing, Williams, & Gil, 1982). The consistencies of these patterns of antisocial behavior from multivariate studies no doubt have influenced recognition of these aggressive and group delinquent types in DSM-III-R.

Salient Symptom Approach

Clinically derived and multivariate approaches used are designed to apply widely across a wide range of disorders rather than exclusively to antisocial behavior. Alternative approaches that focus exclusively on antisocial behavior have been proposed as well.

One approach has been to identify salient symptoms that may yield reliable and clinically meaningful ways of segregating types of conduct disorder. The approach is illustrated in the work of Patterson (1982), who has distinguished antisocial children whose primary symptom is aggression (*aggressors*) from those whose primary symptom is stealing (*stealers*). Aggressors have a history of fighting and engaging in assaultive behavior; stealers have a history of repeated theft and contact with the courts. Although these characteristics often go together, subpopulations of "pure" aggressors or stealers can be readily identified.

Several studies have suggested the utility of distinguishing aggressors and stealers. For example, aggressive children have been found to engage in significantly more aversive and coercive behaviors in their interactions in the home and are less compliant with parents' requests than are children who steal (Patterson, 1982; Reid & Hendriks, 1973). Also, parents of stealers show greater emotional distance in relation to their children (e.g., lack of responding, less disapproval, fewer commands) than do parents of aggressors (Patterson, 1982).

Additional evidence suggests that families of aggressors and stealers respond differently to treatment. Parent-management training has been effective in altering the coercive child–parent interactions that sustain deviant behavior among aggressors. However, coercive child–parent interactions apparently are not a central characteristic of family life among stealers. Although parents of stealers can be trained to apply parent-management techniques, they are less likely to continue to apply them over time than are parents of aggressors. Other studies have shown that the prognosis of antisocial children may vary as a function of whether they have been identified as aggressors or stealers. For example, subsequent contact with the courts several years later is significantly more likely for children previously identified as stealers than for those identified as aggressors (Moore, Chamberlain, & Mukai, 1979).

Interestingly, the salient symptom approach has not neglected the fact that many children are likely to be both aggressors and stealers. Indeed, the combination of salient symptoms may be significant in its own right. "Mixed"-symptom children show characteristics of both types and are especially at risk for child abuse (Patterson, 1982). Thus the approach provides preliminary evidence regarding different salient symptom patterns.

Overt–Covert Types of Antisocial Behavior

Expansion of the aggressor–stealer dimension has suggested a broader focus on delineating subtypes. Antisocial behavior can be examined according to a bipolar dimension of overt and covert behavior (Loeber, 1985). *Overt behaviors* consist of those antisocial acts that are confrontational, such as fighting, arguing, and temper tantrums. *Covert behaviors*, on the other hand, consist of concealed acts such as stealing, truancy, lying, and fire setting.

Loeber and Schmaling (1985a) analyzed a large number of studies that evaluated antisocial behavior of school-age children. Statistical analyses of the grouping of antisocial behaviors across studies supported the dimension of overt and covert behavior. Figure 7.1 shows the behaviors that are associated with each point on the dimension. The data indicated that overt behaviors tend to cluster together. This means that the presence of one overt behavior was likely to be associated with other overt behaviors. Similarly, the presence of a particular covert behavior is likely to be associated with other covert behaviors. As evident in the figure, some behaviors, such as disobedience and sassiness, tend to be present with both types of antisocial behavior.

Given the complexity and diversity of antisocial behaviors, one would expect that some children are likely to perform both overt and covert behaviors (i.e., reflect

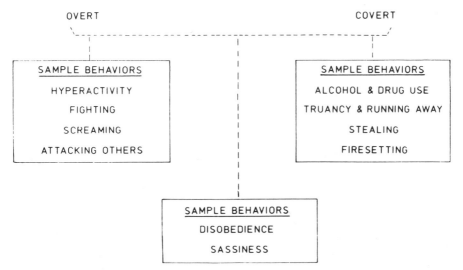

Figure 7.1. Overt–covert behavior as a dimension for delineating subtypes of antisocial behavior. (From Loeber & Schmaling, 1985, "Empirical Evidence for Overt and Covert Patterns of Antisocial Conduct Problems: A Meta-Analysis," *Journal of Abnormal Child Psychology*, *13*, pp. 337–352. Adapted by permission.)

a "mixed" set of behaviors). Evidence suggests that mixed types of children are distinguished from "purer" types by more severe family dysfunction and poorer long-term prognoses, as reflected in subsequent contact with police and careers of antisocial behavior (Loeber & Schmaling, 1985b; McCord, 1980). Thus children whose antisocial behavior is diverse or mixed (overt and covert) may be at high risk for long-term dysfunction (Robins, 1978).

General Comments

There are commonalities among clinically derived, multivariate, and other approaches. Obviously, each approach recognizes a constellation of antisocial behaviors among children and adolescents. Also, there are some consistencies in the subtyping of antisocial behavior. Although debate remains regarding fine delineations of antisocial behavior, each approach has suggested the importance of distinguishing an aggressive type (e.g., fighting) from a delinquent type (e.g., criminal behavior, running away, lying). The characteristics, prognoses, and developmental sequence of different types of conduct disorder remain to be fully elaborated. As for oppositional disorder, the constellation remains to be identified. It may be difficult to separate Oppositional from Conduct Disorder in multivariate studies because the latter entails the former.

CURRENT ISSUES AND FUTURE PROSPECTS

Many questions about the etiology, diagnosis, assessment, and treatment of Conduct Disorder remain. Nevertheless, the discreteness of the behaviors and their stability lead to the conclusion that there is a clear dysfunction. The status of oppositional deviant disorder is not as well developed or studied. Here fundamental questions about the syndrome and the utility or need to incorporate this into psychiatric diagnosis are far from resolved.

Among the many current questions and issues, a few issues related to diagnosis and assessment warrant special comment. Major advances have been made in the diagnosis of conduct disorder and other disorders more generally. For example, in the third edition of the DSM, criteria for invoking diagnoses have been better specified than in previous editions. A further advance with DSM-III-R is the integration of research findings in the subtypes of Conduct Disorder. The delineation of group and solitary aggressive types adheres more closely to the results from empirical evaluations of antisocial behavior than did DSM-III.

The development of salient symptom approaches to identify subtypes is an important step in need of further testing. Evidence suggests that there are types of children who can be identified (e.g., aggressors, stealers) but also that there are mixed and diffuse types. A diagnostic system that adequately handles conduct disorder may need to recognize the fact that the symptom picture in many cases is mixed.

An important diagnostic issue that remains to be addressed is the need for operational criteria for reaching diagnoses of conduct and oppositional disorders (Kazdin, 1988). *Operational criteria* refer to the specific measurement strategies and cutoff scores on these measures that can be used to identify diagnostic groups (cf. Loney, 1983). The current method of attaining psychiatric diagnoses for children is to interview the parent and the child regarding the child's dysfunction. The development of standardized diagnostic instruments is an advance that is not to be treated lightly. On the other hand, significant problems remain that have been largely ignored. For example, discrepancies between parent and child in identifying symptoms are quite common (see Achenbach, McConaughy, & Howell, 1987; Herjanic & Reich, 1982). As yet, there are no consistent methods for integrating information from parent and child.

There is a need for further development of assessment techniques in the area. Several measures have been developed and very carefully evaluated to examine the full spectrum of child and adolescent psychopathology. Prominent among these are the Child Behavior Checklist (Achenbach & Edelbrock, 1983) and the Behavior Problem Checklist (Quay & Peterson, 1979). Assessment techniques are needed to focus more intensively and exclusively on antisocial behavior and conduct problems. Elaboration of the full gamut of symptoms in individual measures may provide more detail and opportunity for subtyping antisocial youths. Assessment techniques focusing on antisocial behavior for children are not well developed (see Kazdin, 1987) and lag behind the development of techniques for other child problems such as childhood depression.

In general, it is important to develop further criteria that will be used to define conduct disorder and the manner in which these criteria will be assessed. To make further advances, there need not be agreement on the many complex questions such as the subtypes of conduct disorder and the organization of symptom patterns. Rather, these questions can be better served by attempts to utilize standardized measures and explicit criteria to select samples for further research.

REFERENCES

Achenbach, T.M., & Edelbrock, C.S. (1981). Behavioral problems and competencies reported by parents of normal and disturbed children aged four through sixteen. *Monographs of the Society for Research in Child Development*, *46*, 188.

Achenbach, T.M., & Edelbrock, C.S. (1983). *Manual for the Child Behavior Checklist and Revised Child Behavior Profile*. Burlington, VT: University Associates in Psychiatry.

Achenbach, T.M., McConaughy, S.H., & Howell, C.T. (1987). Child/adolescent behavioral and emotional problems: Implications of cross-informant correlations for situational specificity. *Psychological Bulletin*, *101*, 213–232.

Alexander, J.F. (1973). Defensive and supportive communications in normal and deviant families. *Journal of Consulting & Clinical Psychology*, *40*, 223–231.

American Psychiatric Association (1980). *Diagnostic and statistical manual of mental disorders* (3rd ed.). Washington, DC: Author.

American Psychiatric Association (1987). *Diagnostic and statistical manual of mental disorders* (3rd ed., rev.). Washington, DC: Author.

Bachman, J.G., Johnston, L.D., & O'Malley, P.M. (1978). Delinquent behavior linked to educational attainment and post-high school experiences. In L. Otten (Ed.), *Colloquium on the correlates of crime and the determinants of criminal behavior*. Arlington, VA: MITRE.

Beach, C.F., & Laird, J.D. (1968). Follow-up study of children identified early as emotionally disturbed. *Journal of Consulting & Clinical Psychology*, *32*, 369–374.

Behar, D., & Stewart, M.A. (1982). Aggressive conduct disorder of children. *Acta Psychiatrica Scandinavica*, *65*, 210–220.

Blashfield, R.K. (1984). *The classification of psychopathology: Neo-Kraepelinian and quantitative approaches*. New York: Plenum.

Carlson, C.L., Lahey, B.B., & Neeper, R. (1984). Peer assessment of the social behavior of accepted, rejected, and neglected children. *Journal of Abnormal Child Psychology*, *12*, 189–198.

Dodge, K.A. (1985). Attributional bias in aggressive children. In P.C. Kendall (Ed.), *Advances in cognitive-behavioral research and therapy* (Vol. 4). Orlando, FL: Academic.

Edelbrock, C.S., & Achenbach, T.M. (1980). A typology of Child Behavior Profile patterns: Distribution and correlates for disturbed children aged 6–16. *Journal of Abnormal Child Psychology*, *8*, 441–470.

Empey, L.T. (1982). *American delinquency: Its meaning and construction*. Homewood, IL: Dorsey.

Farrington, D.P. (1978). The family backgrounds of aggressive youths. In L.A. Hersov, M. Berger, & D. Shaffer (Eds.), *Aggression and anti-social behaviour in childhood and adolescence*. Oxford: Pergamon.

Feldman, R.A., Caplinger, T.E., & Wodarski, J.S. (1983). *The St. Louis conundrum: The effective treatment of antisocial youths*. Englewood Cliffs, NJ: Prentice-Hall.

Freedman, B.J., Rosenthal, L., Donahoe, C.P., Schlundt, D.G., & McFall, R. (1978). A social–behavioral analysis of skills deficits in delinquent and nondelinquent boys. *Journal of Consulting & Clinical Psychology*, *46*, 1448–1462.

Gaffney, L.R., & McFall, R.M. (1981). A comparison of social skills in delinquent and nondelinquent adolescent girls using a behavioral role-playing inventory. *Journal of Consulting & Clinical Psychology*, *49*, 959–967.

Gersten, J.C., Langner, T.S., Eisenberg, J.G., Simcha-Fagan, D., & McCarthy, E.D. (1976). Stability in change in types of behavioral disturbances of children and adolescents. *Journal of Abnormal Child Psychology*, *4*, 111–127.

Gilbert, G.M. (1957). A survey of "referral problems" in metropolitan child guidance centers. *Journal of Clinical Psychology*, *13*, 37–42.

Glueck, S., & Glueck, E. (1950). *Unravelling juvenile delinquency*. Cambridge, MA: Harvard University Press.

Glueck, S., & Glueck, E. (1959). *Predicting delinquency and crime*. Cambridge, MA: Harvard University Press.

Glueck, S., & Glueck, E. (1968). *Delinquents and nondelinquents in perspective*. Cambridge, MA: Harvard University Press.

Goldstein, H.S. (1984). Parental composition, supervision, and conduct problems in youths 12 to 17 years old. *Journal of the American Academy of Child Psychiatry*, *23*, 679–684.

Graham, P. (1979). Epidemiological studies. In H.C. Quay & J.S. Werry (Eds.), *Psychopathological disorders of childhood* (2nd ed.). New York: Wiley.

Group for the Advancement of Psychiatry, Committee on Child Psychiatry (1966). *Psychopathological disorders in childhood: Theoretical considerations and a proposed classification* (Vol. 6). New York: Author.

Hanson, C.L., Henggeler, S.W., Haefele, W.F., & Rodick, J.D. (1984). Demographic, individual, and family relationship correlates of serious and repeated crime among adolescents and their siblings. *Journal of Consulting & Clinical Psychology, 52*, 528–538.

Herjanic, B., & Reich, W. (1982). Development of a structured psychiatric interview for children: Agreement between child and parent on individual symptoms. *Journal of Abnormal Child Psychology, 10*, 307–324.

Hetherington, E.M., & Martin, B. (1979). Family interaction. In H.C. Quay & J.S. Werry (Eds.), *Psychopathological disorders of childhood* (2nd ed.). New York: Wiley.

Hewett, L.E., & Jenkins, R.L. (1946). *Fundamental patterns of maladjustment: The dynamics of their origin.* Springfield, IL: State of Illinois.

Hood, R., & Sparks, R. (1970). *Key issues in criminology.* London: Weidenfeld & Nicholson.

Huesmann, L.R., Eron, L.D., Lefkowitz, M.M., & Walder, L.O. (1984). Stability of aggression over time and generations. *Developmental Psychology, 20*, 1120–1134.

Jessor, R., & Jessor, S.L. (1977). *Problem behavior and psychological development: A longitudinal study of youth.* New York: Academic.

Kazdin, A.E. (1985). *Treatment of antisocial behavior in children and adolescents.* Homewood, IL: Dorsey.

Kazdin, A.E. (1987). *Conduct disorder in childhood and adolescence.* Newbury Park, CA: Sage.

Kazdin, A.E. (1988). The diagnosis of childhood disorders: Assessment issues and strategies. *Behavioral Assessment, 10*, 67–94.

Kendall, P.C., & Braswell, L. (1985). *Cognitive behavioral therapy for impulsive children.* New York: Guilford.

Ledingham, J.E., & Schwartzman, A.E. (1984). A 3-year follow-up of aggressive and withdrawn behavior in childhood: Preliminary findings. *Journal of Abnormal Child Psychology, 12*, 157–168.

Lessing, E.E., Williams, V., & Gil, E. (1982). A cluster-analytically derived typology: Feasible alternative to clinical diagnostic classification of children? *Journal of Abnormal Child Psychology, 10*, 451–482.

Lewis, D.O., Shanok, S.S., Pincus, J.H., & Glaser, G.H. (1979). Violent juvenile delinquents: Psychiatric, neurological, psychological, and abuse factors. *Journal of the American Academy of Child Psychiatry, 18*, 307–319.

Loeber, R. (1985). Patterns and development of antisocial child behavior. In G.J. Whitehurst (Ed.), *Annals of child development* (Vol. 2). New York: JAI.

Loeber, R., & Dishion, T.J. (1983). Early predictors of male delinquency: A review. *Psychological Bulletin, 94*, 68–99.

Loeber, R., & Dishion, T.J. (1984). Boys who fight at home and school: Family conditions influencing cross-setting consistency. *Journal of Consulting & Clinical Psychology, 52*, 759–768.

Loeber, R., & Schmaling, K.B. (1985a). Empirical evidence for overt and covert patterns of antisocial conduct problems: A meta-analysis. *Journal of Abnormal Child Psychology, 13*, 337–352.

Loeber, R., & Schmaling, K.B. (1985b). The utility of differentiating between mixed and pure forms of antisocial child behavior. *Journal of Abnormal Child Psychology, 13,* 315–335.

Loney, J. (1983). Research diagnostic criteria for childhood hyperactivity. In S.B. Guze, F.J. Earls, & J.E. Barrett (Eds.), *Childhood psychopathology and development.* New York: Raven.

Loney, J., Kramer, J., & Milich, R. (1981). The hyperkinetic child grows up: Predictors of symptoms, delinquency, and achievement at follow-up. In K. Gadow & J. Loney (Eds.), *Psychosocial aspects of drug treatment for hyperactivity.* Boulder, CO: Westview.

Loney, J., Langhorne, J., & Paternite, C. (1978). An empirical basis for subgrouping the hyperkinetic/minimal brain dysfunction syndrome. *Journal of Abnormal Psychology, 87,* 431–441.

MacFarlane, J.W., Allen, L., & Honzik, M.P. (1954). *A developmental study of the behavior problems of normal children between 21 months and 14 years.* Berkeley: University of California Press.

McCord, J. (1980). Patterns of deviance. In S.B. Sells, R. Crandall, M. Roff, J.S. Strauss, & W. Pollin (Eds.), *Human functioning in longitudinal perspective.* Baltimore: Williams & Wilkins.

McCord, W. (1982). *The psychopath and milieu therapy: A longitudinal study.* New York: Academic.

McCord, W., McCord, J., & Howard, A. (1961). Familial correlates of aggression in nondelinquent male children. *Journal of Abnormal & Social Psychology, 62,* 79–93.

McCord, W., McCord, J., & Zola, I.K. (1959). *Origins of crime.* New York: Columbia University Press.

Mednick, S.A., & Hutchings, B. (1978). Genetic and psychophysiological factors in asocial behavior. In R.D. Hare & D. Schalling (Eds.), *Psychopathic behaviour: Approaches to research.* Chichester: Wiley.

Moore, D.R., Chamberlain, P., & Mukai, L.H. (1979). Children at risk for delinquency: A follow-comparison of aggressive children and children who steal. *Journal of Abnormal Child Psychology, 7,* 345–355.

Nye, F.I. (1958). *Family relationships and delinquent behavior.* New York: Wiley.

O'Donnell, D.J. (1985). Conduct disorders. In J.M. Weiner (Ed.), *Diagnosis and psychopharmacology of childhood and adolescent disorders.* New York: Wiley.

Offord, D.R. (1982). Family backgrounds of male and female delinquents. In J. Gunn & D.P. Farrington (Eds.), *Abnormal offenders: Delinquency and the criminal justice system.* Chichester: Wiley.

Patterson, G.R. (1982). *Coercive family process.* Eugene, OR: Castalia.

Patterson, G.R. (1986). Performance models for antisocial boys. *American Psychologist, 41,* 432–444.

Prinz, R., Connor, P., & Wilson, C. (1981). Hyperactive and aggressive behaviors in childhood: Intertwined dimensions. *Journal of Abnormal Child Psychology, 9,* 191–202.

Quay, H.C. (1986a). Classification. In H.C. Quay & J.S. Werry (Eds.), *Psychopathological disorders of childhood* (3rd ed.). New York: Wiley.

Quay, H.C. (1986b). A critical analysis of DSM-III as a taxonomy of psychopathology in childhood and adolescence. In T. Millon & G. Klerman (Eds.), *Contemporary issues in psychopathology.* New York: Guilford.

Quay, H.C., & Peterson, D.R. (1979). *The Revised Behavior Problem Checklist: Rationale and development*. Unpublished manuscript, University of Miami and Rutgers State University.

Reid, J.B., & Hendriks, A.F.C.J. (1973). Preliminary analysis of the effectiveness of direct home intervention for the treatment of predelinquent boys who steal. In L.A. Hamerlynck, L.C. Handy, & E.J. Mash (Eds.), *Behavior change: Methodology, concepts and practice*. Champaign, IL: Research Press.

Robins, L.N. (1966). *Deviant children grown up*. Baltimore: Williams & Wilkins.

Robins, L.N. (1978). Sturdy childhood predictors of adult antisocial behavior: Replications from longitudinal studies. *Psychological Medicine, 8*, 611–622.

Robins, L.N. (1981). Epidemiological approaches to natural history research: Antisocial disorders in children. *Journal of the American Academy of Child Psychiatry, 20*, 566–580.

Robins, L.N., West, P.A., & Herjanic, B. (1975). Arrests and delinquency in two generations: A study of Black urban families and their children. *Journal of Child Psychology & Psychiatry, 16*, 125–140.

Rutter, M., Cox, A., Tupling, C., Berger, M., & Yule, W. (1975). Attainment and adjustment in two geographical areas: I. The prevalence of psychiatric disorder. *British Journal of Psychiatry, 126*, 493–509.

Rutter, M., & Giller, H. (1983). *Juvenile delinquency: Trends and perspectives*. New York: Penguin.

Rutter, M., Tizard, J., & Whitmore, K. (Eds.). (1970). *Education, health and behaviour*. London: Longmans.

Sears, R.R., Maccoby, E., & Levin, H. (1957). *Patterns of child rearing*. New York: Harper & Row.

Shamsie, S.J. (1981). Antisocial adolescents: Our treatments do not work——Where do we go from here? *Canadian Journal of Psychiatry, 26*, 357–364.

Stewart, M.A., DeBlois, C.S., Meardon, J., & Cummings, C. (1980). Aggressive conduct disorder children. *Journal of Nervous & Mental Disease, 168*, 604–610.

Sturge, C. (1982). Reading retardation and antisocial behaviour. *Journal of Child Psychology & Psychiatry, 23*, 21–31.

Wadsworth, M. (1979). *Roots of delinquency: Infancy, adolescence and crime*. New York: Barnes & Noble.

West, D.J. (1967). *The young offender*. London: Duckworth.

West, D.J. (1982). *Delinquency: Its roots, careers and prospects*. Cambridge, MA: Harvard University Press.

West, D.J., & Farrington, D.P. (1973). *Who becomes delinquent?* London: Heinemann.

Williams, J.R., & Gold, M. (1972). From delinquent behavior to official delinquency. *Social Problems, 20*, 209–229.

Wilson, H. (1980). Parental supervision: A neglected aspect of delinquency. *British Journal of Criminology, 20*, 203–235.

World Health Organization (1979). *International classification of diseases, injuries, and causes of death* (9th ed.). Geneva: Author.

CHAPTER 8

Anxiety Disorders of Childhood or Adolescence

CYNTHIA G. LAST

DEFINITION

Anxiety disorders of childhood or adolescence is a diagnostic category that first was introduced in the third edition of the *Diagnostic and Statistical Manual of Mental Disorders* (American Psychiatric Association, 1980). The category includes three specific diagnoses: separation anxiety disorder, avoidant disorder, and overanxious disorder. While anxiety is considered to be the central feature for this entire diagnostic group, the specific focus of the anxiety differs among the three disorders. In the case of separation anxiety and avoidant disorders, the anxiety is focused on specific situations, while in overanxious disorder anxiety it is generalized to a variety of situations.

According to DSM-III, the hallmark of separation anxiety disorder is excessive anxiety concerning separation from major attachment figures (e.g., parents) and/or from home or other familiar surroundings. There are nine specific criteria for the diagnosis, of which at least three must be met:

1. Unrealistic worry about possible harm befalling major attachment figures or fear that they will leave and not return
2. Unrealistic worry that an untoward calamitous event will separate the child from a major attachment figure, for example, the child will be lost, kidnapped, killed, or be the victim of an accident
3. Persistent reluctance or refusal to go to school in order to stay with major attachment figures or at home
4. Persistent reluctance or refusal to go to sleep without being next to a major attachment figure or to go to sleep away from home
5. Persistent avoidance of being alone in the home and emotional upset if unable to follow the major attachment figure around the home
6. Repeated nightmares involving the theme of separation

7. Complaints of physical symptoms on school days, for example, stomachaches, headaches, nausea, vomiting

8. Signs of excessive distress on separation, or when anticipating separation, from major attachment figures, for example, temper tantrums or crying, pleading with parents not to leave

9. Social withdrawal, apathy, sadness, or difficulty concentrating on work or play when not with a major attachment figure

In addition to meeting three of these symptoms, the disturbance must be at least 2 weeks in duration. Further, as an exclusion criterion DSM-III notes that if the child is 18 years of age or older he or she does not meet the criteria for agoraphobia.

In avoidant disorder of childhood or adolescence, anxiety is focused on contact with unfamiliar persons, resulting in persistent avoidance or shrinking from both adults and peers. More specifically, the diagnostic criteria for the disorder include: (1) persistent and excessive shrinking from contact with strangers; (2) desire for affection, acceptance, and generally warm and satisfying relations with family members and other familiar figures; and (3) avoidant behavior sufficiently severe to interfere with social functioning in peer relationships. In addition to meeting all three of these criteria, the child must be at least 2½ years of age. Further, if the child is 18 years of age or older, he or she does not meet the criteria for avoidant personality disorder. Finally, the duration of the disturbance must be at least 6 months.

By contrast to the two diagnoses just described, the essential feature of overanxious disorder is excessive worry and fearful behavior that is not limited to a specific situation or object. According to DSM-III, the child must meet at least four of the following seven criteria:

1. Unrealistic worry about future events

2. Preoccupation with the appropriateness of the individual's behavior in the past

3. Overconcern about competence in a variety of areas, for example, academic, athletic, social

4. Excessive need for reassurance about a variety of worries

5. Somatic complaints, such as headaches or stomachaches, for which no physical basis can be established

6. Marked self-consciousness or susceptibility to embarrassment or humiliation

7. Marked feelings of tension or inability to relax

The symptoms must have persisted for at least 6 months. In addition, if the child is 18 or older, he or she does not meet the criteria for generalized anxiety disorder. Finally, the disturbance cannot be due to another mental disorder such as separation anxiety disorder, avoidant disorder, phobic disorder, obsessive–compulsive disorder, depressive disorder, schizophrenia, or pervasive developmental disorder.

HISTORICAL BACKGROUND

Neither separation anxiety disorder nor avoidant disorder of childhood or adolescence was included in previous versions of the DSM, although overanxious disorder (overanxious reaction) was specified as a diagnostic category for children and adolescents in DSM-II (APA, 1968). given the fairly recent inclusion of these disorders in our classification system, epidemiological data are not yet available on them, although such data are available on the prevalence of anxiety *symptoms*. Orvaschel and Weissman (1984), in their review of the literature in this area, conclude that anxiety symptoms (i.e., fears, phobias, worries) are quite prevalent in children of all ages and both sexes, with rates estimated to range from 2 to 43% of the population.

Although there has been relatively little empirical research conducted on these three childhood anxiety disorders, the clinical literature over the years generally has supported the existence of at least two of the disorders. Numerous clinical studies and case reports prior to the appearance of DSM-III in 1980 have appeared that refer to separation anxiety as a clinically significant phenomenon in both children and adolescents (e.g., Berg, Nichols, & Pritchard, 1969; Broadwin, 1932; Chazan, 1962; Eisenberg, 1958; Freud, 1950; Gittelman-Klein & Klein, 1971, 1973; Hersov, 1960, 1972; Johnson, Falstein, Szurek, & Svendson, 1941; Kahn & Nursten, 1962; Klein, 1964; Partridge, 1939; Smith, 1970; Warren, 1948). While most of the literature preceding DSM-III classified these children as having school phobia, rather than separation anxiety per se, it has been noted that a large number of children who are phobic of school have clinically significant levels of separation anxiety (Berg, 1980; Bowlby, 1975; Eysenck & Rachman, 1965; Gittelman-Klein & Klein, 1980; Ollendick & Mayer, 1985; Smith, 1970), with rates estimated to range from 30 to 90% of this population (see Gittelman & Klein, 1984). Similarly, the clinical literature on overanxious disorder has supported its existence as a diagnostic entity (e.g., Hewitt & Jenkins, 1946; Jenkins, 1964, 1969; Jenkins, NurEddin, & Shapiro, 1966; Lewis, 1954; Shamsie, 1968; Suh & Carlson, 1977). By contrast, to our knowledge no reports have appeared on children or adolescents who present with the clinical features of avoidant disorder, although it is clear to most clinicians that such shy and avoidant children indeed do exist.

Since the appearance of DSM-III, a number of trials have been conducted to assess the reliability of the childhood disorders contained in the manual, including the childhood anxiety disorders. Studies conducted during the late 1970s and early 1980s, in general, showed only fair reliability for the diagnostic category anxiety disorders of childhood or adolescence. However, more recently, a large scale test–retest reliability study of these disorders conducted by Last, Hersen, Kazdin, Finkelstein, and Strauss (1987) showed excellent rates of agreement for separation anxiety disorder (kappa = .81) and overanxious disorder (kappa = .82), and moderately high agreement for avoidant disorder (kappa = .64).

In regard to the validity of the three diagnoses, investigation only recently has been undertaken. In their study of separation anxiety disorder and overanxious disorder, Last, Hersen, Kazdin, Finkelstein, and Strauss (1987) found the two disorders to differ significantly on several dimensions, including age, social class, and presence of a coexisting anxiety disorder. In comparing children with separation anxiety to those children who met DSM-III criteria for a phobic disorder of school, Last, Francis, Hersen, Kazdin, and Strauss (1987) found that the two groups of children significantly differed in regard to their sex distribution, pubertal status, and socioeconomic backgrounds. In addition, the two groups of children differed in their symptomatology, comorbidity, and maternal psychiatric illness. In a study of comorbidity among childhood anxiety disorders, Last, Strauss, and Francis (in press) found children who had a primary diagnosis of separation anxiety disorder to have different patterns of comorbidity than children with a primary diagnosis of overanxious disorder. Finally, in an examination of self-reported fears on the Fear Survey Schedule for Children–Revised (Ollendick, 1983), Last, Francis, and Strauss (1987) found statistically significant differences in the types of fears endorsed by children diagnosed as having separation anxiety disorder and those diagnosed as having overanxious disorder.

Taken together, the findings from these studies preliminarily support the validity of separation anxiety disorder and overanxious disorder as two distinct diagnostic entities. Future research in this area is necessary to confirm the findings from Last and colleagues. In addition, investigation of the validity of avoidant disorder as a separate childhood anxiety disorder clearly is warranted.

CLINICAL PICTURE

Children with *separation anxiety disorder* usually are referred to a mental health setting by their parents who are distressed by their child's reluctance or inability to be separated from them. In most cases, the child has difficulty with separation from his or her mother. However, there are instances in which the child is fearful of being away from the father, siblings, or other significant individuals to whom the child is attached. In young children with this disorder, clinging behavior is common. Upon presentation at a mental health setting, the child may refuse to have the parent or parents leave him or her to meet with the clinician. When anticipating separation, young children may tantrum, cry, or scream. At the extreme end of this type of behavior, the child may threaten suicide or make suicidal gestures (e.g., "If you leave me, I'm going to throw myself out of the window").

School reluctance or refusal is characteristic of the disorder, although not required by DSM-III for a diagnosis. Last, Francis, Hersen, Kazdin, and Strauss (1987) have noted that approximately three-quarters of children who meet criteria for the diagnosis of separation anxiety disorder show school reluctance or avoidance. Concomitant with school reluctance or avoidance are somatic complaints, where the child complains of various and often vague physical symptoms in order to avoid going to school. Somatic complaints also can occur in the context of other situations where separation is anticipated. Although separation anxiety disorder is rarer in adolescents than in children (see *Epidemiology*), adolescents with the disorder almost always present with school reluctance or avoidance and somatic complaints (see Last, Francis, & Strauss, in press).

Many younger children with separation anxiety "shadow" the individual from whom they are afraid to be separated. More specifically, they will follow the parent around the house, always being in close proximity (i.e., two steps behind). During middle childhood and adolescence, these children often are reluctant or refuse to sleep away from home, for example, at a friend's house, or to go to sleep-away camp. Repeated nightmares regarding separation themes (i.e., being kidnapped, killed, the death of a parent, etc.) sometimes are reported in younger children with the disorder. Nightmares almost never are reported by adolescents with the disorder.

Worrying that focuses on the theme of separation is common to both children and adolescents with separation anxiety disorder. These worries may take the form of fears of getting kidnapped, being in an accident, or getting killed, or the death of a major attachment figure. The child may worry about something happening to himself or herself, or the worries may be focused on what will happen to the parent. In many instances, both types of worries exist. It is quite common for these youngsters to refuse to be alone in the home, even when of an age where such behavior is expected and usual. In prepubertal children with the disorder, sadness, apathy, or difficulty concentrating may be experienced when the child is separated from his or her parent.

By contrast, the hallmark of *overanxious disorder* is unrealistic worry about future events. In a recent study by our group, we found that more than 95% of children with overanxious disorder meet this specific diagnostic criterion (see Strauss, Lease, Last, & Francis, 1987). In addition to worrying about future events, it is quite common for children with this disorder to have unrealistic worries about the appropriateness of their behavior in the past. This is particularly true for adolescents, who almost always show this problem.

Excessive and/or unrealistic concerns about competence are characteristic of overanxious children. They have been noted to be "perfectionistic," wanting to excel in all facets of their lives: that is, academic performance, social interaction, sports, and so on. As in separation anxiety disorder, somatic complaints are common. However, in the case of overanxious disorder, the somatic complaints are not linked to any particular situation but rather appear to occur "spontaneously" or when the child is "tense." Somatic complaints often take the form of headaches, stomachaches, back pains, or a general feeling of malaise. These children tend to be markedly self-conscious and usually have difficulty speaking out loud in a group setting, such as at school. They also may be embarrassed when other people talk about them, even if the comments are of a positive nature. Because of their excessive worries and insecurities, children and adolescents with overanxious disorder often excessively and repeatedly seek reassurance from significant others. The reassurance-seeking behavior can be in relationship to their academic performance, social interaction, their competence at sports or other hobbies or activities, and their appearance. Finally, generalized tension and an inability to relax are characteristic. The tension may be expressed as "nervous habits," such as nail biting, foot tapping, hair pulling, and fidgeting.

Upon presentation at a mental health setting, parents of overanxious children often will state: "My child is a worry wart and a nervous wreck." Because these children are usually quiet and well behaved, it is unusual for school personnel to be the referral source for this type of anxiety disorder. More often, it is the child or the parents who identify this problem and seek help.

In avoidant disorder, the child is fearful about being around unfamiliar people. In most instances, the unfamiliar people include both children and adults, although we have seen cases where the child is more fearful around one or the other. This fear leads to avoidance behavior where the youngster is extremely reluctant to enter situations where there is someone he or she does not know. Children of this type generally are warm and loving with family and other people whom they know well. Avoidant-disordered children should be distinguished from children who are "slow to warm up," for children with avoidant disorder virtually never "warm up."

Avoidant disorder usually is readily apparent from the child's verbal and physical behavior during a psychiatric interview. In extreme cases, the child may refuse to speak at all or crouch behind a piece of furniture. Avoidant disorder, by contrast to overanxious disorder, often is brought to mental health attention by school personnel. The discomfort of these children in the school setting is most apparent to the teachers who observe them on a daily basis. Children with avoidant disorder typically have few or no friends since their ability to interact with new acquaintances is severely limited.

ASSOCIATED FEATURES

Children with separation anxiety disorder usually present with specific fears in addition to their separation anxiety, such as of the dark, ghosts, bumblebees, and so on, which may or may not be of phobic proportion. Approximately one-third of children with the disorder will show a concurrent overanxious disorder that almost always is secondary to a primary separation anxiety disorder. Although the separation anxiety disorder, in such cases, typically is the presenting problem and the one that requires immediate intervention, it is not uncommon for the overanxious disorder to have preceded the onset of the separation anxiety disorder. Studies by Last and colleagues suggest that approximately one-third of children who present with separation anxiety disorder show a coexisting major depression. In these cases, the major depression almost always antedates the onset of the separation anxiety disorder by several months. It is rare for such patients to have serious suicidal symptomatology; however, in a number of cases, we have seen children who will make suicidal threats in an attempt to avoid or escape a separation situation. It should be noted that children with separation anxiety usually do not have interpersonal difficulties. Generally such children are well liked by their peers and reasonably socially skilled.

Children with overanxious disorder often present with specific fears that are of phobic proportion. The fears may be either simple or social according to DSM-III criteria. Although not one of the DSM-III diagnostic criteria for the disorder, children with overanxious disorder may refuse to attend school because of their anxiety in the school setting. In addition to school avoidance, it is not uncommon to see these children avoid engaging in other age-appropriate activities in which there are demands for performance (i.e., sports, musical instruments, etc.). Obsessional self-doubt is sometimes observed in children with overanxious disorder, which can serve to exacerbate their worries about the future and past. On presentation, some children with overanxious disorder will appear as "little adults"; that is, they will act and appear older than their chronological age. Approximately one-third of children with the disorder meet DSM-III criteria for concurrent major depression.

Children with avoidant disorder typically are very unassertive and lack self-confidence. In adolescence, normal heterosocial and heterosexual activities are avoided. Avoidant disorder rarely occurs alone. In almost all cases, the child will have an additional concurrent anxiety disorder (usually overanxious disorder).

COURSE AND PROGNOSIS

For the most part, separation anxiety has an acute onset. The onset often occurs after a major stressor, such as moving to a new neighborhood and a new school, the death of a family member, or illness of a relative. The onset of the disorder also has been noted to occur following prolonged vacations from school, such as after Christmas or summer vacation. Sometimes the disorder develops after prolonged physical illness where, despite evidence that the illness no longer exists, the child will continue to complain of the symptoms in an attempt to stay home. It also has been noted that at certain developmental transitions, the incidence of the disorder increases, such as entering elementary school or moving from elementary school into junior high school. There are few data on the course of the disorder, although it appears that, without intervention, it may wax and wane according to the life stressors and developmental transitions that are present. It is not uncommon for a child who presents with the disorder at 10, 11, or 12 years of age to have a history of problems upon entering kindergarten or first grade. Without treatment, the prognosis of the disorder also is unknown. Currently, Last and colleagues are conducting follow-up studies of these children to determine more specifically both their course and prognosis.

By contrast to separation anxiety disorder, overanxious disorder appears to be a more chronic (though somewhat milder) disorder. Upon presentation at a mental health setting, it is typical for these children to have a several-year history of the disorder without remission. Although the disorder does not appear to remit spontaneously, it may be exacerbated during times of intense stress or developmental transitions. The outcome or prognosis of the disorder is unknown at this time, but preliminary evidence suggests that overanxious disorder in childhood or adolescence may predispose the individual to developing generalized anxiety disorder as an adult.

As in overanxious disorder, children and adolescents with avoidant disorder usually have a long history of difficulties that do not appear to remit spontaneously. The avoidant behavior may be exacerbated when the child is under sufficient stress or during significant developmental transitions. Without intervention, the problematic behaviors may proceed into college years. Sometimes the forced social exposure that occurs in college years is sufficient to remedy the condition. Although no data currently are available on the prognosis of the disorder, preliminary evidence suggests that these children and adolescents may be at risk for developing social phobia or avoidant personality disorder in adulthood.

IMPAIRMENT

Separation anxiety, in most cases, severely impairs the child's ability to function independently. He or she is unable to go places or stay at home without being accompanied by a major attachment figure. In three-quarters of the patients seen at our clinic for this disorder, school reluctance or refusal also has been observed. Where prolonged school refusal exists, the child obviously is hampered in further academic and social development.

In general, overanxious disorder is less impairing than separation anxiety disorder, except in cases where the overanxious child refuses to go to school. In such cases, similar hampering of academic and social development occurs.

Children with avoidant disorder are, by definition, showing impairment in their social interactions with peers and adults. It is rare for such children to avoid school, and they usually do not suffer from academic problems.

COMPLICATIONS

Children with separation anxiety disorder may seek help from medical practitioners because of their somatic complaints. This can involve frequent physical examinations and elaborate and costly medical procedures. Once organic causes are ruled out, however, medical practitioners usually will refer the child to a mental health setting for assistance. Similarly, children with overanxious disorder may repeatedly visit physicians for their somatic complaints. The most serious complication of avoidant disorder is the failure to form social bonds outside of the immediate family unit. Such inability to form friendships and attachments outside of the family can result in the child's feeling isolated and dysphoric.

EPIDEMIOLOGY

No data currently are available on the prevalence or sociodemographic characteristics of separation anxiety disorder, overanxious disorder, and avoidant disorder in the general population. However, data are available on each of the three disorders from our clinical research setting (see Last, Hersen, Kazdin, Finkelstein, & Strauss, 1987).

Separation anxiety disorder is one of the most common anxiety disorders that we see at our Child and Adolescent Anxiety Disorder Clinic. During the first 18 months in which our clinic was open, we evaluated 91 children, of whom 47% ($N = 43$) met DSM-III criteria for separation anxiety disorder. Further examination of these children indicated that the vast majority are under the age of 13 (91%), with the mean age being 9.1 years. The sex distribution of the disorder is roughly equivalent for boys and girls. The vast majority (86%) of the children seen with the disorder are Caucasian. Finally, it should be noted that 75% of these children come from families of low socioeconomic status (Hollingshead ratings of 4 or 5).

Our clinic data indicate that overanxious disorder is as common as separation anxiety disorder, with 52% ($N = 47$) of our patient sample meeting DSM-III criteria for the disorder. However, in approximately one-half of these patients, overanxious disorder was concurrent with and secondary to a primary separation anxiety disorder. By contrast to separation anxiety disorder, children with overanxious disorder usually are over the age of 13 (69%), with the mean age being 13.4 years. The disorder is equally common in boys and girls. All of the cases evaluated during the 18-month period just described have been Caucasian. It is interesting to note that overanxious children usually (80%) come from families of middle to high socioeconomic status.

Preliminary and unpublished data on avoidant disorder suggest that this childhood anxiety disorder is rarer than separation anxiety or overanxious disorders. Over the past 3 years, we have collected information on 22 children with this disorder. These data suggest that avoidant disorder can occur at any age, with a mean age of 12.7 and equal incidence below and above 13 years of age. The disorder appears to be more prevalent in females (73%), and in Caucasians (94%). Socioeconomic status is equally divided between upper and lower strata, as is not the case for separation anxiety and overanxious disorders.

FAMILIAL PATTERN

In a recent study by Last, Hersen, Kazdin, Francis, and Grubb (1987), the mothers of children with separation and/or overanxious disorder were administered structured diagnostic interviews to assess current and lifetime psychopathology. Results from the study indicated that the vast majority (83%) of mothers of children with these disorders had a lifetime history of an anxiety disorder. This rate significantly differed from that of a psychopathological control group of children. Moreover, it was interesting to observe that approximately one-half of the mothers of the anxious children presented with an anxiety disorder at the same time their children were seen at our clinic for an anxiety problem. Contrary to expectation, although the rates of affective disorders (and major depression) were higher in the mothers of the anxious children, comparisons between the anxious children and the control group were not statistically significant.

Previous research has shown that children of adult anxiety patients are at an increased risk for developing anxiety disorders (Harris, Noyes, Crowe, & Chaudhry, 1983; Weissmann, Leckman, Merikangas, Gammon, & Prusoff, 1984). However, the investigation just cited is the first to demonstrate clearly that the converse of this finding also is true, at least for the mothers of these children. Currently, we are conducting a family study of all first- and second-degree relatives of our separation-anxious and overanxious child patients. These results will give us a more comprehensive understanding of the familial nature of these disorders.

To date, we have collected psychiatric histories on 11 mothers of children diagnosed as having avoidant disorder. These preliminary data show that 91% of these children's mothers have a lifetime history of an anxiety disorder. Moreover, 64% had a *current* anxiety disorder: that is, at the time at which they were interviewed. Further examination of the psychiatric histories of these mothers and comparisons to psychopathological and normal control groups currently are under way.

DIFFERENTIAL DIAGNOSIS

Separation anxiety disorder should be distinguished from developmentally normal concerns about separation that often occur in very young children. Clinical judgment must be used to distinguish between a normal developmental phase and an excessive and pathological reaction. Separation anxiety disorder should be distinguished from a phobic disorder of school, which is quite common in adolescence. In a phobic disorder of school, the anxiety is focused on some aspect of the school environment and not generalized to a number of other settings, while in separation anxiety disorder the anxiety is about being separated from a major attachment figure or home, and school is but one of many settings in which the child is fearful. Separation anxiety disorder also should be distinguished from agoraphobia with panic attacks. Agoraphobia with panic attacks is relatively rare in children under the age of 18. In addition, in agoraphobia with panic attacks, the youngster is fearful of leaving the home because of incapacitation from panic attacks, not because of separation concerns. Although separation-anxious and agoraphobic individuals may show similar patterns of behavior, closer inspection will indicate that separation-anxious children are reluctant to leave the home alone because of concerns about separation, while agoraphobic children are reluctant to leave the home alone because of concerns about having a panic attack. Truancy as part of a conduct disorder should be distinguished from anxiety about attending school due to separation issues. In conduct disorder when the child refuses school, he or she rarely returns to the home setting; rather, such children usually stay out either alone or with friends, as is not the case with separation-anxious children.

Overanxious disorder should be differentiated from social phobia. Social phobia usually is marked by a relatively circumscribed situation that is feared and avoided, such as speaking in public, using public restrooms, writing in front of others, and so on. In overanxious disorder, the fears and concerns cover a variety of situations and settings. Moreover, avoidant behavior is not a criterion for overanxious disorder, while it is considered to be the hallmark of phobic disorders. The disorder also should be distinguished from generalized anxiety disorder, which usually occurs only in adulthood. As the child enters adulthood, however, overanxious disorder may become generalized anxiety disorder. Children with attention deficit disorder with hyperactivity may appear to be fidgety and restless, similar to children with overanxious disorder. However, in attention deficit disorder with hyperactivity, the child does not show the worrying that is characteristic of overanxious disorder.

Avoidant disorder is distinguished from social phobia by the types of fears and avoidance the child exhibits. If the child specifically is afraid of interacting with unfamiliar people, the diagnosis of avoidant disorder should be used. If avoidant disorder persists, the diagnosis of avoidant personality disorder may then be applicable, if the child meets the additional criteria for this personality disorder.

CLINICAL MANAGEMENT: RESEARCH FINDINGS

While numerous case studies and clinical reports have described the treatment of "school phobia," reports in the literature on separation anxiety disorder only recently have begun to emerge. In large part this is due to the fact that the disorder was not included in the DSM classification system until the third version was published in 1980. Case reports on the treatment of separation anxiety disorder typically have described a behavioral approach consisting of graduated in vivo exposure. The exposure can be either therapist-assisted or self-initiated, with the assistance of parents and school personnel. In some cases, additional cognitive procedures have been used as an adjunct to exposure treatment in order to aid in decreasing anticipatory anxiety and in increasing exposure duration. Despite the apparent success of these procedures, to our knowledge no controlled group studies have appeared in the literature.

Imipramine hydrochloride has been used successfully as an adjunct in the treatment of separation anxiety disorder. In the first controlled study of this medication, Gittelman-Klein and Klein (1971) found imipramine, administered in conjunction with a multidiscipline treatment program, to be superior to placebo. However, the criteria for diagnosing these children were unclear, and it appears that many children who were phobic of school rather than having separation anxiety per se were included as subjects in the study. In addition, children were not excluded from participation if they had significant depressive symptomatology, which makes interpretation of findings somewhat unclear. In the later study by Berney and colleagues (1981), the effect of clomipramine was assessed in the treatment of school-phobic children. Contrary to findings by Gittelman-Klein and Klein (1970), this double-blind trial failed to demonstrate any significant effects of the drug. However, once again it is unclear what percentage of this group of school-refusing children had separation anxiety. Moreover, as the investigators themselves note, the dose level of imipramine used by Gittelman-Klein and Klein was higher than the dosage of clomipramine used by Berney and colleagues, which could account for their results.

In our clinical experience we have found graduated in vivo exposure to be the treatment of choice for separation-anxious children. In very chronic and intractable cases, and also in cases where panic is of extreme proportion, we have sometimes found it necessary to use imipramine as an adjunct to behavioral treatment. While we have been very successful in our use of behavioral treatment, either alone or administered concurrently with imipramine, empirical investigation on the relative efficacy of these two treatment approaches remains to be done. Currently we are evaluating this question in a double-blind study.

No reports on the treatment of overanxious disorder have appeared to date. From our clinical experience we have found that the most successful avenue is to administer these children a combined cognitive–behavioral treatment package consisting of relaxation training, exposure, and cognitive therapy. In this way we attempt to deal with the physiological, behavioral, and cognitive concomitants of the disorder.

Much as is the case with overanxious disorder, the treatment of avoidant disorder has not been described in the literature to date. In our clinical practice, we have been treating the disorder with social skills training. It is unclear whether avoidant children lack the social skills necessary for interacting effectively with unfamiliar people, or whether their excessive level of anxiety interferes with their inability to use the skills that they have already acquired. By administering social skills training, both problems are dealt with simultaneously, in that such training teaches skills that the child may be deficient in *and* enforces graduated exposure. In addition, we have found the use of cognitive techniques to be helpful in some cases, particularly for those children who have high levels of anticipatory anxiety.

From the brief summary just given of the state of the art in the treatment of childhood anxiety disorders, it is clear that extensive research is necessary in order clearly to determine the treatment of choice for these disorders. However, in the absence of such investigations we have made some suggestions based on the available literature and our clinical experience.

DSM-III-R

In DSM-III-R (1987), the diagnostic criteria for the three anxiety disorders of childhood or adolescence essentially have remained the same. In fact, separation anxiety disorder is the only disorder of the three that has been altered at all, with changes being of a relatively minor nature. These changes include: (1) dividing criterion 8 into two separate criteria, one of which is excessive distress *when anticipating* separation, the other of which is excessive distress *during* separation; (2) deleting criterion 9 from the criteria for the disorder; and (3) specifying that onset of the disorder must be before 18 years of age.

Whether changes in the diagnostic criteria for separation anxiety disorder will affect significantly the classification of these children remains to be determined.

REFERENCES

American Psychiatric Association (1968). *Diagnostic and statistical manual of mental disorders* (2nd ed.). Washington, DC: Author.

American Psychiatric Association (1980). *Diagnostic and statistical manual of mental disorders* (3rd ed.). Washington, DC: Author.

American Psychiatric Association (1987). *Diagnostic and statistical manual of mental disorders* (3rd ed., rev.). Washington, DC: Author.

Berg, I. (1980). School refusal in early adolescence. In L. Hersov & I. Berg (Eds.), *Out of school*. New York: Wiley.

Berg, I., Nichols, K., & Pritchard, C. (1969). School phobia—Its classification and relationship to dependency. *Journal of Child Psychology & Psychiatry, 10*, 123–141.

Berney, T., Kolvin, I., Bhate, S.R., Garside, R.F., Jeans, J., Kay, B., & Scarth, L. (1981). School phobia: A therapeutic trial with clomipramine and short-term outcome. *British Journal of Psychiatry, 138*, 110–118.

Bowlby, J. (1975). *Attachment and loss: Vol. 1. Attachment*. London: Hogarth Press.

Broadwin, I.T. (1932). A contribution to the study of truancy. *American Journal of Orthopsychiatry, 2*, 253–259.

Chazan, M. (1962). School phobia. *British Journal of Educational Psychology, 32*, 200–217.

Eisenberg, L. (1958). School phobia: A study in the communication of anxiety. *American Journal of Psychiatry, 114*, 712–718.

Eysenck, H.J., & Rachman, S.J. (1965). The application of learning theory to child psychiatry. In J. Howells (Ed.), *Modern perspectives in child psychiatry*. Edinburgh: Oliver & Boyd.

Freud, S. (1950). The analysis of phobia in a five-year-old boy. In *Collected papers* (Vol. 3). London: Hogarth Press.

Gittelman, R., & Klein, D.F. (1984). Relationship between separation anxiety and panic and agoraphobic disorders. *Psychopathology, 17*(Suppl. 1), 56–65.

Gittelman-Klein, R., & Klein, D.F. (1971). Controlled imipramine treatment of school phobia. *Archives of General Psychiatry, 25*, 204–207.

Gittelman-Klein, R., & Klein, D.F. (1973). School phobia: Diagnostic considerations in the light of imipramine effects. *Journal of Nervous & Mental Disorders, 156*, 199–215.

Gittelman-Klein, R., & Klein, D.F. (1980). Separation anxiety in school refusal and its treatment with drugs. In L. Hersov & I. Berg (Eds.), *Out of school*. New York: Wiley.

Harris, E.L., Noyes, R., Crowe, R.R., & Chaudhry, D.R. (1983). Family study of agoraphobia: Report of a pilot study. *Archives of General Psychiatry, 40*, 1061–1064.

Hersov, L.A. (1960). Persistent non-attendance at school. *Journal of Child Psychology & Psychiatry, 1*, 130–136.

Hersov, L.A. (1960). Refusal to go to school. *Journal of Child Psychology & Psychiatry, 1*, 137–145.

Hersov, L.A. (1972). School refusal. *British Journal of Medicine, 3*, 102–104.

Hewitt, C.E., & Jenkins, R.L. (1946). *Fundamental patterns of maladjustment: The dynamics of their origin*. Springfield: State of Illinois.

Jenkins, R.L. (1964). Diagnosis, dynamics, and treatments in child psychiatry. *Psychiatry Research Reports, American Psychiatric Association, 18*, 91–120.

Jenkins, R.L. (1966). Psychiatric syndromes in children and their relation to family background. *American Journal of Orthopsychiatry, 36*, 450–457.

Jenkins, R.L., NurEddin, E., & Shapiro, I. (1966). Children's behavior syndromes and parental responses. *Genetic Psychological Monographs, 74*, 261–329.

Johnson, A.M., Falstein, E.I., Szurek, S.A., & Svendson, M. (1941). School phobia. *American Journal of Orthopsychiatry, 11*, 702–711.

Kahn, J.H., & Nursten, S.P. (1962). School refusal: A comprehensive view of school phobia and other failures of school attendance. *American Journal of Orthopsychiatry, 32*, 707–718.

Klein, D.F. (1964). Delineation of two-drug-responsive anxiety syndrome. *Psychopharmacologica, 5*, 397–408.

Last, C.G., Francis, G., Hersen, M., Kazdin, A.E., & Strauss, C.C. (1987). Separation anxiety and school phobia: A comparison using DSM-III criteria. *American Journal of Psychiatry, 144*, 653–657.

Last, C.G., Francis, G., & Strauss, C.C. (1987). *Fears in anxiety disordered children and adolescents*. Manuscript submitted for publication.

Last, C.G., Hersen, M., Kazdin, A.E., Finkelstein, R., & Strauss, C.C. (1987). Comparison of DSM-III separation anxiety and overanxious disorders: Demographic characteristics and patterns of comorbidity. *Journal of the American Academy of Child & Adolescent Psychiatry, 26*, 527–531.

Last, C.G., Hersen, M., Kazdin, A.E., Francis, G., & Grubb, H.J. (1987). Psychiatric illness in the mothers of anxious children. *American Journal of Psychiatry, 144*, 1580–1583.

Last, C.G., Strauss, C.C., & Francis, G. (in press). Comorbidity among childhood anxiety disorders. *Journal of Nervous & Mental Disease.*

Lewis, H. (1954). *Deprived children*. London: Oxford University Press.

Ollendick, T.H. (1983). Reliability and validity of the Revised Fear Survey Schedule for Children (FSSC-R). *Behavior Research & Therapy, 21*, 685–692.

Ollendick, T.H., & Mayer, J.A. (1985). School phobia. In S.M. Turner (Ed.), *Behavioral treatment of anxiety disorders*. New York: Plenum.

Orvaschel, H., & Weissman, M.M. (1986). Epidemiology of anxiety disorders in children: A review. In R.Gittelman (Ed.), *Anxiety disorders in children*. New York: Guilford.

Partridge, J.M. (1939). Truancy. *Journal of Mental Science, 85*, 45–81.

Shamsie, S.J. (Ed.). (1968). *Adolescent psychiatry*. Pointe Claire, Quebec: Shering.

Smith, S.L. (1970). School refusal with anxiety: A review of sixty-three cases. *Canadian Psychiatric Association Journal, 126*, 815–817.

Strauss, C.C., Lease, C.A., Last, C.G., & Francis, G. (in press). Developmental differences between children and adolescents with overanxious disorder. *Journal of Abnormal Child Psychology.*

Suh, M., & Carlson, R. (1977). Childhood behavior disorder—A family typology. *The Psychiatric Journal of the University of Ottawa, 2*, 84–88.

Warren, W. (1948). Acute neurotic breakdown in children with refusal to go to school. *Archives of Disease in Childhood, 23*, 266–272.

Weissman, M.M., Leckman, J.F., Merikangas, K.R., Gammon, G.D., & Prusoff, B.A. (1984). Depression and anxiety disorders in parents and children: Results from the Yale Family Study. *Archives of General Psychiatry, 41*, 845–852

CHAPTER 9

Phobic Disorders

CYD C. STRAUSS AND GRETA FRANCIS

DEFINITION

The third edition of the *Diagnostic and Statistical Manual of Mental Disorders* (American Psychiatric Association, 1980) presents a subgroup of anxiety disorders called phobic disorders. Phobic disorders are defined in the DSM-III as *persistent and irrational fears* of specific objects, activities, or situations that lead to a *strong desire to avoid* the feared stimulus. According to DSM-III, the fear is *recognized by the individual to be excessive or unreasonable* given the actual threat or danger to the individual when exposed to the situation. The fear significantly affects the individual's life such that he or she is *distressed about having the fear* or *the fear interferes with the individual's social, occupational, or role functioning*. If neither of these criteria is met, the fear is not considered to be a clinically diagnosable phobia. For example, a person may become quite fearful when actually in contact with snakes, but he or she may rarely encounter snakes in day-to-day activities. Therefore, the individual may not be bothered by the fear, it would not seem to impair his or her adjustment in any substantial manner, and consequently this fear would not be considered a phobia.

Thus it is important to differentiate normal *fears* that are commonly found in childhood and adolescence from *phobias* that are more intense, distressing, and persistent. A fear is a normal reaction to a genuine threat that discontinues once the feared stimulus is removed. Researchers have found that children and adolescents experience a variety of transient fears as a normal part of development (e.g., Graziano, DeGiovanni, & Garcia, 1979; Jersild & Holmes, 1935). In fact, Miller, Barrett, and Hampe (1974) included a developmental criterion, in addition to those presented in the DSM-III, to define a phobia occurring in childhood or adolescence. These authors noted that fears in children must not be age or stage specific in order to be considered clinical phenomena, based on their findings and those obtained by other researchers (Agras, Chapin, & Oliveau, 1972) that many childhood fears remit spontaneously. Graziano and colleagues (1979) similarly suggested that fears are clinically meaningful only when their intensity or duration is greater than found in most children. These definitions of phobias indicate that normative data for fears should be taken into account when defining and diagnosing phobias in childhood and adolescence.

Three subtypes of phobic disorders are described in DSM-III: social phobia, agoraphobia, and simple phobia. Social and simple phobias typically are related to specific stimuli, whereas agoraphobia tends to be more generalized and pervasive.

Social phobias are characterized by a persistent, irrational fear and compelling desire to avoid a situation in which the individual is exposed to possible scrutiny or evaluation by others. The child or adolescent is afraid that he or she may act in a manner that will be humiliating or embarrassing. As with all phobias, the individual is distressed about having the problem and perceives the level of fear to be excessive or unreasonable. According to DSM-III, social phobias cannot be due to another mental disorder, such as major depression or avoidant personality disorder.

The primary feature of agoraphobia consists of marked anxiety associated with being alone or in public places in which escape would be difficult or help might be unavailable in case the individual becomes incapacitated. Avoidance behavior becomes increasingly problematic, as the individual's normal activities are constricted and his or her life is dominated by fear and avoidance. In order to meet DSM-III criteria for agoraphobia, symptoms cannot be due to major depression, obsessive–compulsive disorder, paranoid personality disorder, or schizophrenia.

Finally, simple phobias are defined as persistent and irrational fears of objects or situations other than those associated with embarrassment or humiliation in social situations (as in social phobias) and with being alone or being in public places away from home (as in agoraphobia). Again, it is recognized by the child or adolescent that the fear is out of proportion to the circumstances and the phobia causes the child distress. A third criterion for the disorder is that the simple phobia cannot be due to another mental disorder, such as schizophrenia or obsessive–compulsive disorder.

HISTORICAL BACKGROUND

Formal psychiatric classification systems have acknowledged the presence of phobic reactions for approximately 35 years. The first edition of the *Diagnostic and Statistical Manual of Mental Disorders* (DSM) (APA, 1952) labeled phobias as psychoneurotic reactions. In 1968, the DSM-II (APA, 1968) changed the name to phobic neuroses. A phobic neurosis was defined as an intense fear of an object or situation recognized as not dangerous, and was characterized by apprehension in the forms of faintness, fatigue, palpitations, perspiration, nausea, tremor, or panic. Furthermore, psychoanalytic theory was clearly evident in the DSM-II, as the phobic reaction was attributed to fears displaced to the phobic object from some other object, of which the patient was unaware. In the DSM-III (1980), all psychoanalytic interpretation was removed, and specific diagnostic criteria for phobias were delineated. In addition, the three subtypes of phobias were differentiated.

CLINICAL PICTURE

Common types of *social phobias* occurring in childhood and adolescence are fears of speaking or performing in front of groups of people, eating or dressing in the presence of others, using public bathrooms, blushing, and writing in public. As stated in the DSM-III, individuals most commonly present with only one social phobia.

Examples of situations producing anxiety and avoidance in *agoraphobia* include fears of being in crowds, on elevators, on bridges, on public transportation, or in tunnels. People with agoraphobia typically require that a familiar person accompany them whenever they leave the home. Agoraphobia often begins with recurrent panic attacks, such that the individual demonstrates anticipatory anxiety of future panic attacks and refuses to enter situations associated with the occurrence of panic attacks. The onset of this disorder most commonly is observed in late adolescence or early adulthood. In fact, in our sample of 171 children and adolescents with anxiety disorders seen in the Child and Adolescent Anxiety Disorder Clinic at Western Psychiatric Institute and Clinic (for ages 5 to 18 years) during a 34-month period, only 3 adolescents were diagnosed with agoraphobia. Due to the low prevalence of this disorder in childhood and adolescence, this phobic disorder subtype will not be discussed further in this chapter, and instead the reader is referred to reviews of adult anxiety disorders that provide extensive research related to this disorder (e.g., Mavissakalian & Barlow, 1981; O'Brien & Barlow, 1984; Tuma & Maser, 1985).

Common *simple phobias* exhibited in the general population of children and adolescents include marked fears of animals, heights, darkness, and thunderstorms (cf. Ollendick, 1979). In our clinic sample of children, types of simple phobias observed were phobias of school, vomiting, needles, dogs, heights, closed places, fire, escalators or elevators, and eating certain foods.

The most common form of either simple or social phobias in clinic samples of children or adolescents is *school phobia*, in which the child shows a phobic reaction to some aspect of the school environment. School phobia can be due to fears of specific objects or situations in the school setting, such as a particular teacher, fights with peers, or vomiting that may occur at school. In this case, the phobia would be conceptualized as a simple phobia. On the other hand, a phobia of school may be related to an exaggerated fear that the child or adolescent may act in a manner at school that would be humiliating or embarrassing to him or her. For example, the child or adolescent may show a persistent fear of, and thus avoid, school because he or she is excessively uncomfortable dressing in front of others in gym, is overly concerned about performing poorly in front of others in the classroom or in gym, or is afraid of eating in front of others at the school cafeteria. These types of phobic responses would be viewed as social phobias. Thus, although the DSM-III does not present a separate diagnosis of school phobia, this particular type of phobic reaction can be diagnosed as either a simple or social phobia of school. Due to the high prevalence of school phobia, we will examine this subtype separately.

ASSOCIATED FEATURES

Most information regarding the factors associated with phobic disorders has been derived from an extensive literature on factors associated with subclinical childhood fears and/or school phobia. We will discuss the relationship between phobic disorders and depression, other fears, intelligence, externalizing behavior problems, low self-esteem, dependence, and concurrent DSM-III anxiety diagnoses.

Depression

Anxiety and depression often have been found to coexist as part of an "internalizing" dimension of childhood psychopathology (e.g., Achenbach & Edelbrock, 1978). However, very little empirical data are available regarding the relationship between depression and specific phobias in children and adolescents. Last and colleagues (Last, Francis, Hersen, Kazdin, & Strauss, 1987) examined concurrent DSM-III diagnoses in a group of 19 school-phobic children and adolescents. They reported that one-third of these children presented with concurrent affective disorders (primarily major depression).

Additional data from our clinic sample of phobic children and adolescents suggest that children with social phobias report significantly more depressive symptoms than do children with simple phobias. On the Children's Depression Inventory (CDI: Kovacs, 1980–1981), the mean score for children with social phobias was 14.3 compared to a mean score of 9.9 for children with simple phobias. Smucker, Craighead, Craighead, and Green (1986) reported the overall mean on the CDI to be a score of 9, and stated that a cutoff score of 19 identified the upper 10% of the population. As such, it appears that, although social phobics report higher CDI scores than do simple phobics, neither group reported significant depressive symptomatology overall.

Subclinical Fears

A plethora of data indicate that multiple mild fears are common in children (e.g., Hagman, 1932; Jersild & Holmes, 1935; Lapouse & Monk, 1959; MacFarlane, Allen, & Honzik, 1954; Miller, Barrett, Hampe, & Noble, 1973). Ollendick (1983) examined the fears of 25 clinic-referred school-phobic children and 25 matched controls using the Fear Survey Schedule for Children–Revised. He found that school-phobic males and females reported significantly higher total fear scores than did male and female controls. In our clinic sample of phobic children and adolescents we have found that school-phobic adolescents report more social–evaluative fears than do separation-anxious adolescents (Francis, Strauss, & Last, 1988).

Intelligence

Ollendick and Mayer (1984) reported that high, average, and low IQ were represented equally among school-phobic children. In addition, they did not find a disproportionate number of learning disabilities in school-phobic children as compared to non–school-phobic children.

Externalizing Behavior Problems

In general, a relationship between childhood phobias and externalizing behavior problems has not been supported in the literature. For example, Lapouse and Monk (1959) found no significant correlation between phobias and other deviant behaviors, such as bed-wetting or temper tantrums. Similarly, MacFarlane and colleagues (1954) reported low correlations between childhood phobias and irritability or temper tantrums. After reviewing the literature on childhood phobias, Graziano and colleagues (1979) suggested that the *intensity* of the phobic reaction may be related to other pathological behavior such as temper tantrums. Currently, this remains an empirical question.

Self-Esteem

Leventhall and Sills (1964) proposed that school-phobic children may overvalue themselves and their achievements. This hypothesis was tested by Nichols and Berg (1970), who found no statistically significant difference in self-evaluation (esteem) between school-phobic (both chronic and acute onset) and normal children. In fact, contrary to Leventhall and Sills' prediction, school-phobic children tended to report lower self-esteem than did normal children.

Dependence

Berg and colleagues (Berg & McGuire, 1971; Berg, Nichols, & Pritchard, 1969) have suggested that school-phobic children are overly dependent on their mothers. These authors found increased dependence, as assessed via self-report, in chronic school refusers. As they did not distinguish between school refusal due to separation anxiety and school refusal due to a phobic reaction to some aspect of school itself, it remains unclear whether children with a phobic reaction to school indeed are more dependent than nonphobic children.

Concurrent DSM-III Anxiety Diagnoses

In our clinic sample of phobic children we have examined the relationship between phobias and concurrent anxiety diagnoses. We found that 72% of school phobics, 78% of simple phobics, and 67% of social phobics received no additional phobia diagnoses. Thus, in general, we did not find multiple phobias in our sample. However, we did find that many of our phobic children presented with additional, nonphobia, anxiety diagnoses. In fact, 38% of school phobics, 50% of simple phobics, and 67% of social phobics presented concurrently with overanxious disorder.

COURSE AND PROGNOSIS

Studies of subclinical fears indicate a change in the number and type of fears over the course of childhood and adolescence (cf. Graziano et al., 1979). Graziano and colleagues (1979) noted that in general the number of fears reported, as well as the percentage of youngsters reporting one or more fears, appears to decline from early childhood to adolescence. Some studies have demonstrated an increase in the number of reported fears between the ages of 9 and 11 (e.g., MacFarlane et al., 1954), with a peak occurring at age 11 (e.g., Chazan, 1962). However, not all studies have obtained significant correlations between number of fears and age (e.g., Croake & Knox, 1973; Lapouse & Monk, 1959).

With regard to variations in types of fears over the course of childhood, Graziano and colleagues (1979) found in their review of the literature that there seems to be an age-related decrease in reported fears of animals, the dark, and imaginary creatures and an increase in school and social anxieties. For example, 80% of children 5 to 6 years old were found to express a fear of animals, whereas 23% of children 13 to 14 reported this fear (Maurer, 1965). On the other hand, realistic fears (e.g., physical danger, natural hazards, school achievement, loss, and social relationship problems) are infrequent in young children but become more common by early adolescence (Bauer, 1976; Maurer, 1965). An epidemiological study conducted by Agras, Sylvester, and Oliveau (1969) substantiated this latter finding. From childhood to adulthood there was a sharp increase in the prevalence of subclinical fears of snakes, crowds, injection, and other realistic fears. However, most of these fears *began* in childhood and persisted into adolescence; thus the increased prevalence of realistic fears in adolescence seems to reflect an accumulation of fears over age rather than a peak onset during the adolescent period.

Age of onset of phobic levels of fear is apparently related to their stability over time. Agras and colleagues (1972) found that phobias for persons under age 20 were far less persistent than for adults. Indeed, 100% of untreated phobias of children and adolescents had remitted within 5 years. On the other hand, there are preliminary data that some fears are more persistent than others. Agras and colleagues (1972) indicated that more specific and focused fears were associated with better long-term outcome.

Different prognoses may in fact be associated with distinct types of anxiety and with varying levels of severity of fearfulness. In particular, follow-up data for school-phobic children have suggested that this form of anxiety is related to later problems in adjustment (Coolidge, Brodie, & Feeney, 1964; Waldron, 1976). In a large-scale study conducted by Berg, Butler, and Hall (1976), school phobia cases that began in adolescence were followed over a 3-year period. One-third showed no remaining symptoms, but one-third had changed little and the remaining third demonstrated other neurotic symptoms. One-half still had serious school attendance problems and 6 of the 125 patients had developed agoraphobia. Moreover, a 10-year follow-up study of 168 school refusers, originally treated in an adolescent inpatient unit, revealed that almost half required additional psychiatric treatment during the follow-up period (Berg & Jackson, 1985).

The importance of age of onset in our understanding of phobic disorders in childhood and adolescence can be seen further in studies of adults with clinical phobias. The less disabling phobias (e.g., simple phobias) tend to have an earlier onset than more disabling ones (e.g., agoraphobia). Sheehan, Sheehan, and Minichiello (1981) found that 31% of adults with simple phobias reported an onset before 9 years of age and 26% reported onset between ages 10 and 19. In contrast, they found that only 4% of adult agoraphobics reported the onset of their disorder before age 9, but 26% reported onset between 10 and 19 years of age. Marks and Gelder (1966) similarly found that adult patients with specific animal phobias reported a mean age of onset of 4.4 years, whereas most adults with specific situation phobias, social anxieties, and agoraphobia reported an onset in adolescence or later.

Other studies of adult agoraphobics have suggested that school phobia may be a significant precursor. Klein (1964) and Berg (1976) found that agoraphobia that begins in late adolescence or early adulthood is often preceded by school phobia in early adolescence. However, two other studies suggest that the relationship between adolescent school phobia and adult anxiety disorders is not a specific one. Berg, Marks, McGuire, and Lipsedge (1974) found that about one-fourth of both adult agoraphobics and adults with other neurotic disorders reported adolescent school phobia. Similarly, Tyrer and Tyrer (1974) found that school phobia was more common in the developmental histories of phobic, anxious, and depressed adults than in those of normal adults, but the three psychiatric groups did not differ in this respect. However, they did find that the risk of later neurotic disorder was greater for female than for male school phobics. These retrospective studies have important limitations and, clearly, more longitudinal data must be obtained.

IMPAIRMENT AND COMPLICATIONS

Social Phobia

Social phobias seldom are incapacitating in childhood and adolescence. Avoidance of phobic situations may cause inconveniences, however. For example, an adolescent's phobic reaction to eating in public places may cause the youngster to postpone meals until alone. A social phobia of using public bathrooms may cause a child not to go to the bathroom throughout the school day. Vacation trips may have to be avoided due to this difficulty.

Sometimes impairment may be more extensive, such that children with social phobias occurring within the school environment may not be able to avoid confrontation with the feared stimulus while at school and consequently may refuse to attend school. For example, a child who cannot avoid dressing in front of others for gym class may not attend school at all.

In rare cases of children or adolescents with social phobias, there may be pervasive disruption to the youngster's life. Children may fear humiliation or embarrassment in many different social situations, so that they eventually avoid multiple social settings in order to avoid scrutiny of their behavior. The avoidance behavior may be pervasive so that the individual's normal activities are increasingly constricted, as in agoraphobia; however, the reason for pervasive avoidance is different for these two anxiety disorder subtypes. In agoraphobia, situations are avoided due to fear that the person will be incapacitated and unable to escape the circumstance; on the other hand, the activities of the social phobic may be limited severely because of intense fear of negative evaluation or humiliation. A person with social phobia may avoid most or all activities outside the home due to an extreme fear of embarrassment in social situations.

Simple Phobia

There is a wide range of impairment for individuals with simple phobias. The extent of impairment is related directly to the degree to which the phobic stimulus is encountered in the person's daily life. A phobia of an object with which the person is rarely in contact (e.g., snakes, fire) may not interfere to any significant degree with the person's functioning. On the other hand, if the feared stimulus is a routine or necessary part of the person's life, there can be major disruption. Examples include an excessive fear of needles for a diabetic requiring daily insulin shots or of elevators for a child whose family lives on the fifteenth floor of an apartment building.

School Phobia

School phobia typically causes considerable disruption to the child's academic and social functioning, since children with this disorder almost always refuse to attend school. Because of frequent school absenteeism the child or adolescent often falls significantly behind in classwork and loses contact with peers. It may be necessary for the child or adolescent to repeat a grade because of high rates of absenteeism. Due to embarrassment associated with excessive absenteeism, school phobics may begin to avoid social interactions outside of the school setting. It is not uncommon for youngsters with school phobia to exhibit major depression secondary to a phobia of school.

EPIDEMIOLOGY

The primary focus of epidemiological research to date has been on simple phobias and school phobia, whereas only one recent study has been reported in the literature concerning the epidemiology of social phobia in childhood and adolescence.

Prevalence

Although the prevalence of common fears in children has been studied fairly extensively, investigations of the rate of clinically meaningful anxiety disorders in children are rare. Estimates of the prevalence of excessive fears or anxieties primarily were obtained prior to the publication of DSM-III and generally ranged from 0.4% in a study assessing the rate of school phobia in a Venezuelan school population (Granell de Aldaz, Vivas, Gelfand, & Feldman, 1984) to 14% in a study of 3-year-old children in a community in the United States (Earls, 1980).

One recent study investigated the prevalence of DSM-III disorders in 792 11-year-old children from the general population in New Zealand (Anderson, Williams, McGee, & Silva, 1987). DSM-III diagnoses were based on information obtained from structured child interviews and standardized parent and teacher questionnaires. These authors determined prevalence rates at different levels, depending on degree of agreement among the three sources of information (child, parent, teacher). When prevalence rates were based on cases for which diagnostic criteria were met by one source without confirming symptoms by other sources (situational), the prevalence rate for simple phobias was found to be 2.4%. Social phobias were less common, with 0.9% of these preadolescent children demonstrating this phobic disorder subtype. Using a more conservative approach to identify phobic disorders, such that diagnostic criteria were met by one source and confirmed by one or both other sources, no children in this sample were diagnosed with simple or social phobias.

Table 9.1 summarizes studies of prevalence rates found for childhood and adolescent fears and phobias. The broad range of prevalence rates found across studies may be due to differing age groups studied, varying criteria used to define fears or phobias, and different methods used to identify and measure fearfulness.

In our clinic sample of children and adolescents referred for evaluation and treatment of anxiety disorders, 31% were diagnosed with phobic disorders. More specifically, 16.9% had a simple or social phobia of school, 10.5% had some other type of simple phobia, and 8.8% were diagnosed with a social phobia other than that of school. Thus the most common type of phobia observed in our clinic sample of anxious children was a phobia of school.

Sex Differences

A fairly consistent finding across studies of community samples of children and adolescents is that girls tend to report more fears and worries than do boys (Abe & Masui, 1981; Anderson et al., 1987; Earls, 1980; Lapouse & Monk, 1958; Richman, Stevenson, & Graham, 1975). The only study directly evaluating the relative prevalence of DSM-III phobic disorders in a community sample (Anderson et al., 1987) showed that the sex ratio (M:F) was 0.6:1 for simple phobia and 0.2:1 for social phobia. It is unclear, however, whether the higher rate of fears reported for girls actually reflects a greater prevalence of fearfulness in girls or a greater willingness by girls and their parents to admit to girls having fears (Graziano et al., 1979).

In addition to findings demonstrating that the number of fears reported by females differs from that found for males in the general population, types of fears reported by each gender appear to differ as well (Abe & Masui, 1981; Lapouse & Monk, 1959; Spiegler & Lambert, 1970). For example, Abe and Masui (1981) found that girls report fears of lightning, going outdoors, blushing, and being looked at, whereas boys report higher levels of a fear of talking.

TABLE 9.1. Prevalence of Fears and Phobias in Children and Adolescents

Investigation or Sample Studied	Fear or Phobia	Prevalence
Simple Fears and Phobias		
Lapouse & Monk (1953) 1600 children 6 to 12 years old in U.S. community sample	"Many fears and worries" (7 or more)	43%
Agras, Sylvester, & Oliveau (1969) 325 adults and children in U.S. community sample	Simple phobias	7.7%
Richman, Stevenson, & Graham (1975) 705 children 3 years old in U.K. community sample	Fears	12.8%
Kastrup (1976) 175 children 5 and 6 years old in Denmark community sample	Fears	3% (boys) 5% (girls)
Earls (1980) 100 children 3 years old in U.S. community sample	Fears	14%
Abe & Masui (1981) 2500 Japanese subjects 11 to 23 years old	Fears	2%–43%
Anderson, Williams, McGee, & Silva (1987) 792 children 11 years old in U.S. community sample	DSM-III simple phobias	2.4% ± 1.1%
School Phobia		
Kennedy (1965) General population estimate	School phobia	1.7%
Baker & Wills (1978) 1300 clinic children greater than 12 years	School phobia	7.6%
Smith (1970) 370 London outpatient clinic children	School phobia	3.8%
Granell de Aldaz, Vivas, Gelfand, & Feldman (1984) 1034 children 3 to 14 years old in Venezuelan community sample	School phobia	0.4–1.5% (range of criteria used)

In our clinic sample of 171 children and adolescents referred with anxiety disorders, females more commonly received DSM-III diagnoses of simple and social phobias than did males, a finding consistent with sex differences observed in the rate of subclinical fears and phobias in community samples. On the other hand, males (71%) more frequently were found to have school phobia than were females (29%). The latter finding is in contrast to previous reports of an equal prevalence of clinically significant school phobia in males and females (Granell de Aldaz et al., 1984; Kennedy, 1965; Smith, 1970). Perhaps the discrepancy between sex ratios found in our clinic sample and those included in previous studies is due to different criteria employed to define school phobia, since our diagnoses of school phobia are based on DSM-III criteria for phobia whereas previous studies have employed alternative defining criteria. It is interesting to note that females in our clinic sample with school avoidance were more likely to be diagnosed with separation anxiety disorder than with simple phobia (Last, Francis, et al., 1987), thus suggesting that anxiety related to school attendance may be equally prevalent in males and females but the source of anxiety may be distinct.

Socioeconomic Status

Some studies report a higher number of fears in low-socioeconomic-status (SES) children (e.g., Croake & Knox, 1973; Lapouse & Monk, 1959), although other investigations do not find a differential rate of fears among different SES groups (e.g., Richman et al., 1975). Types of fears have consistently been found to differ for children from low-SES and high-SES families. For example, Angelino, Dollins, and Mech (1956) found that lower-SES boys feared switchblades, whippings, robbers and killers, guns, and other stimuli associated with violence, whereas higher-SES boys feared car accidents, getting killed, juvenile delinquents, and disaster. Low- and high-SES girls also were found to differ in the kinds of fears they reported. Data regarding the relationship between phobic disorders and SES are not yet available for clinic populations of children and adolescents.

FAMILIAL PATTERNS

Most available information regarding the familial patterns of childhood phobias is based on clinical descriptions of the family relationships of children with school phobia. For example, Hersov (1960) described three types of family patterns for school phobia: (1) Type I—an overindulgent mother and a passive father; (2) Type II—an overcontrolled mother and a passive father; and (3) Type III—an overindulgent mother and a firm father. Each family pattern was thought to be associated with a different kind of school-phobic child. That is, the Type I child was demanding at home and passive at school; the Type II child was obedient at home and timid at school; and the Type III child was willful at home and friendly at school. Unfortunately, however, no empirical studies have examined Hersov's family subtypes.

Recently, empirical investigations have examined the relationship between child and family psychopathology. Researchers have begun to look at both the parents of school-phobic children and the children of anxiety-disordered parents. Studies of the parents of school-phobic children have reported inconsistent findings. Gittelman-Klein (1975) interviewed the parents of school-phobic children and hyperactive children. She reported no differences between the groups in the rates of major depression or simple phobias in parents. However, the parents of school-phobic children had higher rates of separation anxiety disorder (19%) than did parents of hyperactive children (2%).

Berg and his colleagues (Berg, Butler, & Pritchard, 1974) examined the hospital records of school-phobic and nonschool-phobic adolescents in order to assess maternal psychopathology. They found no increase in anxiety disorders in the mothers of school-phobic adolescents as compared to the mothers of nonschool-phobic adolescents.

A small number of studies have discovered a relationship between parent and child phobias. Bandura and Menlove (1968) found that parents and their children frequently shared a common phobia of dogs. They examined the presence of dog phobias in the parents of children with and without dog phobias. The parents of nonphobic children rarely showed any fear of dogs, while more than half of the parents of children with dog phobias themselves had this phobia. Similarly, Solyom, Beck, Solyom, and Hugel (1974) diagnosed phobias in 30.9% of the mothers of their sample of phobic children. This rate was significantly higher than that found in the mothers of nonphobic control children (7.7%). No relationship was reported between paternal and child phobias.

More recently, Last and colleagues (Last, Francis, et al., 1987) interviewed the mothers of children with specific phobias of school and children with separation anxiety disorder. They reported that the mothers of both groups of children presented similarly high lifetime histories of anxiety disorders. However, mothers of school-phobic children were less likely to evidence lifetime histories of affective disorders. Only 14% of the mothers of school-phobic children had histories of affective disorders as compared to 63% of the mothers of separation-anxious children.

Other researchers have assessed the children of anxious parents (e.g., Berg, 1976; Buglass, Clarke, Henderson, Kreitman, & Presley, 1977). Again, both positive and negative findings have been reported. Berg (1976) examined the children of a large group of agoraphobic mothers. He found that 14% of the children of agoraphobic mothers had school phobia. This rate was higher than would be expected in the general population. In contrast, Buglass and colleagues (1977) studied the children of a small group of agoraphobic mothers and nonagoraphobic mothers. They found no cases of school phobia in any of the children.

In summary, equivocal findings have been reported both from studies of the parents of school-phobic children and from studies of the children of anxiety-disordered parents. However, these findings are suggestive of familial factors that need to be examined further.

DIFFERENTIAL DIAGNOSIS

Social Phobia

Social phobias in children and adolescents need to be differentiated from *normal fears* of embarrassment frequently experienced in this age group. For example, it is not uncommon for children and adolescents to express discomfort associated with public speaking. However, the persistence of extreme anxiety in the feared circumstance and compelling desire to avoid such situations are not present in nonphobic children and adolescents. In addition, children and adolescents with normal levels of social fears rarely indicate that they are distressed about having the fear and seldom describe the fear to be excesssive relative to that of their peers.

Social phobias also need to be distinguished from overanxious disorder in childhood and adolescence. As discussed in DSM-III, social phobias tend to involve a circumscribed stimulus that the individual fears and tends to avoid, and people generally have only one social phobia. Children diagnosed with overanxious disorder may also show extreme discomfort associated with situations involving possible scrutiny by others, but they do not necessarily display avoidance behavior; instead they tend to have a pervasive discomfort associated with multiple situations in which their behavior may be evaluated (e.g., school performance, social interactions with peers, performance in gym). In addition, children and adolescents with overanxious disorder demonstrate additional symptoms that are not present in youngsters with social phobias, such as an excessive need for reassurance, somatic complaints, and marked feelings of tension or an inability to relax.

Social phobia and avoidant disorder also must be differentiated in children and adolescents. Avoidant disorder diagnoses are reserved for those children and adolescents who become very fearful of, and thus have a compelling desire to avoid, social situations involving unfamiliar persons. Children with avoidant disorder may be overconcerned with possible embarrassment and humiliation when around strangers. Social phobia should not be diagnosed when the anxiety is limited to interactions with strangers.

Children and adolescents with major depression, schizophrenia or obsessive–compulsive disorder may exhibit anxiety and avoidance of social interactions. Social phobia should not be diagnosed when the phobia is due to any of these disorders. Finally, simple phobias also involve an excessive fear and avoidance of a circumscribed stimulus, but a fear of social situations involving possible scrutiny, humiliation, and embarrassment is not present.

Simple Phobia

As in diagnoses of social phobias, simple phobias are not diagnosed when the fear is considered developmentally appropriate and is not in excess of that experienced by same-age peers. There is no significant distress about having the fear in children and adolescents with subclinical fears.

In overanxious disorder, the individual has multiple fears and worries, and anxiety is not restricted to a single stimulus or situation as in simple phobias. The predominant feature of overanxious disorder is excessive worrying about a variety of past and future events, and it does not necessarily involve avoidance behavior. Furthermore, children with a simple phobia do not show the whole constellation of symptoms associated with overanxious disorder.

Simple phobias also should not be diagnosed when certain activities are avoided in response to delusions, as in schizophrenia. In addition, a simple phobia should not be diagnosed when the anxiety and avoidance are associated with obsessive–compulsive disorder, such as when a child avoids situations in which he or she fears contamination from dirt or germs.

School Phobia

Children with school phobia need to be differentiated from nonphobic children who state that they do not like school. It is common in the general population for children to express lack of interest in school or dislike for school, but anxiety is absent in nonphobic children. Also, mild levels of anxiety are characteristic of children who are entering a new school, and temporary demonstration of anxiety and reluctance is not considered clinically meaningful.

In addition, simple or social phobias of school often must be distinguished from school refusal associated with separation anxiety disorder, major depression, and conduct disorder or oppositional disorder. In separation anxiety disorder, the child or adolescent avoids school because of a fear of being separated from a major attachment figure (usually the mother) or from home, rather than because of a fear stemming from some aspect of the school environment. Children who refuse to go to school due to separation anxiety disorder usually will show distress in other situations in which they must be separated from a major attachment figure (e.g., are unable to stay home when the mother goes visiting, are unable to play with other children away from home, are unable to sleep away from home).

Children and adolescents with major depression may be reluctant to attend school or resistant because they are experiencing decreased interest or motivation, fatigue and lethargy, and a diminished ability to concentrate. Children who refuse to go to school due to major depression do not report anxiety or fear about going to school and do not experience physical symptoms in the mornings before school, as do children with simple or social phobias of school.

Children and adolescents who do not attend school because of conduct disorder or oppositional disorder (i.e., truancy) do not go to school simply because they do not want to go and do not report symptoms of anxiety or depression related to school attendance. These children will typically show other conduct problem behaviors, such as excessive lying, frequent fighting, stealing, running away from home, and so on.

CLINICAL MANAGEMENT: RESEARCH FINDINGS

A small number of excellent review articles are available summarizing the clinical and research literature on the treatment of childhood fears and phobias (e.g., Graziano et al., 1979; Hatzenbuehler & Schroeder, 1978; Ollendick & Mayer, 1984). Graziano and colleagues (1979) and Hatzenbuehler and Schroeder (1978) reviewed studies of childhood phobias other than school phobia. In contrast, Ollendick and Mayer (1984) reviewed only studies of school phobia. For purposes of clarity, we will discuss the treatment of school phobia separately.

First we will discuss the treatment of childhood phobias other than school phobia. It is important to note that the vast majority of the treatment literature for childhood phobias consists of uncontrolled case reports of the treatment of mild to moderate fears in nonreferred children. Very few controlled single-case or group studies exist. Although the need for more rigorous experimentation is apparent, we are able to gain some knowledge of the efficacy of certain therapeutic techniques based on currently available data. Treatment studies of childhood fears and phobias typically have employed systematic desensitization, modeling, and/or cognitive–behavioral techniques.

A number of researchers have examined the use of desensitization procedures in the treatment of childhood phobias. Most published studies of desensitization have included the concurrent use of operant, contingency management techniques. In general, the evidence for the use of desensitization procedures in the treatment of childhood phobias is equivocal. Both positive and negative results have been reported. For example, Miller and colleagues (1972) and Kelley (1976) found that desensitization produced no changes above and beyond what was seen in a waiting list control group. In contrast, positive results have been reported using complex desensitization plus modeling plus contingency management approaches (e.g., Leitenberg & Callahan, 1973; Mann, 1972; Mann & Rosenthal, 1969). Therefore, Graziano and colleagues (1979) concluded that the efficacy of desensitization approaches alone for the treatment of childhood phobias has not been established.

The most widely researched treatment approach for childhood simple phobias has been modeling. Typically, the use of modeling requires that the fearful child first observe a model demonstrating approach to the feared object or situation, followed by the child himself or herself attempting approach. A number of procedural variants can be employed, including videotaped versus live models, single versus multiple models, similar versus dissimilar models, and modeling with and without additional interventions (e.g., desensitization). Graziano and colleagues (1979) concluded that modeling is an effective treatment for childhood phobia, particularly when used in conjunction with graduated exposure and when live, similar models are included. A number of potentially important variables in the use of modeling in the treatment of childhood phobias have been examined empirically only recently. For example, Kornhaber and Schroeder (1975) suggested that the use of mastery versus coping models may influence treatment outcome and maintenance. In addition, some have questioned whether modeling techniques are practical for the treatment of childhood social phobias (Graziano et al., 1979). In this regard, some investigators have reported good results for the use of videotaped modeling with socially withdrawn or fearful children, who may bear some resemblance to socially phobic children (O'Connor, 1969). However, Gelfand (1978) cautioned that a substantial number of studies have failed to show positive results with modeling alone as a treatment for social withdrawal. Moreover, the actual similarity between social withdrawal and social phobia has not been assessed empirically.

Finally, there is some promising evidence for the use of cognitive techniques to treat childhood phobias. Kanfer, Karoly, and Newman (1975) compared the use of coping and competency self-statements (e.g., "I am a brave boy/girl"), fear-reduction self-statements (e.g., "The dark is a fun place to be"), and neutral self-statements (e.g., "Mary had a little lamb") in the treatment of fear of the dark in 5- and 6-year-old nonclinic children. Coping and competency self-statements were found to be the most effective in decreasing anxiety and avoidance. Clearly, more investigations of this cognitive treatment procedure are needed in clinic-referred populations of phobic children.

In her review of treatment studies of childhood phobias, Harris (1983) concluded:

> Modeling techniques have been most carefully studied and have the best empirical support while systematic desensitization, with a more limited data base, has not been convincingly shown to be effective, and cognitive behavioral approaches, although interesting, are in a preliminary state of development. (p. 528)

Other researchers have reached similar conclusions (e.g., Graziano et al., 1979).

The treatment of school phobia has been attempted using many of the same procedures described earlier. Ollendick and Mayer (1984) reviewed the school phobia literature and discussed the use of exposure (i.e., desensitization or flooding), operant procedures, and modeling. Almost all the available studies of the treatment of school phobia are uncontrolled case studies. Thus conclusions regarding treatment efficacy are tentative.

Desensitization treatment of school phobia has been reported to be successful in a number of case studies. For example, Garvey and Hegrenes (1966) used *in vivo* desensitization to treat successfully an adolescent with school phobia. Their hierarchy progressed gradually from sitting in a car in front of the school to being present in the full classroom. Of note, the authors also had the therapist accompany the adolescent through the hierarchy; therefore, desensitization plus modeling more fully describes this treatment.

Blagg and Yule (1984) compared the use of flooding, psychotherapy, and inpatient hospitalization in their treatment study of school refusal. The authors reported that flooding was more successful than psychotherapy or inpatient hospitalization in increasing school attendance. As the authors included both school refusal due to separation anxiety and school refusal due to a phobia of school, the efficacy of flooding for phobias of school per se is not clear.

Desensitization procedures also have been used in conjunction with pharmacotherapy. Specifically, Gittelman-Klein and Klein (1971) conducted a controlled double-blind placebo study of the treatment of school refusal and separation anxiety. The authors compared a multifaceted psychosocial intervention (which included *in vivo* exposure) with and without imipramine. Results indicated that imipramine plus psychosocial treatment was superior to placebo plus psychosocial treatment in facilitating return to school. Again, the efficacy of imipramine plus psychosocial treatment specifically for children with a phobia of school is not known, as phobic and separation-anxious children were not differentiated in this study.

Contingency management procedures also have been used successfully in the treatment of school phobia (e.g., Ayllon, Smith, & Rogers, 1970; Hersen, 1970; Rines, 1973). Typically these procedures require that the reinforcement value of school attendance is increased while the reinforcement value of staying at home is decreased. For example, teacher, parent, or peer approval of school atttendance may be used in conjunction with a rule against television watching if the child is at home during the school day.

Ollendick and Mayer (1984) reported that there are no studies of the use of modeling alone to treat school phobia. Modeling has been used concurrently with desensitization as described earlier in the Garvey and Hegrenes (1966) study. The use of parent or therapist models in conjunction with graduated exposure does appear to be an effective treatment.

In sum, treatment studies of childhood phobias, even with their methodological limitations, are suggestive of a number of viable treatment approaches including systematic desensitization plus modeling, modeling alone, and contingency management. Although empirical evaluations of the efficacy of cognitive therapy in the treatment of childhood phobias are few in number, this approach does show promise.

Furthermore, certain variables may influence both the selection and outcome of treatment. For example, age of onset appears to be an important variable in selecting treatment and predicting outcome for school-phobic children. Kennedy (1965) reported that for young children with an abrupt onset of school avoidance the most effective treatment approach was forcing the child to return to school as quickly as possible. In contrast, for older children with a lengthy history of school avoidance, often the most effective treatment approach was graduated exposure. Similarly, Atkinson, Quarrington, and Cyr (1985), in their review of the treatment of school refusal, reported that age is an important predictor of sustained impairment. That is, they found that older school phobics were more severely impaired in both the long and the short term. Further assessment of variables that may predict response to treatment (e.g., presence of concurrent diagnoses in the child, family interaction patterns) would facilitate the selection of specific treatment methods for individual children.

DSM-III-R

The major changes in the phobia diagnoses in the DSM-III-R (APA, 1987) involve specifying additional diagnostic criteria for simple and social phobias. The essential features of phobias according to the DSM-III were: (1) persistent fear *and* compelling desire to avoid; (2) marked distress *and* recognition that the fear is excessive or unreasonable; and (3) not due to another psychiatric disorder. In contrast, the diagnostic criteria for both simple and social phobias according to DSM-III-R include the following: (1) persistent fear; (2) during some phase of the disturbance, exposure to the feared object or situation almost always produces an immediate anxiety response; (3) the object or situation is avoided, *or* endured with dread; (4) occupational or social functioning is impaired *or* the person has marked distress because of the fear; (5) recognition that the fear is excessive or unreasonable. As in DSM-III, the phobic stimulus must be unrelated to other psychiatric disorders.

REFERENCES

Abe, K., & Masui, T. (1981). Age-sex trends of phobic and anxiety symptoms in adolescents. *British Journal of Psychiatry, 138,* 297–302.

Achenbach, T.M., & Edelbrock, C.S. (1978). The classification of child psychopathology: A review and analysis of empirical efforts. *Psychological Bulletin, 85,* 1275–1301.

Agras, W.S., Chapin, H.H., & Oliveau, D.C. (1972). The natural history of phobia. *Archives of General Psychiatry, 26,* 315–317.

Agras, W.S., Sylvester, D., & Oliveau, D. (1969). The epidemiology of common fears and phobias. *Comprehensive Psychiatry, 10,* 151–156.

American Psychiatric Association (1952). *Diagnostic and statistical manual of mental disorders.* Washington, DC: Author.

American Psychiatric Association (1968). *Diagnostic and statistical manual of mental disorders* (2nd ed.). Washington, DC: Author.

American Psychiatric Association (1980). *Diagnostic and statistical manual of mental disorders* (3rd ed.). Washington, DC: Author.

American Psychiatric Association (1987). *Diagnostic and statistical manual of mental disorders* (3rd ed., rev.). Washington, DC: Author.

Anderson, J.C., Williams, S., McGee, R., & Silva, P.A. (1987). DSM-III disorders in preadolescent children. *Archives of General Psychiatry, 44*, 69–76.

Angelino, H., Dollins, J., & Mech, E.V. (1956). Trends in the "fear and worries" of school children as related to socioeconomic status and age. *Journal of Genetic Psychology, 89*, 263–276.

Atkinson, L., Quarrington, B., & Cyr, J.J. (1985). School refusal: The heterogeneity of a concept. *American Journal of Orthopsychiatry, 55*, 83–101.

Ayllon, T., Smith, D., & Rogers, M. (1970). Behavioral management of school phobia. *Journal of Behavior Therapy & Experimental Psychiatry, 1*, 125–138.

Bandura, A., & Menlove, F. (1968). Factors determining vicarious extinction of avoidance behavior through symbolic modeling. *Journal of Personality & Social Psychology, 8*, 99–108.

Bauer, D.H. (1976). An exploratory study of developmental changes in children's fears. *Journal of Child Psychology & Psychiatry, 17*, 69–74.

Berg, I. (1976). School phobia in children of agoraphobic women. *British Journal of Psychiatry, 128*, 86–89.

Berg, I., Butler, A., & Hall, J. (1976). The outcome of adolescent school phobia. *British Journal of Psychiatry, 128*, 80–85.

Berg, I., Butler, A., & Pritchard, J. (1974). Psychiatric illness in the mothers of school-phobic adolescents. *British Journal of Psychiatry, 125*, 466–467.

Berg, I., & Jackson, A. (1985). Teenage school refusers grow up: A follow-up study of 168 subjects, ten years on average after inpatient treatment. *British Journal of Psychiatry, 147*, 366–370.

Berg, I., Marks, I., McGuire, R., & Lipsedge, M. (1974). School phobia and agoraphobia. *Psychological Medicine, 4*, 428–434.

Berg, I., & McGuire, R. (1971). Are school phobic adolescents overdependent? *British Journal of Psychiatry, 119*, 167–168.

Berg, I., Nichols, K., & Pritchard, C. (1969). School phobia—Its classification and relationship to dependency. *Journal of Child Psychology & Psychiatry, 10*, 123–141.

Blagg, N.R., & Yule, W. (1984). The behavioral treatment of school refusal—A comparative study. *Behaviour Research & Therapy, 22*, 119–127.

Buglass, D., Clarke, J., Henderson, A.S., Kreitman, N., & Presley, A.S. (1977). A study of agoraphobic housewives. *Psychological Medicine, 7*, 73–86.

Chazan, M. (1962). School phobia. *British Journal of Educational Psychology, 32*, 209–217.

Coolidge, J., Brodie, R., & Feeney, B. (1964). A ten-year follow-up study of sixty-six school-phobic children. *American Journal of Orthopsychiatry, 34*, 675–684.

Croake, J.W., & Knox, F.H. (1973). The changing nature of children's fears. *Child Study Journal, 3*, 91–105.

Earls, F. (1980). Prevalence of behavior problems in three-year-old children. A cross-national replication. *Archives of General Psychiatry, 37*, 1153–1157.

Francis, G., Strauss, C.C., & Last, C.G. (1988). *Social anxiety in school phobic adolescents.* Unpublished manuscript.

Garvey, W.P., & Hegrenes, J.R. (1966). Desensitization techniques in the treatment of school phobia. *American Journal of Orthopsychiatry, 36,* 147–152.

Gelfand, D.M. (1978). Behavioral treatment of avoidance, social withdrawal, and negative emotional states. In B.B. Wolman, J. Egan, & A.O. Ross (Eds.), *Handbook of treatment of mental disorders in childhood and adolescence.* Englewood Cliffs, NJ: Prentice-Hall.

Gittelman-Klein, R. (1975). Psychiatric characteristics of the relatives of school phobic children. In D.V.S. Sankar (Ed.), *Mental health in children* (Vol. 1). Westbury, NJ: PJD Publications.

Gittelman-Klein, R., & Klein, D. (1971). Controlled imipramine treatment of school phobia. *Archives of General Psychiatry, 25,* 204–214.

Granell de Aldaz, E., Vivas, E., Gelfand, D.M., & Feldman, L. (1984). Estimating the prevalence of school refusal and school-related fears: A Venezuelan sample. *Journal of Nervous & Mental Disease, 172,* 722–729.

Graziano, A., DeGiovanni, I.S., & Garcia, K. (1979). Behavioral treatment of children's fears: A review. *Psychological Bulletin, 86,* 804–830.

Hagman, E. (1932). A study of fears of children of preschool age. *Journal of Experimental Education, 1,* 110–130.

Harris, S.L. (1983). Behavior therapy with children. In M. Hersen, A.E. Kazdin, & A.S. Bellack (Eds.), *The clinical psychology handbook.* New York: Pergamon.

Hatzenbuehler, L., & Schroeder, H. (1978). Desensitization procedures in the treatment of childhood disorders. *Psychological Bulletin, 85,* 831–844.

Hersen, M. (1970). Behavior modification approach to a school-phobia case. *Journal of Clinical Psychology, 26,* 128–132.

Hersov, L.A. (1960). Persistent nonattendance at school. *Child Psychology & Psychiatry, 1,* 130–136.

Jersild, A.T., & Holmes, F.B. (1935). Methods of overcoming children's fears. *Journal of Psychology, 1,* 75–104.

Kanfer, F., Karoly, P., & Newman, A. (1975). Reduction of children's fear of the dark by competence-related and situational threat-related verbal cries. *Journal of Consulting & Clinical Psychology, 43,* 251–258.

Kelley, C.K. (1976). Play desensitization of fear of darkness in preschool children. *Behavior Research & Therapy, 14,* 79–81.

Kennedy, W. (1965). School phobia: Rapid treatment of 50 cases. *Journal of Abnormal Psychology, 70,* 285–289.

Klein, D.F. (1964). Delineation of two drug responsive syndromes. *Psychopharmacologica, 3,* 397–408.

Kornhaber, R., & Schroeder, H. (1975). Importance of model similarity on extinction of avoidance behavior in children. *Journal of Consulting & Clinical Psychology, 43,* 601–607.

Kovacs, M. (1980/81). Rating scales to assess depression in school-aged children. *Acta Paedopsychiatry, 46,* 437–457.

Lapouse, R., & Monk, M.A. (1958). An epidemiologic study of behavior characteristics in children. *American Journal of Public Health, 48,* 1134–1144.

Lapouse, R., & Monk, M.A. (1959). Fears and worries in a representative sample of children. *American Journal of Orthopsychiatry*, *29*, 803–818.

Last, C.G., Francis, G., Hersen, M., Kazdin, A.E., & Strauss, C.C. (1987). Separation anxiety and school phobia: A comparison using DSM-III criteria. *American Journal of Psychiatry*, *144*, 653–657.

Last, C.G., Hersen, M., Kazdin, A.E., Finkelstein, R., & Strauss, C.C. (1987). Comparison of DSM-III separation anxiety and overanxious disorders: Demographic characteristics and patterns of comorbidity. *Journal of American Academy of Child Psychiatry*, *26*, 527–531.

Leitenberg, H., & Callahan, E. (1973). Reinforced practice and reduction of different kinds of fears in adults and children. *Behavior Research & Therapy*, *11*, 19–30.

Leventhall, T., & Sills, M. (1964). Self-image in school phobia. *American Journal of Orthopsychiatry*, *34*, 685–695.

MacFarlane, J.W., Allen, L., & Honzik, M.P. (1954). *A developmental study of the behavior problems of normal children between twenty-one months and fourteen years.* Berkeley: University of California Press.

Mann, J. (1972). Vicarious desensitization of test anxiety through observation of videotaped treatment. *Journal of Counseling Psychology*, *19*, 1–7.

Mann, J., & Rosenthal, T.L. (1969). Vicarious and direct counterconditioning of test anxiety through individual and group desensitization. *Behavior Research & Therapy*, *7*, 359–367.

Marks, I.M., & Gelder, M.G. (1966). Different ages of onset in varieties of phobia. *American Journal of Psychiatry*, *123*, 218–221.

Maurer, A. (1965). What children fear. *Journal of Genetic Psychology*, *106*, 265–277.

Mavissakalian, M., & Barlow, D.H. (1981). *Phobia: Psychological and pharmacological treatment.* New York: Guilford.

Miller, L.C., Barrett, C.L., & Hampe, E. (1974). Phobias of childhood in a prescientific era. In A. Davids (Ed.), *Child personality and psychopathology: Current topics.* New York: Wiley.

Miller, L.C., Barrett, C.L., Hampe, E., & Noble, H. (1972). Comparison of reciprocal inhibition, psychotherapy, and waiting list control for phobic children. *Journal of Abnormal Psychology*, *79*, 269–279.

Nichols, K.A., & Berg, I. (1970). School phobia and self-examination. *Journal of Child Psychology & Psychiatry*, *11*, 133–141.

O'Brien, G.T., & Barlow, D.H. (1984). Agoraphobia. In S.M. Turner (Ed.), *Behavioral theories and treatment of anxiety.* New York: Plenum.

O'Connor, R.D. (1969). Modification of social withdrawal through symbolic modeling. *Journal of Applied Behavior Analysis*, *2*, 15–22.

Ollendick, T.H. (1979). Fear reduction techniques with children. In M. Hersen, R. Eisler, & P. Miller (Eds.), *Progress in behavior modification* (Vol. 8.). New York: Academic.

Ollendick, T.H. (1983). Reliability and validity of the Revised Fear Survey Schedule for Children (FSSC-R). *Behavior Research & Therapy*, *21*, 685–692.

Ollendick, T.H., & Mayer, J. (1984). School phobia. In S.M. Turner (Ed.), *Behavioral treatment of anxiety disorders.* New York: Plenum.

Richman, N., Stevenson, J.E., & Graham, P.J. (1975). Prevalence of behaviour problems in 3-year-old children: An epidemiological study in a London borough. *Journal of Child Psychology & Psychiatry, 16*, 277–287.

Rines, W.B. (1973). Behavior therapy before institutionalization. *Psychotherapy: Theory, research and practice, 10*, 281–283.

Sheehan, D.V., Sheehan, K.E., & Minichiello, W.E. (1981). Age of onset of phobic disorders: A reevaluation. *Comprehensive Psychiatry, 6*, 544–553.

Smith, S. (1970). School refusal with anxiety: A review of 63 cases. *Canadian Psychiatric Association Journal, 15*, 257–264.

Smucker, M.R., Craighead, W.E., Craighead, L.W., & Green, B.J. (1986). Normative and reliability data for the Children's Depression Inventory. *Journal of Abnormal Child Psychology, 14*, 25–39.

Solyom, I., Beck, P., Solyom, C., & Hugel, R. (1974). Some etiological factors in phobic neurosis. *Canadian Psychiatry Association Journal, 19*, 69–78.

Spiegler, M., & Lambert, R. (1970). Some correlations of self-reported fear. *Psychological Reports, 26*, 691–695.

Tuma, A.H., & Maser, J.D. (1985). *Anxiety and the anxiety disorders.* Hillsdale, NJ: Erlbaum.

Tyrer, P., & Tyrer, S. (1974). School refusal, truancy, and adult neurotic illness. *Psychological Medicine, 4*, 416–421.

Waldron, S. (1976). The significance of childhood neurosis for adult mental health: A follow-up study. *American Journal of Psychiatry, 133*, 532–538.

CHAPTER 10

Obsessive–Compulsive Disorder

RICHARD WOLFF

DEFINITION

Major considerations of any discussion of obsessive–compulsive disorder in children include the facts that this disorder is not equivalent to obsessive personality, that the clinical picture presented by children is largely identical to that presented by adults, that the disorder is of unknown etiology, that only recently have the clinical and the research literature shown a uniformity in definition, that there is no one form of treatment demonstrating superiority, and that the earliest reports of the difficulty in successfully treating this highly intractable condition remain true today.

DSM-III has three criteria for diagnosis of obsessive–compulsive disorder. The syndrome is made up of either obsessions or compulsions; they are a significant source of distress or they interfere with role functioning; and they are not due to another mental disability (e.g., schizophrenia or depression) (APA, 1980).

In this regard, obsessions are defined as egosyntonic, recurrent thoughts expressed as senseless or repugnant, which the individual attempts to ignore or suppress.

The essential elements of DSM-III and DSM-III-R's (APA, 1987) definition of compulsions are repetitive, seemingly powerful behaviors performed according to certain rules or in stereotyped fashion. The behavior is designed to protect from or to prevent a future event, but it is either excessive in rate or unconnected in any realistic way to the desired outcome. The individual, especially in adult populations, recognizes the senselessness of the compulsion and tries to resist it. Pleasure is not derived from the performance of the act.

The present definition differs little from that offered by Lewis (1935) over half a century ago. He defined the essential elements of the syndrome as the experience of an inner compelling force, internal resistance to it, and the retention of insight.

Although this early definition bears close similarity to that in the current *Diagnostic and Statistical Manual* (APA, 1987), the intervening literature bears little uniformity. Most often, those articles are concerned with a definition as it relates to the clinical picture presented by the experimental subjects. Obsessive–compulsive disorder (OCD) in children is rare, which does not easily lead to large-scale or ongoing populations. Thus several investigators have made one report on the treatment of the disorder and define the term to suit their needs. With the notable exceptions of

Marks and Foa with adults, and Rapoport with children, there has not been continued and ongoing research by a consistent group. The other existing reports fall largely into one of three categories.

Retrospective reviews of hospital and outpatient clinic records often cite the OCD diagnosis as being used in treatment without any form of validation. Subsequently, retrospective reviews have disqualified a large percentage of these patients, for the clinical record does not contain sufficient information to validate that diagnosis (e.g., Judd, 1965). Second, there are reports in the current treatment literature where diagnosis has been successfully treated, but the behavior of the subject or patient group is not related to any standardized definition (e.g., Dalton, 1983; Fine, 1973). Finally, several reports, which are largely in the behavioral literature, focus on only one aspect of the behavior. Although this behavior is the primary presenting problem, the overall effect of social and/or role functions, as well as the DSM-III criteria of diagnosis, is not taken into account (e.g., Campbell, 1973).

Current reports attempt to quantify subjective aspects of the diagnosis category by employing at least one, but often several, assessment measures. Self-report is common in adults (e.g., Wolff, 1977), but it is probably less reliable with children where additional reports from parents and teachers have also been employed (e.g., Ownby, 1983).

Although limited assessments are characteristic of clinical settings, experimental investigations typically use multiple assessments to define the parameters of the term. Boulougouris, Rabavilas, and Stefanis (1977) illustrated multiple physiological measures in a pre/posttreatment design. Perhaps the most extensive and exacting methods have been reported by Flament, Rapoport, Berg, and Kilts (1985) in illustrating assessment of 12 variables (which included rating scales by clinicians and clients, EKG, and sleep EEG). That report stands as a model for comprehensive assessment in measuring this disorder.

In terms of defining the term relative to performance on a standardized test, only two such devices are available for this disorder. The Maudsley Obsessional-Compulsive Inventory (Rachman & Hodgson, 1980) and the Leyton Obsessional Inventory (Cooper, 1970) have been developed, but both have been constructed for assessment of adults. Berg, Rapoport, and Flament (1980) have developed a child version of the Leyton. This is a card-sorting rating scale to quantify subjective reports of feelings and behavior. The child version of the Leyton has been criticized by Clark and Bolton (1985) in that it failed to distinguish between OCD and anxious adolescents. However, the basis of their report was the result of a very small sample, 11 OCD and 10 anxiety patients, and further studies are necessary. Neither of these inventories appears in the treatment literature with any frequency.

The distinction between OCD and obsessive personality was originally made by Freud (1908/1963, cited in Pollak, 1979), and that distinction has functionally been maintained by all subsequent investigators. In reviewing the literature on obsessive personality, Pollak (1979) concludes that individuals with predominantly obsessive–compulsive personality are considered asymptomatic for obsessive–compulsive disorder. Rather, obsessive–compulsive personality is considered a constellation of traits, defenses, and frequent elements of a life-style. Observable, frequent behaviors meeting the DSM-III criteria are not present. This distinction was first scientifically demonstrated through the factor-analytic methods of Sandler and Hazani (1960), and their findings have been consistently replicated. Slade's (1974) factor-analytic investigation concluded that separate factors accounted for obsessional traits and symptoms. In offering a contemporary and uniform definition of the disorder, DSM-III has maintained the essential elements of the disorder that were first suggested more than half a century ago. While the majority of articles in the treatment literature do not relate to that or any other uniform definition, some investigations, such as that of Flament, Rapoport, Berg, and Kilts (1985), are a shining example of pointing to an objective methodology for further refining the term.

HISTORICAL BACKGROUND

OCD is hardly a recent phenomenon, for Shakespearian audiences were acquainted with the disorder in the form of Lady Macbeth's hand-washing ritual. However, in spite of a long history, it is only in the past decade that potentially effective treatments have been reported.

Benson (1975) has reported a medieval French monk's attempt to reduce behavioral excesses, and Bear and Minichiello (1986) have stated that it was Lainert who first attempted to cure this disorder as a psychiatric condition more than 100 years ago. Here an approximation of a differential reinforcement of other (DRO) procedure of memorizing songs replaced the obsessive thoughts, and a 2-year follow-up indicated the patient was free of the distressing thoughts.

Janet (1903) provided a detailed account of his treatment of OCD in a 5-year-old boy, which is generally considered the first report of the disorder. Later, he provided a report of 14 adults who were "accidentally cured" by major life changes in their personal living conditions (Bear & Minichiello, 1986).

The case of the Rat Man (Freud, 1950) states the classic psychoanalytic position regarding the description and treatment of OCD. This case relates the symptoms to difficulties in the anal stage, conflicts with authority, and an eventual poor prognosis. However, it is Hall's (1935) report that is considered the first modern account of childhood OCD. A later report by Bender and Schlinder (1940) described five cases of "impulsions," but the essential elements of the criteria suggested 5 years earlier by Hall were not employed, and it is not clear whether or not these presenting problems could be classified as OCD.

During the middle portion of this century, several theoretical articles and case reports appeared in the psychoanalytic and psychodynamic literature. However, very little of these discussions has been maintained, which may be a result of the generally poor prognosis of these reports. In fact, in a retrospective review, Berman (1942) found that only six cases had been admitted to a major psychiatric hospital during a 7-year period, and his follow-up in 3 to 5 years determined that two were schizophrenic, one was severely disturbed and obsessional, and the remaining three remained mildly disturbed. Later reports by Judd (1965) and Hollingsworth, Tanguay, Grossman, and Pabst (1980) confirmed these findings of infrequent incidents and poor prognosis.

The rarity of this disorder has made large-scale or factorial designs most difficult. With the development of research–treatment programs by Marks in England and Foa in the United States, working with adult populations, and Rapoport at NIMH, focusing on children and adolescents, an understanding of the development of this disorder, its mechanisms, and, it is to be hoped, effective treatments has just begun.

CLINICAL PICTURE

In milder forms of the disorder, the clinical picture of the OCD child or adolescent appears to be quite normal, for ruminative thoughts are not directly observable, and compulsive behaviors are often, at least in the early stages of the disorder, practiced in privacy. However, at the other end of the spectrum, long-term hospitalization may be necessary (Bolton, Collins, & Steinberg, 1983), with the prognosis for recovery remaining poor (Rasmussen & Tsuang, 1986). Although the disorder is reported to have been evidenced as early as 3 or 4, most investigators set the typical age of onset at between 10 and 14 (Berg et al., 1980; Rasmussen & Tsuang, 1986). However, there is no upper age limit or developmental stage associated with onset.

With children and adolescents, boys predominate. Hollingsworth and colleagues' (1980) study reported the proportion of boys to girls was three to one. That finding has been confirmed by Berg and colleagues (1982; 83% male), Flament, Rapoport, Berg, Sceery, and colleagues (1985; 74% male), and Rapoport and colleagues (1981; 78% male). However, reports with adults often show a preponderance of females (Rasmussen & Tsuang, 1986; $N = 44$ adults, 36% male).

The mechanism of onset is unclear, for it may be either insidious or acute. Acute onset has been reported following psychological (Loeb, 1986), physical (McKeon, McGuffin, & Robinson, 1984), or birth (Capstick & Seldrup, 1977) trauma. Some reports of development following head injury are remarkable. McKeon and colleagues (1984) have reported three such cases in a consecutive series, but their numbers are small. In the majority of cases, there is no evidence of either head injury or birth trauma. Further, with detailed questioning, what appears to have been a precipitating event of psychological trauma is less powerful in both its place in time and the behavioral influence than was first reported. Currently, there is no known cause of this disorder (Rapoport, 1982).

OCD children may present with symptoms of anxiety and/or depression. Anxiety usually is associated with practicing the ritual or roadblocks to its performance or stems from a wish to perform and not perform the motoric or cognitive ritual. Because anxiety is always a feature of this syndrome, it is not considered a useful criterion in diagnosis. Depression was found in more than 100 of the 119 OCD adults in Welner, Reich, and Robins's (1976) investigation, and the probability of depression remains high with children (Rapoport, 1982). To a lesser degree, the patient may present the picture of Gilles de la Tourette's syndrome or anorexia. Nee, Caine, Eldridge, and Ebert (1980) found that 34 of 50 consecutive Tourette's syndrome patients met DSM-III criteria for OCD. The relationship with anorexia is occasionally reported, but it is infrequent and unclear.

The belief that OCD is a disorder of children possessing superior intelligence has not been substantiated by the evidence. In a study of 27 children 10 to 18 years old, Flament and Rapoport (1984) determined the Full Scale WISC-R IQ to be 105.9 (SD = 12.9). Although approximately one quarter of the subjects did show significant subtest scatter, neither the WISC-R nor the Bender-Gestalt showed signs of organicity. Further, except when the child was acutely ill, the Peabody Individual Achievement scores were within grade levels. A near identical finding was also determined in a later investigation (Berg et al., 1982), and similar results have been found in adult patients (Flor-Henry, Yeudall, Koles, & Howarth, 1979; Insel, Donnelly, & Lalaken, 1983). The earlier association with superior intelligence may have been based on a clinical impression rather than obtained IQ scores.

EEG abnormalities in this group have been determined to be uncommon, mild, and nonspecific (Flament & Rapoport, 1984). Also, neither ordinal birth position, size of the sibship, nor loss of a parent before age 15 is a related factor (Rasmussen & Tsuang, 1984).

Factors relating to a premorbid personality have been discussed, but the picture is not clear. The families of origin may have a tendency for cleanliness or orderliness, but overt forms of the disorder are not evident in other family members or necessarily in the premorbid functioning of the patient. These children present attributes and behavioral problems typical of the normal range. They are often shy and unassertive, but they are not withdrawn or severely introverted. An attachment to a parent is often a principal feature, and in single-parent families, whether through death or divorce, the remaining parent does seem to become overinvolved in the disorder, which is not to the betterment of the child (Flament & Rapoport, 1984; Rasmussen & Tsuang, 1984).

The primary presenting complaint is usually a combination of compulsive rituals and obsessive thoughts. The sample of 27 children and adolescents in the NIMH study presented fears of contamination as well as rituals focusing on washing, cleaning, and avoidance touching. Compulsions typically center on defending against unwanted events, while obsessive thoughts center on counting or repeating words or phrases (Flament & Rapoport, 1984).

The degree of incapacitation in children is similar to that of adults, in that the entire range of interventions may be necessary. However, in spite of the severity or incapacitation, there is usually no evidence of a thought disorder.

ASSOCIATED FEATURES

Since OCD is a rare condition, there has not been a large population of subjects to study and report associated features. Some investigations have been conducted with small samples, and the results are useful but not definitive. Since the disorder in children is virtually identical to that of adults, valid interpretations for children can be made from the adult literature. Depression, anxiety, and Tourette's syndrome are the most frequently reported asssociated features.

Depression is commonly noted as an associated feature in all group studies. In a study of nine adolescents (age range 13 to 17, mean 14.2 years) Rapoport and colleagues (1981) determined that depressive symptoms were common to all subjects and were most severe with children exhibiting the earliest onset. Depression may occur months or years after onset.

With adults, a major investigation of 149 OCD patients was conducted by Welner and colleagues (1976), and more than 100 of those subjects evidenced depression as either a concomitant or secondary symptom. Interestingly, only 30 subjects (20%) presented OCD as the only disorder. Similar findings have been made with a child population by Rapoport and colleagues (1981) and with adults by Lewis (1935) and Insel, Donnelly, and Lalaken (1983). When OCD appears secondary to depression, the OCD behaviors are eliminated when the depressive symptoms are successfully treated. But the reverse is not true, for with primary OCD, those symptoms will remain when the secondary depression has been alleviated (Elkins, Rapoport, & Lidsky, 1980).

The most notable factor in this regard is the lack of a thought disorder in spite of the severity of the psychopathology (Rapoport et al., 1981). Sleep disorders have been studied in OCD children, but the abnormalities may be a function of the associated depression (Rapoport et al., 1981).

The relationship to anxiety is similar to that of depression, in that there is almost always an associated condition. OCD is classified as an anxiety disorder, but it is distinct from other forms of anxiety (e.g., separation anxiety, generalized anxiety, etc.). There is a similarity to phobic anxiety that is seen relative to the central issue of the disorder (e.g., proximity to dirt, inability to check, etc.). Intensity and degree of incapacitation are related to the current level of stress, which may wax and wane.

Nee, Caine, Eldridge, and Ebert (1980) found that 34 of 50 Tourette's syndrome patients met DSM-III criteria for OCD. The frequency was even higher with those who had a family history of tics (Montgomery, Clayton, & Freidhoff, 1982; Nee, Polinsky, & Ebert, 1980).

There are a number of other reports focusing on neurological disease resulting from trauma that have been associated with OCD. Flor-Henry and colleagues (1979) employed 28 neurological tests with OCD adults and determined a relationship with frontal lobe dysfunction. However, this finding was not replicated in a study of 27 OCD children and adolescents using comparable assessment measures (Rapoport et al., 1981). An association with cerebral pathology resulting from abnormal birth events was reported by Capstick and Seldrup (1977) and McKeon, McGuffin, and Robinson (1984). Additionally, Barton (1954) suggests that diabetes insipidus often accompanies OCD. These relationships remain fruitful areas of investigation, yet evidence is currently inconclusive.

One of the most consistent and remarkable findings is that OCD is not associated with thought or major affective disorders regardless of the severity of the psychopathology (Rapoport et al., 1981).

Studies of family pathology and of twins have produced interesting but also nonconclusive results (Beech, 1984; Elkins et al., 1980; Rapoport et al., 1981).

COURSE AND PROGNOSIS

OCD has been described as a rare yet malignant disorder. Although typical onset for children is between the ages of 10 and 14, most patients develop the symptoms before age 25 (Politt, 1957). Kringlen (1965) reported that more than half of his 91 subjects had been classified as OCD before the age of 20, with one-fifth having exhibited the disorder before onset of puberty. A similar finding was reported by Beech (1974), who determined that one-third of the subjects studied had manifested the syndrome before the age of 15. The actual time of onset is unclear, for some cases report sudden onset, while in others there is no clear marking point reported by either the child or the family. In Judd's (1965) classic paper, onset was related to clear and discernible precipitating events. However, Hollingsworth and colleagues (1980) presented 15 of 17 cases where OCD symptoms were related to frightening yet less specific events.

In most of the reports surveyed, acute onset is not reported. Children with OCD are characteristically secretive, and the intensity of their distresss may go unnoticed until later stages. Flament and Rapoport (1984) conducted detailed, multiple-session interviews with patients and family members concerning these precipitating events. It was their conclusion that the events were of uncertain significance to the patient, that there was not consistent agreement within the family concerning the event and the onset of the disorder, and that the severity of the illness seemed out of proportion to the event. They concluded that the reports of nonphysical or traumatic events were unconvincing. Although there was consistency regarding age of onset, there is no clear answer to the question of acute or insidious onset. And it is likely that the condition occurs as a result of several factors through several mechanisms. Once developed, the disorder bears remarkable resemblance to the picture presented by adults. During adolescence, some changes in the topography of the behavior may occur. Checking may be refocused on issues of contamination; counters often develop sexual preoccupations (Wolff & Rapoport, 1988). However, there is no evidence of symptom substitution with either children (Bear & Minichiello, 1986) or adults (Foa & Steketee, 1977). Hospitalization is rare, with occurrence in child populations being estimated at 1% (Judd, 1965).

Once the condition has developed, the child may be secretive about it, which prevents therapeutic intervention, and most child OCD patients do not seek treatment until they reach their mid-twenties. Often there is a gap of 10 to 20 years between onset and treatment (Rasmussen & Tsuang, 1984).

In adults, the most common obsession is fear of contamination followed by thoughts relating to sexual issues or exactness. Compulsions may be of a single or multiple behavior, and they are often related to checking, cleaning, or washing (Rasmussen & Tsuang, 1984). With children, similarly, obsessions center about functionally meaningless thoughts warding off danger to self or others. Rituals, too, may be demonstrated as a method of warding off the effects of the above or may be related to washing or cleaning (Rapoport, Elkins, Langer, Sceery, Buschbaum, and colleagues, 1981).

Prognosis has always been considered unfavorable. Freud (1955) discussed the difficulty in successfully providing an effective treatment, and he considered the prognosis to be poor. Although optimistic reports of psychoanalytic treatment (Bornstein, 1949), problem-solving therapy (O'Connor, 1983), family therapy (Fine, 1973), and other systems have been made, the eventual rate of success has been low.

Factors related to an unfavorable prognosis include the belief that elements of the disorder are necessary and that bad things will happen to the patient if he or she does not perform them, noncompliance with the treatment program (Foa & Steketee, 1977), and a diagnosis of schizotypal personality disorder (Bear & Minichiello, 1986). In fact, Rachman and Hodgson (1980) state that any abnormal personality factor is predictive of a poor prognosis. Factors related to a positive outcome are mild symptoms, short duration, and a healthy premorbid personality (Goodwin, 1977).

With adults, the prognosis is generally considered to be poor (Skoog, 1965), and treatment leading to a "much improved" category ranges from 20 to 70% (Black, 1974; Kringlen, 1965; Marks, 1981). The report of Hollingsworth and colleagues (1980) is especially interesting, for they located 15 of the 17 patients in his retrospective review. Ten of these subjects agreed to participate in a follow-up, structured interview. Three of the 10 denied any current obsession or compulsion. The remaining seven related that the condition continued but to a degree much improved over the pretreatment levels. Of this group, one had been hospitalized for depressive and suicidal ideation, while another had decompensated into an acute schizophrenic reaction that had been resolved.

A review of the outcome with children (Elkins et al., 1980) concluded that 50% of childhood OCD patients may not make substantive recovery.

IMPAIRMENT

The degree of impairment may cover the entire range of possibilities from undiagnosed (Flament, Rapoport, Whitaker, Berg, & Sceery, 1985) to long-term hospitalization (Apter, Bernhout, & Tyang, 1984). There are no data to indicate the relative percentages of the OCD population that exist at any point along this continuum.

Rasmussen and Tsuang (1986) discussed the condition within a framework of episodic, continuous, and deteriorative categories. Levels of impairment are related to the patient's present position on this continuum.

The episodic classification describes individuals who have recurring episodes of obsessions or compulsions lasting longer than 6 months. Episodes are usually linked to an affective disorder, but they continue as a form of the patient's life-style. Between episodes, the child functions in a rather normal manner. The continuous classification also shows episodic swings, but between episodes (which usually last 3 to 12 months) the individual remains impaired. Social and role functions are possible within the family. Members of the deteriorative category exhibit an intense and stable pattern of OCD that limits or prevents social and occupational function. Episodes are not present.

Episodic and continuous forms of the disorder show a greater relationship to stress, but the deteriorative category does not. The current level of impairment is related to both the intensity of the disorder and interaction with the current stressors. Waxing and waning of the intensity and subsequent impairment are common.

COMPLICATIONS

The relationship of OCD to other disorders has been discussed, but associated conditions are not complications. Major complications relate to compliance.

Unlike bulimia or anorexia, this disorder is not directly observable (e.g., counting). Therapeutic alliance with the child, which may not be present in the initial stages of treatment, is certainly necessary. In fact, quantitative and qualitative aspects of self-report data improve as a function of rapport with the therapist.

Apter and colleagues (1984) report a complete failure in eight cases of hospitalized OCD adolescents using what was described as a form of behavior therapy. The form of treatment centered on "enjoining" the subjects from performing rituals and asking them to think of something else in place of the obsessional thought. When possible, student nurses and other staff were assigned to watch the patients and encourage them to perform an alternative behavior. No comments concerning rate of compliance are given, and motivation for treatment is not discussed. The methodology is not of the form of response prevention customarily employed, and the total failure is not typical. Difficulties with compliance are also reported by Ong and Leng (1979) in the treatment of a hand-washing ritual with a 13-year-old girl. Continuous monitoring could not be provided, and the girl secretively sought other faucets on the hospital ward.

Patient compliance is a major factor in the treatment of any disorder, and with OCD, compliance on the part of the family is especially important. However, neither measures nor estimates of patient motivation for treatment or degree of child and family compliance are contained in the treatment reports.

Some children believe that obsessions and compulsions are necessary or inherently worthwhile. Obviously, in these cases, motivation is low or nonexistent with a resultant poor prognosis.

With children, the behavior exists largely in the home environment; therefore, compliance on the part of the parents is essential in delineating the parameters of the behavior and assessing and treating it. For a variety of reasons (e.g., believing the problem is not serious or will be outgrown), the parents may not be compliant. Enlistment of family members in the assessment and treatment phases of the disorder is recommended and correlated with an improved prognosis.

EPIDEMIOLOGY

As can be expected with any rare disorder, epidemiological studies have been few. The first report by Berman (1942) reviewed more than 3000 records of pediatric cases at a large psychiatric hospital admitted during a 7-year period. Only 6 true cases could be found. A similar retrospective review was performed on the records of 405 in- and outpatients at UCLA (Judd, 1965). Although 34 cases had been diagnosed as OCD during treatment, only 5 (1.50%) met the diagnostic criteria. A comparable procedure was followed by Hollingsworth and colleagues (1980) in reviewing 8367 child in- and outpatients during a 26-year period. Only 50 cases were diagnosed as OCD, and using Judd's criteria, 33 were disqualified. The remaining 17 resulted in a prevalence rate of 0.002.

Other investigations have surveyed the general as opposed to the psychiatric populations. Weissman, Myers, and Harding (1978) surveyed 511 members of a New Haven community and determined that none exhibited OCD. A rural–urban comparison was reported by Blaxter and colleagues (1985), who studied primarily alcohol and drug problems in the Piedmont area of North Carolina. Although children were not the focus of this study, the findings produced nonsignificant results (i.e., the frequency of OCD was higher for rural than for urban populations).

An additional comment concerning OCD in the general population relates to Rasmussen and Tsuang's (1986) attempt to generate subjects for a research project through television coverage and newspaper advertisements. They failed to obtain a single response.

The most ambitious undertaking in this regard was by Flament, Rapoport, Whitaker, Berg, and Sceery (1985), who surveyed more than 5000 students in a New Jersey school district. Psychiatric interviews with children scoring highest on the screening device were included. The findings established a minimal prevalence rate of 0.33 in the general adolescent population. Although this rate is higher than that in other published reports, the authors suggest that it may, in fact, be low. They point to a rate of 0.60 as closer to the true frequency due to the secrecy of the children completing the questionnaire, the possibility that severely disabled children were not participating in the school program, and the fact that a single symptom, such as hand washing, may not have produced a high screening score.

FAMILIAL PATTERN

Family patterns of psychopathology in general and of OCD in particular have been an area of extreme interest and concern throughout the history of this disorder. Parental psychopathology has been reported by Lewis (1935), Kanner (1957), Kringlen (1965), and Adams (1977). Hollingsworth reported a prevalence rate of OCD in parents as 20%, and Lewis (1935) determined the rate in siblings to be 21%. However, Rosenberg's (1967) investigation of first-degree relatives of 144 OCD patients yielded a prevalence rate of less than 1%. A major review of familial psychopathology and obsessionality was conducted by Rasmussen and Tsuang (1984) in which papers published over the last 50 years were considered. This survey included the families of 532 patients. Some of the articles contained in their review did not specify the form of data collection. Since both Judd and Hollingsworth discarded several diagnosed cases because the chart did not validate the diagnosis, the validity of all of these cases may be questioned. Nonetheless, the most prominent finding was that first-degree relatives of adult OCD patients had a higher than normal incidence of psychiatric disorders in general and of obsessive–compulsive disorder in particular.

More recently, an in-depth study of family members of 10 adult patients (ages 18 to 45) has been conducted by Hoover and Insel (1984). Personal, in-depth, family interviews were conducted with a total of 174 family members, including 20 parents, 30 siblings, 3 offspring, and 131 other relatives of the second and third degree. In some cases, interviews occurred over months, and they focused on psychiatric disorders, habits, attitudes, and eccentricities. When information concerning the mental health of the relative could not be determined, that relative was excluded. Some relatives were demanding with themselves and others, some were considered to be "house-proud," and many families tended to have isolated social activities while living in an environment that emphasized orderliness and cleanliness. However, none could be classified as OCD.

The finding was confirmed by Flament and Rapoport (1984) in a study of the families of 27 child and adolescent OCD patients. None of the parents displayed either OCD or perfectionism to the point that it interfered with their social or occupational functions. Sibling dysfunction was present in these troubled families, but the incidence of OCD was not impressive.

Although the role and function of families in the development, maintenance, and treatment of the childhood disorder must be assessed, this area of inquiry is obviously not completely understood.

When viewing the reports of family psychopathology sequentially, the role of the family seems to be decreasing. The differing findings can be understood by considering the refinements in methodology of data collection. The Rasmussen and Tsuang (1984) survey of the literature over a 50-year period contained articles that stated neither a criterion nor a basis on which the information was obtained. Perhaps it was the subjective impression of the therapist. By contrast, the methods employed by Hoover and Insel (1984) were specified and are replicable.

With children, the effects of parental modeling and parental consequences for the OCD behaviors are a major area of concern in understanding the development of this disorder and its assessment and treatment. Obviously, at this time the role of the family is not clearly understood.

DIFFERENTIAL DIAGNOSIS

To meet the DSM-III criteria of obsessive–compulsive behavior, there must be an inner compelling force to act, a resistance to this force, and the retention of insight.

The disorder cannot, of course, be attributable to other mental or neurological dysfunctions.

OCD can be distinguished from rituals that are part of normal development (Gesell & Ilg, 1943). Such rituals may focus on bedtime routines or avoiding sidewalk cracks, but here role functions are not disrupted, and they are not a major source of personal distress. Additionally, complex rituals are frequently modeled by professional athletes. Since this modeling has consequences that are immediate and periodically positive, it is expected that some children will be affected by the model. These samples of behavior are largely elicited only by specific stimuli, and they do not interfere with the child's life in any detrimental fashion.

The distinction between OCD and either Tourette's syndrome or anxiety is not as simple. However, with Tourette's, there is often a preoccupation with actual emission of swear words. There is also a motoric tic that is not present in OCD. Further, the OCD behavior is customarily a more complex behavior than the tic.

The distinction from anxiety, especially phobic anxiety, is less obvious. A child with a cleanliness disorder may act in a phobic manner in the presence of unclean or contaminated objects. Although the anxiety may have a potential to generalize, Rapoport (1982) believes that the distinction is not necessary, for severe OCD always has some phobic anxiety.

Depression is always a feature in adult (Welner et al., 1976) and adolescent (Rapoport, 1981) cases. To make a diagnosis of OCD, depression must be secondary or a concurrent condition. Interestingly, although trichotillomania in both children and adults resembles several characteristics of the OCD patient, it is not an associated condition. Children with thought disorders, schizophrenia, autism, or mental retardation may display signs of OCD; the presenting picture, however, does not meet OCD criteria. With anorexia, the diagnosis is made on the basis of weight loss and other criteria.

As an aid to practitioners, the NIMH group has formulated a step-by-step procedure to aid in differential diagnosis (Rapoport, 1982). Factors to be considered here are the details of the pattern of symptomatology, the senselessness of the acts, disruption to normal living patterns, and an expressed effort to get through the day. Other forms of psychopathology must be ruled out. The family's response to the problem, and their similarities to it, should be assessed, and a thorough medical history should be conducted as well. Previous psychiatric history and its effect on the family are recommended areas of innvestigation.

CLINICAL MANAGEMENT—RESEARCH FINDINGS

A review of the literature indicates that functionally all reported forms of treatment have shown a positive effect, but at this point in time there is no singular treatment of choice.

Psychoanalysis was the first of the currently existing treatments, and although it has been historically related to the disorder, the outcome after extended treatment is not good (Bornstein, 1949; Loeb, 1986).

Supportive therapy has been reported to be beneficial (Rapoport, 1982), but neither supportive psychotherapy nor peer support groups have data validating the efficacy of treatment.

Although psychodynamic psychotherapy is related to the early theoretical explanations of the disorder, again, there is no data base to support it as an effective treatment.

Due to the role of the family in the disorder, family therapy would appear to be a suitable approach, and there are case reports of successful treatment (e.g., Fine, 1973). This literature is composed largely of clinical case studies without controls or specified procedures. Thus once again there is no basis on which to evaluate this form of treatment. Involvement of the family in the treatment process is, however, recommended (Wolff & Rapoport, 1988).

Behavior therapy has demonstrated the most carefully planned protocols featuring controls in the form of groups or the individual as his or her own control, specified and replicable procedures, multiple objective assessments, and often a follow-up period of 1 to 3 years. However, the most scientific of these investigations has been with adult subjects. The child literature is composed largely of single-case studies (e.g., Zikis, 1983) or a collection of case studies (e.g., Bolton, Collins, & Steinberg, 1983). Even using the most liberal definitions of the term, a recent review of the behavioral literature of childhood OCD could identify only 13 articles in the behavioral literature (Wolff & Rapoport, 1988). The type of experiment discussed by Marks (1981) or Foa (Foa & Goldstein, 1978; Foa, Steketee, Grayson, Turner, & Latimer, 1984) has yet to be conducted with children. Nonetheless, behavior therapy has been shown to be effective with adults and case studies with children and holds promise for the future.

In the child OCD literature, behavior therapy is most often employed as a major component in a comprehensive treatment program. A form of response prevention is most frequently employed.

Bolton and colleagues (1983) employed response prevention as a major component in their treatment of 15 hospitalized adolescents and determined that 82% of their subjects demonstrated improvement. The period of hospitalization, however, ranged from 1 week to 2 years. Ong and Leng (1979), as well as Zikis (1983), reported similar successful results.

Thought stopping has been applied as the sole treatment and as an element of treatment programs. It does appear to be a suitable treatment for ruminations, and a positive treatment effect has been reported by Campbell (1973) and Ownby (1983). Systematic desensitization was reported only once with children, and in that situation it was one of six treatments applied (Phillips & Wolpe, 1981).

Treatment by family therapy often includes a behavioral component, for in addition to working with related family issues, family members are enlisted as cotherapists in applying the treatment program in the home (Dalton, 1983).

While many articles list a single form of treatment in the title, Friedman and Silvers (1977) describe a multimodal approach consisting of insight-oriented, group, family, and behavioral therapy. Treatment by functional analysis of the behavior is applied to a group of case studies using multiple behavioral approaches (Queiroz, Motta, Madi, Sossai, & Boren, 1981).

Drug treatment has been applied in clinical and research settings, where several positive effects have been shown (Marks, 1981), with Chlorimipramine showing the greatest positive effect in adults (Insel et al., 1983). Using sophisticated experimental designs with multiple valid and reliable assessment measures, Chlorimipramine has been effective also with children and adolescents (Flament, Rapoport, Berg, & Kilts, 1985; Flament, Rapoport, Berg, Sceery et al., 1985; Rapoport et al., 1981; Warneke, 1985). Obviously, a classic study waiting to be conducted would focus on a large group of OCD children in a factorial design assessing the effects and interaction of Chlorimipramine and behavior therapy with multiple controls. However, given the rarity of the disorder, that unplanned study may never occur. At the present time, treatment relying on a combination of all of the measures outlined earlier and designed to meet the needs of the individual patient would be most suitable. In this regard, an ideal treatment program suggested by Hoover and Insel (1984) would include medication, a behavioral program, conjoint sessions (if applicable), multifamily groups, and individual therapy for family members, including the patient.

DSM-III-R

Since the current standard definition employs most of the present knowledge concerning the disorder and the literature review notes an absence of criticism of it, functionally no changes are indicated at this time.

REFERENCES

Adams, P.L. (1972). Family characteristics of obsessive children. *American Journal of Psychiatry, 128,* 1414–1417.

American Psychiatric Association. (1980). *Diagnostic and statistical manual of mental disorders* (3rd ed.). Washington, DC: Author.

American Psychiatric Association. (1987). *Diagnostic and statistical manual of mental disorders* (3rd ed., rev.). Washington, DC: Author.

Apter, A., Bernhout, E., & Tyang, S. (1984). Severe obsessive-compulsive disorder in adolescence: A report of eight cases. *Journal of Adolescence, 7,* 349–358.

Barton, R. (1954). Diabetes insidipus, obsessional neurosis, and hypothalamic dysfunction. *Proceedings of the Royal Society of Medicine, 47,* 276–277.

Bear, L., & Minichiello, W. (1986). Behavior therapy for obsessive–compulsive disorder. In M. Jenike, L. Bear, & W.E. Minichiello (Eds.), *Obsessive compulsive disorders.* Littleton, MA: PSG.

Beech, L. (1974). *Obsessional states.* London: Methuen.

Bender, L., & Schlinder, P. (1940). Impulsions. *Archives of Neurology & Psychiatry, 44,* 990–1008.

Benson, H. (1975). *The relaxation response.* New York: William Morrow.

Berg, C., Behar, D., Cox, C., Fedio, P., Gillin, J., Ludlow, C., Rapoport, J., Sceery, W., & Zahn, T. (1982). *OCD in childhood*. Paper presented at the Annual Meeting of the American Psychological Association, Washington, DC.

Berg, C., Rapoport, J., & Flament, M. (1980). The Leyton Obsessional Inventory—Child Version. *Journal of the American Academy of Child Psychiatry*, *25*, 84–91.

Berman, L. (1942). The obsessive–compulsive neurosis in children. *Journal of Nervous & Mental Disease*, *95*, 26–39.

Black, A. (1974). The natural history of obsessional neurosis. In H.R. Beech (Ed.), *Obsessional states*. London: Methuen.

Blaxter, D., George, L., Landerman, R., Pennybacker, M., Melville, M., Woodbury, M., Manton, K., Jordon, K., & Locke, B. (1985). Psychiatric disorders: A rural/urban comparison. *Archives of General Psychiatry*, *42*, 651–656.

Bolton, D., Collins, S., & Steinberg, D. (1983). The treatment of OCD in adolescence: A report of fifteen cases. *British Journal of Psychiatry*, *142*, 456–464.

Bornstein, L. (1949). The analysis of a phobic child. *Psychoanalytic Study of the Child*, *3–4*, 181–226.

Boulougouris, J., Rabavilas, A., & Stefanis, C. (1977). Psychophysical responses in obsessive–compulsive patients. *Behaviour Research & Therapy*, *15*, 221–230.

Brown, F. (1942). Heredity in the psychoneuroses. *Proceedings of the Royal Society of Medicine*, *38*, 785–790.

Campbell, L. (1973). A variation of thought-stopping in a twelve-year-old boy: A case report. *Journal of Behavior Therapy & Experimental Psychiatry*, *4*, 69–70.

Capstick, H., & Seldrup, J. (1977). Obsessional states: A case study in the relationship between abnormalities occurring at the time of birth and the subsequent development of obsessional symptoms. *Acta Psychiatrica Scandinavica*, *56*, 427–431.

Clark, D., & Bolton, D. (1985). An investigation of two self-report measures of obsessional phenomena in obsessive–compulsive adolescents: Research note. *Journal of Child Psychology & Psychiatry*, *26*, 429–437.

Cooper, J. (1970). The Leyton Obsessional Inventory. *Psychological Medicine*, *1*, 48–64.

Dalton, P. (1983). Family treatment of an obsessve–compulsive child: A case report. *Family Process*, *22*, 99–108.

Elkins, R., Rapoport, J., & Lipsky, A. (1980). Obsessive compulsive disorder of childhood and adolescence. *Journal of the American Academy of Child Psychiatry*, *19*, 511–524.

Fine, S. (1973). Family therapy and a behavioral approach to childhood obsessive–compulsive neurosis. *Archives of General Psychiatry*, *28*, 695–697.

Flament, M., & Rapoport, J. (1984). Childhood obsessive–compulsive disorder. In T.R. Insel (Ed.), *Obsessive compulsive disorder*. Washington, DC: American Psychiatric Press.

Flament, M., Rapoport, J., Berg, C., & Kilts, C. (1985). A controlled trial of Clomipramine in childhood obsessive–compulsive disorder. *Psychopharmacology Bulletin*, *21*, 150–152.

Flament, M., Rapoport, J., Berg, C., Sceery, W., Kilts, C., Mellstrum, B., & Linnoila, M. (1985). Clomipramine treatment of childhood obscssive–compulsive disorder. *Archives of General Psychiatry*, *42*, 977–983.

Flament, M., Rapoport, J., Whitaker, A., Berg, C., & Sceery, W. (1985). *Obsessive–compulsive disorders in adolescents: An epidemiological study*. Paper presented at the thirty-second meeting of the American Academy of Child Psychiatry, San Antonio.

Flor-Henry, P., Yeudall, L., Koles, Z., & Howarth, B. (1979). Neuropsychological and power spectral EEG investigations of the obsessive–compulsive syndrome. *Biological Psychiatry, 14*, 119–130.

Foa, E. (1979). Failure in treating obsessive–compulsives. *Behaviour Research & Therapy, 17*, 169–176.

Foa, E., & Goldstein, A. (1978). Continuous exposure and complete response prevention in the treatment of obsessive–compulsive neurosis. *Behavior Therapy, 9*, 821–824.

Foa, E.B., & Steketee, G. (1977). Emergent fears during treatment of three obsessive compulsions: Symptom substitution or deconditioning? *Journal of Behavior Therapy and Experimental Psychiatry, 8*, 353–358.

Foa, E., Steketee, G., Grayson, J. (1985). Imaginal and in vivo exposure: A comparison with obsessive–compulsive checkers. *Behavior Therapy, 11*, 292–302.

Foa, E., Steketee, G., Grayson, J., Turner, R., & Latimer, P. (1984). Deliberate exposure and blocking of obsessive–compulsive rituals: Immediate and long-term effects. *Behavior Therapy, 15*, 450–472.

Freud, S. (1955). Obsessions and phobias: Their psychical mechanisms and their aetiology. In J. Strachey (Ed.), *Collected Papers I* (Standard Edition, pp. 128–137). London: Hogarth.

Freud, S. (1955). The disposition of obsessional neurosis. In J. Strachey (Ed.), *Collected Papers I*. London: Hogarth.

Friedmann, C., & Silvers, F. (1977). A multimodality approach to in-patient treatment of obsessive-compulsive disorder. *American Journal of Psychotherapy, 31*, 450–465.

Gesell, A., & Ilg, F. (1943). *Infant and child in the culture today.* New York: Harper & Row.

Goodwin, A., Guze, S., & Robins, E. (1969). Follow-up studies in obsessional neurosis. *Archives of General Psychiatry, 20*, 182–187.

Goodwin, D., & Guze, S. (1979). *Psychiatric diagnosis.* London: Oxford University Press.

Grimshaw, L. (1965). The outcome of obsessional disorder. *British Journal of Psychiatry, 111*, 1051–1056.

Hall, M. (1935). Obsessive–compulsive states in childhood. *Archives of Diseases of Children, 10*, 49–59.

Hollingsworth, C., Tanguay, P., Grossman, L., & Pabst, P. (1980). Long-term outcome of obsessive compulsive disorder in childhood. *Journal of the American Academy of Child Psychiatry, 19*, 134–144.

Hoover, C., & Insel, T. (1984). Families of origin in obsessive compulsive disorder. *The Journal of Nervous & Mental Disease, 172*, 207–215.

Insel, T., Donnelly, E., & Lalaken, N. (1983). Neurological and neuropsychological studies of patients with obsessive–compulsive disorder. *Biological Psychiatry, 18*, 741–751.

Insel, T., Murphy, D., Cohen, R., Alterman, I., Kilts, C., & Linnoila, M. (1983). Obsessive–compulsive disorder: A double-blind trial of Clomipramine and Clorcyline. *Archives of General Psychiatry, 40*, 605–612.

Janet, P. (1903). *Les Obessions et la Psychiastrenie* (Vol. I). Paris: Felix Alean.

Judd, J. (1965). Obsessive–compulsive neurosis in children. *Archives of General Psychiatry, 40*, 136–143.

Kanner, L. (1957). *Child psychiatry.* Springfield, IL: Charles C Thomas.

Kringlen, E. (1965). Obsessional neurosis: A long-term follow-up. *British Journal of Psychiatry*, *111*, 709–722.

Lewis, A. (1935). Problems of obsessional illness. *Proceedings of the Royal Society of Medicine*, *29*, 325–336.

Loeb, L. (1986). Traumatic contributions in the development of an obsessional neurosis in an adolescent. *Adolescent Psychiatry*, *13*, 201–217.

Marks, I. (1981). Review of behavioral psychotherapy: I. Obsessive–compulsive disorders. *American Journal of Psychiatry*, *138*, 584–592.

McKeon, J., McGuffin, P., & Robinson, P. (1984). Obsessive–compulsive neurosis following head injury: A report of four cases. *British Journal of Psychiatry*, *144*, 190–192.

Montgomery, M.A., Clayton, P.I., & Friedhoff, A.J. (1982). Psychiatric illness in Tourette syndrome patients and first degree relatives. *In* A.L. Friedhoff and T.N. Chase (Eds.), *Advances in Neurology*. New York: Raven.

Nee, L., Caine, E., Eldridge, R., & Ebert, M. (1980). Gilles de la Tourette's syndrome: Clinical and family study of 50 cases. *Annals of Neurology*, *7*, 41–49.

O'Connor, J. (1983). Why I can't get hives: Brief strategy therapy with an obsessional child. *Family Process*, *22*, 201–209.

Ong, S., & Leng, V. (1979). The treatment of an obsessive–compulsive girl in the context of Malaysian Chinese culture. *Australian & New Zealand Journal of Psychiatry*, *13*, 255–259.

Ownby, R. (1983). A cognitive behavioral intervention for compulsive handwashing with a thirteen-year-old boy. *Psychology in the Schools*, *20*, 219–222.

Phillips, D., & Wolpe, S. (1981). Multiple behavior techniques in a severe separation anxiety of a 12-year-old. *Journal of Behavior Therapy & Experimental Psychiatry*, *12*, 329–332.

Politt, J. (1957). The natural history of obsessive states: A study of 150 cases. *British Medical Journal*, *1*, 194–198.

Pollak, J. (1979). Obsessive–compulsive personality: A review. *Psychological Bulletin*, *86*, 225–241.

Queiroz, L., Motta, M., Madi, M., Sossai, D., & Boren, J. (1981). A functional analysis of obsessive–compulsive problems with related therapeutic procedures. *Behaviour Research & Therapy*, *19*, 377–388.

Rachman, S., & Hodgson, R. (1980). *Obsessions and compulsions*. Englewood Cliffs, NJ: Prentice-Hall.

Rapoport, J. (1982). Childhood obsessive–compulsive disorder. In D. Shaffer, A. Ehrhardt, & L. Greenhill (Eds.), *Diagnosis and treatment in pediatric psychiatry*. New York: Macmillan.

Rapoport, J., Elkins, R., Langer, D., Sceery, W., Buschbaum, M., Gillin, J., Murphy, D., Zahn, T., Lake, R., Ludlow, C., & Mendelson, W. (1981). Childhood obsessive–compulsive disorder. *American Journal of Psychiatry*, *138*, 1545–1554.

Rasmussen, S., & Tsuang, M. (1984). The epidemiology of obsessive compulsive disorder. *Clinical Psychiatry*, *45*, 450–457.

Rasmussen, S., & Tsuang, M. (1986). Clinical characteristics and family history in DSM-III obsessive compulsive disorder. *American Journal of Psychiatry*, *143*, 317–322.

Rosenberg, C. (1967). Familial aspects of obsessional neurosis. *British Journal of Psychiatry*, *113*, 405–413.

Rutter, M., Tizard, J., & Whitmore, K. (1970). *Education, health, & behavior*. London: Longmans.

Sandler, J., & Hazari, A. (1960). The "obsessional": On the psychological classification of the obsessional character and symptoms. *British Journal of Medical Psychology*, *33*, 113–122.

Shapiro, A., Shapiro, E., Bauun, R., & Sweet, R. (1978). *Gilles de la Tourette's syndrome*. New York: Raven.

Skoog, G. (1965). Onset of anancastic conditions. *Acta Psychiatrica Scandinavica Supplement*, *41*, 184–192.

Slade, P. (1979). Psychometric studies in obsessional illness and obsessional personality. In H.R. Beech (Ed.), *Obsessional states*. London: Methuen.

Warneke, L. (1985). Intravenous chlorimipramine in the treatment of obsessional disorder: Case report. *Journal of Clinical Psychiatry*, *46*, 100–103.

Weissman, M., Meyers, J., & Harding, P. (1978). Psychiatric disorders in a U.S. urban community. *American Journal of Psychiatry*, *135*, 459–462.

Welner, A., Reich, T., & Robins, E. (1976). Obsessive–compulsive neurosis: Record follow-up and family studies. *Comprehensive Psychiatry*, *17*, 527–539.

Wolff, R. (1977). Systematic desensitization and negative practice to alter the aftereffects of a rape attempt. *Journal of Behavior Therapy & Experimental Psychiatry*, *8*, 423–425.

Wolff, R., & Rapoport, J. (1988). Behavioral treatment of childhood obsessive–compulsive disorders. *Behavior Modification*, *12*, 252–266.

Zikis, P. (1983). Treatment of an 11-year-old ritualizer and tiqueur girl with in vivo exposure and response prevention. *Behavioural Psychotherapy*, *11*, 75–81.

CHAPTER 11

Schizoid Disorders of Childhood and Adolescence

SULA WOLFF

The intriguing group of conditions to be described pose many nosological questions. In contrast to early infantile autism, a perplexing variety of names have been assigned to them by successive workers: Asperger's autistic psychopathy (Asperger, 1944, 1979; Wing, 1981); the psychoanalysts' borderline states (Ekstein & Wallerstein, 1956; Geleert, 1967; Singer, 1960) and severe disturbances of ego development (Weil, 1953); Wolff's schizoid personality disorder of childhood (Wolff & Barlow, 1979; Wolff & Chick, 1980; see also Jenkins, 1968; Jenkins & Glickman, 1946); more recently, since the advent of DSM-III and DSM-III-R (American Psychiatric Association, 1980, 1987), pervasive developmental disorder and schizotypal personality disorder of childhood (Nagy & Szatmari, 1986); and, finally, childhood schizophrenia (Cantor & Kestenbaum, 1986).

The following questions arise:

First, is there a single syndrome with a common etiology but with different clinical manifestations, or are we concerned with a group of conditions sharing some features but possibly differing in causation and outcome?

Second, are these childhood disorders continuous with the adult personality disorders described in the older psychiatric literature as schizoid personality disorder (Bleuler, 1954; Kasanin & Rosen, 1933; Kretschmer, 1925; Nannarello, 1953) and as pesudoneurotic schizophrenia (Hoch & Polatin, 1949), then as schizophrenic spectrum disorders (Kety, Rosenthal, Wender, Schulsinger, & Jacobsen, 1975; Rosenthal, 1975), and more recently in DSM-III as schizotypal, paranoid, schizoid, and possibly also borderline personality disorders?

Third, are the conditions to be thought of, as is envisaged for the new *International Classification of Diseases* (ICD-10) (WHO, 1987), as pervasive developmental disorders beginning in childhood, allied to early infantile autism, or are they more helpfully regarded as personality disorders? In DSM-III they might be classed as either.

Fourth, what, if any, are the genetic links between this group of disorders and the schizophrenias on the one hand and early infantile autism on the other, conditions so far regarded as genetically distinct?

Fifth, although severely affected children are clearly disturbed in many ways, and may have a variety of secondary psychiatric symptoms as a result of their social and cognitive impairments, very little is known about people who may have mild schizoid or schizotypal traits. Are we dealing with a group of personality traits that, as Claridge believes (Claridge, 1985; Claridge & Broks, 1984), are common in mild form in the general population so that disturbed people are merely those who have these traits in a severe form; are we dealing with a group of categorical disorders whose presence spells pathology; or are we concerned with categorical conditions that may be present so mildly that they then form part of normal personality variation but can be severe enough to cause trouble? In other words, are the conditions that concern us here to be ascribed to personality or developmental traits, to categorical features, or to a mixture of the two?

Sixth, what if any are the relationships of schizoid and schizotypal features in childhood with special giftedness, inventiveness, or genius?

Seventh, what is the relationship between these disorders and aggressive and antisocial conduct in childhood and adult sociopathy?

DEFINITION

Both the childhood and personality disorder sections of DSM-III represent considerable advances and are likely to contribute in a major way to the revision of the ICD. But the boundaries drawn in DSM-III between schizoid disorder and pervasive developmental disorder among the clinical conditions specific to childhood and schizotypal, schizoid, paranoid, borderline, and avoidant categories in the adult personality disorder section are as yet unlikely to reflect accurately those of the corresponding clinical syndromes (see Bemporad & Schwab, 1986). It is also unlikely that the proposed categorizations in ICD-10 of schizoid disorder of childhood (which includes Asperger's syndrome) with the pervasive developmental disorders among the disorders specific to childhood, of schizotypal disorder with the schizophrenias, and of paranoid and schizoid personality disorders in the personality disorder section will in the long term be found satisfactory.

DSM-III Criteria

Schizoid Disorder of Childhood and Adolescence

In this system this disorder is to be differentiated from avoidant disorder, schizophrenia, pervasive developmental disorders, and undersocialized, nonaggressive conduct disorder. The diagnostic criteria are: (1) no close friends of the same age other than a relative or similarly isolated child; (2) no apparent interest in making friends; (3) no pleasure from the usual peer interactions; (4) general avoidance of nonfamilial social contacts, especially with peers; (5) no interest in activities that involve other children (such as team sports or clubs); (6) duration of at least 3 months; (7) not due to pervasive developmental disorder, conduct disorder, undersocialized, non-aggressive, or any psychotic disorder such as schizophrenia; (8) if 18 or older, does not meet the criteria for schizoid personality disorder.

Clinically, the conditions discussed in this chapter and reported in the literature as Asperger's syndrome (not mentioned in DSM-III) or schizoid personality disorder of childhood would meet all these criteria except the last two but would also include criteria listed in DSM-III as defining other diagnostic categories.

Several of the more severely affected children described by Asperger, by Wing, and by myself would fulfill DSM-III criteria for childhood-onset pervasive developmental disorder, with the full syndrome, with the residual state, or in an atypical form (see Chapter 13 of this volume). In addition, as the more recent literature indicates, many of these children could be classified as having a childhood onset of one or more of the adult types of personality disorder defined in DSM-III as schizotypal, schizoid, or paranoid. For the sake of completeness, these definitions are here briefly outlined.

Schizotypal Personality Disorder

This disorder should comprise at least four of the following features as characterizing the individual's long-term functioning and causing significant social or occupational impairment or subjective distress: magical thinking; ideas of reference; social isolation; recurrent illusions; odd speech; inadequate rapport; suspiciousness; and undue social anxiety.

Schizoid Personality Disorder

This disorder is characterized by emotional coldness; indifference to praise or criticism or the feelings of others; no more than one or two close friends including family members; but without eccentricities of speech, behavior, or thought as in schizotypal personality disorder. (This exclusion seems odd when in fact in this diagnostic system more than one diagnosis is allowed.)

Paranoid Personality Disorder

This disorder is defined as characterized by *pervasive and unwarranted suspiciousness and mistrust* as indicated by at least three of the following: expectations of trickery or harm; hypervigilance; guardedness; avoidance of accepting blame when this is warranted; questioning the loyalty of others; intense, narrowly focused searching for confirmation of bias; overconcern with hidden meanings; pathological jealousy; *hypersensitivity* consisting of at least two of the following: easily slighted and offended; exaggeration of difficulties; readiness to counterattack; inability to relax; and *restricted affectivity* with at least two of the following: appearance of being cold and unemotional; taking pride in objectivity; lack of a sense of humor; absence of tender, sentimental feelings.

DSM-III-R Criteria

According to the recently revised edition, DSM-III-R (APA, 1987), the personality disorder categories may, as before, be applied to children and adolescents in "unusual circumstances" in which maladaptive personality traits appear to be stable. The exception is antisocial personality disorder, where it is now recommended that the category Conduct Disorder be applied to the young person because many conduct-disordered children outgrow their disturbances. The specific category of schizoid disorder of childhood or adolescence has now been omitted.

As in DSM-III, the personality disorders in DSM-III-R are to be recorded on Axis II of the multiaxial classification.

Schizotypal Personality Disorder

This disorder, a pervasive deficit in interpersonal relatedness with peculiarities of ideation, appearance, and behavior, is now defined by at least five of the following: ideas of reference; illusions; eccentric behavior or appearance; no (or only one) close friends apart from first-degree relatives; odd speech; inappropriate affect; suspiciousness or paranoid ideation.

Schizoid Personality Disorder

This disorder, a pervasive pattern of indifference to social relationships and a restricted range of emotional experience and expression, is characterized by at least four of the following: neither desires nor enjoys close relationships; almost always chooses solitary activities; rarely experiences strong emotions; shows little wish for sexual experiences with another person; is indifferent to praise and criticism; has no (or only one) close friends apart from first-degree relatives; displays constricted affect.

Paranoid Personality Disorder

This disorder, a pervasive and unwarranted tendency to interpret the actions of others as deliberately demeaning or threatening, is indicated by at least four of the following: expects without sufficient basis to be exploited or harmed by others; questions the loyalty or trustworthiness of others; reads hidden demeaning or threatening meanings into benign remarks or events; bears grudges; hesitates to confide in others because of unwarranted fears that the information will be used against him or her; is easily slighted and quick to react with anger; questions, without cause, the fidelity of his or her sexual partner.

The more specific DSM-III-R categories of disorders of childhood and adolescence are now subsumed under the heading "Disorders Usually First Evident in Infancy, Childhood, or Adolescence." Those resembling Asperger's syndrome and our own, somewhat broader, concept of schizoid disorders of childhood again appear on Axis II under the general heading "Pervasive Developmental Disorders." This broad category is characterized by impairment of the development of reciprocal social interaction, of communication skills (verbal and nonverbal), and of imaginative activity, with often a restricted repertoire of repetitive activities. Autistic disorders are no longer defined as necessarily beginning before 30 months. The term "pervasive developmental disorder not otherwise specified" is to be used when the criteria for autistic disorder, schizophrenia, schizotypal, or schizoid personality disorder are not met. Some people in this category will have a markedly restricted behavioral repertoire; others will not. The DSM-III criterion of onset after 30 months and before 12 years has been omitted.

It is clear that there is a great deal of overlap within each of the recent classifications, DSM-III, DSM-III-R, ICD-9, and ICD-10, between the definitions of diagnostic categories in this clinical domain, and that little is known about the reliability and validity of these categories (Tyrer & Ferguson, 1987). Therefore, this chapter does not confine itself to any one of these diagnostic schemes. Instead, it starts from the descriptions of the children, young people, and adults as they appear in the literature and in clinical practice.

The term *schizoid personality disorder* (see Tyrer & Ferguson, 1987) throughout is used in a broad sense to include conditions that have also been described as Asperger's syndrome, childhood-onset pervasive developmental disorders, and schizoid, paranoid, or schizotypal personality disorders. The children and young people to be described most often, but by no means invariably, fulfill the criteria for schizotypal personality disorder and, unlike children with pervasive developmental disorders, they are not usually lacking in imaginative activity.

HISTORICAL BACKGROUND

Hans Asperger, the German pedopsychiatrist working in Vienna, published his professorial thesis *Autistic Psychopathy of Childhood* in 1944, not then aware of Kanner's (1943) first description of early infantile autism the year before. Asperger presented four case histories with much literary skill. His account of the syndrome was based on 200 such children seen over 10 years. Because his definitive paper is not readily available in English, a full summary is presented here.

Not every child showed every symptom, yet they had many common features. These persisted throughout life, with some recognizable from the second year. There were universal abnormalities of gaze, impeding emotional contact, as well as poverty of facial expression and gesture. Stereotyped, repetitive movements were common. Speech and voice were often unnatural, like a caricature, inviting ridicule. Asperger described a peculiar autistic intelligence, with the balance between inventiveness and imitative learning weighted toward the former. Gifted autistic psychopaths expressed themselves in highly creative language using uncommon words they would rarely have heard, as well as neologisms. They perceived and thought about the world in new ways, with unusual achievements in restricted fields of special interest. These might be biology, chemistry, poisons, calculations, machinery, or art. While the children assessed themselves and others with surprising accuracy, their basic abnormality was a "disturbance of interactive relationships with others"

(p. 117). Asperger mentions prominent scientists who had autistic features, and suggests that these were associated with an increased facility for abstract thinking.

Affected children ranged from those with originality close to genius through inhibited, unproductive individuals cut off from reality to mentally retarded robotlike children with severe disturbances of affective contact. The last group included children with stereotypic habits and useless skills, like calendrical calculation or an exact memory for railway timetables.

He stressed the children's difficulties in meeting environmental demands, especially at school, so that some very clever children failed in reading, spelling, or arithmetic, unless this furthered their special interest. Asperger was not as aware as recent workers have been (Wing, 1981; Wolff & Chick, 1980) of the specific developmental disorders often associated with the syndrome. He saw the disorder as especially painful for parents, who complained of their children's lack of feeling. Some reported their offspring to be malicious, deliberately aiming to hurt others. Some children voiced sadistic impulses with ominous detachment, for example, to "plunge a knife into the mother's heart and watch the blood flow" (p. 124). Because they did not readily imitate their elders, they had to learn socially appropriate behavior laboriously through articulated rules. Negativism and angry outbursts were common. The children were loners, often reacting in crowded playgrounds with outbursts of rage or tears. They were both over- and insensitive, and sometimes very distressed in strange surroundings. They lacked humor except for puns. Relations with inanimate objects were also unusual, with the formation of specific attachments and collections.

As for the future, Asperger found gifted people to have excellent work adjustments, and considered that, except for the mentally handicapped who might lead a hobo life, with self-neglect and social ostracism as eccentrics, social adaptation often improved with age. Yet the basic personality features endured, and intimate inter-personal relationships remained impaired. Sexual interest might be lacking even in adult life, while some children developed early, fixed patterns of sexual deviancy.

The sex incidence puzzled Asperger. No girl had the complete syndrome, and a number of affected girls were postencephalitic. Yet many mothers had the full picture. He thought the condition might not show itself fully in girls before puberty, and he developed the notion, no longer acceptable, that the condition represented an extreme of male modes of thinking and feeling, with abstract processes pre-dominating.

He firmly held to a genetic causation, because in every case the syndrome or some of its traits were found in biological relatives. Fathers were often professional men or manual workers with intellectual interests. Some families contained artists or scientists in a number of generations. Asperger mentioned similarities with schizophrenia and considered the syndrome a possible preschizophrenic state. Yet apparently only a single case of his developed this psychosis, and he was unsure whether there was an excess of schizophrenia in the children's families. He asserted that the condition was not a process but a personality disorder, and likened it both to Kretschmer's schizothymia and Jung's introversion. He did not mention delinquency.

Only one psychoanalytic author will be cited: Annemarie Weil (1953), because of her illuminating description of "certain severe disturbances of ego development"

(p. 271). She stressed the need to distinguish affected children from neurotics. Abnormalities start early, but the children are most easily recognized during latency because they lack the reasonableness and attempts at control and integration that normally characterize this age period. She too mentioned high intelligence, special talents, and both over- and insensitivity. She referred to a "strongly tainted" (p. 272) heredity, with psychoses and "prepsychotic narcissistic, bizarre" (pp. 272–273) personalities among the relatives. She listed three types of clinical problems: (1) poor social adaptation with extreme, aloof withdrawal, a need for omnipotent control, and paranoid reactions, with ambivalence to others and excessive imitation, for example, of adult speech; (2) management problems with disproportionate outbursts of anger, impulsive unpredictability, and sadomasochism; and (3) neurotic symptoms of anxiety, obsessions and compulsions, restlessness, and autoerotic habits such as rocking. In later life, some of Weil's children became psychotic, but most improved, with "superficial socialization" (p. 276) but persistent deficits of personality structure. As adults, their disorders were described as latent schizophrenia or borderline states.

Wing (1981) reported on 34 patients aged 5 to 35, with what she preferred to call Asperger's syndrome, regarding the condition not as a personality disorder but as allied to early childhood autism. The main feature she stresses is "impairment of two-way social interactions" (p. 116). She refers to some bizarre antisocial behavior. Some of her children were slow to talk, while others were slow to walk and clumsy. Hers was not a child psychiatric population, she did not see any especially gifted people, and mild cases were excluded.

More recently, Nagy and Szatmari (1986) presented a chart review of 20 children fulfilling DSM-III criteria for schizotypal personality disorder: 18 boys and 2 girls. None met DSM-III criteria for infantile autism, but 18 met the criteria for pervasive developmental disorders if onset after 30 months is excluded as a criterion. Eight had experienced thought disorder and/or delusions and/or hallucinations, usually after puberty, and two were hospitalized with a DSM-III diagnosis of schizophrenia.

The Edinburgh Studies

Our own work aimed to validate the syndrome objectively, at first by using psychological tests to differentiate schizoid children from autistics and normals, and later by setting up predictive and consensual validation studies. In addition, the particular association between schizoid personality and antisocial conduct has been explored.

The first 11 children diagnosed as schizoid were described in 1964 before Van Krevelen's English-language accounts of Asperger's work became well known in the United Kingdom (Van Krevelen, 1963; Van Krevelen & Knipers, 1962). All were boys. Their difficulties could not be understood in terms of their life experiences, even after repeated interviews. All had had preschool difficulties, but these became a problem only on starting school. Although of average or above-average abilities, all the children failed socially at school and eight also educationally. Seven, all of high intelligence, were outgoing and communicative; four were withdrawn and uncommunicative. In eight cases one of the parents had schizoid traits and in two others a more distant relative was affected.

Barlow (Wolff & Barlow, 1979) compared small, matched groups of schizoid, autistic, and normal children on a series of psychological tests. The schizoids were atypical in that, to match the autistics, intellectually more able children had to be excluded. Schizoids were intermediate in functioning between normals and autistics. They shared autistic children's stereotypy, some of their linguistic handicaps, and their lack of perceptiveness for meaning. But they lacked the autistics' perserveration, were more poorly motivated for tasks involving cognition and memory (as if distractred from within), and, when describing people on two different tests, they used "psychological" constructs less often than normal and even autistic children.

For the predictive validation study, five core characteristics of the syndrome were postulated, at least for boys, on the basis of clinical experience. These were: (1) solitariness; (2) impaired empathy and emotional detachment; (3) increased sensitivity; (4) rigidity of mental set; and (5) an unusual or odd style of communicating (Wolff & Chick, 1980). Some 10 years after the initial referral, a research psychiatrist interviewed the 22 oldest and most typically schizoid boys as well as a control group of other male clinic attenders, matched for age, year of referral, IQ, and socioeconomic background, blind to the original diagnoses. The interview was structured and contained items designed to tap the postulated core features as well as enabling overall diagnoses of personality and psychiatric status to be made. Of the 22 subjects diagnosed as schizoid in childhood and 22 controls, 18 and 1, respectively, were diagnosed definitely schizoid at follow-up; 2 probands and 1 control were diagnosed doubtfully schizoid; and in 2 probands and 20 controls schizoid personality was judged definitely absent. The core characteristics also differentiated significantly between the groups as follows: four out of five measures for solitariness; self- and interviewer's ratings of impaired empathy as well as a rating of emotional detachment; sensitivity, but only when real handicaps or other stigmatizing features were allowed for; two out of three measures for rigidity (single-minded pursuits of special interests and obsessionality); and all measures for unusual communication.

The two groups did not differ from general population norms on Eysenck's Extraversion or Neuroticism scales, suggesting that schizoidness should not be equated with introversion. A photographs test for psychological construing, however, used also in the comparative study of schizoid, autistic, and normal children, differentiated significantly between the schizoid young adults and their matched controls, and was specifically associated with ratings of impaired empathy (Chick, Waterhouse, & Wolff, 1979). This provides some concurrent, experimental validation of the syndrome.

In a *consensual validation study* (Cull, Chick, & Wolff, 1984), for all 44 subjects, case histories were written, based on the interviews with the subjects themselves and on structured interviews with their mothers conducted by a research psychologist also blind to the diagnosis. These accounts were given to two independent, general psychiatrists for rating of personality disorders, personality characteristics, and psychiatric illness (before the advent of DSM-III). Agreement on the presence of schizoid personality with a consensus diagnosis reached by the research psychiatrists after the diagnostic code had been broken was 88% for one general psychiatrist and 72% for the other.

CLINICAL PICTURE

Because the phenomena that concern us here are not as yet universally recognized in child psychiatric practice, five case reports follow to give the reader an impression of the range of psychopathology to be defined, categorized, and, if possible, explained. These cases illustrate the difficulties there are in drawing boundaries between schizoid personality disorder and infantile autism, schizophrenia, specific developmental disorders, and sociopathy; and in knowing whether the children's conditions grouped together under the term *schizoid* are most helpfully considered as a single category or as multiple diagnostic groups.

CASE HISTORY I

Case I: Schizoid personality disorder (withdrawn, inhibited type) associated with mild mental retardation and elective mutism. Differential diagnosis: early infantile autism.

Referred: Age 10 with educational failure, solitariness, and elective mutism at school. Poor concentration. Draws pictures rapidly when under stress. IQ 66–72 with commensurate educational attainments.

History: Normal birth. Walked and talked at 12/12. Toilet trained soon after. "Slow in wanting to speak, although not in beginning to speak." Always preferred solitary, unimaginative play. Copied what others did. Crib-rocked as toddler; head-banged till age 10. When he was 5, mother left the family for reasons never understood by father and other children. All children brought up by father, but with regular visits to mother.

Family history: Professional family. Youngest child. Father and siblings have no schizoid traits. Mother (not personally seen) described by oldest daughter in later years as perfectionistic, erratic, tending to "pontificate" and to theorize about God and the planets, outgoing with friends, but not very understanding of other people, for example, her children. A second marriage also ended in divorce.

Assessment at 10: Neurologically normal. Fixed, blank facial expression with gaze avoidance. Immobile and lacking in drive. Voice high pitched and monotonous. Speech difficult to understand. No echolalia. Special interests: sewage systems and trains.

Progress: Became happier in a small school for mildly handicapped children. Remained withdrawn and anxious till age 15, with limited initiative and restricted interests. IQ then 73–85.

Follow-up at 20: Still living with father. Left school at 17. Has worked steadily as jobbing gardener for 2½ years. Said: "I am not happy working with other people.

I feel rushed. I like doing jobs on my own." Still plays with model railway and draws a lot. Now also interested in Georgian architecture.

Follow-up at 29: In same job. Lives with older sister; in regular contact with all members of the family. Joined rambling club and art classes. Has two friends he visits, both elderly men. No sexual experiences; considers marriage is not for him. Produces conventional oil paintings, copied from photographs; but also more original and very detailed pen and ink drawings, largely from memory, depicting old houses and city scenes, landscapes, and airplanes. The last are accompanied by written descriptions, copied from magazines, with many spelling errors. Now more outgoing, with clear speech and only a hint of gaze avoidance, but with a fixed smile, and still with markedly limited (and naive) facial expressions and restricted body movements.

Differentiation from early infantile autism: No delay in language acquisition; no typically autistic language abnormalities; no obsessive, repetitive behavior. (Artistic gifts have persisted. In autistic children they often wane at puberty.)

CASE HISTORY II

Schizoid personality disorder (outgoing) with specific developmental language and learning delays, in boy of good intelligence who later developed acute paranoid schizophrenia.

Referred: At 10 because of poor schoolwork, reluctance to mix with other children, and rocking movements. IQ: V 95, P 121. Verbally confused and long-winded. Good reading comprehension; poor accuracy; 3 years retarded in spelling. School psychologist commented on inappropriate wandering about the room during interview.

History: Normal birth. Insisted on feeding from one breast only. Walked at 18/12; toilet trained "late"; spoke "well by 2." Rocked since infancy. Always shy with other children. Always had food fads. Concentrated only on what interested him, recently ancient ruins and castles. Always obstinate. Severe measles at 4; rubella at 5½. Difficulty falling asleep.

Family history: Father, businessman with monosymptomatic phobia totally preoccupying his inner life for years: ruminative, self-preoccupied, with little feeling for the emotional needs of others. His symptom has a delusional quality. Mother warm, supportive of father and other children. One brother had transient language delay.

Initial assessment: Handsome boy with markedly impaired emotional contact. Looked warm and friendly but revealed himself as detached and remote. Had, and knew he had, word-finding difficulties ("I get all muddled up with my words"). Used odd expressions; rocked constantly.

At 17: Hospitalized because of sudden onset of schizophrenia; believed he had been hypnotized by some Chinese boys at school who were influencing his thoughts and made him think of jumping off a high building.

Follow-up at 26: On long-term neuroleptics. Living with parents and working in father's business. No friends. Still very handsome. Constant shaking of knees. Highly sensitive but lacking in empathy. Much socially inappropriate behavior and talk. Overtalkative and preoccupied with his schizophrenic illness and "paranoia."

Unusual thought processes; definite ideas of reference. Blames himself for his illness, but also for not always being kind to his siblings, and for having sexual thoughts about a girl in the neighborhood. Mentioned as his main, but not exclusive, interests: Roman history, coin collecting, and the Bible.

CASE HISTORY III

Schizoid personality disorder (outgoing) in highly intelligent boy who became an exceptionally gifted scientist.

Referred: At 14 because of school failure and "living in a fantasy world." His room at boarding school is littered with paper and apparently useless objects. Teachers report him as untidy, lazy, but also intellectually quick and resourceful. Bottom of class in all subjects except math and science. School essays consist of repetitive, macabre, and cruel themes.

History: Normal birth. Disliked mother holding him but was a sociable baby, early talker, and good at constructional play. Had a series of "compulsions": squeaking; fist banging. Difficulty falling asleep at night. Liked children at 2½, but made a terrible scene on first day at school and never liked it there. Hated ball games. At 5 invented an island on the ocean floor, peopled with imaginary inhabitants. Other children then enjoyed hearing about this. But at 14, when still preoccupied with these tales, he kept them to himself to avoid teasing from other boys. Friendless since middle childhood. Had abiding and all-consuming interest in electronics. Happiest alone.

Family history: Mother saw him as "introverted," like herself. She used to paint but gave this up abruptly on marriage. Decribed maternal grandfather as like her son: "brilliant, but eccentric and hard to live with." This caused maternal grandparents to separate during her childhood. Father and siblings not seen, but described by mother then as warm, sociable, and outgoing.

When first seen: Described himself as "square, different from other people," unable to "fit in." This worried him. WISC IQ:V 140, P 128.

Progress: His personality difficulties were explained to his teachers, with advice to reduce the pressures for conformity and build on his special interests. He was allowed to start an electronics club. His academic progress was excellent and he survived at the same school till he entered the university.

Follow-up at 28 years: Working as scientist at a most prestigious university. Had obtained three degrees. Reported he had never had a close friend and was as solitary as ever. Dressed all in black, with hair totally covering his eyes. When someone knocks on his door, he does not answer. Did enjoy a drama group he had joined temporarily; there he could "let himself go." Visits parents, but rarely talks to them. Still writes reams of rambling stories involving the occult, with much use of neologisms and metaphor. Ideally, he would want to live in this invented world, containing a professor, skeletons, and skulls. Yet he also longs for company.

Follow-up at 37 years: Now happily married with two children. Still working very successfully. He said: "I'm still much the same. Basically I'm a private person." He thought his oldest daughter resembled him: "She has the same sort of sinister bent. She likes dark and strange things. . . ." He now described one brother, less able than himself, as a solitary drifter, taking "low-level courses in psychology and massage." He can understand this brother; and of his maternal grandfather he said: "If we'd been contemporaries, we'd have got on rather well."

CASE HISTORY IV

Schizoid personality (outgoing) in intelligent girl with "borderline" and sociopathic traits.

Referred: At 11, shortly after father's death of a heart attack, because of awkward, self-willed behavior, and domination over her mother. Refused a routine tuberculin test at school, ran out of the room shouting she wanted to die. Previously had hit a teacher who was encouraging her to join in a game. Persistently hostile to elderly grandmother.

Past history: Normal birth and milestones. Demanding, cuddly baby. Fearless toddler, then mixing well with other children. Became solitary on starting school; withdrew from group activities; initially good school achievements declined.

Family history: Only child. Sensitive, emotionally responsive mother. Father never seen. No unusual personality traits described by mother.

Initial assessment: Big child. Highly communicative with marked lack of guardedness. Revealed a recurrent wish to die; also paranoid ideas. Wanted her environment to fit in with her needs. WISC IQ: V 115, P 103, especially gifted at math.

Progress: At 13 developed depressive symptoms with suicidal ideas. Brief psychiatric admission improved her mood state and sociability temporarily. Soon after, while staying with relatives, frightened a cousin with a book about "sex with medieval torture," and with a sheath knife with which she damaged some curtains.

At 16: Left school against educational advice. Unemployed. Grandmother joined the household. Patient told mother, "You chose her instead of me" and left home. Ran off to London. Came home weeks later, dirty, and with stories her mother could not believe.

At 17: Still unemployed; asked for career advice. After full psychological assessment (WAIS IQ: V 133, P 95) and consultations with career officers, at a time of full national employment, she refused all jobs open to the untrained, because of the low wages, but also all training that might last more than a week.

At 18: Still unemployed, she complained of a fly phobia in response to pressure from the employment agency to take a job. Because of her distress, hospital admission was arranged. Within a day she ran off and was once more lost to her mother, this time for 10 weeks.

Follow-up interview with mother at 23: Still unemployed, solitary, living with mother more peaceably (grandmother has died). Mild phobic symptoms remain and personality features are unchanged.

CASE HISTORY V

Schizoid personality disorder (inhibited) in boy of average ability with severe developmental expressive dysphasia in early and middle childhood, and subsequent sociopathy.

Initial referral: To neurologist, speech therapist, and psychologist at 4, because of speech delay.

First psychiatric referral: At 9 with temper outbursts, head banging, and verbal and physical attacks on other children at school in response to minor frustration. Attended special remedial school with small classes. Reported to isolate himself totally from others and to be unhappy.

History: Normal birth and motor milestones. Said "Mom" and "Dad" at 12/12 but then no more till 4½. Had comprehension difficulties till 2. Sociable at nursery school and up to about 6 years. Afterward always solitary and subject to explosive temper outbursts. General intellectual ability: average.

Family history: Skilled working-class family. Father and two sisters also had slow language development. Father is a conscientious, warm man. Mother, a nurse, subject to depressions, is sometimes vague in her talk and mildly out of touch emotionally. Family relationships have been good.

Initial assessment: Normal comprehension. Severe expressive dysphasia. Detached emotionally, avoiding eye contact; very objective in describing himself. Prefers to be alone. Left handed. Clumsy writer; good reader; poor speller.

Progress: At 10, very ritualistic about his belongings, especially books. Gets distressed (throws chairs) if his arrangements are interfered with. Paroxysmal rages at school continue, with bloodthirsty language and threats to kill the others. Said to be calculating and callous in his verbal and nonverbal attacks. Also oversensitive to slights, and suspicious. IQ: V 105, P 113. Spelling age 6.7; reading age 9.9. Has difficulty remembering names. A behavioral approach, initiated at school to cope with his outbursts, succeeded, to his own satisfaction. He remained in his small, structured, special school.

At 13: Still withdrawn and uncommunicative although language skills are much better. Behavior at school remains tolerable. He has had to transfer to senior school. No appropriate day school was available and he entered a special boarding school.

At 15: Big, physically mature. Gets on well with parents and has job delivering papers during weekends at home. Otherwise little drive or interests except in "the occult." Reads "uncensored" books, such as encyclopedias and the *Reader's Digest*, and "censored" books, by which he means sexy magazines.

At 15½: Began to become aggressive and assaultative again at school. Said, "I'm bored and I start annoying other people for no reason at all." Attacked a staff member and had to be restrained. Admitted no feeling of guilt: "It must have been the circumstances; I got bored. There's nothing at the school to fit my needs . . . you're left to your own imagination. There's no program." He longed for a "rota," and reacted especially badly to the self-exploratory group discussions instituted for school dropouts. Parents now very worried "in case the next time there'll be a death."

At 16: Feels school staff have it in for him. They find him egotistical, unable to see anyone else's viewpoint. They view some of his behavior as "bizarre," for example, when he argues with the TV newscaster. Became preoccupied with accidents and violent scenes, amassing in his room at home newspaper accounts of a violent criminal. Remained suspicious, dressed in black leather, and was once seen with a belt and padlock around his neck. Advice to the school to allow him to miss group discussions was not followed, and after one of these sessions he injured another boy with scissors, was charged, convicted, and put on probation. Transferred to special training center run on humanistic lines, but parents continue to worry especially because, for the first time, he physically attacked his father.

The impressions gained from our total cohort of 115 boys and 35 girls diagnosed on clinical grounds as having schizoid personality disorder (a sex ratio of 3.3:1) are that almost all had been referred during the school years. All had had difficulties in social and educational adjustment at school, and most were failing scholastically despite average or superior abilities. The presenting symptoms varied, ranging from school refusal to aggressive outbursts.

The features shared by the whole group were: (1) emotional detachment and solitariness (perhaps less marked for the girls) in addition to one or more of the following features; (2) lack of empathy for the feelings of others at times amounting to callousness; (3) sensitivity with occasional suspiciousness and paranoid ideation; (4) lack of adaptability to social demands with obstinacy and apparent willfulness (some children had obsessional patterns, and many had long-lasting circumscribed interests or preoccupations); and (5) odd ideation with metaphorical use of language and marked lack of guardedness. An unusual fantasy life was reported by a sizable minority. In addition, some had odd facial expressions (sometimes with gaze avoidance), odd body posture and movements, and unusual or manneristic voices. A very few children had had transient hallucinations and delusions under stress.

Their mean intelligence was higher than average, as was their socioeconomic background, so that for our follow-up studies it was difficult to find clinic controls to match them. In respect to social class, the schizoid children resembled autistic children referred to our child psychiatric service (Wolff, Narayan, & Moyes, 1988).

ASSOCIATED FEATURES

In our series, as in Asperger's and Wing's, some children had associated *developmental delays*, a minority had evidence of *cerebral dysfunction*, and a few were *intellectually retarded*.

In the cohort of 22 we followed up after 10 years, 2 of the schizoid young men turned out to be *gifted*: one became an artist and one a brilliant scientist. None of the controls had distinguished themselves in this way. Asperger too stressed the giftedness of some of the children he saw and of their parents. And in mentally handicapped schizoid and autistic children the phenomenon of *idiot savant* (see Hermelin & O'Connor, 1986; Scheerer, Rothmann, & Goldstein, 1945) is not uncommon. Robinson and Vitale (1954) described 3 cases of children who in retrospect belong to the schizoid/Asperger group, with circumscribed interest patterns: One knew a lot about nuclear fission; one about space; and the third had memorized all the local trolley bus and subway routes. I share Asperger's view that the particular cognitive and social features of schizoid personality foster the single-minded pursuit of original thought and action, unhampered by perceived needs for social conformity or by regard for extraneous concerns (Wolff, 1984). To this extent the genetic predisposition to schizoid personality may be biologically advantageous, promoting cultural innovation in scientific, artistic, or political spheres. This feature of the schizoid personality may also account for the excess of gifted and creative people among the relatives of schizophrenics (Karlsson, 1970), and for the association of allusive thinking on an object-sorting test (also found to characterize schizophrenics and their relatives) with creativity (Tucker, Rothwell, Armstrong, & McConaghy, 1982).

A substantial minority of our schizoid boys were withdrawn and uncommunicative, and the incidence of *elective mutism* was high: 4 among our first 30 cases. A majority of schizoid children were communicative and outgoing, and it is our impression, requiring confirmation, that this was so especially for the girls.

While the incidence of *conduct disorders* was no higher than in other clinic attenders, stealing was less often a feature of schizoid boys (Wolff & Cull, 1986), and in these, conduct disorder was not, as in the controls, related to family disruption and socioeconomic disadvantage. Instead, it was associated with an unusual fantasy life. In our total cohort of 145 schizoid children seen in 20 years, serious antisocial conduct was not rare (occurring in 29 out of 111 boys and in 13 out of 34 girls). It took the form of inexplicable and sometimes frightening aggression in the boys and of fraudulent behavior with pathological lying in both boys and girls (Wolff & Cull, 1986). Among adult criminals there is likely to be a subgroup with the clinical features of schizoid personality going back to childhood. These offenders may engage in more dangerous, more repetitive, more violent, and less comprehensible crimes (see Kozol, Boucher, & Garofalo, 1972). Mawson, Grounds, and Tantum (1985) have recently described a violent offender in a maximum security hospital with a clear-cut Asperger syndrome since early childhood, and Hollander and Turner (1985) identified one-third of serious juvenile, especially aggressive, offenders as having borderline, schizotypal, or paranoid personality disorders as well as an excess of developmental delays.

COURSE AND PROGNOSIS

Our 10-year follow-up confirmed Asperger's impression that the condition is very stable over time, the essential features present in childhood being recognizable in early adult life. In an ongoing further follow-up study, when the oldest subjects are now in their thirties, our tentative impression is that the more gifted people are now less solitary, some having married, but their basic personality characteristics remain distinct. On the other hand, some of the less able and withdrawn people, while often working satisfactorily, remain single and excessively dependent on their families.

IMPAIRMENT

The social and cognitive handicaps of schizoid children, as already indicated, impair their social and educational functioning at school. Unless special allowances are made for them, secondary emotional and behavioral disorders of a varied range are common.

COMPLICATIONS

An unexpected finding of the follow-up of our oldest male schizoids (Wolff & Chick, 1980) was the significantly increased rate of later psychiatric morbidity, especially depression and suicidal thoughts or actions, compared with the matched clinic controls.

By the time of this follow-up, a diagnosis of schizophrenia had been made in 2 of the 22 schizoid cases but in none of the controls.

While schizoid youngsters referred to a clinic are no more prone to display anti-social conduct than other psychiatrically disturbed children, their delinquency is less comprehensible and more likely to take the form of aggression or pathological lying.

EPIDEMIOLOGY

Nothing is as yet known about the prevalence of this condition in the general population. One major difficulty here is to define the boundary between normal variations of personality and pathology.

Most of the work has been based on clinic populations of referred children, and the picture of schizoid personality that emerges, while of immediate clinical relevance, may be biased. The sex incidence, for example, may in part be a referral artifact. The clinical picture may well be different and milder in girls, with schizoid withdrawal and solitariness less common.

FAMILIAL PATTERN

All authors have stressed the constitutional nature of the disorder and its familial incidence, but there has been no systematic study of the incidence of either schizoid personality disorder or schizophrenia in the biological relatives of affected children. Van Krevelen (1963) reported two families who had both a child with early infantile autism and a child with Asperger's syndrome.

DIFFERENTIAL DIAGNOSIS

In most cases the distinction between schizoid personality disorder and *early infantile autism* is not in doubt (see Nagy & Szatmari, 1986). Onset is in middle childhood, and the characteristic language abnormalities, the gross impairment of sociability, and the aimless repetitive behavior of autism are lacking. Yet children have been described with features that could fit both syndromes (Bosch, 1970). It is the author's impression that well-functioning autistic adolescents and young adults are more flexible, more eager to adapt socially, and more open to social skills training than schizoid young people of the same intellectual level, who remain more rigid and egocentric and expect the world to accommodate to them.

Schizoid children do not have the symptoms necessary for a diagnosis of *schizophrenia*, although they may be at greater risk than the general population for developing this illness in later life.

ETIOLOGICAL SPECULATIONS

If it should turn out that the characteristics of schizoid children grown up are indistinguishable from those of adults with schizophrenic spectrum disorders, then a genetic link with schizophrenia must be entertained. About one-half of schizophrenic patients have abnormal premorbid personalities (Bleuler, 1978), and Slater (1953) described biological relatives of schizophrenics as having eccentric tendencies, lack of feelings, and anergic and paranoid traits, which resemble the features of our schizoid children. Moreover, Bleuler (1978) recorded the offspring of schizophrenic patients as secretive, cold, unpredictable, and bizarre. Yet even if the premorbid personality traits of 50% of schizophrenic patients were equivalent to schizoid personality disorder (Asperger's syndrome), this tells us nothing of the magnitude of the increased risk of later schizophrenia in affected children. It may be quite small. At a mean age of 22 years, 2 of our 22 schizoid young men had been given a diagnosis of schizophrenia, as had a similar proportion of Nagy and Szatmari's (1986) schizotypal children.

Further slight evidence for a link between schizophrenia and schizoid personality disorder in childhood comes from Zeitlin's (1986) study of psychiatrically disturbed adults who had been referred to a psychiatric clinic as children. Of 14 adult schizophrenics, 4 had been given the same diagnosis in childhood, but 8 of the remaining 10 had had symptoms of conduct disorder with or without emotional or developmental disorders also. Two more specific features had characterized these 8 children, suggesting that they fell into the schizoid/Asperger group: social isolation from peers and the clinicians' recorded description of their behavior as incongruous or unpredictably odd.

O'Neal and Robins, as long ago as 1958, had compared the characteristics of referred children who later became schizophrenic with those of future healthy adults. In both groups childhood conduct disorders were common but the future schizophrenics more often engaged in physical aggression and pathological lying, just as did our own antisocial schizoid children. Odd, paranoid ideas, a cold and unaffectionate temperament, and sleep disorders were also common among future schizophrenics. O'Neal and Robins stressed the importance of recognizing prepsychotic antisocial children, to avoid penal dispositions in favor of psychiatric treatment. Ricks and

Berry (1970) in a similarly conceived study described the characteristics of future schizophrenics seen in a child guidance clinic as social withdrawal, psychoticlike behavior, obsessive thinking, rigidity, abnormal speech output, abnormal gait, low capacity for empathy with peers, and acting-out behavior. Neurological impairment was common.

Support for a genetic link between schizophrenia and schizoid personality disorder of childhood should come from the clinical descriptions of "high-risk" children. Erlenmeyer-Kimling, Kestenbaum, Bird, and Hilldoff (1984), for example, found the offspring of schizophrenic mothers to differ from children of healthy parents in their aggressiveness, withdrawal, poor relationships with teachers, distractibility, and conceptual and cognitive deficits. The trouble with many of these studies is that high- and low-risk children were compared not clinically, but on rather nonspecific physiological, cognitive, temperamental, and social variables without clear hypotheses as to what patterns of personality or cognitive deficits were likely to distinguish the groups (see Watt, 1984).

In contrast, in a less-well-controlled follow-up of 12 infants of schizophrenic and 12 of nonschizophrenic mothers, Fish (1984) found 5 cases of DSM-III schizotypal or schizoid personality disorder and one of paranoid personality disorder among the high-risk children but none among the controls. One of her subjects, fulfilling DSM-III criteria for schizotypal personality disorder, later developed an acute schizophrenia (Fish, 1986). In the most carefully carried out prospective study of high-risk children, Parnas, Schulsinger, Schulsinger, Mednik, and Teasdale (1982) found that by the age of 33 there was a marked excess both of schizophrenia and of DSM-III schizotypal personality disorder among the offspring of schizophrenic mothers compared with the offspring of healthy parents. The premorbid characteristics distinguishing schizophrenic and schizotypal high-risk children from those who at 33 were not disturbed were: incoherence; pathological associations; incongruous facial expressions; abnormal emotional rapport; difficulty in making friends; tenseness; and poor cognitive performance at 15 years of age. Shyness and withdrawal, as in other studies (Michel, Morris, & Sorbler, 1957; Morris, Escoll, & Wexler, 1956), did not predict later schizophrenia or schizotypal disorder.

In a recent controlled study of parents of autistic children and parents of children with other handicaps (Wolff et al., 1988), we found more parents of autistics, especially fathers, to have mild schizoid traits and also, despite matching for socioeconomic status and no significant difference in tested intelligence, to have higher educational achievements. We speculate that, despite the hereditary differentiation between childhood autism and schizophrenia, these conditions may share a genetic predisposition to schizoid personality traits, as well as having further necessary genetic characteristics, specific for each.

Many questions remain unanswered: those relating to the possible genetic links with autism and schizophrenia; to the sex incidence of the condition; to its associations with specific developmental delays (which are thought to be sex linked), and with organic cerebral damage; to the possible association of schizoid traits with giftedness and high social class; and to the effects of schizoid personality disorder on marriage and fertility rates in men and women of different intellectual and social levels. It is possible that, like schizophrenics, schizoid women marry and procreate more readily than schizoid men in all social classes; but that, while schizoid traits are a handicap to marriage and sexual relations among relatively dull and socially disadvantaged men, they may be prized in husbands of superior intelligence among middle and upper social classes.

Despite the puzzle of this condition, often so stressful especially for the parents, the clinician's role is clear.

CLINICAL MANAGEMENT

The condition or group of conditions described needs to be recognized for the following reasons:

1. The personality handicaps of affected children are largely constitutional, and also very long lasting. It compounds the difficulties of families if psychiatric and psychological interventions are based on an erroneous assumption of a psychogenic etiology and on unrealistic expectations for change.
2. The child, the parents, and the teachers are helped if the child's basic personality characteristics are openly acknowledged and understood as part of his or her nature, likely to persist. Allowances have to be made for schizoid children, especially at school. They cope better and with fewer secondary emotional and behavioral symptoms when there is little pressure for gregarious conformity.
3. In families with such a child, as indeed ideally in all families, family dysfunction should be evaluated from the point of view of how much it reflects constitutional personality features of child or parent(s), and how much it expresses the family members' reactions to adverse life experiences. Rado, who incidentally used the term *schizotypal* to stand for *schizophrenic phenotype*, as long ago as 1953 proposed that maladaptations be viewed from both a biological and a psychodynamic perspective. Almost all descriptions of schizoid children stress how commonly one or both parents have similar personality traits. The limited freedom of affected people for change needs to be acknowledged, even if, in the children, this is masked by apparent willfulness. Costly, ineffective psychotherapeutic interventions, likely to increase the pain of child and parents, must be avoided.
4. The nature of the child's condition should determine the psychiatric and educational treatments. Schizoid children with ego deficits, as the psychoanalytic literature makes clear, respond badly to intrusive, interpretive psychotherapy. Instead, a long-term, supportive approach, with the therapist as an "auxiliary ego," can be helpful. Schizoid children also respond to behavioral approaches, including social skills training. At times of stress and during brief episodes of psychotic decompensation, major tranquilizers are helpful.
5. At school, schizoid children often cope better in small, structured classes with permission, if necessary, to avoid group games and noisy activities in

a crowded playground. The child's obstinate refusal to work at subjects other than those of his or her chosen interest can be circumvented by using these interests and any special gifts he or she may have as an initial basis for the educational program, extending this gradually to other fields.

6. As with all children with long-term handicaps, professionals should be available for consultation about treatment and education as the child's needs change in the course of childhood and especially during the transition from school to work. An optimistic stance is warranted because, once school pressures for conformity are at an end, life adjustment often improves.

7. In schizoid young people who become delinquent, psychiatrists can helpfully provide evidence for the courts about the underlying personality disorder, to avoid the deterioration likely to occur if the offender is sent to an ordinary penal setting. Two of the author's 20 seriously antisocial schizoid boys are known to have killed themselves after admission of one to an approved school and the other to prison.

CONCLUSIONS

It remains unclear whether the phenomena here described form a single or multiple syndrome(s). Affected children certainly have enough in common to be thought of as falling into a single category for the purpose of clinical management, at least until greater diagnostic certainty is achieved. Whether or not schizoid personality disorder of childhood is equivalent to the adult personality disorders variously labeled as schizoid, schizotypal, and borderline is currently being studied. A second follow-up of a larger cohort of schizoid children, boys and girls, is under way, using our own interview schedule for schizoid personality as we had defined it, as well as Gunderson's diagnostic interview for borderlines (Gunderson, Kolb, & Austin, 1981) and the Baron schedule for schizotypal personality disorder (Baron, Asnis, & Gwen, 1981). This study should also tell us whether schizoid girls are different from schizoid boys, the hypothesis being that there will be more subjects with DSM-III schizotypal and even borderline features among the girls, and more with DSM-III schizoid characteristics among the boys.

The clinical phenomena of schizoid personality disorder of childhood may well represent a group of heterogeneous conditions. Some cases could be classified as pervasive developmental disorders and others as adult personality disorders with onset in childhood. In the present state of knowledge it seems counterproductive to adhere to rigid specifications of multiple subcategories. Instead, affected children can be helpfully classified as having either a pervasive developmental disorder (if severely affected, resembling autistic children but with a later onset) or as falling within the schizotypal/schizoid/paranoid group of adult personality disorders (if more mildly affected). The criteria for such categorization should be flexibly based on the detailed clinical descriptions of Asperger, Wing, and Wolff, recognizing that within this broad syndrome individual children will differ considerably from one another.

It is our impression, requiring confirmation, that a number of our schizoid young people, especially girls, develop features of borderline personality disorder in later life when under stress. The features characterizing this disorder in DSM-III seem to be complications rather than essential personality traits, and it may be preferable not to use this category for the conditions described in this chapter.

REFERENCES

American Psychiatric Association. (1980). *Diagnostic and statistical manual of mental disorders* (3rd ed.). Washington, DC: Author.

American Psychiatric Association. (1987). *Diagnostic and statistical manual of mental disorders* (3rd ed., rev.). Washington, DC: Author.

Asperger, H. (1944). Die Autistischen Psychopathen im Kindesalter. *Archiv für Psychiatrie und Nervenkrankheiten, 177,* 76–137.

Asperger, H. (1979). Problems of infantile autism. *Communication, 13,* 45–52.

Baron, M., Asnis, L., & Gruen, R. (1981). Schedule for interviewing schizotypal personalities. *Psychological Research, 4,* 213–228.

Bemporad, J.R., & Schwab, M.E. (1986). The DSM-III and clinical child psychiatry. In T. Millon & G.L. Klerman (Eds.), *Contemporary directions in psychopathology: Towards the DSM-IV.* New York & London: Guilford.

Bleuler, M. (1954). The concept of schizophrenia: Correspondence. *American Journal of Psychiatry, 11,* 382–383.

Bleuler, M. (1978). *The schizophrenic disorders.* New Haven: Yale University Press.

Bosch, G. (1970). *Infantile autism: a clinical and phenomenological anthropological investigation taking language as a guide* (D. Jordan & I. Jordan, Trans.). Berlin & New York: Springer.

Cantor, S., & Kestenbaum, C. (1986). Psychotherapy with schizophrenic children. *Journal of the American Academy of Child Psychiatry, 25,* 623–630.

Chick, J., Waterhouse, L., & Wolff, S. (1979). Psychological construing in schizoid children grown up. *British Journal of Psychiatry, 135,* 425–430.

Claridge, G. (1985). *Origins of mental illness: Temperament, deviance and disorder.* Oxford & New York: Basil Blackwell.

Claridge, G., & Broks, P. (1984). Schizotypy and hemisphere function: I. Theoretical considerations and measurement of schizotypy. *Personality & Individual Differences, 5,* 633–648.

Cull, A., Chick, J., & Wolff, S. (1984). A consensual validation of schizoid personality in childhood and adult life. *British Journal of Psychiatry, 144,* 646–648.

Ekstein, R., & Wallerstein, J. (1956). Observations on the psychotherapy of borderline and psychotic children. *Psychoanalytic Study of the Child, 15,* 37–46.

Erlenmeyer-Kimling, L., Kestenbaum, C., Bird, H., & Hilldoff, U. (1984). Assessment of the New York High Risk Project subjects in sample A who are now clinically deviant. In

N.F. Watt, E.J. Anthony, L.C. Wynne, & J.E. Rolf (Eds.), *Children at high risk of schizophrenia*. Cambridge: Cambridge University Press.

Fish, B. (1984). Pandysmaturation. In N.F. Watt, E.J. Anthony, L.C. Wynne, & J.E. Rolf (Eds.), *Children of high risk of schizophrenia*. Cambridge: Cambridge University Press.

Fish, B. (1986). Antecedents of acute schizophrenic break. *Journal of the American Academy for Child Psychiatry, 25*, 595–600.

Geleert, E.R. (1967). Borderline states in childhood and adolescence. *Psychoanalytic Study of the Child, 13*, 279–295.

Gunderson, J., Kolb, J., & Austin, V. (1981). The diagnostic interview for borderlines. *American Journal of Psychiatry, 138*, 896–903.

Hermelin, B., & O'Connor, N. (1986). Idiot savant calendrical calculators: Rules and regularities. *Psychological Medicine, 16*, 885–893.

Hoch, P.H., & Polatin, P. (1949). Pseudoneurotic forms of schizophrenia. *Psychiatric Quarterly, 23*, 248–276.

Hollander, H.E., & Turner, F.D. (1985). Characteristics of incarcerated delinquents: Relationship between developmental disorders, environmental and family factors, and patterns of offence and recidivism. *Journal of the American Academy of Child Psychiatry, 24*, 221–226.

Jenkins, R.L. (1968). The varieties of children's behavior problems and family dynamics. *American Journal of Psychiatry, 124*, 1440–1445.

Jenkins, R.L., & Glickman, S. (1946). The schizoid child. *American Journal of Orthopsychiatry, 16*, 255–261.

Kanner, L. (1943). Autistic disturbances of affective contact. *The Nervous Child, 2*, 217–250.

Karlsson, J.L. (1970). Genetic association of giftedness and creativity with schizophrenia. *Hereditas, 66*, 177–181.

Kasanin, J., & Rosen, Z.A. (1933). Clinical variables in schizoid personalities. *Archives of Neurology & Psychiatry, 30*, 538–566.

Kety, S.S., Rosenthal, D., Wender, P.H., Schulsinger, F., & Jacobsen, B. (1975). Mental illness in the biological and adoptive families of adopted individuals who have become schizophrenic: A preliminary report based on psychiatric interviews. In R.R. Fieve, D. Rosenthal, & H. Brill (Eds.), *Genetic research in psychiatry*. Baltimore: Johns Hopkins University Press.

Kozol, E., Boucher, R.J., & Garofalo, R.F. (1972). The diagnosis and treatment of dangerousness. *Crime & Delinquency, 18*, 371–392.

Kretschmer, E. (1925). *Physique and character*. London: Kegan Paul, Trench and Trubner.

Mawson, D.C., Grounds, A., & Tantum, D. (1985). Violence and Asperger's syndrome. *British Journal of Psychiatry, 147*, 566–569.

Michel, C.M., Morris, D.P., & Sorbler, E. (1957). Follow-up studies of shy withdrawn children: II. Relative incidence of schizophrenia. *American Journal of Orthopsychiatry, 27*, 331–337.

Morris, D.P., Escoll, P.S., & Wexler, R. (1956). Aggressive behavior disturbance of childhood: A follow-up study. *American Journal of Psychiatry, 112*, 991–997.

Nagy, J., & Szatmari, P. (1986). A chart review of schizotypal personality disorders in children. *Journal of Autism & Developmental Disorders, 16*, 351–367.

Nannarello, J.J. (1953). Schizoid. *Journal of Nervous & Mental Disease, 118*, 237–249.

O'Neal, P., & Robins, L.N. (1958). Childhood patterns predictive of adult schizophrenia: A 30-year follow-up study. *American Journal of Psychiatry, 115*, 385–391.

Parnas, J., Schulsinger, F., Schulsinger, H., Mednik, S.A., & Teasdale, T.W. (1982). Behavioral precursors of schizophrenia spectrum: A prospective study. *Archives of General Psychiatry, 39*, 658–664.

Petty, L.K., Ornitz, E.M., Michelman, D.D., & Zimmermann, E.G. (1984). Autistic children who became schizophrenic. *Archives of General Psychiatry, 41*, 129–135.

Rado, S. (1953). Dynamics and classification of disordered behavior. *American Journal of Psychiatry, 110*, 406–416.

Ricks, D.F., & Berry, J.C. (1970). Family and symptom patterns that precede schizophrenia. In M. Roff & D.F. Ricks (Eds.), *Life history research in psychopathology*. Minneapolis: University of Minnesota Press.

Robinson, J.F., & Vitale, L.J. (1954). Children with circumscribed interest patterns. *American Journal of Orthopsychiatry, 24*, 755–766.

Rosenthal, D. (1975). The genetics of schizophrenia. In R.R. Fieve, D. Rosenthal, & H. Brill (Eds.), *Genetic research in psychiatry*. Baltimore: Johns Hopkins University Press.

Scheerer, M., Rothmann, E., & Goldstein, K. (1945). A case of "idiot savant": An experimental study of personality organization. *Psychological Monographs, 58*, 1–63.

Singer, M.B. (1960). Fantasies of a borderline patient. *Psychoanalytic Study of the Child, 15*, 310–356.

Slater, E. (1953). Quoted in Slater, E., & Roth, M. (1977), *Clinical psychiatry* (3rd ed.). London: Bailliere, Tindall and Casell.

Tucker, P.K., Rothwell, S.J., Armstrong, M.S., & McConaghy, N. (1982). Creativity, divergent and allusive thinking in students and visual artists. *Psychological Medicine, 12*, 835–841.

Tyrer, P., & Ferguson, B. (1987). Editorial: Problems in the classification of personality disorders. *Psychological Medicine, 17*, 15–20.

Van Krevelen, D. Arn. (1963). On the relationship between early infantile autism and autistic psychopathy. *Acta Paedopsychiatrica, 30*, 303–323.

Van Krevelen, D. Arn., & Knipers, C. (1962). The psychopathology of autistic psychopathy. *Acta Paedopsychiatrica, 29*, 22–31.

Wallace, M. (1986). *The silent twins*. Harmondsworth, Middlesex: Penguin.

Watt, N.F. (1984). In a nutshell: The first two decades of high-risk research in schizophrenia. In N.F. Watt, E.J. Anthony, L.C. Wynne, & J.E. Rolf (Eds.), *Children at high risk of schizophrenia*. Cambridge: Cambridge University Press.

Weil, A.P. (1953). Certain severe disturbances of ego development in childhood. *Psychoanalytic Study of the Child, 8*, 271–287.

Wing, L. (1981). Asperger's syndrome: A clinical account. *Psychological Medicine, 11*, 115–129.

Wolff, S. (1964, August). *Schizoid personality disorder in childhood*. Paper presented at the Sixth International Congress of Psychotherapy, London.

Wolff, S. (1984). Schizoid personality. In J. Wortis (Ed.), *Mental retardation and developmental disabilities* (Vol. 13). New York: Plenum.

Wolff, S., & Barlow, A. (1979). Schizoid personality in childhood: A comparative study of schizoid, autistic and normal children. *Journal of Child Psychology & Psychiatry, 20*, 29–46.

Wolff, S., & Chick, J. (1980). Schizoid personality in childhood: A controlled follow-up study. *Psychological Medicine, 10*, 85–100.

Wolff, S., & Cull, A. (1986). "Schizoid" personality and antisocial conduct: A retrospective case note study. *Psychological Medicine, 16*, 677–687.

Wolff, S., Narayan, S., & Moyes, B. (1988). Characteristics of parents of autistic children: A controlled study. *Journal of Child Psychology & Psychiatry, 29*, 143–153.

World Health Organization (1987). *I.C.D.-10 1986 draft of chapter V: Mental, behavioural and developmental disorders*. Geneva: WHO Division of Mental Health.

Zeitlin, H. (1986). *The natural history of psychiatric disorder in children*. Maudsley Monographs No. 29. Oxford: Oxford University Press.

CHAPTER 12

Autism

EDWARD M. ORNITZ

DEFINITION

Autism is a severe developmental disorder of behavior that is not accompanied by demonstrable neurologic signs, consistent neuropathology, biochemical or metabolic changes, or genetic markers. Multiple etiologies are suggested by the association with autism of many pre-, peri-, and neonatal conditions that putatively are likely to insult fetal or neonatal brain function. Such conditions account for about one quarter of all cases. In the remaining cases, potential etiologic factors have not been identified, although some evidence from family studies suggests a subgroup with a genetic component.

At least 4 out of 10,000 children are afflicted, and about 80% of those afflicted are mentally retarded. The onset is usually within the first 30 months of life. Most patients remain severely disabled and require care throughout their lives. Longevity is within the normal range.

The behavioral syndrome is unique, consisting of specific disturbances of: (1) relating to people; (2) communication and language; (3) response to objects; (4) sensory modulation; and (5) motility. The complete syndrome is usually observed, or described retrospectively by the parents, before 5 years of age. During later childhood and adolescence, the clinical picture may change. For the majority of patients who are verbally impaired, some continue to appear primarily autistic and others more retarded; a higher-functioning verbal minority manifest symptoms of various personality disorders or, occasionally, a schizophrenic thought disorder.

1. The *disturbances of relating to people* include, for example, emotional remoteness, lack of eye contact, and indifference to affection.

2. The *disturbances of communication and language* include the absence of both verbal and nonverbal communicative intent, severe delays in the acquisition of language, and deviant forms of language, such as delayed echolalia, pronoun reversal, and aprosodic speech.

3. The *disturbances of response to objects* include, for example, stereotypic ordering and arranging of toys without regard to their function, intolerance of change in surroundings and routines, rituals, and the absence of imaginative play.

4. The *disturbances of sensory modulation* involve all sensory modalities, and the faulty modulation is manifest as both under- and overreactivity to sensory stimuli. The latter is often associated with a tendency to seek out and induce sensory input, for example, visual scrutiny of spinning objects.

5. The *disturbances of motility* include, for example, hand flapping and whirling, and may provide such input through proprioceptive and kinesthetic channels.

DSM-III (APA, 1980) fails to include the disturbances of sensory modulation and motility in the diagnostic criteria for autism while including these behaviors in an otherwise similar diagnostic entity called childhood-onset pervasive developmental disorder (COPDD). DSM-III insists that the onset of infantile autism must occur before 30 months of age while the onset of COPDD must occur after 30 months of age. The inadequacies of this distinction are discussed throughout this chapter.

The DSM-III diagnostic criteria for infantile autism are:

1. Onset before 30 months
2. Pervasive lack of responsiveness to other people (autism)
3. Gross deficits in language development
4. If speech is present, peculiar speech patterns such as immediate and delayed echolalia, metaphorical language, pronominal reversal
5. Bizarre responses to various aspects of the environment, for example, resistance to change, peculiar interest in or attachments to animate or inanimate objects.

DSM-III criteria 2 through 5 are congruent with criteria 1 through 3 in this chapter's definition of autism.

HISTORICAL BACKGROUND

Although isolated cases were reported earlier, the syndrome of autism was first formally described in a group of 11 children by Kanner (1943) under the heading "Autistic Disturbances of Affective Contact." In 1944, Kanner adopted the term *early infantile autism*, drawing attention to the fact that the autistic behavior develops in early infancy. This term and its synonyms—*childhood autism, infantile autism*, and *autistic child*—have become the most commonly accepted way of referring to this condition. It is also occasionally referred to as Kanner's syndrome.

The term *atypical development* (Putnam, Rank, Pavenstedt, Andersen, & Rawson, 1948; Rank, 1949, 1955; Reiser, 1963) has been used to describe patients whose symptoms may have been less severe.

The term *symbiotic psychosis* had been used to describe children whose way of relating appeared superficially to be the opposite of an autistic way of relating (Mahler, 1952, 1965). The children, rather than being aloof and remote, would cling tenaciously to the parent. Since such behavior can be found transiently or intermittently in autistic children who are otherwise completely emotionally detached, this term does not describe an independent disorder.

The term *pseudo-retarded* or *pseudo-defective* was used at a time when considerable emphasis was placed on the differential diagnosis between mental retardation and childhood autism. It was thought that the retardation was only apparent—an artifact of inability to relate to tasks and communicate (Bender, 1947, 1956). Since later studies demonstrated that the majority of autistic children are in fact permanently retarded (Lockyer & Rutter, 1969; Rutter, Greenfeld, & Lockyer, 1967), this term is no longer applicable.

The more general but less-well-defined term *infantile psychosis* and its synonyms—*childhood psychosis* and *early onset psychosis*—had been used extensively (Brown, 1969; Havelkova, 1968; Kolvin, 1971; Kolvin, Ounsted, Humphrey et al., 1971; Lockyer & Rutter, 1969; Reiser, 1963; Rutter, 1965, 1967; Rutter & Lockyer, 1967; Rutter et al., 1967). Since autism has been classified by DSM-III and DSM-III-R as a developmental disorder (APA, 1980, 1987) and is no longer considered a psychosis, these terms are no longer acceptable synonyms.

A final term that has received wide usage as a diagnostic label for this group of children is *childhood schizophrenia* (Alderton, 1966; Bender, 1947, 1956; Bender & Freedman, 1952; Bender, Freedman, Grugett, & Helme, 1952; Creak, 1961; DeMyer, Churchill, Pontius, & Gilkey, 1971; Fish, Shapiro, Campbell, & Wile, 1968; Goldfarb, 1961, 1963; Lowe, 1966). The use of this term has created some semantic confusion and much diagnostic controversy in the literature concerned with autistic children, since many students of this illness emphasized that autism is phenomenologically quite distinct from schizophrenia (Kolvin, Ounsted, Humphrey et al., 1971; Rutter, 1965, 1967; Wing, 1966), while others described a continuum of symptoms relating the two syndromes (Bender, 1956, 1971; Brown & Reiser, 1963; Havelkova, 1968). Kanner himself had at one time described autism as "the earliest possible manifestation of childhood schizophrenia" which would never "at any future time have to be separated from the schizophrenias" (1949, pp. 419–420), while in other writings he emphasized "the 'uniqueness' or 'unduplicated nature' of autism" (1943, 1971, p. 141). This nosologic uncertainty was reflected in DSM-II (APA, 1968), which provided the category of schizophrenia, childhood type, and no category for autism, and DSM-III (1980), which provides the category of infantile autism and does not recognize childhood schizophrenia as a disorder distinct from schizophrenia in adults. Both the distinctions and the relationships between autism and schizophrenia are discussed in appropriate sections of this chapter.

CLINICAL PICTURE

It is helpful to think of several categories or subclusters of symptoms when making the diagnosis of childhood autism. These symptom subclusters include: (1) disturbances of relating to people; (2) disturbances of communication and language; (3) disturbances of response to objects; (4) disturbances of sensory modulation; and (5) disturbances of motility.

Disturbances of Relating to People

Behaviors indicative of an early failure to develop interpersonal relationships include poor or deviant eye contact (Hutt & Ounsted, 1966; McConnell, 1967; Wolff & Chess, 1964), delayed or absent social smile, delayed or absent anticipatory response to being picked up (Kanner, 1943; Kanner & Lesser, 1958), apparent aversion to physical contact, a tendency to react to another person's hand or foot rather than to the person (Kanner & Lesser, 1958), lack of interest in playing games with others, and a general preference for being alone (Wing, 1966; Wolf, Wenar, & Ruttenberg, 1972). The disturbed interpersonal relationships may be more subtle and in milder cases and older autistics are manifested as a persistent aloofness. Recent work has focused on the primacy of the autistic disturbances of social relating (Fein, Pennington, Markowitz, Braverman, & Waterhouse, 1986) and has stressed the inability of autistic children to share interest with another person in a toy or an activity (Sigman & Mundy, in press) and of older autistics to have empathy for the feelings and interests of others (Sigman, Ungerer, Mundy, & Sherman, 1987).

Disturbances of Communication and Language

Early language development is usually characterized by muteness or echolalia (Bender, 1947; Cunningham & Dixon, 1961; Kanner, 1943; Shapiro, Fish, & Ginsberg, 1972; Wolff & Chess, 1965). Speech is usually noncommunicative and there is an absence or paucity of nonverbal communication. Facial expression, gesture, and even pointing are not used to communicate in the majority of patients. These deficits in nonverbal *indicating behaviors* distinguish autistic from nonautistic mentally retarded children in quantitative studies (Mundy, Sigman, Ungerer, & Sherman, 1986; Sigman, Mundy, Sherman, & Ungerer, 1986). If communicative speech does develop it is atonal and arrhythmic, lacks inflection, and fails to convey emotion (Goldfarb, 1961). This poverty of the tonal and affective qualities of speech in young autistic children is paralleled in older autistic children by a restriction of spontaneity and originality of communication (Cunningham, 1966; Frith, 1971).

Disturbances of Response to Objects

In young autistic children, the use of inanimate objects may be limited to flicking, twirling, or spinning them. There is a tendency to order and arrange objects in a constant manner, the child seeming to want to maintain an unvarying sameness in his or her environment (DeMyer, Mann, Tilton, & Loew, 1967; Eisenberg & Kanner, 1956; Kanner, 1943; Kanner & Lesser, 1958). With increasing age, these tendencies are manifest in a rigidity and inflexibility in the use of play material (Frith, 1971, 1972) and in the development of repetitive activities and ritualistic use of objects. Autistic children have severe deficiencies in the use of representational and symbolic play (Sigman & Mundy, in press; Sigman et al., 1987) and fail to invest toys and other objects with imagination.

Disturbances of Sensory Modulation

The inability to modulate sensory input adequately is most prominent in younger autistic children (Bergman & Escalona, 1949; Goldfarb, 1961, 1963; Ornitz, 1973, 1974). All sensory modalities are affected and the faulty modulation of sensory input may be manifest as both a lack of responsiveness and an exaggerated reaction to sensory stimuli (Goldfarb, 1961, 1963) along with sensory self-stimulation.

Hyporeactivity to auditory stimuli is apparent in the disregard of both verbal commands and loud sounds. Sudden sounds that would elicit an impressive startle reaction in normal children may elicit no response whatsoever in some autistic children (Anthony, 1958). Visually, the children may ignore new persons or features in their environment and may walk into objects as if they did not see them. Objects placed in the hand may be allowed to fall away as if they had no tactile representation. Painful stimuli (bumps, bruises, cuts) are often ignored.

Contrasting starkly to the hyporeactivity are decidedly exaggerated reactions to the same sensory stimuli. The children may show both heightened *awareness* (distraction by background stimuli of marginal intensity) and heightened *sensitivity* to sensory stimulation that they seek out and induce. Some of the disturbances of motility seem to provide intense sensory stimulation. They may rub, bang, or flick at their ears or grind their teeth, and scratch, tap, or bang surfaces to induce auditory input. Visually, they regard their own writhing hand and finger movements or their more vigorous hand flapping, and they scrutinize the fine detail of surfaces. There are also brief episodes of intense staring. They rub surfaces in response to fine textural differences. They seek out vestibular stimulation (Bender, 1947, 1956) by whirling, rocking, and swaying, or by head rolling. Hand flapping provides proprioceptive input.

Contrasting with the pursuit of sensory stimuli is the paradoxical distress induced by stimuli in all sensory modalities. Autistic children may become agitated by the sound of sirens, vacuum cleaners, or barking dogs, and they may cup their hands over their ears to shut out these intense sounds as well as mild sounds such as the crinkle of paper (Bergman & Escalona, 1949; Goldfarb, 1963). Sudden changes in illumination or confrontation with an unexpected object may elicit the same fearful reactions to visual stimuli. In the tactile modality there may be severe intolerance for certain fabrics, for example, wool, and a preference for smooth surfaces. During the first two years, rough-textured table foods often evoke distress. There may be aversion to vestibular stimulation induced by rough-and-tumble play or even riding in an elevator.

The disturbances of sensory modulation have not been incorporated into DSM-III, where they receive only casual mention as associated symptoms. This omission may be due to two factors. The first is insufficient observation of the preschool autistic child, since the autistic disturbances of both motility and sensory modulation occur primarily between the ages of 24 and 60 months (Fig. 12.1). The second problem has been the manner of conceptualizing the observed behavior. For example, underreactivity and overreactivity to sound were considered symptoms of the language disturbance (Rutter & Lockyer, 1967), and more recently behaviors such as preoc-

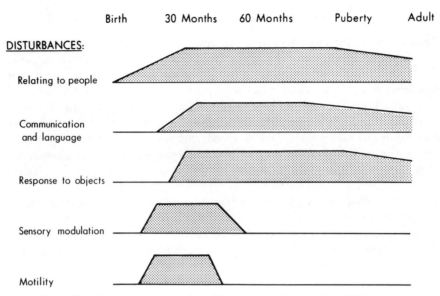

Figure 12.1. Schematic representation of developmental changes in autistic behavior.

cupation with noises, textures, or spinning objects, ignoring noises, and failure to notice painful stimuli were grouped with "responses to the environment" or "affective responses" (Volkmar, Cohen, & Paul, 1986), obscuring the recognition of such behaviors as deviant responses to sensory input: that is, collectively as a disturbance of sensory modulation. Additional obfuscation occurred when DSM-III (APA, 1980) mandated a differential diagnosis between infantile autism and childhood onset pervasive developmental disorder (COPDD) on the dubious basis of age of onset (specified as later than 30 months) while including disturbances of sensory modulation (hyper- or hyposensitivity to sensory stimuli) along with other symptoms of infantile autism (oddities of motor movement, monotonous voice, resistance to change) among the diagnostic criteria for COPDD. However, hyper- and hyposensitivities to sensory stimuli may occur in children diagnosed autistic with onset prior to 30 months of age (Ornitz, Guthrie, & Farley, 1977, 1978). DSM-III-R has removed the distinction based on age of onset but has failed to include the disturbances of motility and sensory modulation as specific symptom clusters in the description of autistic disorder. Instead, DSM-III-R mentions a few such symptoms: for example, "hand flicking or twisting, rocking, spinning" and "repetitive feeling of texture of materials, or spinning wheels of toy cars," under the category of "a markedly restricted repertoire of activities and interests" (p. 39).

Examination of 74 autistic children who were between 16 and 75 months old (45.2 ± 12.6 months) at the time of psychiatric evaluation showed that autistic disturbances of motility and sensory modulation were absent during the examinations (31% of the children were examined on one occasion, 36.5% on two occasions, and 32.5% on three or more occasions) in only 12.2 and 5.4% of the cases, respectively (Ornitz et al., 1977). The behavioral profiles for the autistic disturbances of motility and sensory modulation were very similar to those for the disturbances of relating to people and response to objects (Fig. 12.2). For the same group of autistic children, parental reports on a developmental inventory indicated that the disturbances of sensory modulation and motility are observed with almost the same frequencies as the disturbances of relating to people and response to objects (Ornitz et al., 1978). Using the identical developmental inventory, and considering behaviors that exemplify under- or overreactivity to sensory stimuli, these findings have been replicated on an independent sample of autistic subjects (Volkmar et al., 1986). Gillberg and Wahlstrom (1985) reported "abnormal responses to auditory stimuli, sometimes seemingly deaf and at other times upset by barely audible sounds" (p. 294) in all 46 autistic children in their population study.

Disturbances of Motility

The deviant motility occurs mainly in younger autistic children. The mannerisms are often complex, ritualistic, and stereotyped, and do not seem to be entirely voluntary, appearing intermittently or continuously (Hutt, Hutt, Lee, & Ounsted, 1965; Ornitz, 1974; Sorosky, Ornitz, Brown, & Ritvo, 1968). Writhing or twisting the fingers and palms in front of the eyes may merge into a repetitive stereotyped wiggling of the fingers or the entire hand. This hand flapping involves a rapid flexion and extension of the fingers or hand or an alternating pronation and supination

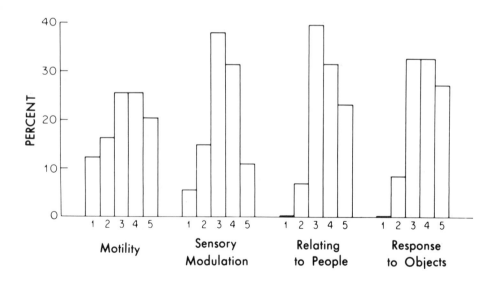

Figure 12.2. The percentage of preschool autistic children showing each of four categories of autistic behavior during developmental examinations. The horizontal scales go from 1 (behavior not present) to 5 (behavior of great clinical significance during the examination).

of the forearm (Aug & Ables, 1971; Ornitz, Brown, Sorosky, Ritvo, & Dietrich, 1970; Ritvo, Ornitz, & LaFranchi, 1968; Sorosky et al., 1968). Toe walking (Colbert & Koegler, 1958) may occur transiently during states of excitement or while running in circles or as the only mode of walking. Movements of the trunk or the entire body include staccato lunging and darting movements, terminated by sudden stops, body rocking, and swaying, often accompanied by head rolling, or head banging, and whirling. In spite of this gross motor activity, autistic children are not necessarily hyperactive, although there are occasional cases in which hyperactivity as a major symptom and autism occur together. In very young autistic children there may be sudden brief episodes of immobility, often associated with posturing of the trunk or extremities, or hyperextension of the back and neck. Abnormal motility can at times be elicited by a rapidly spinning child's top, flickering light displays, or similar visual stimuli.

Summary

The clinical picture of autism is complex. It is however, a unique behavioral syndrome that consists of particular clusters of symptomatology (Ornitz, 1973; Ornitz et al., 1977, 1978). The disturbances of *relating to people, communication and language*, and *response to objects* have been recognized as essential elements of the autistic syndrome in most descriptive schemes. They are congruent with the *triad* of autistic symptomatology, consisting of impairments of reciprocal social relationships, verbal and nonverbal communication, and the ability to play creatively and use imagination, which is currently accepted as the definition of autism (Rutter, 1985; Wing, 1981; Wing & Gould, 1979). Less attention has been paid to the disturbances of *sensory modulation and motility*. They are, however, prominent components of the behavioral syndrome in the preschool autistic child (Bergman & Escalona, 1949; Ornitz, 1969, 1973; Ornitz & Ritvo, 1976), affecting all sensory modalities, and the faulty modulation is manifest as either underreactivity or over-reactivity to sensory stimuli. The latter is often associated with inducing sensory input (Ornitz, 1974), and some of the motility disturbances may provide such input.

ASSOCIATED FEATURES

The major pathologic conditions found in association with autism are mental retardation, organic brain syndromes (with or without seizures), and a history of abnormal pre-, peri-, and neonatal events.

Mental Retardation

Autistic children not only will not, but actually cannot, perform many tasks (Alpern, 1967). The notion that autistic children have a primary affective deficiency (Anthony,

1962) and good cognitive potential (Kanner & Lesser, 1958) has given way to the recognition that the cognitive deficiency in autism is every bit as real as in mental retardation (Rutter & Bartak, 1971; Rutter, Bartak, & Newman, 1971), and that approximately 75% of autistic children can be expected to perform throughout life at a retarded level (Rutter, 1970). Mental retardation and autism clearly coexist (Goldberg & Soper, 1963).

Organic Brain Syndromes

Autism does not follow the clinical course of a degenerative organic process (Kanner, 1949), although typical autistic behavior does occur in association with the mental deterioration in girls with Rett syndrome, a progressive encephalopathy (Al-Mateen, Philippart, & Shields, 1986; Hagberg, Aicardi, Dias, & Ramos, 1983; Olsson & Rett, 1985; Zappella, 1985). In 23% of an unselected sample of autistic children (Ornitz et al., 1977), autism does occur, however, in association with epileptic (particularly infantile spasms), neurostructural, anoxic, traumatic, infectious (particularly congenital rubella [Chess, 1977]), herpes simplex encephalitis (Delong, Bean, & Brown, 1981), and cytomegalovirus (Markowitz, 1983; Stubbs, 1978) disease, and toxic, metabolic, and hormonal diseases with the potential to impair the function of the pre-, peri-, and neonatal nervous system (Deykin & MacMahon, 1980; Finnegan & Quarrington, 1979; Garreau, Barthelemy, Sauvage, Leddet, & Lelord, 1984; review in Ornitz, 1983; Ornitz et al., 1977).

Seizure Disorders

The alterations in consciousness associated with seizure disorders are occasionally confused with the behavior of young autistic children; momentary posturing and staring may simulate petit mal epilepsy. In most cases, however, autism and a seizure disorder may coexist (Creak, 1963; Deykin & MacMahon, 1979; Kolvin, Ounsted, & Roth, 1971). In early infancy, there is an association with infantile spasms (Riikonen & Amnell, 1981; Taft & Cohen, 1971). In late childhood and adolescence, seizure disorders are more likely to occur as autistic children become older (Rutter et al., 1967; Rutter et al., 1971).

Prenatal, Perinatal, and Neonatal Events

There is an excess of mothers 35 years or older at the time of birth of autistic children (Gillberg & Gillberg, 1983; Tsai & Stewart, 1983). There is an excess of firstborn autistic children in families with small sibships (Creak & Ini, 1960; Deykin & MacMahon, 1980; Kanner, 1954; Kolvin, Ounsted, Richardson, & Garside, 1971; Lotter, 1967; Rutter & Lockyer, 1967; Tsai & Stewart, 1983; Wing, 1966). When all abnormal pre-, peri-, and neonatal factors are considered together, there appears to be a signficant association with childhood autism (Deykin & MacMahon, 1980; Finnegan & Quarrington, 1979; Gillberg & Gillberg, 1983; Gittelman &

Birch, 1967; Kolvin, Ounsted, & Roth, 1971; review in Ornitz, 1983; Taft & Goldfarb, 1964; Ward & Hoddinott, 1965).

COURSE AND PROGNOSIS

Course

Autistic behavior may occur from birth or begin after a period of relatively normal development up to the age of 18 to 24 months. The onset usually occurs before 30 months of age (Kolvin, Ounsted, Humphrey et al., 1971; Rutter, 1967). However, later onsets, from 4 to 14 years of age, of autism have been reported; these late onsets in previously nonautistic children have been in association with acute encephalopathies (Delong et al., 1981; Gillberg, 1986; Weir & Salisbury, 1980). The subsequent clinical picture is the same regardless of the exact age at onset of the first symptoms. Very careful history taking may elicit symptoms that did indeed occur during the first year of life but that were forgotten, overlooked, or denied by the parents due to either anxiety about their child's development or unfamiliarity with normal development.

The Neonatal Period

The mother may be convinced that the newborn baby is different from her other babies but she cannot articulate the subtle nature of the strange behavior. The infant may cry infrequently or seem not to need companionship or stimulation. He may become limp or rigid when held. He is often described as a "very good baby" who never fusses, or he may be intensely irritable and overreactive to any form of stimulation (Dudziak, 1982; Ornitz, 1973).

The First Half Year

During the first half year of life it becomes apparent that the baby fails to notice the coming or going of the mother. Responsive smiling and the anticipatory response to being picked up may not occur. Often a baby who is unresponsive to toys, such as a bird mobile, may be paradoxically overreactive to sounds produced by the vacuum cleaner, for example. The earliest vocalizations—cooing and babbling— may not appear or may be considerably delayed (Ornitz, 1973).

The Second Half Year

During the second 6 months, the baby may refuse solid foods. Without intervention some autistic children remain on pureed baby foods for years. Toys are cast or flicked away or simply dropped out of hand. Motor milestones such as sitting and walking may be delayed (Ornitz et al., 1977). The autistic baby is unaffectionate. When picked up the baby may become either limp or stiff, and when put down not seem to care. The autistic baby often fails to show "stranger anxiety" and may not play peek-a-boo and pat-a-cake (Ritvo & Provence, 1953). At 12 months, the baby does not wave bye-bye responsively and syllables are not combined into polysyllabic sounds and words. Occasionally the child develops a few words and then ceases to use them. There is neither verbal nor nonverbal communication; the child neither points nor looks toward a desired object. Peculiar reactions to sensory stimuli develop. The autistic baby may become agitated by sounds to which he or she is completely oblivious on other occasions. Changes in illumination, textures, and sensations induced by change in position may also evoke distress (Ornitz, 1973).

The Second and Third Years

During the second and third years, the child seeks stimulation in all sensory modalities and often engages in peculiar mannerisms that provide such stimulation, for example, tooth grinding, scratching surfaces, staring, rubbing, and stroking (Ornitz, 1973). Unusual repetitive and stereotyped mannerisms include regarding his or her own hand movements, hand flapping, persistent toe walking (Colbert & Koegler, 1958), excessive body rocking, swaying, head banging (Green, 1967), head rolling, and whirling without becoming dizzy (Ornitz, 1973). Often in response to some stimulus, for example, a spinning top, the child will suddenly run in circles on the toes, whirl, make staccatolike lunging and darting movements, and vigorously flap the hands. Toys are ignored or arranged in idiosyncratic patterns without regard to function or meaning. There is little or no imagination, fantasy, or role taking in play (DeMyer et al., 1967). Preoccupation with spinning objects may preclude other forms of play. There is indifference to human contact. The autistic child does not look at the adult when he or she wants something but moves the adult's hand toward the desired object (Ornitz, 1973).

The Fourth and Fifth Years

During the fourth and fifth years, the child may remain mute or speech may be limited to a few inconsistently used words. When speech does occur, it is often limited to delayed echolalia. This is a parrotlike imitation of the speech of others occurring out of social context and having little or no communicative value. There may be misuse of the personal pronouns (the substitution of *you* or *he* for *I* or *me*).

Middle Childhood

Some of the children may continue to manifest most of the symptoms already described. In others, the symptoms of autism become less evident and new features develop, suggesting either alternative or secondary diagnostic considerations. With increasing age, the unusual responses to sensory stimulation and the bizarre motility patterns become less apparent. The disturbed relating is more likely to continue beyond the sixth year, and its severity tends to be in proportion to its severity during the first five years. The same is true of the language disturbances, and if language has not been used consistently for communication by age 5, then it is unlikely that more advanced speech development will occur. When this is the case, intellectual development remains at a standstill, and if the responses to sensory stimulation and the bizarre motility patterns abate, then the child begins to look less autistic and more retarded. If the child does develop communicative speech by the fifth birthday, communication is very literal, affect tends to be flat, and verbal communication does not lead to emotional involvement with others. The child remains aloof and emotionally detached. In some cases the child's communications appear to be characterized by loose, irrelevant, and tangential thinking, and if the child has developed any degree of fantasy life the expressed fantasies tend to be bizarre and may be confused with reality. Less frequently, in some autistic children there may be impulsivity and lack of emotional control, coupled with restlessness, irritability, and hyperactivity.

Puberty and Adolescence

Puberty may be associated with deterioration, including disruptive behavior, self-destructive behavior, and exacerbation of aloofness and resistance to change (Gillberg & Schaumann, 1981). In other autistic youngsters, particularly those who are high functioning and verbal, depression is a frequent problem (Gillberg, 1984a).

Adulthood

The majority of autistics who are also retarded live in institutional settings. The minority who are not retarded maintain strict routines and rituals, lack any inner fantasy life, and are socially inept and unable to engage in social reciprocity (Rutter, 1985). A study of 14 such patients revealed the persistence of stereotyped movements, concrete thinking, flat affect, aprosodic speech, and perseverative interests (Rumsey, Rapoport, & Sceery, 1985). High-functioning autistic adults show poverty of speech, poverty of speech content, perseveration, and affective flattening (Rumsey, Andreasen, & Rapoport, 1986). Very few autistic adults are competitively employed or capable of independent living (Kanner, 1971). There are, however, rare reports of exceptional patients who have achieved success (Grandin & Scariano, 1986).

Prognosis

In approximately 7 (Creak, 1963) to 28% (Rutter, 1970) of autistic children who are not epileptic in early childhood, a seizure disorder develops later. Approximately 75% of autistic children are and remain mentally retarded (Havelkova, 1968; Rutter, 1970). Those autistic children who have seizures or other indications of organic brain damage tend to be the more retarded, with the greatest language delay (Gittelman & Birch, 1967; Rutter, 1970). Failure to use language for communication by the age of 5 implies a very poor prognosis for further intellectual and personality development (Eisenberg, 1956; Eisenberg & Kanner, 1956; Fish et al., 1968; Havelkova, 1968; Rutter et al., 1967), as does failure to use toys appropriately (Brown, 1960). Thus the autistic child who is close to the fifth birthday and is not using communicative speech (the speech may be limited to echolalia), does not play appropriately with toys, and appears intellectually retarded has a poor prognosis and is likely to require lifelong institutional care (Eisenberg, 1957).

For the minority of autistic children who show relatively normal intelligence and who develop communicative speech before the age of 5 years the outlook is different. Many of these children appear introverted, passive, withdrawn, and schizoid (Brown & Reiser, 1963). Although not having delusions or hallucinations, some develop

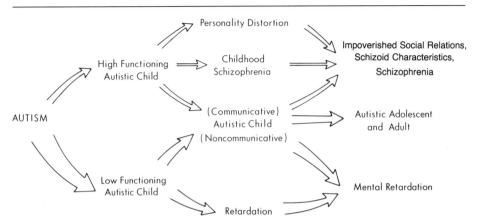

Figure 12.3. Schematic representation of the clinical course of autism and its diagnosis sequelae in relation to the level of functioning. The thickness of the arrows gives a rough impression of the relative frequency of the different courses of development.

severe disturbances of reality testing such as are seen in borderline states (Bender, 1956; Bender et al., 1952; Havelkova, 1968). Several series of cases (Brown, 1969; Brown & Reiser, 1963; Petty & Ornitz, in preparation; Petty, Ornitz, Michelman, & Zimmerman, 1984) and several individual case reports (Darr & Worden, 1951; Noll & Benedict, 1981; Ornitz, 1969; Ornitz & Ritvo, 1968) document a transition from infantile autism to a frank schizophrenia. Those autistic children who are able to live in society and to obtain employment represent a minority of the autistic population (Kanner, Rodriguez, & Ashenden, 1972). They usually have significant residual personality and cognitive impairments (Brown, 1969), remain aloof and literal, lacking social judgment and empathy (Gajzago & Prior, 1974), and exhibit "a lack of social perceptiveness perhaps best characterized as a lack of *savoir faire*" (Eisenberg & Kanner, 1956, p. 559).

Reviews of outcome studies suggest that between 5 and 17% of autistic children may achieve "normal or near normal social life and satisfactory functioning at school or work" (Lotter, 1978, p. 479), although only 1 or 2% become completely normal (DeMyer, Hingtgen, & Jackson, 1981).

Figure 12.3 suggests some of the variations in the clinical course of autism and the several possible outcomes.

IMPAIRMENT

The issue of the degree of impairment, that is, the severity of the disorder, in autism has generated controversy and confusion regarding the limits to which the diagnosis of autism should be applied. The failure adequately to consider the issue of impairment confounds studies of prevalence and influences the extent to which subgroups based on variations in behavior, such as Asperger's syndrome, are proposed. These problems are considered further in later sections.

The issue can be stated simply: Is autism an all-or-nothing syndrome or does it occur, like most medical and psychiatric conditions, with varying degrees of severity from very severe to very mild?

The language of DSM-III has contributed to the impression that autism is an all-or-nothing syndrome. The intent in classifying autism as a *pervasive* developmental disorder was to emphasize a serious abnormality in the developmental process (Rutter, 1985), to separate autism from both the psychoses (particularly childhood schizophrenia) and the *specific* developmental disorders (e.g., developmental language disorder), and to emphasize the *pervasiveness* of the disorder: that is, distortions in *multiple* basic functions, particularly social relationships, language and communication, and all responses to the environment. However, the use of the adjective *pervasive* again in the major diagnostic criterion for autism ("*pervasive* lack of responsiveness to other people"), coupled with the use of adjectives such as *gross* to describe other diagnostic criteria ("*gross* deficits in language development"), and the statement of impairment ("The disorder is extremely incapacitating, and special education facilities are almost always necessary") have become obstacles to recognition of mild manifestations of the autistic behavioral syndrome. Yet such cases do exist, and their reality in the face of the categorical language of DSM-III has generated either vague descriptive statements such as "mental retardation accompanied by some autistic features" (Rutter, 1985, p. 546) and "autisticlike disorders" or the retention of separate diagnostic entities such as Asperger's syndrome.

Recently, a number of investigators have addressed the existence of mild manifestations of autism. In a carefully designed epidemiologic study, Wing and Gould (1979) found that subgroups of children formed on the basis of severity of social impairment did not differ on the speech and behavioral abnormalities associated with autism and "formed a continuum of severity rather than discrete entities" (p. 26). Wing (1981) also observed that in the Wing and Gould (1979) study, while impairments of two-way social interaction, communicative language, and imaginative play tend to cluster together, "each aspect of this triad [which defines autism] can occur in varying degrees of severity, and in association with any level of intelligence as measured on standardized tests" (p. 123). Empirical studies of DSM-III nosology of the pervasive developmental disorders (PDD) suggest that distinctions between infantile autism and both atypical PDD (Rescorla, 1986) and childhood-onset PDD (Dahl, Cohen, & Provence, 1986) probably refer to degrees of severity rather than to different behavioral characteristics. The responses of parents on a developmental inventory completed when their autistic children were younger than 6 years of age indicated that, while almost all children showed severe disturbances of social relating, a substantial number also exhibited varying degrees of social relatedness (Ornitz et al., 1978). Using the same developmental inventory for a well-diagnosed group of older autistics, this finding was recently replicated (Volkmar et al., 1986). A recent study of preschool autistic children revealed evidence of attachment to their mothers and discrimination between their mothers and strangers (Sigman & Ungerer, 1984).

Clearly, autism is not an all-or-nothing syndrome. Its symptoms occur, as is true with most medical and psychiatric disorders, with varying degrees of severity. There seems to be no reason to use terms such as "autisticlike disorder" or "mental retardation with autistic features." The propriety of creating or retaining nosologic subgroups such as Asperger's syndrome or childhood-onset PDD is addressed in the section on differential diagnosis.

A definitive study of the issue of *degrees of severity* is yet to be done. Such a study will need to quantify the joint contributions of the severity of the associated mental retardation and the severity of the autistic behaviors per se to the total degree of severity. The phrase "high-functioning autistic child" is frequently used to describe milder cases of autism without considering why the patient is able to function at a higher level. "High functioning" may be attributed to milder autistic symptomatology in some cases and milder associated mental retardation in others.

COMPLICATIONS

The serious complications of autism tend to occur at the time of puberty and during early adolescence. These include an increasing incidence of seizures and severe behavior outbursts characterized by regressive, impulsive, and aggressive behavior and depression (Gillberg, 1984a).

Rutter (1970) reported that 28% of his cases developed seizures for the first time during adolescence. Deykin and MacMahon (1979) found that about 20% of a series of 183 autistic children developed seizures, with the peak onset between 11 and 14 years. The risk of seizures is greater in the more retarded autistics (Rutter, 1983).

Puberty and early adolescence are frequently accompanied by disruptive behavior, destructive and sometimes violent lashing out against both property and persons, self-mutilation, unprovoked rages, exacerbations of autistic aloofness, hand flapping, and compulsive rituals, and loss of acquired skills and adaptive behaviors (Gillberg & Schaumann, 1981). This behavior is often unmanageable at home and requires hospitalization (Rutter, 1970).

Depression occurs frequently in the milder higher-functioning autistics during adolescence when their increasing capacity for self-awareness leads to severely diminished self-esteem. I have known several of these very distressed patients who have attempted suicide, sometimes successfully. Similar cases have been reported under the rubrics of Asperger's syndrome (Wing, 1981) or schizoid personality (Wolff & Chick, 1980). Suicide is a serious risk in the mild autistic adolescent.

EPIDEMIOLOGY

The accepted prevalence of autism has been 4 to 5 cases per 10,000. This figure is based on epidemiologic studies reported from England (Lotter, 1966; Wing, Yeates, Brierley, & Gould, 1976), Denmark (Brask, 1970), Japan (Hoshino, Kumashiro, Yashima, Tachibana, & Watanabe, 1982), and Sweden (Bohman, Bohman,

Bjorck, & Sjoholm, 1983; Gillberg, 1984b) prior to 1984, using established epidemiologic survey techniques and stringent diagnostic criteria for autism (Table 12.1). Two of these studies delineated autistic subgroups based on severity (Lotter, 1966; Wing et al., 1976). Comparison of the last three columns in Table 12.1 indicates the dependence of prevalence estimates on the extent to which a continuum of severity of autism is accepted as opposed to an all-or-nothing definition of the disorder as discussed in the section on impairment. When cases with "some autistic features" are included, some of the earlier prevalence estimates increase to 8 cases per 10,000 (Lotter, 1966; Wing et al., 1976).

Further consideration of the Camberwell population (Wing et al., 1976) identified 74 socially impaired children, most of whom also showed mutism or echolalia, and repetitive stereotyped behaviors (Wing & Gould, 1979). This triad of symptomatology defines autism. Wing and Gould separated their cases into those who at interview showed elaborate repetitive routines and those who did not. The former group were those who had a history of typical autism (prevalence 4.9 per 10,000). The latter group had a prevalence of 16.3 per 10,000. Together the total prevalence of children with the triad of symptomatology consistent with the definition of autism was 21.2 per 10,000. Subgrouping of these same 74 socially impaired children by severity of social impairment gave prevalence rates (per 10,000) of 10.6 for the most impaired, 5.7 for the next subgroup, and 4.9 for the least impaired. All three subgroups contained children with the history of typical autism. These results reinforce the concept that autism occurs along a continuum of severity and that when milder cases are recognized, the prevalence is considerably higher than previously stated.

Since 1983, several studies from Japan (Ishii & Takahashi, 1983; Matsuishi et al., in press; Sugiyama & Abe, 1986), using stringent diagnostic criteria and epidemiologic techniques equal or superior to the earlier studies both in Japan (Hoshino et al., 1982) and elsewhere (Bohman et al., 1983; Brask, 1970; Gillberg, 1984b; Lotter, 1966; Wing et al., 1976), have reported prevalences of about 16 per 10,000. As with Lotter's (1966), Hoshino and colleagues' (1982), Bohman and colleagues' (1983), and Gillberg's (1984b) studies, these three recent studies have screened *all* children, including all those in schools for normal children. The Sugiyama and Abe (1986) study is of particular interest since 92% of a total population of 12,263 children were given well child health examinations at 18 months of age. At this time, screening for behavioral disturbance resulted in direct examinations of 139 of these children *prior to 36 months of age*. Diagnoses of autism in 20 of these children were confirmed by follow-up examinations between 3 and 6 years of age.

The recent increased prevalence estimates cannot be attributed to different diagnostic criteria. Possible explanations include increased appreciation of milder cases and/ or an actual increase in the prevalence of autism, perhaps due to increased fetal salvage, increasing the pool of viable but damaged infants out of which cases of autism might develop.

Technical issues affecting prevalence estimates in some studies include case solicitation rather than epidemiologic screening (Steinhausen, Gobel, Breinlinger, & Wohlleben, 1986) and screening using less than optimal screening criteria or nomenclature such as "childhood schizophrenia" (Treffert, 1970), resulting in underestimation of prevalence. Hoshino and colleagues (1982) noted prevalence differences between urban and rural areas, suggesting differences in case recognition. The influence of the age range of the population seems to have affected some studies but not others. Hoshino and colleagues (1982) and Bohman and colleagues (1983) found higher prevalences in children 4 to 11 years old than in younger and older children. Hoshino and colleagues attributed lower prevalences below 5 years of age and between 12 and 18 years of age to greater difficulty in case recognition. However, Gillberg (1984b) observed no differences associated with age between 4 and 18 years of age.

FAMILIAL PATTERN

Family Characteristics

Earlier descriptions of the parents as strongly preoccupied with abstractions and emotionally cold (Kanner, 1949) and more balanced appraisals describing the parents as being unusually "perplexed" and ineffective in communicating with their child (Goldfarb, Levy, & Meyers, 1972; Meyers & Goldfarb, 1961) have been refuted by careful studies of parental child-rearing behavior (Cantwell, Baker, & Rutter, 1978; DeMyer et al., 1972; Kolvin, Garside, & Kidd, 1971; Rutter & Bartak, 1971; Rutter et al., 1971).

Genetics

Older reviews of the literature on concordance for autism in twins (Ornitz, 1973; Rutter, 1967) and more recent comparisons of mono- and dizygotic twins (Folstein & Rutter, 1977; Ritvo, Freeman, Mason-Brothers, Mo, & Ritvo, 1985) suggest a genetic determinant in some cases of autism. For nontwin siblings of autistic children, the generally accepted occurrence of autism is 2 to 3% (Folstein, 1985). Shell, Campion, Minton, Caplan, and Campbell (1984) report that 2.4% of the 284 siblings in families of 174 autistic children were diagnosed autistic, and a very few families have three autistic children. Spence developed an autosomal recessive inheritance model to account for the distribution of autistic cases in 46 families with multiple incidence (two or three autistic siblings) of autism (Ritvo, Spence, Freeman, Mason-Brothers, Mo, & Marazita, 1985). In addition, there is an increase in cognitive–linguistic deficiencies in the siblings of autistic children (August, Stewart, & Tsai, 1981; Bartak, Rutter, & Cox, 1975; Minto, Campbell, Green, Jennings, & Samit, 1982), suggesting a possible genetic factor common to two related phenotypic expressions. Genetic factors are unlikely, however, to account for the majority of cases (Hanson & Gottesman, 1976).

Autosomal chromosomal abnormalities in autistic children occur but are quite rare and variable and may be associated with minor dysmorphic features (Jayakar et al., 1986; Mariner et al., 1986). Occasional sex chromosomal abnormalities also

TABLE 12.1. Prevalence Studies of Autism

Author	Year	Place	Screening	Age Range (Years)	Population
Lotter	1966	Middlesex, U.K.	Queried all children's schools and other facilities using questionnaire re autistic behaviors	8–10	78,000
Brask	1970	Aarhus, Denmark	Reviewed case notes on all children in mental health and pediatric facilities	2–14	46,000
Treffert	1970	Wisconsin, U.S.A.	Queried mental health facilities re diagnosis of "childhood schizophrenia"	3–12	899,750
Wing et al.	1976	Camberwell, U.K.	Interviewed teachers of each child at all mental health facilities	5–14	25,00
Wing & Gould	1979	Camberwell, U.K.	As in Wing et al., 1976	0–15	35,000
Hoshino et al.	1982	Fukushima, Japan	Queried all schools and mental health and pediatric facilities re autistic behavior	0–18 5–11	609,848 217,626
Bohman et al.	1983	Västerbotten, Sweden	Queried personnel in all schools and mental health facilities re "psychotic behavior"	0–20	69,000
Ishii & Takahasi	1983	Toyota, Japan	Queried all primary schools re suspected cases of autism	6–12	34,987
Gillberg	1984	Gothenburg, Sweden	Queried all physicians in well-child clinics, facilities for mentally retarded, and medical facilities	4–18	128,584
Sugiyama & Abe	1986	Nagoya, Japan	Queried public health nurses during 18-mth old well child examinations; examined all children with unusual behavior	1½–3	12,263
Steinhausen et al.	1986	West Berlin, F.R.G.	Autistic children solicited from university clinic and treatment programs	0–15	279,616
Matsuishi et al.	in prep.	Kurume, Japan	Examined all records from all schools, including normal schools, special education, and mental health facilities	4–12	32,834

Diagnostic Criteria for Autism	Subgroups	Prevalence Each Subgroup	(Number per 10^4)	
			A + B	All Cases
Profound lack affect. Preservation sameness.	A. These features very severe	2.0	4.5	7.8
	B. These features milder	2.5		
	C. Some autistic features	3.3		
Not described.	No subgroups			4.3
Inability to relate. Speech problems. Need for sameness. Exclude any evidence of organicity.	A. These features pronounced	0.8	2.5	3.1
	B. Some of these features	1.7		
	C. Some of these features and organicity	0.6		
Social withdrawal. Elaborate repetitive behavior.	A. These features pronounced	2.0	4.8	8.0
	B. Less elaborate repetitive behavior	2.8		
	C. Some autistic features	3.2		
Impaired social interaction. Repetitive behavior. Abnormalities of language and symbolic activity.	A. With "elaborate repetitive routines"	4.9	21.2	21.2
	B. Without "elaborate repetive routines"	16.3		
Kanner's diagnostic criteria.	0. to 18 years old	2.33		2.33
	5 to 11 years old	4.96		4.96
Social impairment. Deviant language. Stereotypic and repetitive activity.	No subgroups			5.6
Autistic social impairments, deviant language, and insistence on sameness.	No subgroups			16.0
Severe impairments of social relating and language. Elaborate repetitive rituals and stereotypes. Insistence on sameness.	A. These features and onset <2½ years	2.0		3.9
	B. These features and onset >2½ years	1.9		
DSM-III diagnostic criteria.	A. Definitely autistic by 18 months	13.0	16.3	21.2
	B. Suspected at 18 months and later confirmed	3.3		
	C. Meet DSM-III criteria temporarily	4.9		
Impairment of social development. Deviant language. Insistence on sameness.	No subgroups			1.9
DSM-III diagnostic criteria.	No subgroups			15.5

have been reported (see review in Mariner et al., 1986). In spite of considerable interest in the possible association with fragile X (August, 1983; Brown et al., 1982; Gillberg, 1983; Gillberg & Wahlstrom, 1985; Meryash, Szymanski, & Gerald, 1982), recent studies have reported relatively low occurrence rates in autistic populations: 0% (Goldfine et al., 1985; Jayakar et al., 1986; Venter, Op't Hof, Coetzee, Van der Walt, & Retief, 1984); 2.5% (Wright, Young, Edwards, Abramson, & Duncan, 1986); 7.3% (McGillivray, Herbst, Dill, Sandercock, & Tischler, 1986); 12.5% (Fisch et al., 1986); 13% (Wahlstrom, Gillberg, Gustavson, & Holmgren, 1986); 13.1% (Brown et al., 1986); and 16% (Blomquist et al., 1985). Thus autism is probably no more related to fragile X than it is related to many of the other associated conditions previously mentioned. On the other hand, just as with congenital rubella (Desmond, Montgomery, Melnick, et al., 1969), there may be a high prevalence of autism (16 to 46%) and autistic behaviors (88 to 96%) among populations of fragile-X syndrome patients (Hagerman, Jackson, Levitas, Rimland, & Braden, 1986).

DIFFERENTIAL DIAGNOSIS

Autism is not mutually exclusive with certain conditions from which it can be differentiated; it frequently coexists with mental retardation, organic brain syndromes, and seizure disorders. Other conditions from which autism can be differentiated, notably schizophrenia and certain personality disorders, may occur as sequelae of an earlier autistic development. Some conditions, for example, Asperger's syndrome, childhood-onset PDD, and atypical PDD, which have been differentiated from autism, probably constitute milder forms of autism. Other conditions clearly require differential diagnosis. These include behavioral disturbances due to environmental deprivation or extremely and chronically stressful environments, some depressive syndromes, elective mutism, developmental language disorders, and major sensory deficits.

Conditions That Do Not Require Differential Diagnosis from Autism

Conditions Occurring in Association with Autism

These conditions, which have been discussed earlier, include mental retardation, some organic brain syndromes, and some seizure disorders.

Conditions Occurring as Sequelae of Autism

Symptoms of personality disorders, particularly schizoid personality and compulsive personality, can be found in higher-functioning verbal autistic adults. The history of a diagnosis of autism and residual autistic behavior are usually sufficient to indicate that these personality developments are sequelae of the earlier autistic development (Rumsey et al., 1985).

Childhood schizophrenia can be diagnosed as early as 5 years of age and is distinguished from autism by the prevailing symptomatology (positive thought disorder and hallucinations), which does not occur in most prepubertal autistic children (Green et al., 1984). Most schizophrenic children do not have an earlier autistic history, and *most* autistic children do not develop schizophrenia. However, in *some* higher-functioning verbal autistic children, typical schizophrenic disorders may develop in early or mid-childhood, adolescence, or adulthood as sequelae to the earlier autistic development (Darr & Worden, 1951; Noll & Benedict, 1981; Petty et al., 1984). Cantor, Evens, Pearce, and Pezzot-Pearce (1982) described a group of children some of whom had autistic symptoms during the first few years of life, who met DSM-III criteria for schizophrenia. A group of high-functioning autistic adults showed the same degree of affective flattening as a group of schizophrenic adults, but did not show positive schizophrenic thought disorders such as derailment (Rumsey et al., 1986).

Conditions That Represent Milder Forms of Autism

ASPERGER'S SYNDROME (AUTISTIC PSYCHOPATHOLOGY).   This syndrome was first described by Asperger (1944) just a year after Kanner's (1943) first description of infantile autism. Until recent years, Asperger's syndrome was described primarily in the German literature, while descriptions of autism were confined to the English literature. This perpetuated treatment of the two syndromes as separate entities. Asperger's description of the syndrome emphasized impairment of reciprocal social interaction, language, and nonverbal communication (including pedantic speech, pronoun reversal, limited gestures and facial expression, and monotonous intonation), and repetitive activities (perseverative observance of spinning objects) and resistance to change. In addition to this clinical picture, there often is a history of lack of normal interest in human company during infancy and deficiency of imaginative play during childhood. Thus Asperger's syndrome and autism share sufficient features to consider them identical syndromes (Wing, 1981), varying mainly along a continuum of severity (Wing & Gould, 1979). Recent case histories (Burgoine & Wing, 1983; Gillberg, 1985; Kerbeshian & Burd, 1986; Mawson, Grounds, & Tantam, 1985; Volkmar, Paul, & Cohen, 1985) support this point of view.

SCHIZOID PERSONALITY.   Wolff and her colleagues (Cull, Chick, & Wolff, 1984; Wolff & Barlow, 1979; Wolff & Chick, 1980) have described a syndrome occurring in childhood characterized by emotional detachment and solitariness, impaired empathy, rigidity, odd ideation, obsessive preoccupations, and abnormalities of verbal communication. They identify this syndrome as being identical with Asperger's syndrome and curiously distinguished it from autism on the grounds that "impaired language development with echolalia; lack of emotional responsiveness with gaze avoidance; ritualistic and compulsive behavior" never occur (Wolff & Chick, 1980, p. 89). In fact, these same characteristics occur in Asperger's syndrome (Wing, 1981). If schizoid personality, as described by Wolff and her colleagues, is indeed identical to Asperger's syndrome, then it is also identical to milder forms of higher-functioning autism. The characteristics of "solitariness, impaired empathy, single-minded pursuit of special interests and abnormalities of verbal communication with verbosity, vague, digressive language" (Cull et al., 1984, p. 646) are also found in those higher-functioning verbal adult autistics who have been less severely impaired in the course of their development. Most important, in a detailed comparison of schizoid and high-functioning autistic children using psychometric tests, Wolff and Barlow (1979), while claiming a difference, state that "schizoid children on the whole were intermediate in their functioning between autistics and normals. They shared autistic children's stereotypy, their tendency to impose patterns, some of their linguistic handicaps and their lack of perceptiveness for meaning" (p. 43). In fact, the only clear difference was that schizoid children "had none of the repetitiveness of autistic children." This description of schizoid children suggests a milder manifestation of autism rather than a distinction between the two groups.

CHILDHOOD-ONSET PERVASIVE DEVELOPMENTAL DISORDER (COPDD). This entity is an invention of DSM-III that does not appear in DSM-III-R. It attempts to differentiate infantile autism from another pervasive developmental disorder with onset in *childhood* rather than *infancy*. In Table 12.2 the capital letters compare the DSM-III criteria for autism and COPDD. The lowercase letters add those symptoms that are commonly seen in young autistic children even though they are not included in DSM-III criteria for autism. It can readily be seen that the *only* criterion that distinguishes the two entities is age of onset. Parental histories (Ornitz et al., 1978; Volkmar et al., 1986) and chart reviews (Dahl et al., 1986) suggest

TABLE 12.2. DSM-III Diagnostic Criteria for Pervasive Developmental Disorders

Infantile Autism	Childhood Onset Pervasive Development Disorder
PERVASIVE LACK OF RESPONSIVENESS	GROSS SUSTAINED IMPAIRED RELATIONSHIPS
GROSS DEFICITS IN LANGUAGE AND PECULIAR SPEECH PATTERNS	ABNORMAL SPEECH, E.G., QUESTIONLIKE MELODY, MONOTONOUS VOICE
RESISTANCE TO CHANGE; RITUALS	RESISTANCE TO CHANGE; RITUALS
PECULIAR INTERESTS OR ATTACHMENTS INCLUDING FASCINATION WITH MOVEMENT Under- and overreactivity to and seeking out of sensory stimuli	UNDER- AND OVERSENSITIVITY TO SENSORY STIMULI
PECULIAR HAND MOVEMENTS Motility disturbances including posturing and hand flapping	ABNORMAL MOTILITY AND POSTURING INCLUDING PECULIAR HAND MOVEMENTS
LACK OF EMOTIONAL INVOLVEMENT	CONSTRICTED OR INAPPROPRIATE AFFECT
head banging	SELF MUTILATION
	EXCESSIVE AND ILLOGICAL ANXIETY
ONSET PRIOR TO 30 MONTHS	ONSET AFTER 30 MONTHS

that DSM-III distinctions between autism and COPDD merely refer to differences in degree of severity, a later *manifest onset* suggesting a milder form of the syndrome.

ATYPICAL PERVASIVE DEVELOPMENTAL DISORDER. This loosely defined DSM-III category to be "used for children with distortions in the development of multiple basic psychologic functions that are involved in the development of social skills and language" is also the wastebasket category ("and that cannot be classified as either Infantile Autism or Childhood Onset PDD") for the DSM-III section on PDD. It disappears in DSM-III-R. It does, however, overlap with groups of children who have been referred to as "atypical" (Brown, 1978; Brown & Reiser, 1963; Rank, 1949; Rescorla, 1986; Sparrow et al., 1986). The group of 100 "atypical" children followed by Brown (1978) showed early autistic behavior and scored high on Kanner's criteria for autism. Substantial numbers of the "atypical" children studied by Rescorla (1986) showed autistic aloofness. Sparrow and colleagues (1986) could differentiate their sample of "atypical" children from autistic children *only* on the bases of higher level of cognitive functioning and less severe social–communicative deficits. Such distinctions suggest again that the "atypical" children represent a milder manifestation of autism.

Conditions That May Require Differential Diagnosis from Autism

Weintraub and Mesulam (1983) have described a group of patients with neurologic and neuropsychologic evidence of right hemisphere dysfunction, emotional and interpersonal difficulties, and pathologic shyness, who, while not considered autistic, shared many features with high-functioning communicative autistics, namely, poor eye contact, deficient use of prosody and gesture, inability to display emotion, poor social perception, and social isolation. Voeller (1986) has described a group of children with neurologic or CT scan evidence of right hemisphere lesions or dysfunction who failed to understand social nuances, had atypical prosody, for example, "monotonous, robot-like intonations" (p. 1007), rocked, and failed to make adequate eye contact. These cases with neurologic evidence of right hemisphere pathology show typical autistic behavior. It will be necessary to evaluate more of these cases before deciding whether it is more useful to include such cases in the differential diagnosis of autism or to consider them an etiologic subgroup that can be added to the ever-increasing listing of associated conditions previously described. I have discussed the possible relationship between right hemisphere dysfunction and the autistic deficiencies in directed attention elsewhere (Ornitz, in press).

Conditions That Do Require Differential Diagnosis from Autism

Environmental Deprivation

The immediate and long-term sequelae of environment deprivation have been well documented both in infants raised in institutions (Provence & Lipton, 1962; Spitz, 1945, 1946) and at home (Coleman & Provence, 1957) when there is deprivation of physical warmth and cuddling and social interaction with a caring adult, absence of novelty, and deficit of sensory input. Deprived infants show delayed development and disturbances of motility, relating, language, and perception. These are the same functions that are adversely affected in autistic children. However, the nature of the individual symptoms is quite different (Ornitz, 1971).

Deprived children suffer a delay in the adaptive use of toys. Autistic children fail to use toys playfully. While deprived children may flick at toys or drop them as do young autistic children, their general interest in toys remains undeveloped; autistic children, in contrast, use toys in bizarre ways, such as spinning them. Deprived infants engage in body rocking and some hand posturing but *not* the tenacious, stereotyped hand flapping, whirling, toe walking, and darting and lunging movements of autistic children. Deprived children adapt poorly to holding but do not become limp or rigid as do autistic children. Deprived children may fail to seek adults out, but instead of avoiding eye contact, they engage in intense visual regarding of adults. While autistic children rarely play games with others, deprived children will participate. Deprived children may show a delay in language acquisition; however, they acquire language if the deprivation is relieved, and their speech is not aprosodic like that of autistic children, nor do echolalia and misuse of pronouns occur. Deprived children do not show the faulty modulation of sensory input seen in autistic children.

When the conditions of deprivation are relieved, the children usually make significant gains. Sequelae include faulty self-regulation of food intake, but not the bizarre food preference of autistic children. There are residual mild deficits in coordination of body movement but not the hand flapping and toe walking seen in autistic children. Residual lags in language development are not accompanied by delayed echolalia. Instead of remaining emotionally detached, children recovering from deprivation show an indiscriminate friendliness.

Anaclitic Depression

The anaclitic depression is accompanied by profound developmental retardation and severe disturbances of relating; therefore it must be distinguished from autism. Anaclitic depression is associated with the interruption after the sixth month of life of an intact mother–infant relationship (Spitz, 1946). The infant reacts by becoming weepy, demanding, and clinging, followed by a period of psychomotor and language retardation, weight loss, and intense wailing. After 2 or 3 months, the child becomes lethargic and apathetic; quiet whimpering and facial rigidity suggest a profound depression. The disturbances of motility and sensory modulation of autism do not occur, and the failure to relate is characterized by apathy and withdrawal rather than the aloofness of the autistic child.

Other Behavioral Disturbances Due to Environmental Influences

Various disturbances of the mother–infant relationship or within the family can induce unusual behavior accompanied by developmental lags in the child. Body rocking and other unusual mannerisms may develop in response to chronic frustration or traumatic emotional experiences. It is to be emphasized that not all bizarre behavior seen in young children implies autism. In the differential diagnosis of autism there must be a thorough assessment of family and mother–infant relationships.

In *elective mutism* the child voluntarily withholds speech, usually in response to a specific pathological family situation or parent–infant interaction. These children will speak fluently under certain limited conditions: for example, only in the presence of other children and never with an adult, or only within, never outside, the family, or only in a whisper.

Deafness and Blindness

In early childhood deafness and blindness can precipitate severe emotional reactions. The combination of such emotional disturbances with the limitations imposed by the sensory deficit can result in a clinical picture that may be confused with autism (Easson, -1971). Since absence or delay of speech acquisition almost always accompanies autism, hearing loss should always be considered. Deafness and autism can also occur together, as in congenital rubella.

Complete or partial blindness can induce disturbed behavior, including mannerisms known as blindisms. These involve gesturing with the hands in front of the face; they usually do not have the stereotypic quality of the hand flapping of autistic children. The blind children show interest in their environment when their visual deficit is recognized and an attempt is made to relate to them through nonvisual means. Autism has been described in association with retrolental fibroplasia but not with other types of visual impairment (Keeler, 1958).

Developmental Dysphasia

In both developmental receptive and expressive dysphasia (Wing, 1966) and in autism there are abnormal responses to sounds, delay in the acquisition of speech, difficulty in its comprehension and use, and sometimes difficulties in articulation (Churchill, 1972; Wing, 1966). As speech is slowly acquired, both dysphasic and autistic children distort and invent words. Because of their difficulty in communicating and being understood, dysphasic children may develop secondary disturbances of relating suggestive of autism. However, dysphasic children do not develop sensory hyper- and hyposensitivities, and they do communicate by nonverbal gestures and expressions (Kanner, 1949). As speech is acquired, dysphasic children rarely show the lack of communicative intent and emotion (de Hirsch, 1967) and the *delayed* echolalia (Fay, 1969; Rutter et al., 1971) of autism. Linguistic processing is different in autism and developmental dysphasia (Arnold & Schwartz, 1983; Bartak et al., 1975).

Rett Syndrome

This progressive encephalopathy in girls (Al-Mateen et al., 1986) is characterized by deterioration of behavior after 7 to 18 months, dementia, loss of purposeful use of the hands and "hand-washing" stereotypic behavior, jerky truncal ataxia, microcephaly, and autistic behaviors (Hagberg et al., 1983). It occurs in atypical forms (Goutieres & Aicardi, 1986; Hagberg & Rasmussen, 1986), and the associated autistic behavior may be indistinguishable from that observed in other cases of autism (Gillberg, 1986; Zappella, 1985), although the variety of stereotypic behaviors is greater in autism than in Rett syndrome (Spiess, Bolthauser, Hanggeli, & Rubl, 1986). For these reasons, Rett syndrome should be suspected in young girls with autistic behavior.

CLINICAL MANAGEMENT

There is no specific treatment for autism, and the earlier observation that no single treatment has withstood the test of time (Ward, 1970) is still true today. Interventions that have been attempted have included family therapy, psychotherapy and counseling for the parents, psychotherapy for the autistic child, behavior modification, speech therapy and signing, various forms of special education, the day treatment center approach, residential treatment, medication with psychotropic drugs, and vitamins.

Since autistic children vary greatly in their intellectual capacity, use, and understanding of speech, general developmental level, age at time of treatment, level of personality development, general severity of the illness, and family circumstances, it is not surprising that some of the approaches just mentioned have been helpful in certain cases of autism but not in others (Wenar & Ruttenberg, 1969). The response to treatment is determined primarily by the degree of impairment and only secondarily by the type of treatment in the individual case (Brown, 1960; Ornitz, 1973). At best, interventions ameliorate but usually do not eliminate symptoms; the children, though improved in a specific respect, remain definitely autistic (Eisenberg, 1957; Ornitz, 1973; Ornitz & Ritvo, 1976).

The best intervention strategy is a flexible one that can be constantly adapted to the changes in developmental level, symptoms, and capacity to communicate and learn, which take place over a period of years (Ornitz & Ritvo, 1976; Schopler, 1982). The parents and the patients both benefit most from an approach that provides long-term management and guidance (Wing, 1966) and recognizes that spontaneous improvements and regressions are likely to outweigh the influence of the most optimistically presented treatment plan.

With these reservations, some interventions will be discussed.

Therapeutic Work with the Parents

Parental counseling (Wing, 1966) is useful when directed both at the very difficult management problems presented by the autistic child and at the guilt and loss of self-esteem engendered in the parents by having a child who does not participate in ordinary parent–child relationships (Rutter & Sussenwein, 1971; Schulman, 1963). Earlier attempts to view and treat the parent as the cause of the child's illness (Call, 1963; Kaufman, Rosenblum, Heims, & Willer, 1957; Rank, 1955; Szurek & Berlin, 1956) have given way to modern treatment approaches that have found the parent, when given proper counseling and support, to be a major asset in the management of the autistic child (Holmes, Hemsley, Rickett, & Likierman, 1982; Schopler, Mesibov, & Baker, 1982; Schopler & Reichler, 1971; Schulman, 1963).

Psychotherapy

In the minority of autistic children who develop communicative speech relatively early in life and who do not suffer from a profound developmental arrest, there is a lack of self-esteem and depression that may be ameliorated by psychotherapy. The effectiveness of such treatment depends on the clarity of the structure provided (Schopler, Brehm, Kinsbourne, & Reichler, 1971).

Behavior Modification

Both greater (Brawley, Harris, Allen, Fleming, & Peterson, 1969; Hewett, 1965; Hingtgen, Coulter, & Churchill, 1967; Lovaas, 1971; Lovaas, Schaeffer, & Simmons, 1965; Lovaas, Schreibman, & Koegel, 1974; Metz, 1965; Ney, Palvesky, & Markely, 1971) and lesser degrees (Churchill, 1969; Fischer & Glanville, 1970) of success in carrying out behavior modification have been claimed.

A follow-up study by the group most highly identified with behavior modification of autistic children (Lovaas, Koegel, Simmons, & Long, 1973) actually shows that relatively minor changes in autistic self-stimulatory behaviors and echolalic speech occurred during the course of therapy. While there were increases in appropriate verbal behavior, social behavior, and play, the best performance in these areas was such that the children would still be considered autistic by any clinical standards (Lovaas et al., 1974).

As with psychotherapy, behavior modification is appropriate for those autistic children with specific symptoms at a specific developmental level. In most cases it can make an unmanageable autistic child more manageable (Davison, 1964; Marshall, 1966; Martin, England, Kaprowy, Kilgour, & Pikel, 1968; Wolf, Risley, & Mees, 1964) and reduce the amount of self-destructive behavior in certain autistic children (Lovaas, 1979; Lovaas et al., 1965; Lovaas & Simmons, 1969; Simmons & Lovaas, 1969; Simmons & Reed, 1969). Although more manageable children are no less autistic, they are more accepted by their families (Runco & Schreibman, 1983). While behavior modification is unlikely to make autistic children more *sociable*, it will make them more *socialized*. The advantages to parents, siblings, teachers, and caretakers are such that behavior modification has become the mainstay of management of autistic children.

Speech Therapy

While autistic children have a language problem (Ruttenberg & Wolf, 1965; Rutter et al., 1971), the failure or delay in speech acquisition cannot be treated as an isolated deficit (Rutter & Sussenwein, 1971). Attempts to develop useful speech through operant conditioning have often been unrewarding. Even though the child may be conditioned to emit words in response to reward, this procedure only occasionally facilitates the use of speech for communication (Howlin, 1981; Rutter & Sussenwein, 1971). Programs that provide language stimulation in the context of encouraging and stimulating increased social relating have demonstrated some meaningful improvement (Bloch, Gersten, & Kornblum, 1980). The use of nonvocal communication techniques, for example, signing, remains an experimental procedure (Kiernan, 1983).

The Therapeutic Milieu and Special Education

Special education is perhaps the most widely practiced intervention with autistic children. The particular procedures and treatment philosophies vary from center to center (Bartak & Rutter, 1971) and generally tend to draw on techniques used in psychotherapy, behavior modification (DeMyer & Ferster, 1962; Fischer & Glanville, 1970; Hudson & DeMyer, 1968; Martin et al., 1968) and speech therapy (Halpern, 1970). Many centers for the special education of autistic children add parent counseling to comprehensive treatment programs and may involve the parents directly in the treatment of their children (Schopler, 1978). Thus special education tends to be eclectic and pragmatic, and when used in conjunction with highly structured behavioral programs (Bartak & Rutter, 1973; Rutter & Bartak, 1973) it constitutes the treatment of choice for autistic children (DeMyer et al., 1981; Schopler et al., 1982).

Medication

Almost every conceivable psychotropic medication has been used with autistic children (Ornitz, 1973). No single medication has made autistic children any less autistic, nor has any medication proven successful in removing any particular symptom.

Autistic children are unusually resistant to conventional sedatives such as chloral hydrate or barbiturates. Antihistamines may provide necessary short-term sedation, for example, ameliorating acute episodes of sleep disturbances. Antidepressants have no use, and stimulants (e.g., methylphenidate) often increase autistic symptoms, particularly stereotypies (Aman, 1982; Ornitz, 1973). Earlier enthusiastic reports about triiodothyronine (Campbell et al., 1972, 1973) were not confirmed in placebo-controlled double-blind crossover studies (Campbell et al., 1978).

The neuroleptics carry the risk of tardive dyskinesia, a neurologic disease characterized by involuntary abnormal movements that are disruptive and disfiguring, involving the face and extremities and in extreme cases the trunk muscles so as to interfere with respiration, and should only be used when their benefits unequivocally outweigh this risk. About 25% of all patients exposed to these drugs develop tardive dyskinesia, and of those who do develop symptoms, only 37% recover when the drug is discontinued (Jeste & Wyatt, 1982). In spite of these facts, the specific occurrence of tardive dyskinesia in autistic and other children (Browning & Ferry, 1976; Campbell, Grega, Green, & Bennett, 1983; Gualtieri & Guimond, 1981; Gualtieri, Quade, Hicks, Mayo, & Schroeder, 1984; Gualtieri, Schroeder, Hicks, & Quade, 1986; Perry et al., 1985; Petty & Spar, 1980), the probable occurrence of a tardive Tourette's syndrome in an autistic patient (Stahl, 1980) and of super-sensitivity psychosis in children (Gualtieri & Guimond, 1981), and the fact that behavioral training can be used successfully in lieu of neuroleptics (Baskett, 1983), some child psychiatrists have persisted in recommending these drugs for autistic children. Although haloperidol has some effect in autistic children (Anderson et al., 1984; Campbell, 1985; Campbell, Anderson, Deutsch, & Green, 1984; Campbell et al., 1982; Campbell, Cohen, & Anderson, 1981), the primary symptom of autism, withdrawal, is only reduced about 10% (Anderson et al., 1984). The benefits are clearly marginal relative to the risk of tardive dyskinesia.

Fenfluramine, structurally similar to amphetamine, with anorexic and stimulant effects, is a potent antiserotonergic drug. Its use in autism was suggested by the presence of elevated blood serotonin in about 30% of autistic children (Hanley, Stahl, & Freedman, 1979; Ritvo et al., 1970). Reports of therapeutic effectiveness, based on small numbers of cases (Geller, Ritvo, Freeman, & Yuwiler, 1982), and the methodologic limitations of a placebo–drug–placebo design (Ritvo, Freeman, Geller, & Yuwiler, 1983; Ritvo et al., 1986) and open studies (Campbell, Deutsch, Perry, Wolsky, & Palij, 1986; Campbell, Perry et al., 1986), have not been replicated in respect to intellectual functioning (August, Raz, & Davis-Baird, 1985; August et al., 1984; Ho, Lockitch, Eaves, & Jacobson, 1986), social responsiveness (August et al., 1985; Ho et al., 1986), communicative skills (Madsen-Beisler, Tsai, & Stiefel, 1986), or disturbances of sensory modulation (August et al., 1985). Fenfluramine does reduce (by about 30%) the autistic motility disturbances (flapping, rocking, whirling) (August et al., 1985; Ritvo et al., 1986; Stubbs, Budden, Jackson, Terdal, & Ritvo, 1986), an effect perhaps related to its similarity to amphetamine in reducing the general activity level (August et al., 1984; August et al., 1985). This nonspecific effect has been associated with lethargy and sleepiness as side effects in a number of the studies just mentioned. A preliminary analysis of a double-blind placebo-controlled parallel study indicated no effect specific to fenfluramine in autistic children (Campbell et al., 1987). No studies have found any relationship between any behavioral effects and fenfluramine's effect on blood serotonin. Thus both the lack of a rationale for using fenfluramine and the failure to replicate earlier therapeutic results suggest that this drug is not a useful therapy for most autistic children.

Initial reports of the therapeutic effectiveness of a combination of vitamin B_6 and magnesium in a double-blind placebo-controlled short-term (2 weeks of therapeutic agents) study (Martineau, Barthelemy, Garreau, & Lelord, 1985) have not yet been replicated in other laboratories or described in long-term therapy.

DSM-III-R

Beginning with the first description of autism (Kanner, 1943), a triad of symptomatology was recognized involving autistic disturbances of: (1) relating to people; (2) communication and language; and (3) response to objects in the environment. Kanner (1943) focused on (1) the condition of "extreme autistic aloneness" (p. 242),

(2) the structural and communicative impairments of language, and (3) the "obsessive desire for the maintenance of sameness" (p. 245) in the environment. More recent reconstructions of the same triad of symptomatology have shifted the emphasis in the autistic disturbance of relating to people from the state of the child to an impairment in the capacity to engage in reciprocal social interactions (Cohen, Paul, & Volkmar, 1986; Rutter, 1985; Wing, 1981; Wing & Gould, 1979). Congruent with this shift in emphasis, there has been an increased emphasis on the impairments in the use of language for social communication (Cohen et al., 1986; Rutter, 1985; Wing, 1981). In respect to the autistic disturbances of response to objects in the environment, the emphasis on preservation of sameness has been supplemented by a recognition of the inability of autistic children to invest objects in their environment with imagination and to engage in play that requires imagination, fantasy, and the capacity to use toys and thoughts symbolically and abstractly to represent things, activities, and roles in real life.

Table 12.3 compares DSM-III and DSM-III-R. The diagnostic criteria are basically similar, but the emphases have shifted in the directions just described. DSM-III-R puts more weight on: (1) the impaired awareness of the existence and feelings of others; (2) the communicative aspects of both verbal and nonverbal language; and (3) the capacity to imagine and play. Although it is not explicitly stated, DSM-III-R implicitly draws attention to impairments in the inner mental life of the autistic patient, that is, the capacity to empathize and to project mental representations onto objects in the environment through imagination, fantasy, and representational play.

As seen in Table 12.3, the most striking change in diagnostic criteria is the elimination of the age-of-onset criterion. There are several important implications of this change. First, there is recognition that autism can occur after the infantile period, as documented earlier in this chapter. Acceptance of later onsets and recognition of autism as a clinical state persisting throughout life are reflected in the change of nomenclature from *infantile autism* to *autistic disorder*. Second, the possibility of later onsets is consistent with the notion of milder degrees of impairment; some milder cases may not be manifest as early in development as more severe cases. Along with the acceptance of autism as occurring along a continuum of severity, DSM-III-R has eliminated some descriptive adjectives such as *pervasive* and *gross* that in the past have focused attention on the more severe cases to the exclusion of milder ones. These issues have been discussed in a previous section.

TABLE 12.3. Comparison of DSM-III and DSM-III-R

DSM-III: Infantile Autism	DSM-III-R: Autistic Disorder
Pervasive lack of responsiveness to others	Qualitative impairment in reciprocal social interaction
Gross deficits in language or peculiar speech, e.g., echolalia, pronominal reversal	Qualitative impairment in communication and imaginative activity
Bizarre responses to the environment, e.g., resistance to change, peculiar interest in objects	Restricted activities and interests
Onset before 30 months	Onset during infancy or childhood

In DSM-III, autism is classified as a pervasive developmental disorder (PDD) along with two other PDDs, childhood-onset PDD and atypical PDD. As discussed earlier in this chapter, childhood-onset PDD was an arbitrary category distinguished from autism almost solely on the basis of age of onset, a criterion no longer in use, and atypical PDD was a wastebasket category, often confused with the notion of atypical psychosis derived from an earlier literature. In DSM-III-R, autism is the only PDD, with either an infantile onset or a childhood onset (after 36 months of age), except for another wastebasket category, PDD "not otherwise specified" (p. 39).

DSM-III-R is ambivalent about the issue of degree of impairment. Although DSM-III-R states that "the degree of impairment varies," by inventing the category "PDD not otherwise specified" to be used when there are impairments in reciprocal social interaction and verbal and nonverbal communication (criteria for autism) but when "the criteria are not met for Autistic Disorder," DSM-III-R also limits autism to very severe cases and relegates the more numerous milder cases to another diagnostic category. DSM-III-R reinforces this association of autism with severity of impairment by stating that autism is seen more than PDD not otherwise specified (PDDNOS) in clinical settings while the reverse is true in the general population. If one thinks about this, it would seem that those with PDDNOS are simply not impaired enough to come to the clinic and be diagnosed autistic.

Neither DSM-III nor DSM-III-R has recognized the autistic disturbances of sensory modulation and motility. These aspects of autistic symptomatology have been described in detail in several sections of this chapter, and the reasons for their inclusion as diagnostic criteria have been given.

REFERENCES

Al-Mateen, M., Philippart, M., & Shields, W.D. (1986). Rett syndrome. A commonly over-looked progressive encephalopathy in girls. *American Journal of Diseases in Children*, *140*, 761–765.

Alderton, H.R. (1966). A review of schizophrenia in childhood. *Canadian Psychiatry*, *11*, 276–285.

Alpern, G.D. (1967). Measurement of "untestable" autistic children. *Journal of Abnormal Psychology*, *72*, 478–486.

Aman, M.G. (1982). Stimulant drug effects in developmental disorders and hyperactivity—Toward a resolution and disparate findings. *Journal of Autism & Developmental Disorders*, *12*, 385–398.

American Psychiatric Association. (1968). *Diagnostic and statistical manual of mental disorders* (2nd ed.). Washington, DC: Author.

American Psychiatric Association. (1980). *Diagnostic and statistical manual of mental disorders* (3rd ed.). Washington, DC: Author.

American Psychiatric Association. (1987). *Diagnostic and statistical manual of mental disorders* (3rd ed., rev.). Washington, DC: Author.

Anderson, L.T., Campbell, M., Grega, D.M., Perry, R., Small, A.M., & Green, W.H. (1984). Haloperidol in the treatment of infantile autism: Effects on learning and behavioral symptoms. *American Journal of Psychiatry*, *141*, 1195–1202.

Anthony, E.J. (1962). Low-grade psychosis in childhood. In B.W. Richards (Ed.), *Proceedings of the London Conference of Scientific Study of Mental Deficiencies* (Vol. 2) (pp. 398–410). London: May & Baker.

Anthony, J. (1958). An experimental approach to the psychopathology of childhood autism. *British Journal of Medical Psychology*, *31*, 221–225.

Arnold, G., & Schwartz, S. (1983). Hemispheric lateralization of language in autistic and aphasic children. *Journal of Autism & Developmental Disorders*, *13*, 129–139.

Asperger, H. (1944). Die 'autistischen Psychopathen' im Kindesalter. *Archiv fur Psychiatrie und Nervenkrankheiten*, *117*, 76–136.

Aug, R.G., & Ables, B.S. (1971). A clinician's guide to childhood psychosis. *Pediatrics*, *47*, 327–338.

August, G.J. (1983). A genetic marker associated with infantile autism. *American Journal of Psychiatry*, *140*, 813.

August, G.J., Raz, N., & Davis-Baird, T. (1985). Affects of fenfluramine on behavioral, cognitive, and affective disturbances in autistic children. *Journal of Autism & Developmental Disorders*, *15*, 97–107.

August, G.J., Raz, N., Papanicolaou, A.C., Baird, T.D., Hirsh, S.L., & Hsu, L. (1984). Fenfluramine treatment in infantile autism. Neurochemical, electrophysiological, and behavioral effects. *Journal of Nervous & Mental Disease*, *172*, 604–612.

August, G.J., Stewart, M.A., & Tsai, L. (1981). The incidence of cognitive disabilities in the siblings of autistic children. *British Journal of Psychiatry*, *138*, 416–422.

Bartak, L., & Rutter, M. (1971). Educational treatment of autistic children. In M. Rutter (Ed.), *Infantile autism—Concepts, characteristics and treatment*. London: Churchill Livingstone.

Bartak, L., & Rutter, M. (1973). Special educational treatment of autistic children: A comparative study: I. Design of study and characteristics of units. *Journal of Child Psychology & Psychiatry*, *14*, 161–179.

Bartak, L., Rutter, M., & Cox, A. (1975). A comparative study of infantile autism and specific developmental receptive language disorder: I. The children. *British Journal of Psychiatry*, *126*, 127–145.

Baskett, S.J. (1983). Tardive dyskinesia and treatment of psychosis after withdrawal of neuroleptics. *Brain Research Bulletin*, *11*, 173–174.

Bender, L. (1947). Childhood schizophrenia. Clinical study of one hundred schizophrenic children. *American Journal of Orthopsychiatry*, *17*, 40–56.

Bender, L. (1956). Schizophrenia in childhood—Its recognition, description and treatment. *American Journal of Orthopsychiatry*, *26*, 499–506.

Bender, L. (1971). Alpha and omega of childhood schizophrenia. *Journal of Autism & Childhood Schizophrenia*, *1*, 115–118.

Bender, L., & Freedman, A. (1952). A study of the first three years in the maturation of schizophrenic children. *Quarterly Journal of Child Behavior*, *4*, 245–272.

Bender, L., Freedman, A., Grugett, A.E., & Helme, W. (1952). Schizophrenia in childhood: A confirmation of the diagnosis. *Transactions of the American Neurological Association*, *77*, 67–73.

Bergman, P., & Escalona, S.K. (1949). Unusual sensitivities in very young children. *Psychoanalytic Study of the Child, 3–4*, 333–353.

Bloch, J., Gersten, E., & Kornblum, S. (1980). Evaluation of a language program for young autistic children. *Journal of Speech & Hearing Disorders, 45*, 76–89.

Blomquist, H.K., Bohman, M., Edvinsson, S.O., Gillberg, C., Gustavson, K.H., Holmgren, G., & Wahlstrom, J. (1985). Frequency of the fragile-X syndrome in infantile autism: A Swedish multicenter study. *Clinical Genetics, 27*, 113–117.

Bohman, M., Bohman, I.L., Bjorck, P.O., & Sjoholm, E. (1983). Childhood psychosis in a northern Swedish county: Some preliminary findings from an epidemiological survey. In H. Schmidt & H. Remschmidt (Eds.), *Epidemiological approaches in child psychiatry II: International Symposium Mannheim 1981* (pp. 164–173). New York: Thieme-Stratton.

Brask, B.H. (1970). A prevalence investigation of childhood psychosis. In *The Sixteenth Scandinavian Congress of Psychiatry*.

Brawley, E.R., Harris, F.R., Allen, K.E., Fleming, R.S., & Peterson, R.F. (1969). Behavior modification of an autistic child. *Behavioral Science, 14*, 87–97.

Brown, J. (1960). Prognosis from presenting symptoms of preschool children with atypical development. *American Journal of Orthopsychiatry, 30*, 382–390.

Brown, J.L. (1969). Adolescent development of children with infantile psychosis. *Seminars in Psychiatry, 1*, 79–89.

Brown, J.L. (1978). Long-term follow-up of 100 "atypical" children of normal intelligence. In M. Rutter & E. Schopler (Eds.), *Autism: A reappraisal of concepts and treatment*. New York: Plenum.

Brown, J.L., & Reiser, D.E. (1963). Follow-up study of preschool children of atypical development (infantile psychosis)—Later personality patterns in adaptation to maturational stress. *American Journal of Orthopsychiatry, 33*, 336–338.

Brown, W.T., Jenkins, E.C., Cohen, I.L., Fisch, G.S., Wolf-Schein, E.G., Gross, A., Waterhouse, L., Fein, D., Mason-Brothers, A., Ritvo, E., Ruttenberg, B.A., Bentley, W., & Castells, S. (1986). Fragile X and autism: A multicenter study. *American Journal of Medical Genetics, 23*, 341–352.

Brown, W.T., Jenkins, E.C., Friedman, E., Brooks, J., Wisniewski, K., Raguthu, S., & French, J. (1982). Autism is associated with the fragile-X syndrome. *Journal of Autism & Developmental Disorders, 12*, 303–308.

Browning, D.H., & Ferry, P.C. (1976). Tardive dyskinesia in a ten-year-old boy. An undesirable sequel of phenothiazine medication. *Clinical Pediatrics, 15*, 955–957.

Burgoine, E., & Wing, L. (1983). Identical triplets with Asperger's syndrome. *British Journal of Psychiatry, 143*, 261–265.

Call, J.D. (1963). Interlocking affective freeze between an autistic child and his "as-if" mother. *Journal of the American Academy of Child Psychiatry, 2*, 2–15.

Campbell, M. (1985). On the use of neuroleptics in children and adolescents. *Psychiatric Annals, 15*, 101–107.

Campbell, M., Anderson, L.T., Deutsch, S.I., & Green, W. H. (1984). Psychopharmacological treatment of children with the syndrome of autism. *Pediatric Annals, 13*, 309–316.

Campbell, M., Anderson, L.T., Small, A.R., Perry, R., Green, W.H., & Caplan, R. (1982). The effects of haloperidol on learning and behavior in autistic children. *Journal of Autism & Developmental Disorders, 12*, 167–175.

Campbell, M., Cohen, I.L., & Anderson, L.T. (1981). Pharmacotherapy for autistic children: A summary of research. *Canadian Journal of Psychiatry*, *26*, 265–273.

Campbell, M., Deutsch, S.I., Perry, R., Wolsky, B.B., & Palij, M. (1986). Short-term efficacy and safety of fenfluramine in hospitalized preschool-aged autistic children: An open study. *Psychopharmacology Bulletin*, *22*, 141–147.

Campbell, M., Fish, B., David, R., Shapiro, T., Collins, P., & Koh, C. (1972). Response to triiodothyronine and dextroamphetamine: A study of preschool schizophrenic children. *Journal of Autism & Childhood Schizophrenia*, *2*, 343–358.

Campbell, M., Fish, B., David, R., Shapiro, T., Collins, P., & Koh, C. (1973). Liothyronine treatment in psychotic and non-psychotic children under 6 years. *Archives of General Psychiatry*, *29*, 602–608.

Campbell, M., Grega, D.M., Green, W.H., & Bennett, W.G. (1983). Neuroleptic-induced dyskinesias in children. *Clinical Neuropharmacology*, *6*, 207–222.

Campbell, M., Perry, R., Polonsky, B.B., Deutsch, S.I., Palij, M., & Lukashok, D. (1986). Brief report: An open study of fenfluramine in hospitalized young autistic children. *Journal of Autism and Developmental Disorders*, *16*, 495–506.

Campbell, M., Small, A.M., Hollander, C.S., Korein, J., Cohen, I.L., Kalmijn, M., & Ferris, S. (1978). A controlled crossover study of triiodothyronine in autistic children. *Journal of Autism & Childhood Schizophrenia*, *8*, 371–381.

Campbell, M., Small, A.M., Palij, M., Perry, R., Polonsky, B.B., Lukashok, D., & Anderson, L.T. (1987). The efficacy and safety of fenfluramine in autistic children: Preliminary analysis of a double-blind study. *Psychopharmacology Bulletin*, *23*, 123–127.

Cantor, S., Evans, J., Pearce, J., & Pezzot-Pearce, T. (1982). Childhood schizophrenia: Present but not accounted for. *American Journal of Psychiatry*, *139*, 758–762.

Cantwell, D.P., Baker, L., & Rutter, M. (1978). Family factors. In M. Rutter & E. Schopler (Eds.), *Autism: A reappraisal of concepts and treatment*. New York: Plenum.

Chess, S. (1977). Follow-up report on autism in children with congenital rubella. *Journal of Autism & Childhood Schizophrenia*, *7*, 69–81.

Churchill, D.W. (1969). Psychotic children and behavior modification. *American Journal of Psychiatry*, *125*, 1585–1590.

Churchill, D.W. (1972). The relation of infantile autism and early childhood schizophrenia to developmental language disorders of childhood. *Journal of Autism & Childhood Schizophrenia*, *2*, 182–197.

Cohen, D.J., Paul, R., & Volkmar, F.R. (1986). Issues in the classification of pervasive and other developmental disorders: Toward DSM-IV. *Journal of the American Academy of Child Psychiatry*, *25*, 213–220.

Colbert, E., & Koegler, R. (1958). Toe walking in childhood schizophrenia. *Journal of Pediatrics*, *53*, 219–220.

Coleman, R.W., & Provence, S. (1957). Environmental retardation (hospitalism) in infants living in families. *Pediatrics*, *19*, 285–292.

Creak, E.M. (1963). Childhood psychosis. *British Journal of Psychiatry*, *109*, 84–89.

Creak, E.M., & Ini, S. (1960). Families of psychotic children. *Journal of Child Psychology & Psychiatry*, *1*, 156–175.

Creak, E.M. (1961). Schizophrenic syndrome in childhood—Progress report of a working party. *Cerebral Palsy Bulletin*, *3*, 501–503.

Cull, A., Chick, J., & Wolff, S. (1984). A consensual validation of schizoid personality in childhood in adult life. *British Journal of Psychiatry, 144*, 646–648.

Cunningham, D.A., & Dixon, C. (1961). A study of the language of an autistic child. *Journal of Child Psychology & Psychiatry, 2*, 193–202.

Cunningham, M.A. (1966). A five-year study of the language of an autistic child. *Journal of Child Psychology & Psychiatry, 7*, 143–154.

Dahl, E.K., Cohen, D.J., & Provence, S. (1986). Clinical and multivariate approaches to the nosology of pervasive developmental disorders. *Journal of the American Academy of Child Psychiatry, 25*, 170–180.

Darr, G.C., & Worden, F.G. (1951). Case report of twenty-eight years after an infantile autism disorder. *American Journal of Orthopsychiatry, 21*, 559–570.

Davison, G.C. (1964). A social learning therapy programme with an autistic child. *Behaviour Research and Therapy, 2*, 149–159.

de Hirsch, K. (1967). Differential diagnosis between aphasic and schizophrenic language in children. *Journal of Speech & Hearing Disorders, 32*, 3–10.

Delong, G.R., Bean, S.C., & Brown, F.R. (1981). Acquired reversible autistic syndrome in acute encephalopathic illness in children. *Archives of Neurology, 28*, 191–194.

DeMyer, M.K., Churchill, D.W., Pontius, W., & Gilkey, K.M. (1971). A comparison of five diagnostic systems for childhood schizophrenia and infantile autism. *Journal of Autism & Childhood Schizophrenia, 1*, 175–189.

DeMyer, M.K., & Ferster, C.B. (1962). Teaching new social behavior to schizophrenic children. *Journal of the American Academy of Child Psychiatry, 1*, 443–461.

DeMyer, M.K., Hingtgen, J.N., & Jackson, R.K. (1981). Infantile autism reviewed: A decade of research. *Schizophrenia Bulletin, 7*, 388–451.

DeMyer, M.K., Mann, N.A., Tilton, J.R., & Loew, L.H. (1967). Toy-play behavior and use of body by autistic and normal children as reported by mothers. *Psychological Reports, 21*, 973–981.

DeMyer, M.K., Pontius, W., Norton, J.A., Barton, S., Allen, J., & Steele, R. (1972). Parental practices and innate activity in normal, autistic and brain damaged infants. *Journal of Autism & Childhood Schizophrenia, 2*, 49–66.

Desmond, M.M., Montgomery, J.R., Melnick, J.L., Cochran, G.C., & Verniaud, W. (1969). Congenital rubella encephalitis. *American Journal of Diseases of Children, 118*, 30–31.

Deykin, E.Y., & MacMahon, B. (1979). The incidence of seizures among children with autistic symptoms. *American Journal of Psychiatry, 136*, 1310–1312.

Deykin, E.Y., & MacMahon, B. (1980). Pregnancy, delivery, and neonatal complications among autistic children. *American Journal of Diseases of Children, 134*, 860–864.

Dudziak, D. (1982). Parenting the autistic child. *Journal of Psychosocial Nursing & Mental Health Services, 20*, 11–16.

Easson, W.M. (1971). Symptomatic autism in childhood and adolescence. *Pediatrics, 47*, 717–722.

Eisenberg, L. (1956). Early infantile autism: 1943–1955. *American Journal of Orthopsychiatry, 112*, 607–612.

Eisenberg, L. (1957). The course of childhood schizophrenia. *Archives of Neurological Psychiatry, 78*, 69–83.

Eisenberg, L., & Kanner, L. (1956). Childhood schizophrenia symposium. *American Journal of Orthopsychiatry*, *26*, 556–566.

Fay, W.H. (1969). On the basis of autistic echolalia. *Journal of Communication Disorders*, *2*, 38–47.

Fein, D., Pennington, B., Markowitz, P., Braverman, M., & Waterhouse, L. (1986). Toward a neuropsychological model of infantile autism: Are the social deficits primary? *Journal of the American Academy of Child Psychiatry*, *25*, 198–212.

Finnegan, J., & Quarrington, B. (1979). Pre-, peri-, and neonatal factors in infantile autism. *Journal of Child Psychology & Psychiatry*, *20*, 119–128.

Fisch, G.S., Cohen, I.L., Wolf, E.G., Brown, W.T., Jenkins, E.C., & Gross, A. (1986). Autism and the fragile X syndrome. *American Journal of Psychiatry*, *143*, 71–73.

Fischer, I., & Glanville, W.K. (1970). Programmed teaching of autistic children. *Archives of General Psychiatry*, *23*, 90–94.

Fish, B., Shapiro, T., Campbell, M., & Wile, R. (1968). A classification of schizophrenic children under five years. *American Journal of Psychiatry*, *124*, 109–117.

Folstein, S.E. (1985). Genetic aspects of infantile autism. *Annual Review of Medicine*, *36*, 415–419.

Folstein, S., & Rutter, M. (1977). Genetic influences and infantile autism. *Nature*, *265*, 726–728.

Frith, U. (1971). Spontaneous patterns produced by autistic, normal and subnormal children. In M. Rutter (Ed.), *Infantile autism—Concepts, characteristics and treatment*. London: Churchill Livingstone.

Frith, U. (1972). Cognitive mechanisms in autism—Experiments with color and tone sequence production. *Journal of Autism & Childhood Schizophrenia*, *2*, 160–173.

Gajzago, C., & Prior, M. (1974). Two cases of "recovery" in Kanner syndrome. *Archives of General Psychiatry*, *31*, 264–268.

Garreau, B., Barthelemy, C., Sauvage, D., Leddet, I., & Lelord, G. (1984). A comparison of autistic syndromes with and without associated neurological problems. *Journal of Autism & Developmental Disorders*, *14*, 105–111.

Geller, E., Ritvo, E.R., Freeman, B.J., & Yuwiler, A. (1982). A preliminary observation on the effect of fenfluramine on blood serotonin and symptoms in three autistic boys. *New England Journal of Medicine*, *307*, 165–169.

Gillberg, C. (1983). Perceptual, motor and attentional deficits in Swedish primary school children. Some child psychiatric aspects. *Journal of Child Psychology & Psychiatry*, *24*, 377–403.

Gillberg, C. (1984a). Autistic children growing up: Problems of puberty and adolescence. *Developmental Medicine & Child Neurology*, *26*, 125–133.

Gillberg, C. (1984b). Infantile autism and other childhood psychoses in a Swedish urban region. Epidemiological aspects. *Journal of Child Psychology & Psychiatry*, *25*, 35–43.

Gillberg, C. (1985). Asperger's syndrome and recurrent psychosis: A case study. *Journal of Autism & Developmental Disorders*, *15*, 389–397.

Gillberg, C. (1986). Autism and Rett syndrome: Some notes on differential diagnosis. *American Journal of Medical Genetics*, *24*, 127–131.

Gillberg, C., & Gillberg, I.C. (1983). Infantile autism: A total population study of reduced optimality in the pre-, peri-, and neonatal period. *Journal of Autism & Developmental Disorders*, *13*, 153–166.

Gillberg, C., & Schaumann, H. (1981). Infantile autism and puberty. *Journal of Autism & Developmental Disorders, 11*, 365–373.

Gillberg, C., & Wahlstrom, J. (1985). Chromosome abnormalities in infantile autism and other childhood psychoses: A population study of 66 cases. *Developmental Medicine & Child Neurology, 27*, 293–304.

Gittelman, M., & Birch, H.G. (1967). Childhood schizophrenia. *Archives of General Psychiatry, 17*, 16–25.

Goldberg, B., & Soper, H.H. (1963). Childhood psychosis or mental retardation—A diagnostic dilemma: I. Psychiatric and psychological aspects. *Canadian Medical Association Journal, 89*, 1015–1019.

Goldfarb, W. (1961). *Childhood schizophrenia*. Cambridge, MA: Harvard University Press.

Goldfarb, W. (1963). Self-awareness in schizophrenic children. *Archives of General Psychiatry, 8*, 47–60.

Goldfarb, W., Levy, D.M., & Meyers, D.I. (1972). The mother speaks to her schizophrenic child: Language in childhood schizophrenia. *Psychiatry, 35*, 217–226.

Goldfine, P.E., McPherson, P.M., Heath, G.A., Hardesty, V.A., Beauregard, L.J., & Gordon, B. (1985). Association of fragile X syndrome with autism. *American Journal of Psychiatry, 142*, 108–110.

Goutieres, F., & Aicardi, J. (1986). Atypical forms of Rett syndrome. *American Journal of Medical Genetics, 24*, 183–194.

Grandin, T., & Scariano, M.M. (1986). Emergence labeled autistic. Novato, CA: Arena.

Green, A.H. (1967). Self mutilation in schizophrenic children. *Archives of General Psychiatry, 17*, 234–244.

Green, W.H., Campbell, M., Hardesty, A.S., Grega, D.M., Padron-Gayol, M., Shell, J., & Erlenmeyer-Kimling, L. (1984). A comparison of schizophrenic and autistic children. *Journal of the American Academy of Child Psychiatry, 23*, 399–409.

Gualtieri, C.T., & Guimond, M. (1981). Tardive dyskinesia and the behavioral consequences of chronic neuroleptic treatment. *Developmental Medicine & Child Neurology, 23*, 255–259.

Gualtieri, C.T., Quade, D., Hicks, R.E., Mayo, J.P., & Schroeder, S.R. (1984). Tardive dyskinesia and other clinical consequences of neuroleptic treatment in children and adolescents. *American Journal of Psychiatry, 141*, 20–23.

Gualtieri, C.T., Schroeder, S.R., Hicks, R.E., & Quade, D. (1986). Tardive dyskinesia in young mentally retarded individuals. *Archives of General Psychiatry, 43*, 335–340.

Hagberg, B., Aicardi, J., Dias, K., & Ramos, O. (1983). A progressive syndrome of autism, dementia, ataxia, and loss of purposeful hand use in girls: Rett's syndrome: Report of 35 cases. *Annals of Neurology, 14*, 471–479.

Hagberg, B., & Rasmussen, P. (1986). "Forme fruste" of Rett syndrome—A case report. *American Journal of Medical Genetics, 24*, 175–181.

Hagerman, R.J., Jackson, A.W., Levitas, A., Rimland, B., & Braden, M. (1986). An analysis of autism in fifty males with the fragile X syndrome. *American Journal of Medical Genetics, 23*, 359–374.

Halpern, W.I. (1970). The schooling of autistic children—Preliminary findings. *American Journal of Orthopsychiatry, 40*, 665–671.

Hanley, H.G., Stahl, S.M., & Freedman, D.X. (1979). Hyperserotonemia and amine metabolites in autistic and retarded children. *Archives of General Psychiatry, 34*, 1–52.

Hanson, D.R., & Gottesman, I.I. (1976). The genetics, if any, of infantile autism and childhood schizophrenia. *Journal of Autism & Childhood Schizophrenia, 6,* 209–234.

Havelkova, M. (1968). Follow-up study of 71 children diagnosed as psychotic in preschool age. *American Journal of Orthopsychiatry, 38,* 846–857.

Hewett, F.M. (1965). Teaching speech to an autistic child through operant conditioning. *American Journal of Orthopsychiatry, 35,* 927–936.

Hingtgen, J.N., Coulter, S.K., & Churchill, D.W. (1967). Intensive reinforcement of imitative behavior in mute autistic children. *Archives of General Psychiatry, 17,* 36–43.

Ho, H.H., Lockitch, G., Eaves, L., & Jacobson, B. (1986). Pediatric pharmacology and therapeutics. *Journal of Pediatrics, 108,* 465–469.

Holmes, N., Hemsley, R., Rickett, J., & Likierman, H. (1982). Parents as cotherapists: Their perceptions of a home-based behavioral treatment for autistic children. *Journal of Autism & Developmental Disorders, 12,* 331–342.

Hoshino, Y., Kumashiro, H., Yashima, Y., Tachibana, R., & Watanabe, M. (1982). The epidemiological study of autism in Fukushima-ken. *Folia Psychiatrica et Neurologica Japonica, 36,* 115–124.

Howlin, P. (1981). The effectiveness of operant language training with autistic children. *Journal of Autism & Developmental Disorders, 9,* 89–105.

Hudson, E., & DeMyer, M.K. (1968). Food as a reinforcer in educational therapy of autistic children. *Behavior Research & Therapy, 6,* 37–43.

Hutt, C., Hutt, S.J., Lee, D., & Ounsted, C. (1965). A behavioral and electroencephalographic study of autistic children. *Journal of Psychiatric Research, 3,* 181–197.

Hutt, C., & Ounsted, C. (1966). The biological significance of gaze aversion with particular reference to the syndrome of infantile autism. *Behavioral Science, 11,* 346–356.

Ishii, T., & Takahashi, O. (1983). The epidemiology of autistic children in Toyota, Japan: Prevalence. *Japanese Journal of Child & Adolescent Psychiatry, 24,* 311–321.

Jayakar, P., Chudley, A.E., Ray, M., Evans, J.A., Perlov, J., & Wand, R. (1986). Fra(2) (q13) and inv (9) (p11q12) in autism: Causal relationship? *American Journal of Medical Genetics, 23,* 381–392.

Jeste, D.V., & Wyatt, R.J. (1982). Therapeutic strategies against tardive dyskinesia. Two decades of experience. *Archives of General Psychiatry, 39,* 803–816.

Kanner, L. (1943). Autistic disturbances of affective contact. *Nervous Child, 2,* 217–250.

Kanner, L. (1944). Early infantile autism. *Journal of Pediatrics, 25,* 221–217.

Kanner, L. (1949). Problems of nosology and psychodynamics of early infantile autism. *American Journal of Orthopsychiatry, 19,* 416–426.

Kanner, L. (1954). To what extent is early infantile autism determined by constitutional inadequacies? *Research Publications—Association for Research in Nervous and Mental Disease, 33,* 378–385.

Kanner, L. (1971). Follow-up study of eleven autistic children originally reported in 1943. *Journal of Autism & Childhood Schizophrenia, 1,* 119–145.

Kanner, L., & Lesser, L.I. (1958). Early infantile autism. *Pediatric Clinics of North America, 5,* 711–730.

Kanner, L., Rodriguez, A., & Ashenden, B. (1972). How far can autistic children go in matters of social adaptation? *Journal of Autism & Childhood Schizophrenia, 2,* 9–33.

Kaufman, I., Rosenblum, E., Heims, L., & Willer, L. (1957). Childhood psychosis: I.

Childhood schizophrenia—Treatment of children and parents. *American Journal of Orthopsychiatry, 27,* 683–690.

Keeler, W.R. (1958). Autistic patterns and defective communication in blind children with retrolental fibroplasia. In P.H. Hoch & J. Zubin (Eds.), *Psychopathology of communication* (pp. 64–83) New York: Grune & Stratton.

Kerbeshian, J., & Burd, L. (1986). Asperger's syndrome and Tourette syndrome: The case of the pinball wizard. *British Journal of Psychiatry, 148,* 731-736.

Kiernan, C. (1983). The use of nonvocal communication techniques with autistic individuals. *Journal of Child Psychology & Psychiatry, 24,* 339–375.

Kolvin, I. (1971). Psychosis in childhood—A comparative study. In M. Rutter (Ed.), *Infantile Autism—Concepts, characteristics and treatment.* London: Churchill Livingstone.

Kolvin, I., Garside, R.F., & Kidd, J.S.H. (1971). Studies in the childhood psychoses: IV. Parental personality and attitude and childhood psychoses. *British Journal of Psychiatry, 118,* 403–406.

Kolvin, I., Ounsted, C., Humphrey, M., McNay, A., Richardson, L.M., Garside, R.F., Kidd, J.S.H., & Roth, M. (1971). Six studies in the childhood psychoses. *British Journal of Psychiatry, 118,* 381–419.

Kolvin, I., Ounsted, C., Richardson, I.M., & Garside, R.F. (1971). Studies in the childhood psychoses: III. The family and social background in childhood psychoses. *British Journal of Psychiatry, 118,* 396–402.

Kolvin, I., Ounsted, C., & Roth, M. (1971). Studies in the childhood psychoses: V. Cerebral dysfunction and childhood psychoses. *British Journal of Psychiatry, 118,* 407–414.

Lockyer, L., & Rutter, M. (1969). A five- to fifteen-year follow-up study of infantile psychosis—III. Psychological aspects. *British Journal of Psychiatry, 115,* 865–882.

Lotter, V. (1966). Epidemiology of autistic conditions in young children: I. Prevalence. *Social Psychiatry, 1,* 124–137.

Lotter, V. (1967). Epidemiology of autistic conditions in young children: II. Some characteristics of the parents and children. *Social Psychiatry, 1,* 163–173.

Lotter, V. (1978). Follow-up studies. In M. Rutter & E. Schopler (Eds.), *Autism: A reappraisal of concepts and treatment.* New York: Plenum.

Lovaas, O. I. (1971). Considerations in the development of a behavioral treatment program for psychotic children. In D.W. Churchill, G.D. Alpern, & M. DeMyer (Eds.), *Infantile autism.* Proceedings of the Indiana University Colloquium. Springfield, IL: Charles C Thomas.

Lovaas, O.I. (1979). Contrasting illness and behavioral models for the treatment of autistic children: A historical perspective. *Journal of Autism & Developmental Disorders, 9,* 315–323.

Lovaas, O.I., Koegel, R., Simmons, J.Q., & Long, J.S. (1973). Some generalization and follow-up measures on autistic children in behavior therapy. *Journal of Applied Behavior Analysis, 6,* 131–166.

Lovaas, O.I., Schaeffer, B., & Simmons, J.Q. (1965). Building social behavior in autistic children by use of electric shock. *Journal of Experimental Research in Personality, 1,* 99–109.

Lovaas, O.I., Schreibman, L., & Koegel, R.L. (1974). A behavior modification approach to the treatment of autistic children. *Journal of Autism & Childhood Schizophrenia, 4,* 111–129.

Lovaas, O.I., & Simmons, J.Q. (1969). Manipulation of self-destruction in three retarded children. *Journal of Applied Behavior Analysis, 2*, 143–157.

Lowe, L.H. (1966). Families of children with early childhood schizophrenia. *Archives of General Psychiatry, 14*, 26–30.

Madsen-Beisler, J., Tsai, L.Y., & Stiefel, B. (1986). The effects of fenfluramine on communication skills in autistic children. *Journal of Autism & Developmental Disorders, 16*, 227–233.

Mahler, M.S. (1952). On child psychosis and schizophrenia: Autistic and symbiotic infantile psychosis. *Psychoanalytic Study of the Child, 7*, 286–305.

Mahler, M.S. (1965). On early infantile psychosis. The symbiotic and autistic syndromes. *Journal of the American Academy of Child Psychiatry, 4*, 554–568.

Mariner, R., Jackson, A.W., Levitas, A., Hagerman, R.J., Braden, M., McBogg, P.M., Berry, R., & Smith, A.C.M. (1986). Autism, mental retardation, and chromosomal abnormalities. *Journal of Autism & Developmental Disorders, 16*, 425–440.

Markowitz, P.I. (1983). Autism in a child with congenital cytomegalovirus infection. *Journal of Autism & Developmental Disorders, 13*, 249–253.

Marshall, G.R. (1966). Toilet training of an autistic eight-year-old through conditioning therapy: A case report. *Behavior Research & Therapy, 4*, 242–245.

Martin, G.L., England, G., Kaprowy, E., Kilgour, K., & Pikel, V. (1968). Operant conditioning of kindergarten-class behavior in autistic children. *Behavior Research & Therapy, 6*, 281–294.

Martineau, J., Barthelemy, C., Garreau, B., & Lelord, G. (1985). Vitamin B6, magnesium, and combined B6-Mg: Therapeutic effects in childhood autism. *Biological Psychiatry, 20*, 467–478.

Matsuishi, T., Shiotsuki, Y., Yoshimura, K., Shoji, H., Imuta, F., & Yamashita, F. (in press). High prevalence of infantile autism in Kurume City. *Journal of Child Neurology*.

Mawson, D., Grounds, A., & Tantam, D. (1985). Violence and Asperger's syndrome: A case study. *British Journal of Psychiatry, 147*, 566–569.

McConnell, O.L. (1967). Control of eye contact in an autistic child. *Journal of Child Psychiatry, 8*, 249–255.

McGillivray, B.C., Herbst, D.S., Dill, F.J., Sandercock, H.J., & Tischler, B. (1986). Infantile autism: An occasional manifestation of fragile (X) mental retardation. *American Journal of Medical Genetics, 23*, 353–358.

Meryash, D.L., Szymanski, L.S., & Gerald, P.S. (1982). Infantile autism associated with the fragile-X syndrome. *Journal of Autism & Developmental Disorders, 12*, 295–301.

Metz, J.R. (1965). Conditioning generalized imitation in autistic children. *Journal of Experimental Child Psychology, 2*, 389–399.

Meyers, D., & Goldfarb, W. (1961). Studies of perplexity in mothers of schizophrenic children. *American Journal of Orthopsychiatry, 3*, 551–564.

Minton, J., Campbell, M., Green, W.H., Jennings, S., & Samit, C. (1982). Cognitive assessment of siblings of autistic children. *Journal of the American Academy of Child Psychiatry, 21*, 256–261.

Mundy, P., Sigman, M., Ungerer, J., & Sherman, T. (1986). Defining the social deficits of autism: The contribution of non-verbal communication measures. *Journal of Child Psychology & Psychiatry, 27*, 657–669.

Ney, P.G., Palvesky, A.E., & Markely, J. (1971). Relative effectiveness of operant conditioning and play therapy in childhood schizophrenia. *Journal of Autism & Childhood Schizophrenia*, *1*, 337–349.

Noll, R.B., & Benedict, H. (1981). Differentiations within the classification of childhood psychosis: A continuing dilemma. *Merrill-Palmer Quarterly*, *27*, 175–195.

Olsson, B., & Rett, A. (1985). Behavioral observations concerning differential diagnosis between the Rett syndrome and autism. *Brain & Development*, *7*, 281–289.

Ornitz, E.M. (1969). Disorders of perception common to early infantile autism and schizophrenia. *Comprehensive Psychiatry*, *10*, 259–274.

Ornitz, E.M. (1971). Childhood autism: A disorder of sensorimotor integration. In M. Rutter (Ed.), *Infantile autism: Concepts, characteristics and treatment*. Edinburgh and London: Churchill Livingstone.

Ornitz, E.M. (1973). Childhood autism: A review of the clinical and experimental literature. *California Medicine*, *118*, 21–47.

Ornitz, E.M. (1974). The modulation of sensory input and motor output in autistic children. *Journal of Autism & Childhood Schizophrenia*, *4*, 197–215.

Ornitz, E.M. (1983). The functional neuroanatomy of infantile autism. *International Journal of Neuroscience*, *19*, 85–124.

Ornitz, E.M. (in press). Autism at the interface between sensory and information processing. In G. Dawson (Ed.), *Autism: Perspectives on diagnosis, nature and treatment*. New York: Guilford.

Ornitz, E.M., Brown, M.B., Sorosky, A.D., Ritvo, E.R., & Dietrich, L. (1970). Environmental modification of autistic behavior. *Archives of General Psychiatry*, *22*, 560–565.

Ornitz, E.M., Guthrie, D., & Farley, A.J. (1977). The early development of autistic children. *Journal of Autism and Childhood Schizophrenia*, *7*, 207–229.

Ornitz, E.M., Guthrie, D., & Farley, A.J. (1978). The early symptoms of childhood autism. In G. Serban (Ed.), *Cognitive defects in the development of mental Illness*. New York: Brunner/Mazel.

Ornitz, E.M., & Ritvo, E.R. (1968). Perceptual inconstancy in early infantile autism. *Archives of General Psychiatry*, *18*, 76–98.

Ornitz, E.M., & Ritvo, E.R. (1976). The syndrome of autism: A critical review. *American Journal of Psychiatry*, *133*, 609–621.

Perry, R., Campbell, M., Green, W.H., Small, A.M., Die Trill, M.L., Meiselas, K., Golden, R.R., & Deutsch, S.I. (1985). Neuroleptic-related dyskinesias in autistic children: A prospective study. *Psychopharmacology Bulletin*, *21*, 140–143.

Petty, L.K., Ornitz, E.M., Michelman, J.D., & Zimmerman, E.G. (1984). Autistic children who become schizophrenic. *Archives of General Psychiatry*, *41*, 129–135.

Petty, L.K., & Spar, C.J. (1980). Haloperidol-induced tardive dyskinesia in a 10-year-old girl. *American Journal of Psychiatry*, *137*, 745–746.

Provence, S., & Lipton, R.D. (1962). *Infants in institutions*. New York: International Universities Press.

Putnam, M.C., Rank, B., Pavenstedt, E., Andersen, I.N., & Rawson, J. (1948). Case study of an atypical two-and-a-half year old. *American Journal of Orthopsychiatry*, *18*, 1–30.

Rank, B. (1949). Adaptation of the psychoanalytic technique for the treatment of young children with atypical development. *American Journal of Orthopsychiatry*, *19*, 130–139.

Rank, B. (1955). Intensive study and treatment of preschool children who show marked personality deviations, or "atypical development," and their parents. In G. Caplan (Ed.), *Emotional problems of early childhood*. New York: Basic.

Reiser, D.E. (1963). Psychosis of infancy and early childhood, as manifested by children with atypical development. *New England Journal of Medicine, 269,* 790–798, 844–850.

Rescorla, L.A. (1986). Preschool psychiatric disorders: Diagnostic classification and symptom patterns. *Journal of the American Academy of Child Psychiatry, 25,* 162–169.

Riikonen, R., & Amnell, G. (1981). Psychiatric disorders in children with earlier infantile spasms. *Developmental Medicine & Child Neurology, 23,* 747–760.

Ritvo, E.R., Freeman, B.J., Geller, E., & Yuwiler, A. (1983). Effects of fenfluramine on 14 autistic patients. *Journal of the American Academy of Child Psychiatry, 22,* 549–558.

Ritvo, E.R., Freeman, B.J., Mason-Brothers, A., Mo, A., & Ritvo, A.M. (1985). Concordance for the syndrome of autism in 40 pairs of afflicted twins. *American Journal of Psychiatry, 142,* 74–77.

Ritvo, E.R., Freeman, B.J., Yuwiler, A., Geller, E., Schroth, P., Yokota, A., Mason-Brothers, A., August, G.J., Klykylo, W., Leventhal, B., Lewis, K., Piggott, L., Realmuto, G., Stubbs, E.G., & Umansky, R. (1986). Fenfluramine treatment of autism: UCLA collaborative study of 81 patients at nine medical centers. *Psychopharmacology Bulletin, 22,* 133–140.

Ritvo, E.R., Ornitz, E.M., & LaFranchi, S. (1968). Frequency of repetitive behaviors in early infantile autism and its variants. *Archives of General Psychiatry, 19,* 341–347.

Ritvo, S., & Provence, S. (1953). Form perception and imitation in some autistic children: Diagnostic findings and their contextual interpretation. *Psychoanalytic Study of the Child, 8,* 155–161.

Ritvo, E.R., Spence, M.A., Freeman, B.J., Mason-Brothers, A., Mo, A., & Marazita, M.L. (1985). Evidence for autosomal recessive inheritance in 46 families with multiple incidences of autism. *American Journal of Psychiatry, 142,* 187–192.

Ritvo, E.R., Yuwiler, A., Geller, E., Ornitz, E.M., Saeger, K., & Plotkin, S. (1970). Increased blood serotonin and platelets in early infantile autism. *Archives of General Psychiatry, 23,* 566–572.

Rumsey, J.M., Andreasen, N.C., & Rapoport, J.L. (1986). Thought, langue, communication, and affective flattening in autistic adults. *Archives of General Psychiatry, 43,* 771–777.

Rumsey, J.M., Rapoport, J.L., & Sceery, W.R. (1985). Autistic children as adults: Psychiatric, social and behavioral outcomes. *Journal of the American Academy of Child Psychiatry, 24,* 465–473.

Runco, M.A., & Schreibman, L. (1983). Parental judgments of behavioral therapy efficacy with autistic children: A social validation. *Journal of Autism & Developmental Disorders, 13,* 237–248.

Ruttenberg, B.A., & Wolf, E.G. (1965). Evaluating the communication of the autistic child. *Journal of Speech & Hearing Disorders, 32,* 314–324.

Rutter, M. (1965). The influence of organic and emotional factors on the origins, nature and outcome of childhood psychosis. *Developmental Medicine & Child Neurology, 7,* 518–528.

Rutter, M. (1967). Psychotic disorders in early childhood. In A.J. Coppen & A. Walk (Eds.), *Recent developments in schizophrenia—A symposium*. London: RMPA.

Rutter, M. (1970). Autistic children: Infancy to adulthood. *Seminars in Psychiatry*, *2*, 435–450.

Rutter, M. (1983). Cognitive deficits in the pathogenesis of autism. *Journal of Child Psychology & Psychiatry*, *24*, 513–531.

Rutter, M. (1985). Infantile autism and other pervasive developmental disorders. In M. Rutter & L. Hersov (Eds.), *Child and adolescent psychiatry: Modern approaches*. London: Basil Blackwell.

Rutter, M., & Bartak, L. (1971). Causes of infantile autism—Some considerations from recent research. *Journal of Autism & Childhood Schizophrenia*, *1*, 20–32.

Rutter, M., & Bartak, L. (1973). Special education treatment of autistic children: A comparative study: II. Follow-up findings and implications for services. *Journal of Child Psychology & Psychiatry*, *14*, 241–270.

Rutter, M., Bartak, L., & Newman, S. (1971). Autism—A central disorder of cognition and language? In M. Rutter (Ed.), *Infantile autism—Concepts, characteristics and treatment*. London: Churchill Livingstone.

Rutter, M., Greenfeld, D., & Lockyer, L. (1967). A five- to fifteen-year follow-up study of infantile psychosis: II. Social and behavioral outcome. *British Journal of Psychiatry*, *113*, 1183–1200.

Rutter, M., & Lockyer, L. (1967). A five- to fifteen-year follow-up study of infantile psychosis: I. Description of sample. *British Journal of Psychiatry*, *113*, 1169–1182.

Rutter, M., & Sussenwein, F. (1971). A developmental and behavioral approach to the treatment of preschool autistic children. *Journal of Autism & Childhood Schizophrenia*, *1*, 376–397.

Schopler, E. (1978). Changing parental involvement in behavioral treatment. In M. Rutter & E. Schopler (Eds.), *Autism: A reappraisal of concepts and treatment*. New York: Plenum.

Schopler, E. (1982). Evolution in understanding and treatment of autism. *Triangle*, *21*, 51–57.

Schopler, E., Brehm, S.S., Kinsbourne, M., & Reichler, R.J. (1971). Effect of treatment structure on development in autistic children. *Archives of General Psychiatry*, *24*, 415–421.

Schopler, E., Mesibov, G., & Baker, A. (1982). Evaluation of treatment for autistic children and their parents. *Journal of the American Academy of Child Psychiatry*, *21*, 262–267.

Schopler, E., & Reichler, R.J. (1971). Developmental therapy by parents with their own autistic child. In M. Rutter (Ed.), *Infantile autism—Concepts, characteristics and treatment*. London: Churchill Livingstone.

Schulman, J.L. (1963). Management of the child with early infantile autism. *American Journal of Psychiatry*, *120*, 250–254.

Shapiro, T., Fish, B., & Ginsberg, G.L. (1972). The speech of a schizophrenic child from two to six. *American Journal of Psychiatry*, *128*, 92–98.

Shell, J., Campion, J.F., Minton, J., Caplan, R., & Campbell, M. (1984). A study of three brothers with infantile autism: A case report with follow-up. *Journal of the American Academy of Child Psychiatry*, *23*, 498–502.

Sigman, M., & Mundy, P. (in press). Symbolic processes in young autistic children. In D. Cicchetti & M. Beeghly (Eds.), *Symbolic development in atypical children*. San Francisco: Jossey-Bass.

Sigman, M., Mundy, P., Sherman, T., & Ungerer, J. (1986). Social interactions of autistic, mentally retarded and normal children and their caregivers. *Journal of Child Psychology & Psychiatry*, *27*, 647–656.

Sigman, M., & Ungerer, J.A. (1984). Attachment behaviors in autistic children. *Journal of Autism & Developmental Disorders*, *14*, 231–244.

Sigman, M., Ungerer, J.A., Mundy, P., & Sherman, T. (1987). Cognition in autistic children. In D.J. Cohen & A.M. Donnellan (Eds.), *Handbook of autism and disorders of atypical development*. Silver Spring, MD: Winston.

Simmons, J.Q., & Lovaas, O.I. (1969). Use of pain and punishment as treatment techniques with childhood schizophrenics. *American Journal of Psychotherapy*, *23*, 23–36.

Simmons, J.Q., & Reed, B.J. (1969). Therapeutic punishment in severely disturbed children. *Current Psychiatric Therapies*, *9*, 11–18.

Sorosky, A.D., Ornitz, E.M., Brown, M.B., & Ritvo, E.R. (1968). Systematic observations of autistic behavior. *Archives of General Psychiatry*, *18*, 439–449.

Sparrow, S.S., Rescorla, L.A., Provence, S., Condon, S.O., Goudreau, D., & Cicchetti, D.V. (1986). Follow up of "atypical" children: A brief report. *Journal of the American Academy of Child Psychiatry*, *25*, 181–185.

Spiess, Y., Bolthauser, E., Hanggeli, A., & Rubl, R. (1986). Rett-syndrom: ein progredientes neurologisches syndrom bei mädchen. *Schweizerische Medizinische Wochenschrift*, *116*, 458–463.

Spitz, R.A. (1945). Hospitalism—An inquiry into the genesis of psychiatric conditions in early childhood. *Psychoanalytic Study of the Child*, *1*, 53–74.

Spitz, R.A. (1946). Hospitalism—A follow-up report. *Psychoanalytic Study of the Child*, *2*, 113–117.

Stahl, S. (1980). Tardive Tourette syndrome in an autistic patient after long-term neuroleptic administration. *American Journal of Psychiatry*, *137*, 1267–1269.

Steinhausen, H.-C., Gobel, D., Breinlinger, M., & Wohlleben, B. (1986). A community survey of infantile autism. *Journal of the American Academy of Child Psychiatry*, *25*, 186–189.

Stubbs, E.G. (1978). Autistic symptoms in a child with congenital cytomegalovirus infection. *Journal of Autism & Childhood Schizophrenia*, *8*, 37–43.

Stubbs, E.G., Budden, S.S., Jackson, R.H., Terdal, L.G., & Ritvo, E.R. (1986). Effects of fenfluramine on eight outpatients with the syndrome of autism. *Developmental Medicine & Child Neurology*, *28*, 229–235.

Sugiyama, T., & Abe, T. (1986). The results and problems of the routine health check-up for one and a half year olds in Nagoya, Japan. *Japanese Journal of Developmental Disabilities*, *8*, 49–57.

Szurek, S.A., & Berlin, I.N. (1956). Elements of psychotherapeutics with the schizophrenic child and his parents. *Psychiatry*, *19*, 1–9.

Taft, L.T., & Cohen, H.J. (1971). Hypsarrhythmia and infantile autism: A clinical report. *Journal of Autism & Childhood Schizophrenia*, *1*, 327–336.

Taft, L.T., & Goldfarb, W. (1964). Prenatal and perinatal factors in childhood schizophrenia. *Developmental Medicine & Child Neurology*, *6*, 32–43.

Treffert, D.A. (1970). Epidemiology of infantile autism. *Archives of General Psychiatry*, *22*, 431–438.

Tsai, L.Y., & Stewart, M.A. (1983). Etiological implications of maternal age and birth order in infantile autism. *Journal of Autism & Developmental Disorders, 13*, 57–65.

Venter, P.A., Op't Hof, J., Coetzee, D.J., Van der Walt, C., & Retief, A.E. (1984). No marker (X) syndrome in autistic children. *Human Genetics, 67*, 107–111.

Voeller, K.K.S. (1986). Right-hemisphere deficit syndrome in children. *American Journal of Psychiatry, 143*, 1004–1009.

Volkmar, F.R., Cohen, D.J., & Paul, R. (1986). An evaluation of DSM-III criteria for infantile autism. *Journal of the American Academy of Child Psychiatry, 25*, 190–197.

Volkmar, F.R., Paul, R., & Cohen, D.J. (1985). The use of Asperger's syndrome. *Journal of Autism & Developmental Disorders, 15*, 437–439.

Wahlstrom, J., Gillberg, C., Gustavson, K.H., & Holmgren, G. (1986). Infantile autism and the fragile X. A Swedish multicenter study. *American Journal of Medical Genetics, 23*, 403–408.

Ward, A.J. (1970). Early infantile autism—Diagnosis, etiology and treatment. *Psychological Bulletin, 73*, 350–362.

Ward, T.F., & Hoddinott, B.A. (1965). A study of childhood schizophrenia and early infantile autism. *Canadian Psychiatric Association Journal, 10*, 377–386.

Weintraub, S., & Mesulam, M.-M. (1983). Developmental learning disabilities of the right hemisphere. *Archives of Neurology, 40*, 463–468.

Weir, K., & Salisbury, D.M. (1980). Acute onset of autistic features following brain damage in a ten-year-old. *Journal of Autism & Developmental Disorders, 10*, 215–225.

Wenar, C., & Ruttenberg, B.A. (1969). Therapies for autistic children. In J.H. Masserman (Ed.), *Current psychiatric therapies*. New York: Grune & Stratton.

Wing, J.K. (1966). Diagnosis, epidemiology, aetiology. In J.K. Wing (Ed.), *Early childhood autism*. Oxford: Pergamon.

Wing, L. (1981). Asperger's syndrome: A clinical account. *Psychological Medicine, 11*, 115–129.

Wing, L., & Gould, J. (1979). Severe impairments of social interaction and associated abnormalities in children: Epidemiology and classification. *Journal of Autism & Developmental Disorders, 9*, 11–29.

Wing, L., Yeates, S.R., Brierley, L.M., & Gould, J. (1976). The prevalence of early childhood autism: Comparison of administrative and epidemiological studies. *Psychological Medicine, 6*, 89–100.

Wolf, E.G., Wenar, C., & Ruttenberg, B.A. (1972). A comparison of personality variables in autistic and mentally retarded children. *Journal of Autism & Childhood Schizophrenia, 2*, 92–108.

Wolf, M., Risley, T., & Mees, H. (1964). Application of operant conditioning procedures to the behavior problems of an autistic child. *Behaviour Research & Therapy, 1*, 305–312.

Wolff, S., & Barlow, A. (1979). Schizoid personality in childhood: A comparative study of schizoid, autistic and normal children. *Journal of Child Psychology & Psychiatry, 20*, 29–46.

Wolff, S., & Chess, S. (1964). A behavioral study of schizophrenic children. *Acta Psychiatrica Scandinavica, 40*, 438–466.

Wolff, S., & Chess, S. (1965). An analysis of the language of fourteen schizophrenic children. *Journal of Child Psychology & Psychiatry*, *6*, 29–41.

Wolff, S., & Chick, J. (1980). Schizoid personality in childhood: A controlled follow-up study. *Psychological Medicine*, *10*, 85–100.

Wright, H.H., Young, S.R., Edwards, J.G., Abramson, R.K., & Duncan, J. (1986). Fragile-X syndrome in a population of autistic children. *Journal of the American Academy of Child Psychiatry*, *25*, 641–644.

Zappella, M. (1985). Rett syndrome: A significant proportion of girls affected by autistic behavior. *Brain & Development*, *7*, 307–312.

CHAPTER 13

Schizophrenia

SHEILA CANTOR†

DEFINITION

Both DSM-III (APA, 1980) and DSM-III-R (APA, 1987) require that children and adolescents meet the same diagnostic criteria as adults before a diagnosis of schizophrenia can be made. Schizophrenia in children and adolescents is thus defined as a syndrome in which there are "characteristic disturbances in several of the following areas: content and form of thought, perception, affect, sense of self, volition, relationship to the external world, and psychomotor behavior" (APA, 1980, p. 182).

The difficulties encountered in adapting these diagnostic criteria to children have been discussed in some detail (Cantor, 1987; Fish & Ritvo, 1978). Four factors in particular seem to mitigate against making a diagnosis of schizophrenia in childhood using DSM-III: (1) The cognitive development of children makes it extremely unlikely that Schneiderian First Rank symptoms will be observed in a child less than 9 years of age; (2) the symptoms of schizophrenia in childhood tend to be Bleulerian rather than Schneiderian (i.e., they frequently involve disturbances in affective expression, associative thinking, and attentional behavior [Cantor, 1987], symptoms that were somewhat deemphasized by DSM-III); (3) the requirement that a "deterioration from a previous level of functioning" be documented makes it unlikely that a diagnosis of schizophrenia will be considered in a preschooler (when autonomous ego functioning has barely begun, how does one state with confidence that "deterioration" has occurred?); and (4) given the stigma attached to a diagnosis of schizophrenia, given the hope attached to the developmental process, given our attachment to children, and given our lack of "objective" data on which to base so serious a diagnosis, clinicians tend to be extremely reluctant to make a diagnosis of schizophrenia in children.

Nevertheless, this chapter attempts to illustrate the ways in which DSM-III schizophrenia can be observed in very young children, albeit that the symptoms that are emphasized in DSM-III (and DSM-III-R) are not necessarily the most

---

† The death of Sheila Cantor (5/3/88) is deeply regretted by all who know her excellent research and clinical work in the area of schizophrenia.

prominent symptoms of schizophrenia in childhood (Cantor, 1987), and a "classical" DSM-III schizophrenia is relatively rare before puberty.

HISTORICAL BACKGROUND

Few diagnoses have generated more controversy than that of schizophrenia. From the time that Bleuler (1911) first insisted that the term *schizophrenia* more accurately described the disease than did the term, then in common use, *dementia praecox* (Kraepelin, 1919), clinical investigators have defined and redefined this syndrome. It would seem that few subjects in psychiatry more closely approximate the fabled elephant and the blind men; that is, the definition offered reflects most accurately the part of the subject with which the definer is in contact.

In child psychiatry, prior to 1970, there were at least five major efforts to define a syndrome identified as childhood schizophrenia: Potter (1933), Bradley (1941), Despert (1947), Bender (1947), and Creak (1964). The most recent definition was by far the most overinclusive, and prompted an indignant Michael Rutter (1972) to suggest that the entire concept of childhhod schizophrenia be reconsidered.

In opting for the elimination of childhood schizophrenia from its diagnostic manual, DSM-III returned to the custom that was observed before Potter (1933). Children and adolescents would be diagnosed using the same criteria as for adults. This position was challenged even before it was published (Fish & Ritvo, 1979) and almost immediately after it appeared in print (Cantor, Evans, Pearce, & Pezzot-Pearce, 1982). There is reason to believe that the failure to recognize schizophrenia in children results in affected children being incorrectly educated with the mentally retarded (Cantor, 1987) and causes significant hardship for their families (Spungen, 1983; Wilson, 1968).

CLINICAL PICTURE

The signs and symptoms of schizophrenia in childhood are, at least to some extent, age dependent (see Tables 13.1–13.4). The older the child, the more like "adult" schizophrenia the clinical picture (Cantor, 1987; Cantor et al., 1982).

This observation holds true even for many of those whose schizophrenia began before puberty. Thus, in a group of 54 "childhood" schizophrenics (i.e., schizophrenics in whom the symptoms of the disease were documented prepubertally), hallucinations were documented in only 25% of preschoolers (6 of 25 children) compared with 64% of adolescents (9 of 14 youngsters). Similarly, delusions were extremely rare in this population during the preschool years (2 of 25 cases), but were fairly frequently developed by these youngsters postpubertally (6 of 114 cases). Paranoia, which in preschool-aged childhood schizophrenics manifested itself as an expression of profound mistrust and animosity toward others, was more frequently articulated by postpubertal childhood schizophrenics (9 of 14 adolescents, compared with 5

TABLE 13.1.   The Symptom Scale

| Symptom | Observed in >50% of the Population | | |
	Preschool ($N = 25$)	Latency ($N = 15$)	Adolescent ($N = 14$)
Constricted affect	+	+	+
Perseveration	+	+	+
Good eye contact when in need	+	+	+
Inappropriate affect	+	+	+
Anxiety	+	+	+
Fragmented thought	+	+	+
Hyperacusis	+	+	−
Monotonous voice	+	+	+
Loose associations	+	+	+
Neologisms	−	−	−
Echolalia	−	−	−
Illogicality	+	+	+
Mannerisms	+	+	+
Grimacing	−	+[a]	+
Perplexity	+	+	+[b]
Autism	−	−	+
Clang associations	−	−	−
Incoherence	+	+	+

[a] Latency >preschool ($p < .05$).
[b] Adolescent >preschool ($p < .005$).

of 25 preschoolers), and was more likely to consist of complex, delusional material (Cantor, 1982).

The Symptom Scale

In 1981, in an effort to determine what clinical signs were associated with schizophrenia in children, two clinical psychologists and I, utilizing score sheets that listed all the symptoms described by Lehmann in the *Comprehensive Textbook of Psychiatry/ II* (Lehmann, 1975), examined a group of 8 schizophrenic children (Cantor, Pearce, Pezzot-Pearce, & Evans, 1981). Each child was examined by two raters (one of

TABLE 13.2.   Associated Symptoms

| Symptom | Observed in >50% of the Population | | |
	Preschool ($N = 25$)	Latency ($N = 15$)	Adolescent ($N = 14$)
Ambivalence	−	−	+[a]
Delusions	−	−	−
Paranoid ideation	−	−	+[b]
Hallucinations	−	−	+[c]
Poverty of speech	−	+	−
Poverty of content of speech	+	+	+

[a] Adolescent >preschool ($p < .004$).
[b] Adolescent >preschool ($p < .05$).
[c] Adolescent >preschool ($p < .04$).

TABLE 13.3.   The Physical Characteristics

Characteristic	50% of Population Show Sign		
	Preschool (N = 25)	Latency (N = 15)	Adolescent (N = 14)
Hypotonia	+	+	+
Brachycephaly	−	+	+
Long hands	−	−	−
Decreased muscle power	+	+	+
Decreased muscle mass	+	+	+
Hypercanthism	+	+	+
Soft velvety skin	+	+	+
Head height	−	+	+
Increased head circumference	−	+	+
Prominent nasal bridge	−	+	−
Deep-set eyes	−	+	−
Short fingers	+	+	−
Lax elbows	+	−	−
Lax metacarpal/pharangeal	+[a]	+	−

[a]Preschool more likely than adolescent ($p < .005$).

the two clinical psychologists and myself) and each symptom was scored as being either present or absent. For a child to be regarded as demonstrating a specific symptom, the symptom had to have been scored as present by *both* of the examiners (who were blind to each other's ratings).

The symptom scale (see Table 13.1) was then constructed to consist of all of the symptoms that had been rated as present in at least 50% of the children. This scale has proven to be a useful tool for examining childhood schizophrenics (Cantor, 1987). With the exception of "neologisms, echolalia, and clang associations, all of the symptoms included in the original symptom scale have continued to be observed in more than 50% of schizophrenic children examined (the N of 54 mentioned earlier).

A severe association defect appears to be characteristic of schizophrenia in childhood, as symptoms such as fragmented thought processing, loose associations, illogicality, incoherence, and poverty of content of speech dominate the clinical picture. Cognitive phenomena such as these were believed by Bleuler to be directly

TABLE 13.4.   Associated Physical Signs

Sign	>50% of Population Show Sign		
	Preschool (N = 25)	Latency (N = 15)	Adolescent (N = 14)
Lordosis	+	+	−
Strabismus	−	−	−
Dysarthria	+	+	−
Flat feet	−	+	−
Loss of flexor tone	−	+[a]	−
No arm swing while walking	−	+	−
Abnormal gait	+	+	+

[a]Latency more likely than preschool ($p < .05$).

attributable to the association defect, which he considered pathognomonic of the schizophrenic process.

For the purpose of making a DSM-III diagnosis of schizophrenia in prepubertal subjects, the clinician will usually need to rely on being able to document the presence of the characteristic disturbance in thought processing and to observe that this disturbance is present in association with constricted or inappropriate affect. We have found that an unstructured play interview, or a structured academic lesson, can provide the most favorable setting for making such observations.

For example, during a free-play period, a 7-year-old schizophrenic boy was overheard quietly chanting to himself the words "sleeping gas" while piling up milk cartons. When asked the meaning of these words he correctly defined them as referring to "a gas that makes you sleepy." When asked why he was chanting these words while at play, he could only shrug and say, "I don't know." This same child, when asked to prepare valentines for his classmates, crawled into a large cardboard box (used by the children as a play area) and produced a series of valentines (see Fig. 13.1) that even he found difficult to rationalize.

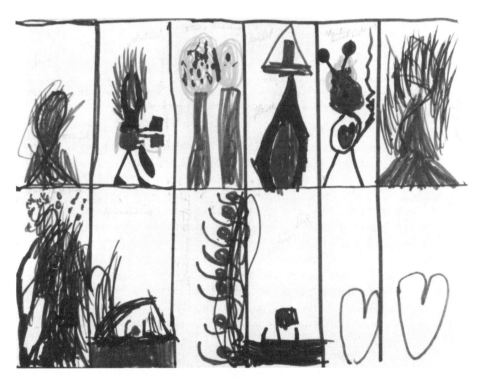

Figure 13.1. The response of a 7-year-old schizophrenic boy to an assignment to "prepare valentines" for his classmates. The child crawled into an empty carton and drew this series of pictures which he insisted were all "valentines." He later explained these pictures to his therapist as follows (reading from left to right, beginning in the upper left-hand corner): "fire"; "electricity, chain saw, ax and hammer"; "two trees kissing"; "rocket with flame"; "martian—burnt his hand"; "fire again—an apartment block"; "swimming"; "swimming contest"; "sinking ship." The last two blocks are obvious valentines.

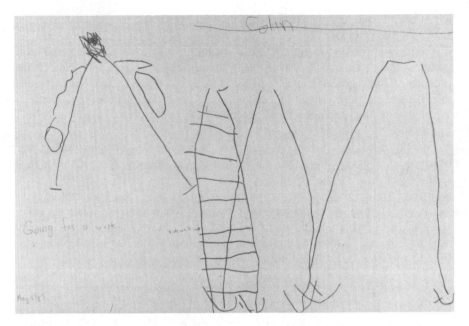

Figure 13.2. The response of a 12-year-old schizophrenic boy who has spent the last 6 years in a classroom for the "trainably mentally handicapped" to being asked to draw a picture of the morning's activities. The boy drew "going for a walk"—a sidewalk and legs. After prompting from the teacher he added the stick figure, which has a head and primitive arms and hands.

The fragmented thought processing of schizophrenic children presents many challenges to those who would be teachers of such children. For example, a 17-year-old schizophrenic girl persistently resisted all attempts to teach her that two halves make a whole. (When two half glasses of water were used to illustrate the point, she insisted that they were still two halves even after they had been poured into a single glass.) A 7-year-old boy, when presented with a picture of a family in a kitchen and asked to identify the function of the room in the picture, replied, "Well . . . there's no sofa in there . . . there's no rug on the floor . . . there's lots of dishes," yet he could not put this information together to correctly identify the room as a kitchen, despite numerous "clues" provided by the teacher.[1] A 12-year-old boy, when asked to draw a picture depicting the day's activity, drew "going for a walk," a picture that consisted of a sidewalk, a head, arms, and legs (see Fig. 13.2).

Disturbances in perceptual and motor functioning are also frequently observed in schizophrenic children (see Tables 13.1, 13.3, 13.4). *Hyperacusis*, or the difficulty screening out extraneous sound (and engaging in selective listening), interferes with the ability of schizophrenic children to attend and learn. A monotonous voice, motor

[1] During a guessing game, if adults attempt to provide a schizophrenic child with "clues," the child's associative dysfunction will lead the child *away* from the correct response.

mannerisms, and facial grimacing are all frequently observed signs of motor dysfunction in this population of children (see Table 13.1).

The most severe symptoms, neologisms, echolalia, and clang associations, are usually found only in the presence of some degree of dementia. These symptoms have been documented in less than 50% of the 54 schizophrenic children examined (Cantor, 1987).

Neologisms were most frequently observed during the preschool years (6 of 25 preschoolers, 3 of 15 latency-aged children, and only 1 of 14 adolescents). Echolalia was a common clinical observation in preschool and latency-aged schizophrenic children (12 of 25 and 7 of 15 cases, respectively), but had diminished considerably by adolescence (2 of 14 cases). Clang associations, which at times formed part or all of the expressive speech of preschool, language-delayed schizophrenic children (11 of 25 cases), were observed less frequently in the latency-aged population (5 of 15 cases) and were uncommon in adolescence (3 of 14) cases.

Autism was regarded as being present if the schizophrenic child or adolescent was preoccupied with internal stimuli or thought processes. This phenomenon was relatively uncommon in the more externally directed preschoolers (10 of 25 cases), slightly more common during latency (7 of 15 cases), and fairly prevalent by adolescence (11 of 14 cases).

The term *perplexity* was used by us to identify the mood of puzzlement so often observed in schizophrenic children, as they struggled to achieve a greater understanding of the external world. It was thus fairly infrequently observed in preschoolers (13 of 25), became far more prevalent during latency (13 of 15 cases), and was consistently observed by adolescence (14 of 14 cases).

Finally, "good eye contact when in need" was included by us in the symptom scale in order to differentiate schizophrenic from autistic children. All schizophrenic children, regardless of age, did make frequent eye contact.

The Associated Symptoms

For the sake of completeness, the "associated symptoms" were subsequently added to our clinical assessments of schizophrenic children (see Table 13.2). Ambivalence, hallucinations, and paranoia were significantly more prevalent after puberty. Poverty of speech was most prevalent among latency-aged children (10 of 25 preschoolers, 10 of 15 latency, 6 of 14 adolescents), although during the phase when they were just acquiring language all the schizophrenic preschoolers could have been deemed to be displaying poverty of speech (therefore we did not score this item during this phase).

The Physical Characteristic Scale

Hypotonic schizophrenia, that is, schizophrenia that is associated with specific physical signs (Cantor et al., 1981), is the form of schizophrenia that is prevalent in prepubertal subjects (Cantor, 1987). At least some of the signs and symptoms characteristic of this type of schizophrenia have also been observed in schizophrenia that began postpubertally (Yardin & Discipio, 1971). A study to determine what proportion of postpubertal schizophrenia is associated with hypotonia is currently in progress.

We have seen a small number of children who have manifested *only* the physical signs associated with hypotonic schizophrenia (i.e., these children had signs of neuromuscular dysfunction in the absence of DSM-III schizophrenia). We have not, thus far, encountered the converse: that is, children with the symptoms of DSM-III schizophrenia who were free of signs of neuromuscular dysfunction.

The neuromuscular signs, such as hypotonia, decreased muscle power, decreased muscle mass, lax elbows, and lax metacarpal/phalangeal joints, all become somewhat less prevalent postpubertally. In general, motor functioning appears to be at its worst during latency (we have now had the opportunity to observe several children who lost postural tone between the ages of 4 and 8), while the "head" signs, such as brachycephaly, increased head circumference, and head height, all tend to increase in prevalence with maturation (Cantor, 1987).

The 14 characteristics that comprise the physical characteristic scale (see Table 13.3) were all observed in 50% or more of the pilot group of 8 schizophrenic children (Cantor et al., 1981). The correlation between the physical characteristic scale score and the symptom scale score has remained statistically significant over 54 cases (Cantor, 1987). This observed association between the physical signs and the symptoms of schizophrenia must, however, be regarded as hypothetical, at least until this association has been confirmed by other medical centers.

Complete instructions on how to use the physical characteristic scale to assess children, as well as the normative data needed for the purpose of comparing these children with the age-appropriate norm, have been provided in the appendix of the textbook *Childhood Schizophrenia* (Cantor, 1987).

The Associated Physical Signs

Most of the associated physical signs (see Table 13.4) were added to our clinical assessment, because documenting their presence provided strong "objective" evidence of hypotonia.

The abdominal muscles of schizophrenic children tend to be very weak, and almost certainly are the major cause of the lordosis so commonly associated with this disorder (19 of 25 preschoolers; 11 of 15 latency; 7 of 14 adolescents). We have also found that schizophrenic children need to be closely monitored for scoliosis, as asymmetrical motor tone results in the development of scoliosis during the latency years in a small percentage of these children.

The dysarthria and strabismus associated with childhood schizophrenia frequently persist into the postpubertal years (6 of 14 adolescents still manifested some dysarthria). There was some tendency for an abnormal gait to correct itself with maturation (21 of 25 preschoolers; 13 of 15 latency; 9 of 14 adolescents), and lack of flexor tone, or the ability of gravity to extend the patient's arm fully when the patient was standing in a relaxed posture, was most frequently observed in latency-aged subjects (5 of 25 preschoolers; 9 of 15 latency; 4 of 14 adolescents).

Growth and Development in Schizophrenic Children

Schizophrenia in childhood interferes dramatically with the developmental process (Cantor, 1987). Although we did not have access to the birth and early developmental history of all of our 54 subjects, we did have a detailed developmental history for at least 29 youngsters, who were less than 10 years old when their parents completed our developmental questionnaire. Table 13.5 presents the results of comparing the questionnaires completed by the parents of 27 male schizophrenics with the questionnaires completed by the parents of 40 "normal" male preschoolers. By parental report schizophrenic males manifested significant developmental deviation (i.e., their behavior was significantly different from that of the control males) in 9 of the 11 areas of functioning examined.

Vegetative Functioning

The feeding difficulties reported by the parents of schizophrenic children included poor suck, resisting or regurgitating solids, and odd food preferences. Of these, only the difficulty adjusting to solid foods was also reported to occur in control children.

Although sleep disturbance was reported with surprising frequency by the parents of control children, difficulty falling asleep at older than 36 months and difficulty staying asleep at older than 36 months were reported significantly more often by the parents of schizophrenic children. Severe nightmares at older than 24 months

TABLE 13.5.   Developmental Dysfunction Associated with Hypotonic Schizophrenia

	Proportion of Population Affected	
Developmental Dysfunction	Controls ($N = 40$)	Schizophrenics ($N = 27$)
Feeding difficulties	0.10	0.44[a]
Sleep disturbance	0.30	0.70
Toilet-training difficulties	0.05	0.41[b]
Atypical social behavior	0.40	0.67
Atypical play behavior	0.10	0.59[c]
Unusual peer behavior	0.08	0.85[d]
Atypical speech development	0.35	0.82[e]
Atypical motor development	0.10	0.58[f]
Motor mannerisms reported	0.23	0.48[g]
Unusual fears reported	0.28	0.89[h]
Unusual behavior noted	0.05	0.41[i]

[a] $p < .005$.
[b] $p < .0005$.
[c] $p < .0001$.
[d] $p < .00001$.
[e] $p < .0005$.
[f] $p < .0001$.
[g] $p < .01$.
[h] $p < .0001$.
[i] $p < .0005$.

were reported only by the parents of schizophrenic children. It is a relatively rare phenomenon, having been reported in only 3 of our 27 schizophrenic children.

The toileting difficulties of schizophrenic children included 5 children who resisted training (and who were not trained until older than 36 months) and 6 children whose parents were completely unsuccessful at training them. (These children were trained in our treatment program.)

Social and Play Behavior

Although a surprising 40% of the control children were reported to be experiencing some "atypical" social behavior, infants who preferred to be left alone occurred only in the schizophrenic population, as did all of those children (with a single exception) who chose to cuddle "hard" transitional objects (e.g., a car, a calculator).

Perseverative play further distinguished the schizophrenic children from the control children (having been described in 12 of 27 schizophrenic children and only 3 of 40 control children). As well, only schizophrenic children were reported to have disliked or been uninterested in toys. Even in schizophrenic children, this was a rare phenomenon (reported in only 3 of 27 children).

Unusual peer behavior was so commonly observed among schizophrenic children, and so rarely noted among control children, that it was one of two factors that could statistically predict group membership (the other factor being unusual behavior). Schizophrenic children were reported to prefer to play alone, provoke fights with peers, and behave in a domineering or hyper manner with peers.

Language and Motor Development

Schizophrenic children differed significantly from the control children in vocalizing little early babble, being slow to imitate parental vocalization, and being able to produce no sentence development by 36 months. They were also significantly more likely to make up words.

The major motor milestones were seldom delayed in schizophrenic children, such delay occurring in only 5 of the 27 index children. The most common motor abnormality nonetheless observed and reported by the parents of schizophrenic children was abnormal gait (e.g., toe walking).

Motor mannerisms were significantly more often reported by the parents of schizophrenic children than by the parents of control children, although no single mannerism was typical of the group of schizophrenic children. Hand flapping was noted in only 2 of the 27 schizophrenic children, while rocking (6 of 27 children) and head banging (5 of 27 children) were far more commonly observed.

Unusual Fears and Unusual Behavior

Schizophrenic children were significantly more likely than the control children to be afraid of loud or sudden noises, moving toys and slides, all humans except significant others, and water.

Unusual behaviors were significantly more frequently reported to occur in the population of schizophrenic children, although no single behavior emerged as characteristic of the group. Unusual behaviors reported included "unusual sensory" (e.g., smelling or compulsive touching of objects), "unusual motor" (e.g., compulsve pacing), lining objects up, obsessions, and paranoid responses (e.g., refusing to eat with others).

COURSE AND PROGNOSIS

Schizophrenia in children is, too often, associated with functional mental retardation, even when the disease stops short of a total dementia (Cantor, 1987). If one considers how difficult it is for the adult schizophrenic to attend to work, to learn, and to function independently, it should not be surprising to note that the interference with these same functions in children—who have not yet achieved mastery and autonomous ego functioning—frequently results in mental retardation.

The signs and symptoms of schizophrenia in childhood are those that are associated with a poor prognosis in adult schizophrenia. The lack of affect, the poverty of speech, the deficit in the associative process, the anergy (which is probably secondary to poor muscle tone), the inability to play (the child's equivalent of anhedonia), and the attentional deficits are all considered to be "negative" symptoms of schizophrenia. These symptoms respond poorly, if at all, to the neuroleptics that are the treatment of choice in adult schizophrenia.

There is very minimal evidence that neuroleptics are of any benefit to children with schizophrenia. I have observed the converse, a negative response to phenothiazines, on several occasions (Cantor, 1987). Childhood schizophrenics are susceptible to tardive dyskinesia. Indeed, movements resembling tardive dyskinesia have developed in a 20-year-old childhood schizophrenic who had received no neuroleptics since she was 14 years old (and whose lifetime dose of phenothiazines was negligible).

There is evidence that schizophrenic children, who have not been identified and who have received little or no treatment, have fared very poorly (Cantor, 1987). Even among adult schizophrenics, the younger the age of onset, the worse the prognosis (Yardin & Discipio, 1971).

Within the population of prepubertal-onset schizophrenics, age of onset does not necessarily predict severity of disorder (Richards, 1951). Our own clinical research has suggested that Group 1 children, or children with high symptom scale scores relative to their physical characteristic scale scores, are more severely impaired in every area of functioning examined than are Group 2 children, or children whose physical characteristic scale score and symptom scale score are more nearly equal (Cantor, 1987). This is consistent with the findings of Richards (1951), who reported that poor prognosis for childhood schizophrenics was associated with severity of illness rather than with age of onset.

Impairment

Most schizophrenic children are not globally impaired, although the most severely affected do appear to be suffering from what Lauretta Bender once described as a pandevelopmental disorder (Bender, 1947).

On objective tests of functioning, such as the Bruininks-Oseretsky Test of Motor Proficiency (1978) or the WISC-R, a characteristic pattern of results tends to emerge (Cantor, 1987; Wechsler & Jaros, 1965). In general, the gross motor functioning of schizophrenic children is more severely affected than the fine motor functioning, and language functioning is more severely impaired than perceptual functioning (Cantor, 1987).

Motor Functioning

The Bruininks-Oseretsky demonstrates very well the difficulty prepubertal schizophrenics experience with gross motor functioning, balance, and bilateral coordination. In contrast, these children often demonstrate little or no impairment on tests of visual motor functioning or fine motor control (Cantor, 1987). Schizophrenic children can be gifted artists and musicians, since these areas of functioning are often only minimally impaired as a result of the disease. (We have had at least one very gifted artist in our treatment program, who drew and printed very skillfully despite a pencil grasp that was little more than a clenched fist [Cantor, 1982].)

Cognitive Functioning

In our group of schizophrenic children, the Performance subtests of the WISC-R tended to show a lesser degree of impairment than did the Verbal subtests (Cantor 1987). For most schizophrenic children tested, inter- and intratest variability have been reported to be the rule rather than the exception (Wechsler & Jaros, 1965; Cantor, 1987). Thought disorder seems to inferfere significantly with the ability of these children to perform the Verbal subtests of the WISC-R, as the Comprehension subtest frequently reveals the extent of the defect in the association process, and the Vocabulary and Similarities subtests often elicit echolalia and idiosyncratic and clang associations (Cantor, 1987).

Social and Adaptive Functioning

Like their adult counterparts, schizophrenic children are totally lacking in appropriate social skills. Spontaneous associative learning, which relies heavily on contextual cues, is rare in these children. Schizophrenic children must therefore be taught how to recognize and respond to social norms self-consciously.

Schizophrenic children perseverate. It is very difficult for such children to adjust to environmental change. Even those children who are not rigid and who demonstrate some ability to adjust may be upset by diverse stimuli and may lack the capacity to adapt readily to the complexity of daily living.

The difficulty schizophrenic children experience with selective attention (i.e., the inability to screen out extraneous sensory stimuli and internal thought and memory intrusions) further compromises the ability of these children to learn. Schizophrenic children often attend equally to all sounds, reacting as readily to the sound of footsteps in the hall as to the teacher's voice. Internal stimuli, such as bodily sensations (the urge to urinate or defecate), memories, and perseverative preoccupations also easily disrupt the learning process in such children.

Difficulties with auditory discrimination and with visual tracking further compromise the ability of schizophrenic children to learn. The former is reflected by the prevalence of word approximations in the speech of young schizophrenics, the latter by the highly impoverished observation skills. Tactile defensiveness may restrict play behavior and limit the child's willingness to take part in "hands-on" learning, thus closing off still another avenue for acquiring information.

Speech delay, which includes a significant deficit in both expressive language and language comprehension skills, further constricts the ability of the schizophrenic child to learn and develop. Such children rarely ask information-seeking questions, an essential aid to learning in the normal child.

Complications

Schizophrenic children frequently demonstrate autonomic instability. Unexplained flushing, bizarre skin eruptions, and strange swellings (most likely extravasations) are encountered within this population of children. It is not uncommon to encounter allergiclike phenomena among these children (e.g., excessive mucous secretion with upper respiratory tract infections, repeated bouts of otitis media, etc.), although there is no increased prevalence of genuine atypy.

Hyperthermia occurs with increased frequency among schizophrenic children (Cantor, 1982, 1987). Schizophrenic children were somewhat more likely than control children to develop hyperthermia in response to an overheated atmosphere. (This was reported to occur in 4 of 27 schizophrenic children compared with 2 of 40 control children.) The children with signs of autonomic instability were the most likely to demonstrate this type of hyperthermia, and had to be protected during the summer months.

The poor motor tone of schizophrenic children makes them vulnerable to motor deformities, such as strabismus, lordosis, scoliosis, kyphosis, dysarthria, flat feet, internally rotated hips and knees, and a grossly abnormal gait. It seems likely that poor postural tone also contributes to variable arousal levels in very young schizophrenics, and that this decrease in alertness adversely affects learning. Lethargy may be yet another complication of hypotonia, and may also predispose to slower development, as lethargic children seldom actively explore their environment.

EPIDEMIOLOGY

There have been few epidemiological studies in contemporary child psychiatry. Perhaps the most famous of these, the Isle of Wight study (Rutter, Graham, & Yule, 1970), would have utilized a more inclusive definition of childhood schizophrenia than is presented here, but applied that diagnosis more conservatively. (Rutter et al. reported that there were no children with schizophrenia in their cohort.) A frequently quoted figure for the prevalence rate of childhood schizophrenia is 4 or 5 per 10,000. This figure more accurately reflects the prevalence rate of infantile autism.

There is general agreement that the sex ratio of male to female for all types of childhood psychosis is 4 or 5 to 1. My own findings do not differ significantly from this figure as the male:female ratio for my 54 subjects was 43:11.

This male:female figure was, however, not evenly distributed, as I was surprised to find that there were few females within the population of preschool (23:2) and latency-aged children (13:2), and a majority of females within the population of adolescent-aged childhood schizophrenics (6:8). This suggests a strange diagnostic bias here in Winnipeg. (All the subjects in this study were referred to me with a presumptive diagnosis of childhood schizophrenia.) I can only speculate that females are less likely than males to be identified during the preschool and latency years, and that the majority of males who had been identified during the preschool years (and who at the time of my research would be postpubertal) had been institutionalized prior to puberty and were therefore not available for inclusion in my adolescent cohort.

In support of this general hypothesis, the majority of females in the adolescent-aged cohort had not been identified prior to age 6. In fact, of the 8 females in the adolescent-aged cohort, 2 had been identified at age 4, 2 at age 6, 1 at age 10, and 2 at age 12. Of the 6 males in the adolescent-aged cohort, 3 were identified during the preschool years, and 3 at age 12. Speech delay was reported in less than one-third of the females in our cohort, as opposed to more than three-quarters of the males. The relatively normal development of speech among females with childhood schizophrenia may account for the later identification of these females by physicians.

Childhood schizophrenia continues to be diagnosed relatively rarely in most medical centers. In many centers a majority of psychotic children are being identified as atypical psychosis, in recognition of the fact that, although these children do not really resemble adult schizophrenics, they are psychotic and they are not autistic. It may be that with the redefinition in DSM-III-R of pervasive developmental disorder some psychotic children will now be diagnosed as pervasive developmental disorder NOS (not otherwise specified).

FAMILIAL PATTERN

The evidence from our sample of schizophrenic children suggests the same pattern of inheritance as has been documented for adult schizophrenia: that is, a dominant gene with limited penetrance. We found it difficult to get an accurate family history from our subjects. In some cases families chose to withhold a positive family history, at least until they had known us for 6 months or longer. In other cases, the family members themselves did not know of any affected relatives. A family member who had been institutionalized some years ago had been forgotten or was not known to the affected child's parents.

Nevertheless, we found a history of schizophrenia that had led to hospitalization among the first- and second-degree relatives of 20% of our patient cohort (10 of 51 cases in whom family history was available). In fact, only 21 of 51 subjects had no history of either schizophrenia, schizotypal personality disorder, or "nervous breakdown."

Schizophrenia was more common in second-degree relatives than in first-degree relatives; that is, the affected relative was more likely to be an aunt or an uncle or a grandparent than a parent or a sibling. We have no explanation for this phenomenon, but we know it is not unique to our medical center. At a meeting some years ago, compatible figures were presented by another medical center (which reported that schizophrenia had occurred in 15% of the second-degree relatives of their patient population, but only 8% of the first-degree relatives).

DIFFERENTIAL DIAGNOSIS

Schizophrenic children must be differentiated from attention-deficit-disordered children, severely learning-disabled children, aphasic children, children with anaclitic depressions, and autistic children.

Differentiating the Schizophrenic Child from the Child with Attention Deficit Disorder (ADD)

The schizophrenic child who is agitated and provocative can be difficult to differentiate from the ADD child. The clinician must take a careful history (inquiring as to whether the child's attention is variable or consistently short, and inquiring as to whether the child's activity level is variable or consistently high active) and observe the child carefully during an unstructured play interview. The schizophrenic child will tend to settle on a perseverative activity if the opportunity presents itself (i.e., if an object that forms the subject of a current preoccupation is in the clinician's office). Formal thought disorder is not characteristic of ADD children, although fragmented perceptions (a not uncommon finding among severe ADD children) may be confused with fragmented thought processing. When present, other characteristics of childhood schizophrenia, such as an aversion to toys, a tendency to ignore peers, psychotic perceptions (hallucinations and visual distortions), psychotic preoccupations (obsessional terrors, paranoid responses [e.g., avoidance of touching and being touched]), and bizarre mannerisms all help to differentiate the schizophrenic child from the ADD child.

Differentiating the Schizophrenic Child from the Severely Learning-Disabled and/or the Aphasic Child

Nonpsychotic preschool children with developmental disabilities can be difficult to differentiate from schizophrenic children. The clinician will need to take a careful history (with special emphasis on social and adaptive development) and may need to observe the child over a prolonged period of time. Nonpsychotic learning-disabled children tend to enjoy more normal personality development (i.e., they may relate well to others and be affectively spontaneous) until the frustration that is associated with their particular deficit begins to exact an emotional toll. Nonpsychotic, developmentally disabled children continue to struggle with external reality. Eating and sleeping disturbances should not accompany nonglobal developmental disabilities, unless the child has been neglected to the point of developing a reactive depression.

Bizarre mannerisms and behaviors should not be associated with nonpsychotic learning disabilities, unless the child has been severely stressed and neglected.

Differentiating the Schizophrenic Child from the Child Who Is Manifesting an Anaclitic Depression

A child with an anaclitic depression is perhaps the easiest child to confuse with a childhood schizophrenic. Affect may appear blunted in children who have been neglected to the point of failure to thrive. Such children may no longer relate normally to adults, may ignore toys, may be lethargic and withdrawn, be delayed in language and motor development, manifest hypotonia, and develop some idiosyncratic belief systems as a result of total neglect. Many of these signs will, however, quickly correct themselves when the child is removed from the malignant environment and a more normal growth pattern resumes. A necessary precondition for the diagnosis of anaclitic depression to be made is for malignant neglect to the point of failure to thrive to be documented.

Differentiating the Schizophrenic Child from the Child with Early Infantile Autism

Most schizophrenic children will enjoy a period of normal development, at least during the first year of life (Cantor, 1987). In addition, the classical definition of schizophrenia used in this chapter limits the diagnosis to a "functional" psychosis; that is, such a diagnosis excludes children with a metabolic defect, a history of organic insult, or a history of birth or postnatal trauma sufficient to explain the symptoms. Both DSM-III and DSM-III-R permit a diagnosis of autism to be made in a child with a definable developmental defect.

Unlike classically autistic children, schizophrenic children do communicate with others, using both verbal and gestural communication. Most preschizophrenic infants like and anticipate being picked up and—when not frightened—are normally curious about their immediate environment. The extreme avoidance of human contact that is characteristic of autism during the preschool years is rarely associated with schizophrenia in early childhood, as most schizophrenic preschoolers, like schizophrenic adults, continue to show affection for their families and seek comfort when they are hurt.

As they mature, untreated schizophrenic children become more oppositional and socially withdrawn, whereas autistic children often become more approachable. Temper tantrums are more often associated with autism in adolescence, with childhood schizophrenia in childhood. Finally, unlike autistic children, childhood schizophrenics often experience the hallucinations and delusions characteristic of postpubertal-onset schizophrenia at some time in their life cycle, most often during late childhood or early to middle adolescence, or during a period of exceptional stress in their lives (Cantor, 1987).

The question of whether early "functional" infantile autism, as originally described by Kanner (1943), is in fact the most severe and earliest manifestation of schizophrenia remains an open one. Initially, Dr. Kanner himself advanced strong arguments in favor of this position (Kanner, 1949). Some published descriptions of mature autistic children (see Cantor, 1987) strongly resemble the simple schizophrenia that was described by Kraepelin (1919), even though the researchers who examined and described "Kanner's children" did not acknowledge such resemblance. This controversy is unlikely to be satisfactorily resolved until a diagnosis of schizophrenia can be confirmed by the clinical chemistry laboratory.

CLINICAL MANAGEMENT

The clinical management of childhood schizophrenia reflects the diagnostic conflict that has dominated the field: There is no definitive clinical management, no "treatment of choice."

There have been therapeutic trials of various shock therapies (both electroconvulsive and chemical [insulin and metrazol]) and of different neuroleptics. Since no two studies employed the same diagnostic criteria, nor exercised adequate internal controls, the results of these studies will not be reviewed here. The interested reader is referred to the detailed historical review by Fish and Ritvo (1979).

Our own approach to the treatment of schizophrenic children has been focused on symptom control and clinical management (Cantor, 1987; Cantor & Kestenbaum, 1986).

Pharmacotherapy

Sedation

In our experience, the approach to pharmacotherapy with schizophrenic children must be one of extreme caution. The earliest symptom the clinician may be called upon to "control" is sleep disturbance. We have found that preschool schizophrenic children show little or no response to the sedative effects of phenothiazines. Antihistamines, such as diphenhydramine, in doses of approximately 2 to 4 mg/Kg, appear to offer the safest and most effective way of sedating a sleepless schizophrenic child.

The Control of Hyperactivity

The hyperactivity that may be associated with schizophrenia during early and middle childhood responds best to remedial education and psychotherapy. The hyperactive schizophrenic child (as well as the lethargic schizophrenic child) requires a therapeutic educational program. Psychoactive stimulants are best avoided, as some schizophrenic children will respond to such stimulants by developing a full-blown psychosis, some will appear clinically depressed, and some will develop a severe sleep disturbance and/or nightmares.

A schizophrenic child may appear to be more manageable as a result of the daily administration of a psychoactive stimulant, but cognitive functioning (including the ability to attend) will not be enhanced. (I suspect deterioration occurs, although a rigorous study of these effects would present ethical problems.) The use of psychoactive stimulants is best avoided in those children who continue to experience a severe attention deficit while taking therapeutic doses of such stimulants. Given the extensive literature documenting the ability of psychoactive stimulants to induce an adult-type psychosis, the medical dictum "primum non nocere" comes to mind.

The Control of Hallucinations and Delusions

The use of phenothiazines in postpubertal or latency-aged childhood schizophrenics who are manifesting the "positive" symptoms of schizophrenia also present special problems. Individuals with childhood or hypotonic schizophrenia, including those of my adult patients who have many signs of motor and perceptual dysfunction, appear to be very sensitive to phenothiazines. I have seen five cases of tardive dyskinesia in such individuals, including one case in a 20-year-old childhood schizophrenic who had received only minimal doses of phenothiazines over a period of 3 years and no medication at all for more than 5 years before the symptoms developed. A telephone consultation with a colleague from Yale has provided evidence of this susceptibility, as he reported the development of tardive dyskinesia in a 17-year-old girl with hypotonic schizophrenia who had only been on phenothiazines for a few weeks.

In addition, childhood schizophrenics appear to be extraordinarily sensitive to the anticholinergic side effects of phenothiazines. I have had three childhood schizophrenics become more psychotic on phenothiazines. Two patients were so sensitive that even the lowest doses of phenothiazines could not be used. The anticholinergic psychosis is readily distinguishable from the patient's steady-state symptoms, as the face becomes flushed, hot, and dry, the pupils are dilated, the patient experiences visual hallucinations, becomes visibly agitated, and is often confused and completely incoherent. Some patients may not sleep until the medication is discontinued, although in one case, at least initially, she slept very well.

Despite these warnings, in some childhood schizophrenics low doses of phenothiazines can and indeed must be used, and will have good therapeutic results. Their use is not recommended before puberty, nor should they be used in conjunction with anti-Parkinsonian agents such as Cogentin. Childhood schizophrenics will stress a clinician's prescribing skills!

Designing a Therapeutic Education Program

Schizophrenic children who are developmentally disabled will require a therapeutic education program. Indeed, the child with schizophrenia who can function in a non–special education setting is the exception, not the rule. Most children with schizophrenia are as unable to function in a regular school setting as their adult namesakes are in a regular work setting.

I have previously described in some detail an optimum therapeutic school setting (Cantor, 1987). As long as childhood schizophrenia remains "incurable," much emphasis should be placed on designing and implementing optimal therapeutic environments.

The Importance of Psychotherapy

More mildly affected schizophrenic children, and many paranoid schizophrenic children, are able to handle a regular curriculum and attend school with other children. These children remain, however, at great risk for developing the more readily recognized postpubertal schizophrenia. Some may mature into personality disorders. Vulnerable children will often form a therapeutic alliance with a psychotherapist, who as "auxiliary" ego nurtures and strengthens the child's rather tenuous understanding of reality. Such a relationship represents preventive child psychiatry at its best (Cantor & Kestenbaum, 1986).

SUMMARY

Childhood schizophrenia has been described as consisting of characteristic motor signs (hypotonia and associated gross motor dysfunction), perceptual signs (oversensitivity to sensory stimulation and difficulty with selective attention), and signs of affective and psychic disturbance (blunting of affect and formal thought disorder). Some emphasis has been placed on developmental issues, including the signs and symptoms that are associated with the preschool years, latency, and adolescence. A plea has been made for the identification of such children and for the designing of adequate treatment facilities. In the absence of such treatment facilities, children with severe childhood schizophrenia will continue to swell the ranks of the mentally retarded, more mildly affected children will stress hospital systems for the insane, and some of the least severely affected will stress the criminal justice system and the substance abuse system.

REFERENCES

American Psychiatric Association. (1980). *Diagnostic and statistical manual of mental disorders* (3rd ed.). Washington, DC: Author.

American Psychiatric Association. (1987). *Diagnostical and statistical manual of mental disorders* (3rd ed., rev.). Washington, DC: Author.

Bender, L. (1947). Childhood schizophrenia: A clinical study of 100 schizophrenic children. *American Journal of Orthopsychiatry, 17,* 40–56.

Bleuler, E. (1950). *Dementia praecox or the group of schizophrenias* (J. Zinkin, Trans.). New York: International Universities Press. (Original work published 1911.)

Bradley, C. (1941). *Schizophrenia in childhood.* New York: Macmillan.

Bruininks, R. (1978). *Bruininks-Oseretsky Test of Motor Proficiency: Examiner's manual.* Circle Pines, MN:. American Guidance Service.

Cantor, S. (1982). *The schizophrenic child*. Montreal: Eden.

Cantor, S. (1987). *Childhood schizophrenia*. New York: Guilford.

Cantor, S., Evans, J., Pearce, J., & Pezzot-Pearce, T. (1982). Childhood schizophrenia: Present but not accounted for. *American Journal of Psychiatry*, 139, 758–762.

Cantor, S., & Kestenbaum, C. (1986). Psychotherapy with schizophrenic children. *Journal of the American Academy of Child Psychiatry*, 25, 623–630.

Cantor, S., Pearce, J., Pezzot-Pearce, T., & Evans, J. (1981). The group of hypotonic schizophrenics. *Schizophrenia Bulletin*, 7, 1–11.

Creak, M. (1964). Schizophrenia syndrome in childhood: Further progress report of a working party. *Developmental Medicine & Child Neurology*, 6, 530–535.

Despert, L. (1947). The early recognition of childhood schizophrenia. *Medical Clinics of North America, Pediatrica*, 680–687.

Fish, B., & Ritvo, E. (1979). Psychoses in childhood. In J. Noshpitz (Ed.), *Basic handbook of child psychiatry*. New York: Basic.

Kanner, L. (1942–1943). Autistic disturbances of affective contact. *Nervous Child*, 2, 217–250.

Kanner, L. (1949). Problems of nosology and psychodynamics of earily infantile autism. *American Journal of Orthopsychiatry*, 19, 416–426.

Kraepelin, E. (1913). *Lectures on clinical psychiatry* (T. Johnston, Trans.). New York: William Wood. (Original work published 1904.)

Kraepelin, E. (1971). *Dementia praecox and paraphrenia*. Huntington, NY: Robert E. Krieger. (Original work published 1919.)

Lehman, H.E. (1975). Schizophrenia: Clinical features. In A.M. Freedman, H.I. Kaplan, & B.J. Sadock (Eds.), *Comprehensive textbook of psychiatry* (Vol. 1, 2nd ed.). Baltimore: Williams & Wilkins.

Potter, H.W. (1933). Schizophrenia in children. *American Journal of Psychiatry*, 12, 1253–1270.

Richards, B.W. (1951). Childhood schizophrenia and mental deficiency. *Journal of Mental Science*, 97, 290–312.

Rumsey, J.M., Andreasen, N.C., & Rapaport, J.L. (1986). Thought, language and communication, and affective flattening in autistic adults. *Archives of General Psychiatry*, 43, 771–777.

Rutter, M. (1972). Childhood schizophrenia reconsidered. *Journal of Autism & Childhood Schizophrenia*, 2, 315–337.

Rutter, M., Graham, P., & Yule, W. (1970). A Neuropsychiatric study in childhood. *Clinics in Developmental Medicine*, 35–36. London: Heinemann.

Spungen, D. (1983). *And I don't want to live this life*. New York: Random House.

Wechsler, D., & Jaros, E. (1965). Schizophrenic patterns of WISC. *Journal of Clinical Psychology*, 3, 288–291.

Wilson, L. (1968). *This stranger my son*. Toronto: Longmans Canada Ltd.

Yarden, P.E., & DiScipio, W.J. (1971). Abnormal movements and prognosis in schizophrenia. *American Journal of Psychiatry*, 128, 317–323.

CHAPTER 14

Bipolar Disorder

MICHAEL STROBER, GREGORY HANNA, AND JAMES McCRACKEN

Juvenile bipolar illness is a rapidly expanding focus of research in psychiatry. Though this work is riding the crest of an advancing state of knowledge of the condition in adults, there remains uncertainty about the phenomenology, incidence, course, differential diagnosis, and management of the illness when it arises early in life. Since large sample studies of children and adolescents are still sparse, we shall, for the purpose of this chapter, consider the literature on adult bipolar illness, when relevant, to put these questions in perspective.

DEFINITION

It is now generally agreed that the differentiation of bipolar from unipolar affective disorder serves important heuristic and clinical purposes. Reviews of descriptive, genetic, neurobiological, and pharmacologic data validating this distinction can be found elsewhere (Belmaker & van Praag, 1980; Post & Ballenger, 1984). Patients with bipolar illness are those in whom alternating cycles of depression and euphoric–hyperactive behavior are the primary and distinctive feature. The mood shifts are usually drastic and accompanied by florid cognitive and behavioral symptoms, although episode duration, cycle length, and the intensity and composition of symptoms are strikingly variable among patients (see Goodwin & Jamison, 1984).

The extremes of mood, behavior, and cognitive functioning that characterize the manic state are listed in Table 14.1; operational diagnostic criteria for mania codified in DSM-III (APA, 1980) are given in Table 14.2. Required are (1) the presence of an elevated, expansive, or irritable mood; (2) a specified number of accessory symptoms; (3) a minimum duration of illness of 1 week; (4) absence of nonaffective psychosis or features suggestive of schizophrenia during intermorbid periods; and (5) absence of known organic etiologies.

Descriptively, mania is a phenomenologically consistent and discriminable syndrome of pathologically excessive mental and physical activity. The patient's premorbid adjustment may be unremarkable, or distinguished by mild depression, episodic mood swings, extraversion, or irritability of variable duration (Kraepelin, 1921). Onset of the acute phase is not uncommonly abrupt, with symptoms peaking in

TABLE 14.1.   The Phenomenology of Mania

Mood

Elated
Expansive
Infectious or humorous
Sometimes petulant or irritable

Behavior–Activity

Impulsive, disinhibited
Decreased sleep
Indefatigable
Socially intrusive
Provocative
Contentious
Hyperactive
Excessive planning or grandiose scheming

Cognition

Flight of ideas
Pressure of speech
Grandiose thought content
Distractibility

From Shopsin (1979).

intensity in a matter of days to weeks. The mood of the patient is usually one of gaiety, exhilaration, or expansiveness, though in some the disturbance shows itself as irritability, belligerence, or an admixture of dysphoria and elation. The manic's infectious wit, quickness of mind, and boundless energy may initially evoke praise and admiration from others, but with increasing severity the behavior proves offensive and self-injurious. Owing to his or her grandiosity, egocentrism, and heightened

TABLE 14.2.   DSM-III Criteria for Manic Episode

A. One or more distinct periods of predominantly elevated, expansive, or irritable mood. The mood is a prominent part of the illness and relatively persistent.
B. Duration of at least 1 week during which at least three of the following symptoms have persisted (four if mood is irritable) and are present to a significant degree:
   1. Increased activity
   2. Pressure of speech
   3. Flight of ideas
   4. Decreased sleep
   5. Distractible
   6. Inflated self-esteem, which may be delusional
   7. Excessive involvement in activities with potentially painful consequences
C. Periods between episodes not dominated by bizarre behavior or mood-incongruent delusions or hallucinations
D. Not superimposed on schizophrenia, schizophreniform disorder, or paranoid disorder.
E. Not due to organic mental disorder or substance abuse.

sense of endurance, the manic downplays any suggestion of disturbance, seems incapable of self-examination, and is unrepentant and emotionally unresponsive to others. Likewise, because of the unrelenting pressure to act, rapidity of thought, and flight of ideas, manic behavior is often senseless and unfocused.

As Kraepelin (1921) originally noted, psychosis is not uncommon during the course of an episode and sometimes obscures these more protean manifestations. Thematic content in manic hallucinations and delusions is usually consonant with the patient's predominant affective state—for example, omnipotent control, supernatural strength, divine inspiration, or grandeur—though it usually lacks the sensory distinctness and implausibility characteristic of schizophrenic psychoses. However, we are reminded by Kraepelin's clinical experience and more recent systematic study (Carlson & Goodwin, 1973) that the severity of untreated episodes can escalate to the point where symptoms of disorientation, perplexity, incoherence, and mood-incongruent psychosis are prominent features.

HISTORICAL BACKGROUND

For decades, child psychiatry has struggled with the question of whether or not disturbances in children and adolescents can be meaningfully drawn together into behaviorally specific diagnostic entities. The debate reflects the influence of historical factors, especially the tension between Kraepelinian approaches to classification and the psychoanalytic frame of reference that viewed syndrome description as too restrictive with children and foreign to the study of developmental processes. Needless to say, since diagnostic conceptualizations in child psychiatry have leaned heavily toward the psychoanalytic view, attempts to establish the limits of differential diagnosis, the frequency of occurrence of clinical syndromes, and continuities with adult disorders have become widely valued concerns only in the past 15 years.

Concerning the affective disorders, the reluctance of clinicians to extend the syndromes of depression, melancholia, and mania downward to children also derives, to some degree, from psychoanalytic and metapsychological theories of their causation (Lewin, 1959). If, as speculated, mania was an attempt to ward off psychic pain produced by a dominant and harsh superego, it followed that children were naturally protected against these regressive states because of the relative immaturity of their ego defenses and intrapsychic structures. In a similar vein, it was routinely argued that, because children and adolescents were developmentally inclined to express underlying mood disturbance differently from adults, traditional diagnostic criteria had little pertinence to this age group.

Nonetheless, these ideas did not completely discourage historical interest in the identification and expression of juvenile manic–depressive states. According to Henderson and Gillespie (1947), circular manic–depressive episodes in children were first described by Esquirol in the middle nineteenth century. In his 1921 treatise, Kraepelin wrote that the susceptibility to manic–depression could affect the mental development of children from very early on in life, and later he (Kraepelin, 1931) cited the case of a 5-year-old boy with a 6-month episode of mania. Bleuler (1934) also held that the onset of illness could be traced back to childhood in some cases. Several individual case reports published during the 1930s and 1940s are noteworthy (Barrett, 1931; Kasanin, 1930; Olkon, 1945; Rice, 1944) for their description of the periodicity of manic and depressive cycles and heavy familial loading of the illness. In the ensuing years, Campbell (1952) described circular patterns of depression, elation, hyperactivity, aggressiveness, and push of speech in children and adolescents that were initially mistaken for physical disease, but that he regarded unequivocally as early manifestations of adult manic–depressive illness. Nonetheless, other influential authorities (Kanner, 1946) still held that the incidence of the illness prior to late adolescence was negligible.

In the first comprehensive account of manic–depressive illness in children, Anthony and Scott (1960) postulated that embryonic forms of mania may exist in very young children as extremes of negativism and cheerfulness, or unverbalized fantasies of omnipotence and inflated self-esteem. In an attempt to resolve diagnostic uncertainties, they proposed 10 criteria that were sufficiently objective to discriminate manic–depression from other childhood psychopathological disorders:

1. Evidence of an abnormal psychiatric state at some time of the illness approximating the classical clinical description
2. Evidence of a positive family history suggesting a manic–depressive diathesis
3. Evidence of an early tendency to a manic–depressive type of reaction as manifested in: (a) a cyclothymic tendency with gradually increasing amplitude and length of oscillations or (b) delirious manic or depressive outbursts
4. Evidence of a recurrent or periodic illness with at least two observed episodes
5. Evidence of a diphasic illness showing swings of pathologic dimension
6. Evidence of an endogenous illness indicating that the phases of the illness alternate with minimal reference to environmental events
7. Evidence of a severe illness as indicated by a need for inpatient treatment, heavy sedation, or electroconvulsive treatment
8. Evidence of an abnormal underlying personality of an extroverted type
9. Absence of features of schizophrenia or organic states
10. The evidence of current, not retrospective assessments

Of the more than 60 purported cases of childhood manic–depression in the literature reviewed by the authors, only 3 were found to satisfy these criteria. To these the authors added a case of their own, a 12-year-old boy with a relapsing biphasic course over a 10-year period.

CLINICAL PICTURE AND ASSOCIATED FEATURES

During the past 30 years there has been no shortage of case descriptions of bipolar illness in children and adolescents (Ballenger, Reus, & Post, 1982; Berg, Hullin,

Allsopp, O'Brien, & MacDonald, 1974; Canino & Youngerman, 1982; Carlson & Strober, 1978; Coll & Bland, 1979; Coryell & Norten, 1980; Dyson & Barcai, 1970; Engstrom, Robbins, & May, 1978; Esman, Hertzig, & Aarons, 1983; Feinstein & Wolpert, 1973; Hassanyeh & Davison, 1980; Horowitz, 1977; Hsu & Starzynsk, 1986; Hudgens, 1974; Kelly, Koch, & Buegel, 1976; Landolt, 1957; McKnew, Cytryn, & White, 1974; Olsen, 1961; Poznanski, Israel, & Grossman, 1984; Sylvester, Burke, McCauley, & Clark, 1984; Thompson & Schindler, 1976; van Krevelen & van Voorst, 1959; Varanka, Weller, Weller, & Fristad, in press; Varsamis & MacDonald, 1972; Warneke, 1975; Weinberg & Brumback, 1976; White & O'Shanick, 1977). The clinical features that have been described in prepubertal children include hyperactivity, intermittent irritability, gregariousness, push of speech, destructiveness, grandiose ideas, mood shifts, and affective dysregulation, intermixed with periods of dysphoria, tearfulness, and lethargy. However, a detailed analysis of these cases by Carlson (1983) concludes that symptom patterns vary by age. In older children, 9 to 12 years of age, euphoria, elation, paranoia, and grandiose delusions are common, whereas irritability and emotional lability are predominant features in younger manics—hyperactivity, push of speech, and distractibility being the most consistently noted abnormalities in both age groups. Maturation also appears to influence the phenomenology of depression in bipolar children. Whereas crying spells, anxiety, and somatic complaints are frequent in younger children, classic melancholic symptoms such as retardation, anhedonia, depressed appearance, alterations in vital functions, and delusions of guilt and persecution become increasingly prevalent in older children, and are highly discriminating features of bipolar depression in adolescence (Akiskal et al., 1983; Strober & Carlson, 1982). Overall, the literature to date suggests that prepubertal bipolar children begin the illness with frequent cycles of brief duration in which dysphoria, hypomania, and agitation are intermixed, and that cyclical extremes of depression and manic excitement become more common with the onset of puberty (DeLong & Aldershof, 1987; Puig-Antich, 1980).

On the other hand, opinion has been sharply divided on whether or not puberty inclines adolescents to a more psychotic or atypical presentation of bipolar illness compared to adults. Landolt (1957, p. 67) described "schizophrenic coloring" of manic episodes in 18 of 60 patients whose illness occurred between 13 and 22 years of age. Similarly, Olsen (1961) reported on a series of 28 patients with onsets between 13 and 19 years of age and concluded that differential diagnosis of their manic state was complicated by the additional presence of hysterical and schizophreniform features. More recently, Ballenger and colleagues (1982) compared the frequency of Schneiderian symptoms and other schizophreniclike phenomena in 9 adolescent bipolars and in 12 patients whose illness began after age 30. Although the two groups did not differ in lithium response or family psychiatric history, a significantly higher frequency of psychotic symptoms was found among adolescent patients. Similar findings have been reported by Rosen, Rosenthal, Van Dusen, Dunner, and Fieve (1983). In contrast, other workers (Carlson & Strober, 1978; Coryell & Norten, 1980; Hassanyeh & Davison, 1980; Horowitz, 1977; Hsu & Starzynski, 1986) have concluded that adolescent bipolars have the same range, intensity, and periodicity of manic and depressive symptoms as adults.

More controversial, yet theoretically intriguing, is the idea that there are lithium-responsive *forme frustes*, or variants, of bipolar illness in young children that may go undetected because full-fledged manias and depressions are not clinically obvious. Davis (1979) believed that the most discriminating diagnostic features in such children included: affective storms and temper outbursts; the absence of clear-cut environmental precipitants; mental, verbal, and motoric hyperactivity; erratic interpersonal relationships; a family history of mood disorder; and absence of abnormal thought content. Other oft-cited characteristics are low frustration tolerance, poor concentration, and intermittent aggressiveness (Dyson & Barcai, 1970; Frommer, 1968); alternating periods of boisterousness and passivity (Annell, 1969); periodic stupor and paranoia (Annell, 1969); and cyclic alternations between extreme vegetative states—that is, "low" periods of unusually sound and lengthy sleep, dysphoria, and reduced dream recall, and "high" periods of increased motor restlessness, excessive appetite and thirst, decreased sleep, and violent imagery in dreams and fantasy (Popper & Famularo, 1983).

Further efforts to elucidate behavioral precursors of bipolar illness have come through the study of behavioral adjustment in the offspring of bipolar parents, who in most cohorts range in age from 6 to 18 (Decina et al., 1983; Gershon et al., 1985; Greenhill & Shopsin, 1979; Kestenbaum, 1979; Klein, Depue, & Slater, 1985; Kuyler, Rosenthal, Igel, Dunner, & Fieve, 1980; Mayo, O'Connell, & O'Brien, 1979; McKnew, Cytryn, Efron, Gershon, & Bunney, 1979; O'Connell, Mays, O'Brien, & Mirsheidaie, 1979; Waters, 1980). However, except for isolated cases of mania and cyclothymia (Gershon et al., 1985; Klein et al., 1985) the wide range of abnormality that has been observed in these offspring raises doubts about the validity of differentiating prebipolar states from other, nonaffective disturbances common to this age group.

In sum, we concur with Waters (1979) that available evidence, limited though it is, indicates the existence of a continuum of bipolar syndromes in children varying in severity and phenotypic resemblance to the adult condition. However, our knowlege of the developmental patterns presaging bipolar illness remains incomplete, and it seems unlikely that a truly accurate identification of the child at risk will be feasible until robust biological and genetic markers of susceptibility are determined.

COURSE AND OUTCOME

Literature on the extended course and prognosis of bipolar illness in adults prior to the introduction of drug therapies has been ably summarized by Zis and Goodwin (1979), Coryell and Winokur (1982), and Goodwin and Jamison (in press). Several points are well established. First, the illness is invariably episodic, which is to say that relatively few patients have a single manic–depressive cycle without relapse; the number of episodes per lifetime in most studies is in the range of four to nine. Second, the average manic episode has a duration of roughly 3 months, with depressions lasting 4 to 6 months on average. Third, as the illness progresses, the interval between episodes (i.e., the cycle length) tends to decrease, until the pattern eventually stabilizes. Clearly, introduction of lithium carbonate has dramatically altered the course and outcome of many patients. In brief, the existing data suggest that relative risks of relapse in untreated bipolar patients are five times those for patients receiving lithium prophylaxis, and that relapse during lithium treatment predicts a more chronic cyclic course. Current estimates (Keller, 1985) put the rate of chronicity in bipolar patients at roughly 20%, and it may even be higher in those who enter treatment in mixed or polyphasic episodes.

Whether there is a difference in the natural history and long-term outcome of bipolar illness when it arises early in life is unclear. A study by Welner, Welner, and Fishman (1979) described the course of 28 adolescents 10 years after hospitalization for primary depression of bipolar illness. At follow-up, 3 of 12 bipolar patients had committed suicide, and the remaining patients were chronically ill with poor social and vocational adjustment. Of the 16 nonbipolar depressives, 11 had episodic courses and 5 had single episodes from which they recovered and remained well. However, Carlson, Davenport, and Jamison (1977) compared 28 bipolar patients whose mean age of onset was 15.8 years with 20 whose mean age of onset was 50.6 years and found no significant differences in episode frequency per year, educational achievement, mortality, family satisfaction, or occupational adjustment.

IMPAIRMENT AND COMPLICATIONS

The most ominous complication of bipolar illness is increased mortality, due mainly to suicide and accidental death. Life table analysis of the Iowa 500 follow-up data by Tsuang (1978; Tsuang & Woolson, 1978; Tsuang, Woolson, & Fleming, 1980) indicates that suicide rates normally peak in the first year after discharge from the index episode, after which the risk decreases. As noted earlier, there is no current evidence that mortality in general, or suicide in particular, is increased in younger bipolar patients.

Regrettably, data concerning the social, academic, and psychological effects of bipolar illness in children and adolescents are virtually absent from the literature. That there is a need to take account of these issues seems undeniable. In a thoughtful paper, Campbell (1953) observed that the development of bipolar illness early in life created in many children pathological insecurity, timidity, fears of social ostracism, and tendencies toward evasion and defense. Following more psychodynamic constructs, Popper and Famularo (1983) described the bipolar child as one who is particularly fearful of abandonment and defends against the wish for dependence through negativism and noncompliance with treatment recommendations.

Episodic drinking, sedative drug use, and concomitant neurologic disorder have also been noted to complicate the course and treatment of bipolar illness in adolescence, and may play a role in provoking mixed episodes and rapid cycling in some. An excellent discussion of this issue can be found in Himmelhoch and Garfinkel (1987).

EPIDEMIOLOGY

Epidemiologic studies undertaken in the last three decades put the lifetime expectancy of bipolar illness at 0.24 to 1.2% (Boyd & Weissman, 1981). Estimates of the annual incidence of new cases in males age 15 and above have ranged from 9.2 to 15.2 per 100,000 and in women from 7.4 to 32.5 per 100,000 (Boyd & Weissman, 1981). Rates do not appear to differ by sex, race, place of residence (urban vs. rural), or religion, but may be increased among individuals of high educational and social achievement levels (Hirschfeld & Cross, 1982).

Early studies of hospital admission records report rates of manic–depressive illness of 2.5% among children 16 years or less (Kasanin & Kaufman, 1929) and 22% among children 14 to 18 with an admitting diagnosis of psychosis (Carter, 1942). However, the accuracy of these figures is doubtful considering historical prejudices against the diagnosis of affective illness prior to late adolescence or early adulthood.

Modern population-based surveys of the lifetime prevalence and annual incidence of bipolar illness in children do not currently exist, though rates increase sharply at the time of puberty with some 15 to 30% of patients experiencing their first attacks by age 19 (Kraepelin, 1921; Loranger & Levine, 1978; Winokur, Clayton, & Reich, 1969).

Regarding nonbipolar depression, several recent studies are informative. In the Isle of Wight study of 10-year-old children, Rutter, Graham, Chadwick, and Yule (1976) found a prevalence of depressive disorder of only 0.14 per 100; however, 9 cases were identified when this cohort was reexamined at age 14 plus an additional 26 with mixed anxiety and depressive features. Overall, new onsets at age 14 were much commoner in females than in males. Two American studies are concordant with these findings in two respects: Both find a rapid increase in the prevalence of depression with puberty along with a predominance of females among adolescent-onset cases compared with male and female rates of roughly the same order during childhood. Cohen, Velez, and Garcia (1985) carried out independent parent and child diagnostic interviews in 757 families randomly selected from two counties in New York. Children ranged in age from 9 to 18 at the time of interview. For the total sample, the prevalence of major depression was 1% when diagnoses were based on interviews with mothers and 1.7% when based on interviews of the children themselves; the prevalence of past episodes of major depression, by the child's report, was estimated at 4.5%. There were no cases of depression among females prior to age 13, whereas depression among males in the cohort was predominantly prepubertal. Age-specific rates of disorder increase steadily in females, from 1.0% at age 13 to 7% at age 19.

Kashani and colleagues (Kashani et al., 1987) investigated the prevalence of major depression among 150 adolescents 14 to 16 years old, representing 7% of all adolescents attending public schools in Columbia, Missouri. Diagnoses based on DSM-III criteria were derived from structured interviews conducted separately with the adolescent and his or her parents, with the additional provision that symptoms were judged sufficiently handicapping to warrant treatment. Of the 150 subjects, 7

(4.7%) met criteria for current or past major depression and an additional 5 (3.3%) met criteria for dysthymic disorder, 10 of the 12 cases being female.

Perhaps the single most important finding in recent epidemiologic studies relevant to juvenile affective illness concerns an apparent rise in the incidence of unipolar and bipolar illness in adolescents. As part of the National Institute of Mental Health Collaborative Program on Depression, rates of depression were determined in more than 2200 first-degree relatives of 523 adults with major depressive disorder (Klerman et al., 1985). For data analysis, relatives were aggregated into six decades of birth strata (before 1910; 1910–1919; 1920–1929; etc.) and life table statistics were used to estimate age-specific probabilities of onset within each of the birth cohorts up to the time of interview. The analysis showed: (1) that risk for depression increased significantly in successive birth cohorts; (2) that first onsets of disorder were occurring earlier in later cohorts; and (3) that in younger individuals differences between females and males in rates of depression were narrowing. Comparable evidence of an increasing incidence of bipolar illness in more recently born offspring of bipolar patients has been reported (Gershon, Hamovit, Guroff, & Nurnberger, 1987). Although an explanation of these trends remains to be clarified, they imply that juvenile affective illness will be an increasingly recognized public health concern.

FAMILIAL PATTERN

The tendency for bipolar illness to run in families has been increasingly recognized during the past 20 years. It is widely accepted that genetic transmission plays a role, but whether it is best understood in terms of autosomal, multifactorial, X-linked, or mixed models of inheritance remains unclear. Moreover, family studies of bipolar probands published during the past two decades indicate a sevenfold variation in morbid risk estimates of bipolar illness (2.5 to 17.7%) among first-degree relatives (Gershon, in press). Although a lack of uniformity in diagnostic procedures can account for some of these inconsistencies, genetic heterogeneity may also explain why risk estimates vary so significantly across studies.

This being so, increasing attention has focused on elucidating the relationship between age at onset of illness in bipolar patients and extent of familial transmission. Results of these studies have been fairly consistent: Relatives of early-onset probands have an appreciably higher lifetime risk for affective disorder compared to relatives of late-onset probands (for review see Gershon, in press), which would seem to favor the existence of a continuum of inherited liability whereby earlier age at onset defines a more severe, genetically deviant subform of the illness (Reich, James, & Morris, 1972; Rice et al., 1987).

In support of this idea, two recent studies have found an unusually high lifetime prevalence of affective illness in the relatives of children and adolescents with bipolar illness. Dwyer and DeLong (1987) studied 249 first- and second-degree relatives of 20 children diagnosed with bipolar illness who ranged in age from 4 to 18. They found the lifetime rate of bipolar illness in parents to be 20%, with 17 of 20 probands (85%) having at least 1 relative with bipolar illness. While these rates are five to eight times greater than those reported in recent studies of first-degree relatives of adult bipolars (2.4% to 3.9%—Andreasen et al., 1987; Coryell, Endicott, Reich, Andreasen & Keller, 1984; Endicott et al., 1985; Gershon et al., 1982; Weissman et al., 1984), the lack of blind diagnosis, reliance on family history data, and the small sample size raise doubts about their interpretation.

More recently, Strober and colleagues (in press) compared lifetime rates of affective illness in the adult relatives of 50 adolescents with bipolar I illness and in the relatives of age-matched schizophrenic controls. All first-degree relatives were personally interviewed and blindly diagnosed, thereby ensuring comparability of our methods with those used in adult family studies. Three major findings were noted. First, familial aggregation of unipolar and bipolar illness was observed only in bipolar probands. Second, the lifetime rate of bipolar I illness in the parents and siblings of these probands was 13.9%, four times that found in the relatives of adult probands. And third, support was obtained for a distinction on genetic and pharmacologic grounds between adolescent bipolars with and without behavioral pathology in their premorbid childhood adjustment. Specifically, first-degree relatives of probands with prepubertal onset of psychiatric disturbance had a greater than threefold increase in the rate of bipolar I disorder compared to relatives of probands who were psychiatrically well prior to onset of their affective symptoms, and also exhibited a significantly poorer response to lithium carbonate. Clearly, a major implication of these findings is that onsets of bipolar illness early in life may indicate a more severe genetic diathesis. If so, family studies of younger patients may shed new light on the nature of predisposing genetic effects, their pathophysiologic expression, and the role played by social factors in the onset and course of the illness.

DIFFERENTIAL DIAGNOSIS

Differentiation from Attention Deficit Disorder with Hyperactivity (ADDH)

Follow-up studies of hyperactive or conduct-disordered children have not found any greater incidence of bipolar illness than in the general population. Nor does lithium carbonate appear to be effective in the treatment of ADDH (DeLong & Aldershoff, 1987; Greenhill, Rieder, Wender, Buchsbaum, & Zahn, 1973). Still this distinction often presents difficulty because symptoms of irritability, pressure to act, inattention, and impulsivity are characteristic of both syndromes, and because full-fledged symptoms of elation are not always present in younger bipolar patients. However, the child with bipolar illness usually has a more pronounced and sustained shift in mood than the child with ADDH; has an increase in *goal-directed* activity; and may intermittently manifest paranoia, stupor, hallucinations, or delusional thinking. Along these lines, Nieman and DeLong (1987) have shown that manic children could be distinguished from those with ADDH on the Personality Inventory for Children in terms of more extreme aggressiveness, psychotic thinking, and hyperactivity.

Differentiation from Schizophrenia

Data on symptom, course, treatment, and family history differences among the psychotic illnesses of childhood and adolescence are sparse. It suffices to say that the differential diagnosis of bipolar and schizophrenic psychosis in young patients is not without significant challenge or complexity. Nonetheless, it bears remembering that both Kraepelin and Bleuler commented on the frequency with which particular abnormalities of behavior and temperament foreshadowed later schizophrenic and affective illness. Along these lines, social withdrawal, oddities in communication, solitary acts of antisocial conduct, and nervousness are often observed in the premorbid adjustment of schizophrenics, but are rare in bipolars, who more commonly exhibit features of a hyperthymic or cyclothymic temperament before onset of their acute symptoms. Clinically, though the two syndromes can overlap to a degree, their differences are notable. Schizophrenia is usually more insidious in its development, more protracted in its course, and invariably dominated by mood-incongruent psychotic ideation and hallucinations. Thus with careful attention to symptom phenomenology, premonitory disturbance, and course of illness, the separation of bipolar from schizophrenic illness can be made with reasonable certainty in many cases.

Differentiation from Unipolar Depression

One question of obvious importance in regard to differential diagnosis is whether or not early and reliable assessment of polarity of illness is feasible in young depressed patients. Two prospective follow-up studies (Akiskal et al., 1983; Strober & Carlson, 1982) have considered this problem by examining the power of clinical, familial, and treatment variables to predict manic switches in adolescents following remission from the depressive episode. Results of the two studies were remarkably consistent: Teenagers with manic outcomes were more likely to have delusions and psychomotor retardation during their index episodes, increased rates of familial bipolar illness, and a somewhat greater susceptibility to tricyclic-induced hypomania than were teenagers with unipolar outcomes. The specificities of these variables were high, ranging from 83 to 100%. Predictive values in the cohort studied by Strober and Carlson (1982) ranged from 42 to 100%, and 72 to 100% in the cohort studied by Akiskal and colleagues (1983).

CLINICAL MANAGEMENT: RESEARCH FINDINGS

The rationale and guidelines for the pharmacotherapy of juvenile bipolar disorder continue to be largely extrapolated from studies of adults. Unfortunately, the available data are sparse and lack scientific rigor. Nevertheless, a summary of available data on lithium carbonate treatment of juvenile bipolar disorder is in order given the frequency of its use. The general usages of lithium in child psychiatry have been comprehensively reviewed elsewhere (Campbell, Perry, & Green, 1984).

A wide variety of case reports beginning in 1959 (Van Krevelen & Van Voorst) have described the potentially beneficial effects of lithium for mania both in children and adolescents (Campbell, Green, & Deutsch, 1985; Youngerman & Canino, 1978). Annell (1969) described improvement on lithium in a diagnostically heterogeneous sample of 12 juveniles, 2 of whom exhibited manic–depressive cycles. Successful use of lithium in treating hypomanic states in a small series of children has also been reported by Frommer (1968). Four late adolescents included in a large study by Van der Velde (1970) of adults with manic–depressive illness were all seen as markedly improved with lithium therapy (Van der Velde, 1970). Horowitz (1977) described 8 adolescents, 7 of whom manifested classic mania with prominent psychotic features; all patients were reported to have experienced complete remissions on lithium alone. Two cases of definite mania in children were among 6 subjects described by Brumback and Weinberg (1977). Each experienced prolonged remissions following initiation of treatment with lithium, whereas the remainder, some of whom had prominent depressive and psychotic symptoms, showed minimal improvement or exacerbations of symptoms. Carlson and Strober (1978) reported that 3 of 6 manic adolescents diagnosed by RDC criteria showed a markedly positive response to lithium, while the remaining 3 demonstrated only partial improvement. At follow-up, which averaged 18 months, lithium appeared to have prophylactic value in the 3 with the best initial response, whereas recurrences were seen in the other 3 cases. Another report of 10 adolescent patients with mania concluded that lithium was effective in 6 of the 7 treated cases, as judged by the significantly shorter duration of episodes in this group compared to the 3 patients not treated with lithium (Hassanyeh & Davison, 1980). And in one of the few studies of prepubertal children to apply DSM-III diagnostic criteria for mania, Varanka and colleagues (in press) found that each of 10 prepubertal children, who also demonstrated prominent psychotic features, was significantly improved on lithium alone beginning an average of 11 days after the start of treatment.

Lithium has also been reported to be strikingly effective in children and young adolescents with cyclic behavioral disorders suggesting bipolar illness (Davis, 1979; DeLong, 1978; DeLong & Aldershoff, 1987) and in psychiatrically ill children of lithium-responsive bipolar parents (DeLong & Aldershoff, 1987; Dyson & Barcai, 1970; McKnew et al., 1981).

Fewer studies have employed randomized, double-blind placebo-controlled methods to assess lithium's effectiveness in children. In one (Gram & Rafaelson, 1972), a diagnostically mixed group of 18 patients were studied, including 2 probably with bipolar illness; both of these children showed significantly greater improvement during the 6-month period on lithium compared to the 6-month period on placebo. Similarly, DeLong and Nieman (1983) found significantly greater overall improvement in 11 manic children during a 3-week period of lithium treatment than during the 3-week period of placebo.

To summarize, the available data on lithium treatment of juvenile bipolar disorders suggests its potential efficacy. However, few double-blind placebo-controlled studies are available, and methods used to document drug effects are poorly described in many of the reports. Also not to be overlooked is the problem of lithium resistance, which has been described in adolescents (Hsu, 1986; Strober et al., in press). Long-term studies of lithium prophylaxis in juvenile bipolar patients do not yet exist.

DSM-III-R

The revision of DSM-III incorporates changes in the diagnostic criteria for manic episodes that are relatively minor. Criteria A and B (see Table 14.2) are retained, with the exception that the 1-week-duration criterion has been deleted. Exclusionary criterion C has been modified slightly, so that patients who exhibit persistence (i.e., more than 2 weeks) of delusions and hallucinations in the absence of prominent mood symptoms are henceforth classified as schizoaffective. Finally, DSM-III-R adds an impairment criterion that stipulates that the patient's mood disturbance be self-injurious, sufficiently severe to cause marked impairment in occupational, role, or interpersonal functioning, or a threat to others. Concerning the diagnosis of cyclothymia, which, as noted previously, is particularly prevalent in the adolescent-age offspring of bipolar patients, DSM-III-R is less stringent than DSM-III, permitting the diagnosis in children and adolescents if symptoms have been present for at least 1 year, in contrast to the 2-year duration criterion for adults.

It remains uncertain whether or not these changes, minor as they are, will significantly change the future direction of clinical and empirical investigation of bipolar illness in children and adolescents. Clearly, there is an urgent need for more systematic study of the natural history of this condition, its genetic underpinnings, and the value of pharmacologic and other treatment modalities in reducing the substantial morbidity and life disruption it produces in young people.

REFERENCES

Akiskal, H.S., Walker, P., Puzantian, V.R., King, D., Rosenthal, T.L., & Dranon, M. (1983). Bipolar outcome in the course of depressive illness: Phenomenologic, familial, and pharmacologic predictors. *Journal of Affective Disorders*, *5*, 115–128.

American Psychiatric Association (1980). *Diagnostic and statistical manual of mental disorders* (3rd ed.). Washington, DC: Author.

American Psychiatric Association (1987). *Diagnostic and statistical manual of mental disorders* (3rd ed., rev.). Washington, DC: Author.

Andreasen, N.C., Rice, J., Endicott, J., Coryell, W., Grove, W.M., & Reich, T. (1987). Familial rates of affective disorder. *Archives of General Psychiatry*, *44*, 461–469.

Annell, A. (1969). Lithium in the treatment of children and adolescents. *Acta Psychiatrica Scandinavica* (Suppl. 207), 19–30.

Anthony, J., & Scott, P. (1960). Manic-depressive psychosis in childhood. *Journal of Child Psychology & Psychiatry*, *1*, 53–72.

Ballenger, J.C., Reus, V.I., & Post, R.M. (1982). The "atypical" clinical picture of adolescent mania. *American Journal of Psychiatry*, *139*, 602–606.

Barrett, A.M. (1931). Manic-depressive psychosis in childhood. *International Clinics*, *3*, 205–211.

Belmaker, R.H., & van Praag, H.M. (1980). *Mania: An evolving concept.* New York: Spectrum.

Berg, I., Hullin, R., Allsopp, M., O'Brien, P., & MacDonald, R. (1974). Bipolar manic-depressive psychosis in early adolescence. *British Journal of Psychiatry, 125,* 416–417.

Bleuler, E. (1934). *Textbook of psychiatry.* New York: Macmillan.

Boyd, J.H., & Weissman, M.M. (1981). The epidemiology of affective disorders. *Archives of General Psychiatry, 38,* 1039–1047.

Brumback, R.A., & Weinberg, W.A. (1977). Mania in childhood: II. Therapeutic trial of lithium carbonate and further description of manic-depressive illness in children. *American Journal of Diseases of Children, 131,* 1122–1126.

Campbell, J.D. (1952). Manic depressive psychosis in children—Report of 18 cases. *Journal of Nervous & Mental Disease,* 116–128.

Campbell, J.D. (1953). Manic-depressive disease in children. *Journal of the American Medical Association, 158,* 154–157.

Campbell, M., Green, W.H., & Deutsch, S.I. (1985). *Child and adolescent psychopharmacology.* Beverly Hills: Sage.

Campbell, M., Perry, R., & Green, W.H. (1984). Use of lithium in children and adolescents. *Psychosomatics, 25,* 95–106.

Canino, I.A., & Youngerman, J. (1982). Lithium use in adolescents: A responder vs a nonresponder. *Journal of Psychiatric Treatments, 4,* 37–40.

Carlson, G.A. (1983). Bipolar affective disorders in childhood and adolescence. In D.P. Cantwell & G.A. Carlson (Eds.), *Affective disorders in childhood and adolescence: An update.* New York: Spectrum.

Carlson, G.A., Davenport, Y.B., & Jamison, K. (1977). A comparison of outcome in adolescent and late onset bipolar manic-depressive illness. *American Journal of Psychiatry, 134,* 919–922.

Carlson, G.A., & Goodwin, F.K. (1973). The stages of mania. *Archives of General Psychiatry, 28,* 221–228.

Carlson, G.A., & Strober, M. (1978). Manic-depressive illness in early adolescence: A study of clinical and diagnostic characteristics in six cases. *Journal of the American Academy of Child Psychiatry, 17,* 138–153.

Cohen, P., Velez, C.N., & Garcia, M. (1985). *The epidemiology of childhood depression.* Presented at the annual meeting of the American Academy of Child Psychiatry, San Antonio.

Coll, P.G., & Bland, R. (1979). Manic depressive illness in adolescence and childhood. *Canadian Journal of Psychiatry, 24,* 255–263.

Coryell, W., Endicott, J., Reich, T., Andreasen, N., & Keller, M. (1984). A family study of bipolar II disorder. *British Journal of Psychiatry, 145,* 49–54.

Coryell, W., & Norten, S.G. (1980). Mania during adolescence. *Journal of Nervous & Mental Disease, 168,* 611–613.

Coryell, W., & Winokur, G. (1982). Course and outcome. In E.S. Paykel (Ed.), *Handbook of affective disorders.* New York: Guilford.

Davis, R.E. (1979). Manic-depressive variant syndrome of childhood: A preliminary report. *American Journal of Psychiatry, 136,* 702–705.

Decina, P., Kestenbaum, C.J., Farber, S., Kron, L., Gargan, M., Sackeim, H.A., & Fieve,

R.R. (1983). Clinical and psychological assessment of children of bipolar probands. *American Journal of Psychiatry, 140,* 548–553.

DeLong, G.R. (1978). Lithium carbonate treatment of select behavior disorders suggesting manic-depressive illness. *Journal of Pediatrics, 93,* 689–694.

DeLong, G.R., & Aldershoff, A.L. (1987). Long-term experience with lithium treatment in childhood: Correlation with clinical diagnosis. *Journal of the American Academy of Child & Adolescent Psychiatry, 26,* 389–394.

DeLong, G.R., & Nieman, G.W. (1983). Lithium induced changes in children with symptoms suggesting manic-depressive illness. *Psychopharmacology Bulletin, 19,* 258–265.

Dwyer, J.T., & DeLong, G.R. (1987). A family history study of twenty probands with childhood manic-depressive illness. *Journal of the American Academy of Child & Adolescent Psychiatry, 26,* 176–180.

Dyson, L., & Barcai, A. (1970). Treatment of lithium-responding parents. *Current Therapeutic Research, 12,* 286–290.

Endicott, J., Nee, J., Andreasen, N., Clayton, P., Keller, M., & Coryell, W. (1985). Bipolar II: Combine or keep separate? *Journal of Affective Disorders, 8,* 17–28.

Engstrom, F.W., Robbins, D.R., & May, J.G. (1978). Manic-depressive illness in adolescence. *Journal of the American Academy of Child Psychiatry, 17,* 514–520.

Esman, A.H., Hertzig, M., & Aarons, S. (1983). Juvenile manic depressive illness: A longitudinal perspective. *Journal of the American Academy of Child Psychiatry, 22,* 302–304.

Feinstein, S.C., & Wolpert, E.A. (1973). Juvenile manic-depressive illness. *Journal of the American Academy of Child Psychiatry, 12,* 123–136.

Frommer, E.A. (1968). Depressive illness in childhood. In A. Coppen & A. Walk (Eds.), *Recent developments in affective disorders.* Kent: Headybros.

Gershon, E.S. (in press). Genetics. In F.K. Goodwin & K.R. Jamison, *Manic depressive illness.* Oxford: Oxford University Press.

Gershon, E.S., Hamovit, J., Guroff, J., Dibble, E., Leckman, J.F., Sceery, W., Targum, S.D., Nurnberger, J.I., Jr., Goldin, L.R., & Bunney, W.L.S., Jr. (1982). A family study of schizoaffective, bipolar I, bipolar II, unipolar, and normal controls. *Archives of General Psychiatry, 39,* 1157–1167.

Gershon, E.S., Hamovit, J.H., Guroff, J., & Nurnberger, J.I., Jr. (1987) Birth cohort changes in manic and depressive disorders in relatives of bipolar and schizoaffective patients. *Archives of General Psychiatry, 44,* 314–319.

Gershon, E.S., McKnew, D., Cytryn, L., Hamovit, J., Schreiber, J., Higgs, E., & Pellegrini, D. (1985). Diagnosis in school-age children of bipolar affective disorder patients and normal controls. *Journal of Affective Disorders, 8,* 283–291.

Goodwin, F.K., & Jamison, K.R. (1984). The natural course of manic-depressive illness. In R.M. Post & J.C. Ballenger (Eds.), *The neurobiology of mood disorders.* Baltimore: Williams & Wilkins.

Gram, L.F., & Rafaelson, O.J. (1972). Lithium treatment of psychotic children and adolescents. *Acta Psychiatrica Scandinavica, 48,* 253–260.

Greenhill, L.L., Rieder, R.O., Wender, P., Buchsbaum, M., & Zahn, T.P. (1973). Lithium carbonate in the treatment of hyperactive children. *Archives of General Psychiatry, 28,* 636–640.

Greenhill, L.L., & Shopsin, B. (1979). Survey of mental disorders in the children of patients with affective disorders. In J. Mendlewicz & B. Shopsin (Eds.), *Genetic aspects of affective illness*. New York: Spectrum.

Hassanyeh, F., & Davison, K. (1980). Bipolar affective psychosis with onset before age 16: Report of 10 cases. *British Journal of Psychiatry*, *137*, 530–539.

Henderson, D.K., & Gillespie, R.D. (1947). *A textbook of psychiatry*. New York: Oxford Medical Publications.

Himmelhoch, J.M., & Garfinkel, M.E. (1986). Sources of lithium resistance in mixed mania. *Psychopharmacology Bulletin*, *22*, 613–620.

Hirschfeld, R.M.A., & Cross, C.K. (1982). The epidemiology of affective disorders. *Archives of General Psychiatry*, *39*, 35–46.

Horowitz, M.M. (1977). Lithium and the treatment of adolescent manic-depressive illness. *Diseases of the Nervous System*, *38*, 480–483.

Hsu, L.K.G. (1986). Lithium-resistant adolescent mania. *Journal of the American Academy of Child Psychiatry*, *25*, 280–283.

Hsu, L.K.G., & Starzynski, J.M. (1986). Mania in adolescence. *Journal of Clinical Psychiatry*, *47*, 596–599.

Hudgens, R.W. (1974). *Psychiatric disorders in adolescence*. Baltimore: Williams & Wilkins.

Kanner, L. (1946). *Child psychiatry*. Springfield, IL: Charles C. Thomas.

Kasanin, J., & Kaufman, M.R. (1929). Study of functional psychoses in childhood. *American Journal of Psychiatry*, *9*, 307–384.

Kasanin, J. (1930). The affective psychoses in children. *American Journal of Psychiatry*, *10*, 897–926.

Kashani, J.H., Carlson, G.A., Beck, N.C., Hoeper, E.W., McAllister, J.A., Corcoran, C.M., Fallahi, C., Rosenberg, T.K., & Reid, J.C. (1987). Depression, depressive symptomatology, and depressed mood among a community sample of adolescents. *American Journal of Psychiatry*, *144*, 931–934.

Keller, M.B. (1985). Chronic and recurrent affective disorder: Incidence, course, and influencing factors. In D. Kemali & G. Racagni (Eds.), *Chronic treatments in neuropsychiatry*. New York: Raven.

Kelly, J.T., Koch, M., & Buegel, D. (1976). Lithium carbonate in juvenile manic-depressive illness. *Diseases of the Nervous System*, *37*, 90–92.

Kestenbaum, C.J. (1979). Children at risk for manic depressive illness: Possible predictors. *American Journal of Psychiatry*, *136*, 1206–1208.

Klein, D.N., Depue, R.A., & Slater, J.F. (1985). Cyclothymia in the adolescent offspring of parents with bipolar affective disorder. *Journal of Abnormal Psychology*, *94*, 115–127.

Klerman, G.L., Lavori, P.W., Rice, J., Reich, T., Endicott, J., Andreasen, N.C., Keller, M.B., & Hirschfield, R.M.A. (1985). Birth-cohort trends in rates of major depressive disorder among relatives of patients with affective disorder. *Archives of General Psychiatry*, *42*, 689–695.

Kraepelin, E. (1921). *Manic depressive insanity and paranoia*. Edinburgh: E. & S. Livingston.

Kraepelin, E. (1931). *Psychiatrie*. Leipzig: Johann Ambrosium Barth.

Kuyler, P.L., Rosenthal, L., Igel, G., Dunner, D.L., & Fieve, R.R. (1980). Psychopathology among children of manic-depressive patients. *Biological Psychiatry*, *15*, 589–597.

Landolt, A.B. (1957). Follow-up studies on circular manic-depressive reactions occurring in the young. *Bulletin of the New York Academy of Medicine*, *33*, 65–73.

Lewin, B.D. (1959). Some psychoanalytic ideas applied to elation and depression. *American Journal of Psychiatry*, *116*, 38–43.

Loranger, A.W., & Levine, P.M. (1978). Age of onset of bipolar illness. *Archives of General Psychiatry*, *35*, 1345–1348.

Mayo, J.A., O'Connell, R.A., & O'Brien, J.D. (1979). Families of manic-depressive patients: Effects of treatment. *American Journal of Psychiatry*, *136*, 1535–1539.

McKnew, D.H., Cytryn, L., Buchsbaum, M.S., Hamovit, J., Lamour, M., Rapoport, J.L., & Gershon, E.S. (1981). Lithium in children of lithium-responding parents. *Psychiatry Research*, *4*, 171–180.

McKnew, D.H., Cytryn, L., Efron, A.M., Gershon, E.S., & Bunney, W.E. (1979). Offspring of patients with affective disorders. *British Journal of Psychiatry*, *134*, 148–152.

McKnew, D.H., Cytryn, L., & White, I. (1974). Clinical and biochemical correlates of hypomania in a child. *Journal of the American Academy of Child Psychiatry*, *13*, 576–585.

Nieman, G.W., & DeLong, R. (1987). Use of the Personality Inventory for children as an aid in differentiating children with mania from children with attention deficit disorder with hyperactivity. *Journal of the American Academy of Child and Adolescent Psychiatry*, *26*, 381–388.

O'Connell, R.A., Mays, J.A., O'Brien, J.D., & Mirsheidaie, F. (1979). Children of bipolar manic-depressives. In J. Mendlewicz & B. Shopsin (Eds.), *Genetic aspects of affective illness*. New York: Spectrum.

Olkon, D.M. (1945). *Essentials of neuro-psychiatry*. Philadelphia: Lea & Febiger.

Olsen, T. (1961). Follow-up study of manic-depressive patients whose first attack occurred before the age of 19. *Acta Psychiatrica Scandanavica* (Suppl.), *162*, 45–51.

Popper, C., & Famularo, R. (1983). Child and adolescent psychopharmacology. In M.D. Levine, W.B. Carey, & R.T. Gross (Eds.), *Developmental behavioral pediatrics*. Philadelphia: Saunders.

Post, R.M., & Ballenger, J.C. (1984). *The neurobiology of mood disorders*. Baltimore: Williams & Wilkins.

Poznanski, E.O., Israel, M.C., & Grossman, J. (1984). Hypomania in a four year-old. *Journal of the American Academy of Child Psychiatry*, *23*, 105–110.

Puig-Antich, J. (1980). Affective disorders in childhood. *Psychiatric Clinics of North America*, *3*, 403–423.

Reich, T., James, J.W., & Morris, C.A. (1972). The use of multiple thresholds in determining the mode of transmission of semi-continuous traits. *Annals of Human Genetics*, *36*, 163–184.

Rice, J., Reich, T., Andreasen, N.C., Endicott, J., Van Eerdwegh, M., Fishman, R., Hirschfeld, R.M.A., & Klerman, G.L. (1987). The familial transmission of bipolar illness. *Archives of General Psychiatry*, *44*, 441–450.

Rice, K.K. (1944). Regular 40 to 50 day cycle of psychotic behavior in a 14 year old boy. *Archives of Neurology & Psychiatry*, *51*, 478–483.

Rosen, L.N., Rosenthal, N.E., van Dusen, P.H., Dunner, D.L., & Fieve, R.R. (1983). Age at onset and number of psychotic symptoms in bipolar I and schizoaffective disorder. *American Journal of Psychiatry*, *140*, 1523–1525.

Rutter, M., Graham, P., Chadwick, O., & Yule, W. (1976). Adolescent turmoil: Fact or fiction? *Journal of Child Psychology and Psychiatry*, *17*, 35–56.

Shopsin, B. (1979). *Manic illness*. New York: Raven.

Strober, M., & Carlson, G. (1982). Bipolar illness in adolescents: Clinical, genetic and pharmacologic predictors in a three- to four-year prospective follow-up. *Archives of General Psychiatry*, *39*, 549–555.

Strober, M., Morrell, W., Burroughs, J., Lampert, C., Danforth, H., & Freeman, R. (in press). A family study of bipolar I disorder in adolescence: Early onset of symptoms linked to increased familial loading and lithium resistance. *Journal of Affective Disorders*.

Sylvester, C.E., Burke, P.M., McCauley, E.A., & Clark, C.J. (1984). Manic psychosis in childhood. *Journal of Nervous & Mental Disease*, *172*, 12–15.

Thompson, R.J., & Schindler, F.H. (1976). Embryonic mania. *Child Psychiatry & Human Development*, *6*, 149–154.

Tsuang, M.T. (1978). Suicide in schizophrenics, manics, depressives, and surgical controls. *Archives of General Psychiatry*, *35*, 153–155.

Tsuang, M.T., & Woolson, J.R.F. (1980). Excess mortality in schizophrenia and affective disorders. *Archives of General Psychiatry*, *35*, 1181–1185.

Tsuang, M.T., Woolson, J.R.F., & Fleming, J.A. (1980). Premature deaths in schizophrenia and affective disorders. *Archives of General Psychiatry*, *37*, 979–983.

Van der Velde, C. (1970). Effectiveness of lithium carbonate in the treatment of manic-depressive illness. *American Journal of Psychiatry*, *127*, 121–127.

van Krevelen, V.D.A., & Van Voorst, J.A. (1959). Lithium in the treatment of a cryptogenetic psychosis in a juvenile. *Acta Paedopsychiatrica*, *26*, 148–152.

Varanka, T.M., Weller, E.B., Weller, R.A., & Fristad, M.A. (in press). Lithium treatment of prepubertal manic children with psychotic features. *Journal of Affective Disorders*.

Varsamis, J., & MacDonald, S.M. (1972). Manic depressive disease in childhood. *Canadian Journal of Psychiatry*, *17*, 279–281.

Warneke, L. (1975). A case of manic depressive illness in childhood. *Canadian Journal of Psychiatry*, *20*, 195–200.

Waters, B.G.H. (1979). Risk to bipolar affective psychosis. In B. Shopsin (Ed.), *Manic illness*. New York: Raven.

Waters, B.G.H. (1980). The outlook for children of manic depressive patients. *American Journal of Psychiatry*, *137*, 1126.

Weinberg, W.A., & Brumback, R.A. (1976). Mania in childhood. *American Journal of Diseases in Children*, *130*, 380–385.

Weissman, M.M., Gershon, E.S., Kidd, K.K., Prusoff, B.A., Leckman, J.F., Dibble, E., Hamovit, J., Thompson, D., Pauls, D.L., & Guroff, J. (1984). Psychiatric disorders in the relatives of probands with affective disorders: The Yale University-National Institute of Mental Health Collaborative Study. *Archives of General Psychiatry*, *41*, 13–21.

Welner, A., Welner, Z., & Fishman, R. (1979). Psychiatric adolescent inpatients: A 10-year follow-up. *Archives of General Psychiatry*, *36*, 698–700.

White, J.H., & O'Shanick, G. (1977). Juvenile manic-depressive illness. *American Journal of Psychiatry*, *134*, 1035–1036.

Winokur, G., Clayton, P.J., & Reich, T. (1969). *Manic-depressive illness*. St. Louis: Mosby.

Youngerman, J., & Canino, I.A. (1978). Lithium carbonate use in children and adolescents. *Archives of General Psychiatry*, *35*, 216–224.

Zis, A.R., & Goodwin, F.K. (1979). Major affective disorder as a recurrent illness. *Archives of General Psychiatry*, *36*, 835–839.

CHAPTER 15

Major Depression

NEAL D. RYAN

In contrast to those of depressive disorders in adults, systematic studies of affective disorders in childhood and adolescence are the product of only about the past dozen years. Therefore, this chapter takes special pains to emphasize areas of research knowledge about the similarities and differences in the manifestations of major depressive disorder with age. In many areas we must fall back on clinical intuition and assumed parallels between child and adult forms of the disorder, since research in child affective disorders remains far behind that in adult disorders.

DEFINITION

Avoiding for the moment the issue of change in symptom pattern of major depression across the life span, the advances in the study of major depression in childhood started with the application of adult diagnostic criteria, RDC and DSM-III (American Psychiatric Association, 1980), to children and adolescents. In retrospect, the approach of using unmodified adult criteria has proven even more felicitous than would earlier have been imagined.

The first DSM-III criterion for major depression is *dysphoric mood or loss of interest or pleasure in all or almost all usual activities and pastimes.* Dysphoric mood is characterized by descriptions of affects such as depressed, sad, blue, hopeless, low, down in the dumps, or irritable according to the DSM-III. The mood disturbance must be prominent and relatively persistent. For children under the age of 6 the dysphoric mood may be inferred from a persistently sad appearance.

It is in the assessment of affect states (in distinction to assessment of behavior) that the child clinician faces the greatest challenge. The best available information is obtained by combining both parent and child reports (Weissman, 1987). The cognitive immaturity of the child can easily result in confusion about chronology and about the presence or absence of various affects. For example, while an adult will know that the term *depressed* is used to describe a range of dysphoric affects, the child may have idiosyncratic words for different dysphoric affects. One school-age child when asked if he was depressed said no. He also denied feeling sad. He did, however, say that he was blue. When he was asked to explain the difference, he stated that he was sad when his grandfather had died and now he was blue and that they were both bad feelings but they were different bad feelings. In other words, this excellent information had described both dysphoric mood and distinct quality of mood but because of his cognitive immaturity he applied the label *blue* to this mood. It's easy for an interviewer who does not dig to miss symptoms like this entirely. Therefore, when interviewing a child about psychiatric symptomatology, one can expect to spend considerably more time to cover the same ground than would be necessary with an adult. The interviewer must ask each question in a number of different ways and must be flexible and willing to use the child's words for particular symptoms.

Criterion B of the DSM-III for major depressive disorder requires at least four of the following symptoms to have been present nearly every day for a period of at least 2 weeks (with the exception that in a child under 6 the criterion requires three of the first four symptoms). These are: (1) poor appetite or significant weight loss (when not dieting) or increased appetite or significant weight gain (in children under 6, consider failure to make expected weight gains); (2) insomnia or hypersomnia; (3) psychomotor agitation or retardation (but not merely subjective feelings of restlessness or being slowed down) (in children under 6, hypoactivity); (4) loss of interest or pleasure in usual activities, or decrease in sexual drive not limited to a period when delusional or hallucinating (in children under 6, signs of apathy); (5) loss of energy, fatigue; (6) feelings of worthlessness, self-reproach, or excessive or inappropriate guilt (either may be delusional); (7) complaints or evidence of diminished ability to think or concentrate, such as slowed thinking, or indecisiveness not associated witth marked loosening of associations or incoherence; and (8) recurrent thoughts of death, suicidal ideation, wishes to be dead, or suicide attempt.

The remaining three critiera (C through E) exclude mood-incongruent delusions or hallucinations or bizarre behavior dominating the clinical picture at a time without prominent affective symptomatology, exclude schizophrenia, schizophreniform disorder, or paranoid disorder, and exclude any organic mental disorder or uncomplicated bereavement.

For children the same symptom severity thresholds are used as are used for adults. However, for the related symptoms in criterion B for major depression the interviewer should keep in mind that in the assessment of weight loss the item is scored as positive if over a period of months the child has failed to gain weight at a time when the weight should have increased to keep up with growth.

Errors are frequently made in assessing the other symptoms by disbelieving the child's report. For example, frequently a child will report insomnia, saying he or she takes 30 minutes or an hour to get to sleep, but the parents will report that they look in and the child is definitely not having trouble going to sleep. It is probably a mistake to believe the parent here. What may well be going on is that indeed the child does have some sleep disturbance and is going in and out of light sleep. There are certainly times when a child's more severe report of a particular symptom is discounted because of a clear and convincing report from a parent, but these should be extremely rare.

Another mistake is the failure to ascertain whether or not a child has partial anhedonia, instead only determining that he or she does not have total anhedonia.

A related problem is the child who has been more dysphoric and depressed in the past and now has a partial improvement. The clinican may not determine this without very astute questioning. The interchange frequently goes something like this: The clinician asks if the child is sad or blue most of the time, the child says that was the case in the past but not now, and the clinician stops. If the clinician continues, frequently what will be discovered is that the child's mood is not normal now, and is not even normal for part of the day now; it is just not as bad as it used to be and the child does not describe that clearly. Especially when interviewing a younger child the clinician has to do a lot of detective work—keeping all potential possibilities in mind and not leaping to premature closure.

HISTORICAL BACKGROUND

Affective disorders were not mentioned in any child psychiatric textbook until 1976 (cf. Puig-Antich, 1985). In contrast to depressive disorder in adults, affective disorders in childhood have been studied for a little more than a decade and a half. The very late recognition of this syndrome in children and adolescents stems from several factors: the idea that children do not have sufficient psychic maturity to be depressed (Rie, 1966); overemphasis on the normal developmental processes of childhood and adolescence; and the concept that psychopathological manifestations and turmoil are normative, at least in adolescence (A. Freud, 1958).

In considering the possibility of childhood depression, the concept of "masked depression" was proposed. This suggested that, while children did not become depressed in the same fashion as adults, the depression would manifest differently, primarily as somatic symptoms, conduct disturbance, enuresis, or encopresis (Cytryn & McKnew, 1972; Glaser, 1967). As originally proposed, this hypothesis was severely limited by the absence of criteria to judge which children with psychiatric disorders were excluded from this group. Subsequently, better symptom assessment has revealed that many children with masked depression meet systematic criteria for depression with proper symptom assessment (Carlson & Cantwell, 1980).

As noted earlier, the application of adult criteria for major depression to children and adolescents showed that a number were identified with symptomatology similar to adult major depression (Carlson & Cantwell, 1982; Puig-Antich, 1982b). Nevertheless, that children and adolescents are found who meet adult criteria for major depression does not in itself mean that this is the same or a related syndrome. Instead we must look to clinical course, genetics, and neurobiology for evidence of continuity of child, adolescent, and adult major depression.

CLINICAL PICTURE

The clinical picture of children and adolescents with major depression is surprisingly similar throughout childhood and adolescence (Ryan et al., 1987) and is similar to the picture in adults, allowing for the effects of cognitive immaturity on the naming of intrapsychic symptoms. Contrary to hypothesis, one study found no relationship between Piagetian cognitive stages and depressive symptomatology in children (Kovacs & Paulauskas, 1984).

Depressed appearance, which meets criterion A for the DSM-III for children under 6, is more frequent in children than in adolescents (Poznanski, 1982; Ryan, 1987). Similarly, somatic complaints are more frequent in younger children. Hallucinations are more common in a younger age group, while delusions are very infrequent. With adolescents, hallucinations become somewhat less frequent, although they still occur, and delusions become much more frequent. Delusions and hallucinations may also have different prognostic significance. Hallucinations in a child with prepubertal depression predicts worse response to tricyclic antidepressants (Puig-Antich et al., 1987), while delusions in adolescents strongly suggest bipolarity.

Surprisingly, the frequency and severity of suicidal ideation also did not vary between children and adolescents with MDD. More than 50% of children and adolescents with MDD had suicidal ideation with a definite suicide plan in one large sample of outpatients (Ryan, 1987). What did differ was the number of suicide attempts and the lethality of suicide attempts. Prepubertal children made few attempts, and those attempts they did make were not as likely to be lethal. What seems to be going on here is that the younger children have equal suicide intent, but simply do not have the cognitive ability to formulate successful suicide plans. For example, children with MDD have described plans including drowning themselves in the bathtub, hanging themselves with a bath towel over the curtain rod, or riding a bicycle down a hill and throwing themselves off into the rocks. On the other hand, adolescents choose a more effective method, such as gunshot or overdose.

In the study of Ryan and colleagues (1987) there was no difference between children and adolescents with MDD in the average overall severity of depressive symptomatology, in the rate of RDC endogenous subtype, or in the severity of the majority of individual depressive symptoms including depressed mood, negative self-image, diurnal variation of guilt, fatigue, impaired concentration, psychomotor retardation, irritability, insomnia, anorexia or increased appetite, and suicidal ideation. Prepubertal children had more somatic complaints, more psychomotor agitation, more frequent separation anxiety, more frequent phobias, and more often had hallucinations. Adolescents had greater hopelessness/helplessness, anhedonia, hypersomnia, weight changes, annd lethality of suicide attempt. The frequent occurrence of depressed appearance in younger children with MDD has been noted by others (Poznanski, 1982) and is permitted as the criterion symptom for depressed mood in childern under 6, by DSM-III. Similarly, the finding of increased somatic complaints in younger children parallels clinical observation and supports the observation of Carlson and Cantwell (1980) that masked depression can be unmasked by proper assessment of other depressive symptoms. In other words, somatic complaints may be a frequent presenting complaint in children with MDD in this age group, but proper symptom assessment will frequently demonstrate a full depressive syndrome.

A principal component analysis of the same data gave a symptom factor structure similar to that found in adult studies, with an endogenous factor (anhedonia, fatigue, psychomotor retardation, social withdrawal, depressed mood, anorexia, decreased weight, diurnal variation, and hypersomnia), a negative cognitions factor (negative self-image, hopelessness/helplessness, suicidal ideation, and brooding/worrying), an anxiety factor (brooding/worring, separation anxiety, insomnia, somatic complaints, hallucinations, and psychomotor agitation) and appetite and weight factor (increased appetite and increased weight vs. decreased appetite and decreased weight), and a disturbed conduct factor (suicidal ideation, psychomotor agitation, conduct disorder, and anger/irritability). The first factor found in the study is similar to adult endogenous factors found in multiple studies (see review by Nelson & Charney, 1981). The third factor, the anxiety factor, also strongly parallels anxiety factors found in multiple studies of adults with major depression.

Among adolescents in this study, duration of MDD episode of greater than 2 years (present in half of the adolescent sample) was very strongly associated with greater severity of suicidal ideation, greater number of suicide attempts, and more serious suicide attempts.

ASSOCIATED FEATURES

Comorbidity is more the rule than the exception in both children and adolescents with MDD. In the study by Ryan and colleagues (1987) of 187 children and adolescents with MDD, separation anxiety with functional impairment occurred in 58% of the children and 37% of the adolescents, phobias with avoidant behavior occurred in 45% of the children and 27% of the adolescents, overanxious disorder occurred in 20% of both subgroups, obsessive–compulsive disorder occurred in 11% of both subgroups, and conduct disorder of sufficient severity to have disruptive effects on school or other outside-the-home functioning was present in 16% of children and 11% of adolescents. The mean numbers of comorbid diagnoses, not counting MDD itself, were 1.5 for the prepubertal children and 1.1 for the adolescents.

Carlson and Cantwell (1980) found that 32% of their depressed children had conduct disorder or attention deficit disorder, and Puig-Antich (1982a) found a 37% rate of diagnosable conduct disorder in prepubertal boys with MDD. Kovacs, Feinberg, Crouse-Novak, Paulauskas, and Finkelstein (1984) found a 33% rate of anxiety disorder and a 7% rate of conduct disorder that predated the onset of MDD in their school-age cohort.

Beginning with adolescence, alcohol and drug abuse are common comorbid diagnoses with MDD. The question then is whether the depression is primary or secondary to the drug and alcohol abuse. In a study of Deykin, Levy, and Wells (1987), examining college students ages 16 to 19 using the DIS (Robbins, Helzer, Crougham, & Ratcliff, 1981), the lifetime prevalence of alcohol abuse or dependence was 8.2%, of substance abuse or dependence was 9.4%, and of major depressive disorder was 6.8%. In this study, adolescents with MDD were 4.5 times more likely to abuse alcohol and 3.3 times more likely to abuse other substances as adolescents without a psychiatric disorder. They were also at increased risk compared to adolescents without a nonaffective psychiatric disorder. Most important, in general, the MDD preceded (by an average of 4.5 years) the onset of alcohol abuse. In half of the subjects with both alcohol abuse and MDD, the MDD preceded even the first exposure to alcohol. Similar findings pertained to MDD and substance abuse.

COURSE AND PROGNOSIS

The best data on the naturalistic longitudinal course of depression in school-age children are from a large study of Kovacs and her colleages (Kovacs, Feinberg, Crouse-Novak, Paulauskas, & Finkelstein, 1984; Kovacs, Feinberg, Crouse-Novak, Paulauskas, Pollock, & Finkelstein, 1984). In their cohort of rigorously assessed and diagnosed school-age children, the mean length of episode for a major depressive disorder was 32 weeks. The mean length of episode for a dysthymic disorder was 68 weeks. The maximal recovery rate for MDD of 92% was reached 1.5 years after the onset of the illness. The other 8% of the children are very unlikely to recover over the subsequent year. The earlier age at onset predicted more protracted recovery from both major depressive disorder and dysthymic disorder.

After an episode of MDD, the risk of a subsequent episode is high. In their study, Kovacs and colleagues (Kovacs, Feinberg, Crouse-Novak, Paulauskas, Pollock, & Finkelstein, 1984) found a cumulative probability of 72% of having a recurrent episode of MDD within 5 years after the onset of the first episode. The children with major depression superimposed on dysthymia, "double depression," had the shortest time to relapse.

In summary, the course of child and adolescent depression appears somewhat similar to the course of adult depression, with recurring depressions being the rule.

IMPAIRMENT

In a study comparing children with MDD, children with nondepressive neurotic disorders (primarily anxiety disorders and phobias), and normal children in terms of their psychosocial functioning, the children with MDD had the worst functioning in all areas (Puig-Antich et al., 1985a, 1985b). Children with MDD had impairment at school, both in academic performance and in teacher–child relationships. However, the school impairments were not specific to children with MDD, as the nondepressed psychiatric controls also showed school impairments. MDD children had marked impairment in the mother–child relationship, as compared to both the nondepressive control and normal control groups: There was significantly less mother–child communication and the relationship was significantly cooler and more distant. The father–child relationship was also impaired, with decreased communication, poorer quality in communication, and more father–child tension and hostility. There were similar impairments in parent–sibling relationships. In general, depressives were less able to have special or "best" friendships, had lower ability to make and maintain positive peer relationships, and were significantly more teased. While there was a tendency for the children with MDD to be more severely affected than nondepressed neurotic children, most of the deficits were not specific to depression but were more general to psychiatrically disturbed children.

Follow-up of the same children after recovery (Puig-Antich et al., 1985b) showed a complete normalization of school functioning but only a partial improvement in the child's intrafamilial and extrafamilial relationships. Moreover, there was a distinct pattern to the recovery, in that moderate deficits in general improved completely, while more severe psychosocial deficits improved only to the level of moderate impairment.

COMPLICATIONS

As is the case with adult disorder, the most serious complication of a major depressive disorder in adolescence (and much more rarely in childhood) is suicide. Suicide is the leading cause of death among adolescents and accounts for 11.8% of the mortality among American youth between the ages of 15 and 24 (Center for Health Promotion and Education, 1985). There is a very strong secular increase in the rate of suicide (Frederick, 1978; Shaffer & Fisher, 1981) in this age group in recent decades. It is paralleled by a similar secular increase in the rate of major depression in young adults (Lavori et al., 1987). While not all adolescent suicides have an affective disorder, both suicide victims and suicidal inpatients have high rates of affective disorder and high rates of family history for affective disorder (Brent et al., in press). Adolescents with bipolar disorder or psychosis may be at particularly high risk for suicide (Otto, 1972; Welner, Welner, & Fishman, 1979). When combined with major depression, other comorbid diagnoses (Brent et al., in press), especially alcohol abuse (Brent et al., in press; Ryan et al., 1987), may cause particularly high risk for suicide attempts and completed suicide.

EPIDEMIOLOGY

Major depressive disorder is rare but exists in the preschool child (Kashani & Carlson, 1987). MDD becomes more frequent with school-age children, with several studies converging on a point prevalence of about 1.8% (Anderson, Williams, McGee, & Silva, 1987; Kashani & Simonds, 1979; Kashani et al., 1983). MDD becomes even more frequent with adolescents with a point prevalence of 4.7% in one study (Kashani et al., 1987). These studies all used clinical interviews. The evidence suggests that a fully structured interview (Nreslau, 1985) and self-report questionnaires are poor in picking up affective psychopathology; they probably have too many false positives and false negatives for screening purposes at least before adolescence.

FAMILIAL PATTERN

Two strategies have been used to examine the pattern of familial transmission of affective disorders in children. One, the "top-down" approach, takes adult probands for major depression and looks at their child and adolescent offspring. The other, the "bottom-up" approach, looks at the adult relatives of child probands with major affective disorder. The age-corrected lifetime morbid risk for major depression in first-degree relatives of adult probands with major depression is between .18 and .30 (Gershon, Bunney, Leckman, van Erdewegh, & Debauche, 1976; Gershon, Targum, Kessler, Mazure, & Bunney, 1977; Gershon et al., 1982; Perris, 1974; Weissman, Kidd, & Prusoff, 1982; Weissman et al., 1984). The two studies examining adolescent probands with major depression found an age-corrected risk in adult relatives of .35 (Strober, unpublished data) and .37 (Puig-Antich, unpublished data) in their adult relatives. The single study looking at the adult relatives of prepubertal children with major depression found an age-corrected morbid risk of .50 (Puig-Antich et al., 1988). The majority of the adult studies were done with the more sensitive family study method, while the adolescent and child studies thus far reported had been done with the family history method, which was less sensitive. This supports even more strongly the conclusion that children and adolescents with depression come from the most heavily affectively loaded families. Studies of the child offspring of adult MDD programs (Gershon et al., 1982; Weissman, Leckman, Merikangas, Gammon, & Prusoff, 1984; Welner, Welner, McCrary, & Leonard, 1977) indicate that the morbid risk for major depression in children and adolescents increases with parental major depression. Only one "top-down" study (Gershon et al., 1985) has failed to find this.

The data, however, also suggest that the families with early onset of major depression also have increased morbid risk for alcoholism and anxiety disorders. This may be due to both assortative mating of the two diagnoses and transmission of common genetic or familial factors increasing morbid risk for multiple disorders.

DIFFERENTIAL DIAGNOSIS

As in the adult disorder, the diagnosis is made only when it cannot be established that an organic factor initiated and maintained the disturbance. In practice, the organic etiologic factors that are important in this age group are most often psychoactive medications, in particular phenobarbital used to treat seizure disorders (Brent, Crumrine, Varma, Allan, & Allman, 1987), exogenous steroids used to treat medical disorders, ongoing alcohol abuse or stimulant withdrawal. Other etiologies that are more important in adults (thyroid disease, Cushing's disease, or cancer of the pancreas) certainly all occur in children or adolescents but are less frequent.

CLINICAL MANAGEMENT: RESEARCH FINDINGS

There are as yet no controlled studies of any psychotherapeutic techniques in either children or adolescents with major affective disorder. While it is likely that techniques with proven efficacy in adult major depression, cognitive–behavioral therapy and interpersonal therapy, will prove to be useful with at least older adolescents, these techniques may not be as readily modifiable to be useful in children or younger adolescents due to their cognitive and psychological immaturity.

Several studies (Geller, Perel, Knitter, Lycaki, & Farooki, 1983; Geller, Cooper, Farooki, & Chestnut, 1985; Preskorn, Weller, & Weller, 1982; Puig-Antich et al., 1987) demonstrate a plasma level–response relationship between tricyclic antidepressants and clinical improvement in major depression in prepubertal children. In prepubertal children one study has failed to find a medication placebo difference (Puig-Antich et al., 1987), while another found superiority of imipramine over placebo (Preskorn, Weller, Hughes, Weller, & Bolte, 1987), particularly in dexamethasone-nonsuppressing children. Therefore, thus far the evidence suggests that tricyclic antidepressants are likely to have a place in the treatment of prepubertal children; however, this is complicated by the high placebo response rate of children in that age group with major depression or other disorders.

The place of tricyclic antidepressants in the treatment of adolescent depression is less clear. One study of amitriptyline versus placebo failed to find any significant difference between the two groups (Kramer & Feguine, 1983). This study, however, was limited by small sample size (10 per cell) and some diagnostic problems. Another study (Ryan et al., 1986) giving a fixed, weight-adjusted dose of imipramine in adolescent depression failed to find a plasma level–response relationship. Thus the evidence for efficacy of tricyclic antidepressants in adolescent major depression is at present much less than at other points in the life span. Open clinical studies suggest that both lithium augmentation (Ryan, Meyer, Dachille, Mazzie, & Puig-Antich, in press) and monoamine oxidase inhibitors (Ryan, Puig-Antich, et al., in press) may have a place in the pharmacological treatment of adolescent MDD, but this remains to be studied in a controlled fashion.

DSM-III-R

The DSM-III-R (APA, 1987) criteria for major depressive syndrome require the presence of at least five out of nine symptoms over a 2-week period, where one of the five symptoms must be either depressed mood (or irritable mood in children or adolescents) or loss of interest or pleasure. Therefore, in terms of the symptom count it essentially parallels DSM-III, which requires one of those two symptoms plus four out of eight other symptoms. Changes, however, have been made in severity thresholds required for some symptoms to be counted as positive. These changes make the category somewhat more restrictive. Changes include requiring that the depressed mood and/or diminished interest or pleasure be "most of the day, nearly every day" (p. 222). Data from studies of children and adolescents in general fail to support this increased threshold. For example, medication efficacy in prepubertal affective illness showed little change by severity or endogenicity of the child (Puig-Antich et al., 1987).

Several minor changes were made to the inclusion criteria that are consistent with child and adolescent data. These include the importance of depressed appearance as a substitute for depressed mood, especially in younger children (Poznanski, Mokros, Grossman, & Freeman, 1985; Ryan et al., 1987) and the use of irritability as a substitute for dysphoric mood in children and adolescents.

The criteria for melancholic subtype were augmented by several criteria that severely complicate their use in children. These are: no significant personality disturbance before first major depressive episode; one or more previous major depressive episodes followed by complete recovery or nearly complete recovery; and previous good response to specific and adequate somatic antidepressant therapy, for example, tricyclics, ECT, MAOIs, lithium. The problem here is that these additional criteria apply poorly to children who will have had few if any lifetime episodes when they are first seen and are unlikely to have had specific treatment, and in whom a personality diagnosis cannot be made because of a current age of less then 18 years.

In summary, research evidence does not as yet support the change from DSM-III to DSM-III-R criteria for the diagnosis of MDD in children or adolescents.

REFERENCES

American Psychiatric Association. (1980). *Diagnostic and statistical manual of mental disorders* (3rd ed.). Washington, DC: Author.

American Psychiatric Association. (1987). *Diagnostic and statistical manual of mental disorders* (3rd ed., rev.). Washington, DC: Author.

Anderson, J.C., Williams, S., McGee, R., & Silva, P.A. (1987). DSM-III disorders in preadolescent children. *Archives of General Psychiatry, 44*, 69–76.

Brent, D.A., Perper, J.A., Goldstein, C.E., Kolko, D.J., Allan, M.J., Allman, C.J., & Zelenak, J. (in press). Risk factors for adolescent suicide: A comparison of adolescent suicide victims with suicidal inpatients. *Archives of General Psychiatry*.

Brent, D., Crumrine, P., Varma, R., Allan, M., & Allman, C. (1987). Phenobarbital treatment and major depressive disorder in children with epilepsy. *Pediatrics, 80*, 909–917.

Breslau, N. (1985). Depressive symptoms, major depression, and generalized anxiety: A comparison of self-reports on CES-D and results from diagnostic interviews. *Psychiatry Residency, 15*, 219–229.

Carlson, G.A., & Cantwell, D.P. (1980). Unmasking masked depression in children and adolescents. *American Journal of Psychiatry, 137*, 445–449.

Carlson, G.A., & Cantwell, D.P. (1982). Suicidal behavior and depression in children and adolescents. *Journal of the American Academy of Child Psychiatry, 21*, 361–368.

Center for Health Promotion and Education. (1985). *Suicide surveillance 1970–1980*. Atlanta: U.S. Department of Health and Human Services, Centers for Disease Control.

Cytryn, L., & McKnew, D.H. (1972). Proposed classification of childhood depression. *American Journal of Psychiatry, 129*, 149–155.

Deykin, E.Y., Levy, J.C., & Wells, V. (1987). Adolescent depression, alcohol and drug abuse. *American Journal of Public Health, 77*, 178–182.

Frederick, C. (1978). Current trends in suicidal behavior in the United States. *American Journal of Psychotherapy, 32*, 172–200.

Freud, A. (1958). Adolescence. *Psychoanalytic Study of the Child, 13*, 255–278.

Geller, B., Cooper, T.B., Farooki, Z.Q., & Chestnut, E.C. (1985). Dose and plasma levels of nortriptyline and chlorpromazine in delusionally depressed adolescents and of nortriptyline in nondelusionally depressed adolescents. *American Journal of Psychiatry, 142*, 336–338.

Geller, B., Perel, J.M., Knitter, E.F., Lycaki, H., & Farooki, Z.Q. (1983). Nortriptyline in major depressive disorder in children: Response, steady-state plasma levels, predictive kinetics, and pharmacokinetics. *Psychopharmacology Bulletin, 19*, 62–65.

Gershon, E.S., Bunney, W.E., Leckman, J.F., van Erdewegh, M., & Debauche, B.A. (1976). The inheritance of affective disorders: A review of data and of hypotheses. *Behavior Genetics, 6*, 227–261.

Gershon, E.S., Hamovit, J., Guroff, J.J., Dibble, E., Leckman, J.F., Sceery, W., Targum, S.D., Nurnberger, J.I., Goldin, L.R., & Bunney, W.E. (1982). A family study of schizoaffective, bipolar I, bipolar II, unipolar, and normal control probands. *Archives of General Psychiatry, 39*, 157–167.

Gershon, E.S., McKnew, D., Cytryn, L., Hamovit, J., Schreiber, J., Hibbs, E., & Pellegrini, D. (1985). Diagnoses in school-aged children of bipolar affective disorder patients and normal controls. *Journal of Affective Disorders, 8*, 283–291.

Gershon, E.S., Targum, S.D., Kessler, L.R., Mazure, C.M., & Bunney, W.E. (1977). In A.G. Steinberg, A.G. Bearn, & A.G. Motulsky (Eds.), *Progress in medical genetics* (Vol. II). Philadephia: W.B. Saunders.

Glaser, K. (1967). Masked depression in children and adolescents. *American Journal of Psychotherapy, 19*, 565–574.

Kashani, J.H., & Carlson, G.A. (1987). Seriously depressed preschoolers. *American Journal of Psychiatry, 144*, 348–350.

Kashani, J.H., Carlson, G.A., Beck, N.C., Hoeper, E.W., Corcoran, C.M., McAllister, J.A., Fallahi, C., Rosenberg, T.K., & Reid, J.C. (1987). Depression, depressive symptoms, and depressed mood among a community sample of adolescents. *American Journal of Psychiatry, 144*, 931–934.

Kashani, J.H., Holcomb, W.R., & Orvaschel, H. (1986). Depression and depressive symptoms in preschool children from the general population. *American Journal of Psychiatry, 143*, 1138–1143.

Kashani, J.H., McGee, R.O., Clarkson, S.E., Anderson, J.C., Walton, L.A., Williams, S., Silva, P.A., Robins, A.J., Cytryn, L., & McKnew, K.H. (1983). Depression in a sample of 9-year-old children. *Archives of General Psychiatry, 40*, 1217–1223.

Kashani, J.H., & Simonds, J.F. (1979). The incidence of depression in children. *American Journal of Psychiatry, 136*, 1203–1205.

Kovacs, M., Feinnberg, T.L., Crouse-Novak, M.A., Paulauskas, S.L., & Finkelstein, R. (1984). Depressive disorders in childhood: I. A longitudinal prospective study of characteristics and recovery. *Archives of General Psychiatry, 41*, 229–237.

Kovacs, M., Feinberg, T.L., Crouse-Novak, M.A., Paulauskas, S.L., Pollock, M., & Finkelstein, R. (1984). Depressive disorders in childhood: II. A longitudinal study of the risk for a subsequent major depression. *Archives of General Psychiatry*, *41*, 643–649.

Kovacs, M., & Paulauskas, S.L. (1984). Developmental stage and the expression of depressive disorders in children: An empirical analysis. In D. Cicchetti & K. Schneider-Rosen (Eds.), *Childhood depression: New directions for child development*. San Francisco: Jossey-Bass.

Kramer, E., & Feguine, R. (1983). Clinical effects of amitriptyline in adolescent depression. *Journal of the American Academy of Child Psychiatry*, *20*, 636–644.

Lavoir, P.W., Klerman, G.L., Keller, M.B., Reich, T., Rice, J., & Endicott, J. (1987). Age-period-cohort analysis of secular trends in onset of major depressions: Findings in siblings of patients with major affective disorder. *Journal of Psychiatric Residency*, *21*, 23–35.

Nelson, J.C., & Charney, D.S. (1981). The symptoms of major depressive illness. *American Journal of Psychiatry*, *138*, 1–13.

Otto, U. (1972). Suicidal acts by children and adolescents: A follow-up study. *Acta Psychiatrica Scandinavica* (Suppl. 233), 1–123.

Perris, C. (1974). The genetics of affective disorders. In J. Mendels (Ed.), *Biological psychiatry*. New York: Wiley.

Poznanski, E.O. (1982). The clinnical phenomenology of childhood depression. *American Journal of Orthopsychiatry*, *52*, 308–313.

Poznanski, E.O., Mokros, H.B., Grossman, J., & Freeman, L.N. (1985). Diagnostic criteria in childhood depression. *American Journal of Psychiatry*, *142*, 1168–1173.

Preskorn, S.H., Weller, E.B., Hughes, C.W., Weller, R.A., & Bolte, K. (1987). Depression in prepubertal children: Dexamethasone nnonsuppression predicts differential response to imipramine vs. placebo. *Psychopharmacology Bulletin*, *23*, 128–133.

Preskorn, S., Weller, E., & Weller, R. (1982). Childhood depression: Imipramine levels and response. *Journal of Clinical Psychiatry*, *43*, 450–453.

Puig-Antich, J. (1982a). Major depression and conduct disorder in prepuberty. *Journal of the American Academy of Child Psychiatry*, *21*, 118–128.

Puig-Antich, J. (1982b). The use of RDC criteria for major depressive disorder in children and adolescents. *Journal of the American Academy of Child Psychiatry*, *21*, 291–293.

Puig-Antich, J. (1985). Affective disorders and suicidality in children and adolescents. In H.I. Kaplan & B.J. Sadock (Eds), *Comprehensive textbook of psychiatry/IV*. Baltimore: Williams & Wilkins.

Puig-Antich, J., Goetz, D., Davies, M., Kaplan, T., Davies, S., Ostrow, L., Asnis, L., Twomey, J., Iyengar, S., & Ryan, N.D. (1988). *A controlled family history study of prepubertal major depressive disorder*. Manuscript submitted for publication.

Puig-Antich, J., Lukens, E., Davies, M., Goetz, D., Brennan-Quattrock, J., & Todak, G. (1985a). Psychosocial functioning in prepubertal major depressive disorders: I. Interpersonal relationships during the depressive episode. *Archives of General Psychiatry*, *42*, 500–507.

Puig-Antich, J., Lukens, E., Davies, M., Goetz, D., Brennan-Quattrock, J., & Todak, G. (1985b). Psychosocial functioning in prepubertal major depressive disorders: II. Interpersonal relationships after sustained recovery from affective episode. *Archives of General Psychiatry*, *42*, 511–517.

Puig-Antich, J., Perel, J.M., Lupatkin, W., Chambers, W.J., Tabrizi, M.A., King, J., Goetz, R., Davies, M., & Stiller, R.L. (1987). Imipramine in prepubertal major depressive disorders. *Archives of General Psychiatry*, *44*, 81–89.

Rie, H.E. (1966). Depression in childhood: A survey of some pertinent contributions. *Journal of the American Academy of Child Psychiatry*, *5*, 653–683.

Robins, L.N., Helzer, J.E., Crougham, J., & Ratcliff, K.S. (1981). National Institute of Mental Health diagnostic interview schedule: Its history, characteristics and validity. *Archives of General Psychiatry*, *38*, 381–389.

Ryan, N.D., Meyer, V.A., Dachille, S., Mazzie, D., & Puig-Antich, J. (in press). Lithium antidepressant augmentation in TCA-refractory non-bipolar major depression in adolescents. *Journal of Child & Adolescent Psychiatry*.

Ryan, N.D., Puig-Antich, J., Rabinovich, H., Fried, J., Ambrosini, P., Meyer, V., Torres, D., Dachille, S., & Mazzie, D. (in press). MAOIs in adolescent major depression unresponsive to tricyclic antidepressants pilot clinical report. *Journal of the American Academy of Child & Adolescent Psychiatry*.

Ryan, N.D., Puig-Antich, J., Ambrosini, P., Rabinovich, H., Robinson, D., Nelson, B., Iyengar, S., & Twomey, J. (1987). The clinical picture of major depression in children and adolescents. *Archives of General Psychiatry*, *44*, 854–861.

Ryan, N.D., Puig-Antich, J., Cooper, T., Rabinovich, P., Ambrosini, M., Davies, M., King, J., Torres, D., & Fried, J. (1986). Imipramine in adolescent major depression: Plasma level and clinical response. *Acta Psychiatria Scandinavica*, *73*, 275–288.

Shaffer, D., & Fisher, P. (1981). The epidemiology of suicide in children and young adolescents. *Journal of the American Academy of Child Psychiatry*, *20*, 545–561.

Weissman, M.M., Gershon, E.S., Kidd, K.K., Prusoff, B.A., Leckman, J.F., Dibble, E., Hamovit, J., Thompson, D., Pauls, D.L., & Guroff, J.J. (1984). Psychiatric disorders in the relatives of probands with affective disorders. *Archives of General Psychiatry*, *41*, 13–21.

Weissman, M.M., Kidd, K.K., & Prusoff, B.A. (1982). Variability in rates of affective disorders in relatives of depressed and normal probands. *Archives of General Psychiatry*, *39*, 1397–1406.

Weissman, M.M., Leckman, J.F., Merikangas, K.R., Gammon, G.D., & Prusoff, B.A. (1984). Depression and anxiety disorders in parents and children. *Archives of General Psychiatry*, *41*, 845–853.

Weissman, M.M., Wickramaratne, P., Warner, V., John, K., Prusoff, B.A., Merikangas, K.R., & Gammon, G.D. (1987). Assessing psychiatric disorders in children. *Archives of General Psychiatry*, *44*, 747–753.

Welner, A., Welner, Z., & Fishman, R. (1979). Psychiatric adolescent inpatients: Eight-to-ten-year follow-up. *Archives of General Psychiatry*, *36*, 698–700.

Welner, Z., Welner, A., McCrary, M.D., & Leonard, M.A. (1977). Psychopathology in children of inpatients with depression: A controlled study. *Journal of Nervous & Mental Disease*, *164*, 408–413.

CHAPTER 16

Dysthymic and Cyclothymic Disorders

MARTIN B. KELLER AND FRANCES M. SESSA

Research studies describing the course and correlates of childhood cyclothymia and dysthymia are beginning to emerge, although the incidence and prevalence of chronic low-grade affective disorders in the general population and in clinical populations are still unknown. This chapter will discuss the diagnosis of cyclothymia and dysthymia in children and present the information that is available on rates of these disorders in children studied in a variety of settings. The boundary issues between dysthymia and major depression, personality disorder, and several of the nonaffective disorders will be discussed, as will the relationship between cyclothymia and bipolar I and bipolar II disorder. Finally, this chapter will describe what is known on the course of these disorders, the frequency of suicide attempts, and the treatment of children and adolescents diagnosed with cyclothymia and dysthymia.

DEFINITION

Cytryn, McKnew, and Bunney (1980) divided childhood depressions into two subtypes: acute and chronic. These subtypes are subsumed under the classification of major depression in DSM-III (APA, 1980) and DSM-III-R (APA, 1987), with severity levels ranging from moderate to severe. They defined acute childhood depression as a single episode that may be associated with severe psychosocial stressors. Chronic childhood depression is defined as recurrent episodes of longer duration with no immediate precipitant.

In DSM-III-R, chronic and intermittent low-grade depressions are diagnosed as dysthymia on Axis I, and are considered to be mood disorders. The criteria for diagnosing dysthymia in children are identical to those for adults except that the minimum duration of dysphoric mood is 1 year for children and adolescents and 2 years for adults. In addition, the child or adolescent is not symptom free for more than 2 consecutive months during the 1-year period. Dysthymia is defined as a persistent or phasic despondency accompanied by at least two of the following symptoms: increased or decreased appetite, insomnia or hypersomnia, low energy or fatigue, low self-esteem, poor concentration or difficulty making decisions, and pessimism or feelings of hopelessness (p. 232). There must be an absence of major depressive episodes during the first year from onset, and psychotic symptoms, manic episodes, and organic factors are exclusion criteria. As in adults, dysthymia in children is distinguished from major depression by reduced number and severity of symptoms and extended episode duration.

In the Research Diagnostic Criteria (RDC) (Spitzer, Endicott, & Robins, 1985), the diagnoses of chronic and intermittent depressive disorder and minor depression of 1 or 2 years' duration resemble the DSM-III-R criteria for dysthymia in adults and children. However, the RDC does not specify any differences between adult and child criteria for these conditions, as is done in DSM-III-R.

Like that of dysthymia, a diagnosis of cyclothymia is considered an Axis I mood disorder in DSM-III-R, whereas in the RDC it is classified as a personality disorder. Cyclothymia is characterized by mild oscillations in mood ranging from euphoric to depressed, where symptoms are not of sufficient number, severity, or duration to meet criteria for a diagnosis of major depression or mania.

In the DSM-III-R, cyclothymia in children is defined as it would be in adults except that the required duration of symptoms is at least 1 year for children and adolescents, compared to 2 years for adults. At least three of the following symptoms are required during hypomanic cycles: decreased need for sleep, inflated self-esteem or grandiosity, increased goal-directed activity or psychomotor agitation, excessive involvement in pleasurable activities with lack of concern for the high potential for painful consequences, more talkative than usual, flight of ideas, and distractibility (p. 217). Additionally, the patient must not be without hypomanic or depressive symptoms for 3 consecutive months. Psychotic symptoms or an organic etiology are exclusion criteria.

Akiskal and colleagues (1985) noted that cyclothymia in their adolescent patients was often characterized by phasic oscillations in the juvenile's activity level.

> [The] cyclothymic disposition was manifested in short-lived subsyndromal mini-episodes of depression and hypomania, alternating in an irregular fashion, which often led to tempestuous life events. In this group, depressive periods tended to dominate the clinical picture, with occasional elevated periods. (p. 999)

Historical Background and Clinical Picture

In the past 5 to 10 years, there has been renewed interest in childhood affective disorders, with increasing acceptance of childhood depression as a valid clinical entity (Cytryn et al., 1984). Despite this interest and the emerging use in children of the methodologic research strategies developed through work with adults, the chronic, less severe forms of major affective disorder (dysthymia, chronic and intermittent depression, minor depression of at least 2 years' duration, sustained hypomania, and cyclothymia) in children have received minimal attention. Nonetheless, the identification of these disorders is important because unrecognized and inadequately treated episodes can lead to severe psychosocial impairment and maladjustment (Akiskal et al., 1985).

Dysthymia and cyclothymia in children are commonly overlooked, since depressive or manic symptoms are often thought to be part of the normal vicissitudes of childhood and adolescence or part of nonaffective psychiatric conditions and personality disorders such as conduct disorder, attention deficit disorder, and borderline or narcissistic personality disorders.

Dysthymia has been long known in adults, although its nosologic status continues to be debated. According to Akiskal and colleagues (1980), dysthymia comprises a heterogeneous group of disorders that merits division into the characterologic and the subsyndromal forms. They have found that the characterologic form of dysthymia is associated with early onset (before age 25) and a history of educational problems. This has been corroborated by some investigators (Klein, 1974) and not by others (Keller & Lavori, 1984). Although such chronic subclinical manifestations of affective disorders are presumed to have their onsets during childhood, their continuity from childhood to adulthood has not yet been demonstrated in prospective longitudinal studies (Kovacs et al., 1984a). Research (Kovacs et al., 1984a) does indicate that dysthymic disorders are protracted in juveniles; however, it is not known whether they represent the same entity as chronic low-grade depressions that are first manifest in adulthood.

The diagnosis of cyclothymia in childhood or adolescence is difficult because the change in mood from depression to euphoria is often seen as an indication of improved emotional health. Also, in adolescence, the diagnosis of cyclothymia can be obscured by what would be considered the turmoil of adolescence. Furthermore, the RDC exclude the diagnosis of cyclothymia prior to the age of 20, which lessened the likelihood that the diagnosis would be made in children or adolescents. In 1987, DSM-III-R established criteria enabling the diagnosis of cyclothymia to be made in children. Much of the research done on cyclothymia in adults has relevance for understanding and studying this disorder in children.

Several studies suggest that cyclothymia may be a mild phenotypic expression of a bipolar genotype, and as such, the identification of cyclothymia in the families of bipolar patients could advance research on the genetic markers and transmissibility of bipolar affective disorder (Cloninger, Reich, & Yokoyama, 1983; Klein, Depue, & Slater, 1986; Turner & King, 1983). Furthermore, adult cyclothymic patients are at risk for developing full-blown affective disorders (Akiskal, Djenderedjian, Rosenthal, & Khani, 1977; Klein & Depue, 1984), and a number of investigators report that cyclothymia may be a precursor of bipolar disorder (Akiskal, 1983; Depue et al., 1981; Klein, Depue, & Slater, 1985, 1986). Although cyclothymia is common in outpatient mental health clinics, it is frequently misdiagnosed (Akiskal et al., 1977; Klein et al., 1986). Moreover, since cyclothymic patients often respond to lithium carbonate, the accurate identification of cyclothymia has important implications for treatment (Klein et al., 1986; Peselow, Dunner, Fieve, & Lautin, 1982; Rounsaville, Sholomskas, & Prusoff, 1980).

COURSE AND PROGNOSIS

Much of the information available on the natural course of dysthymia comes from the prospective, longitudinal study of Kovacs and colleagues (1984a, 1984b). In that study (1984a) of school-age depressed children, ages of onset for dysthymia range from 6 to 13 years old. These data suggest that dysthymia has an earlier age of onset than major depression in children. The average duration of dysthymia is significantly longer than that of major depression in children. Dysthymic disorder has an average episode length of 3 years, compared to 32 weeks for a major depressive episode (Kovacs et al., 1984a). The median time to recovery from dysthymia in childhood is 3.5 years (Kovacs et al., 1984a). The time to recovery from major depression is significantly faster than recovery from dysthymia. A 92% recovery rate is reached 1.5 years from the onset of a major depressive episode, while for child dysthymics it takes 6.5 years to reach an 89% recovery rate (Kovacs et al., 1984a). Kovacs and colleagues (1984a) also report that a younger age of onset predicts a more protracted episode of dysthymia.

In children, Kovacs and colleagues did not find differences in the cumulative probability of recovery from the dysthymia or major depressive disorder in patients with and without a superimposed major depressive disorder (Kovacs et al., 1984a). This is in contrast to the data on adult depression, which indicate that patients are more likely to recover from a major depressive episode if it is superimposed on a chronic underlying depressive disorder than if there is no underlying dysthymia (Keller & Shapiro, 1982). Kovacs and colleagues (1984a) also found no significant differences in the recovery rates of dysthymic children with and without a coexisting anxiety disorder.

We could not find any reports on the probability of relapse in children who recover from a dysthymic disorder. This is in large part due to the very slow recovery rate from the dysthymia. In Kovacs and colleagues' study (1984a), this led to a short duration of observation in which they were at risk to develop another episode.

After 40 months from the onset of dysthymia, 50% of the patients will develop a major depressive episode (Kovacs et al., 1984a). Within 5 years from the onset of dysthymia, 69% of the children will have their first episode of major depression (Kovacs et al., 1984a). Eleven percent of Kovacs and colleagues' (1984a) cohort of dysthymic children with a superimposed major depression developed the major depressive disorder within 1 year from the onset of the dysthymia. The majority, however, have more protracted episodes of the chronic underlying disorder prior to the onset of the major depression. Furthermore, 38% of the children with major depression have an underlying dysthymia (Kovacs et al., 1984b).

Shorter well intervals and a higher probability of relapse between episodes of major depression are predicted by the presence of a double depression in children. Forty-three percent of the dysthymic children in Kovacs and colleagues' (1984a) study developed a new episode of major depression during the first year at risk, and by the end of 4 years, 54% of children with dysthymia, compared to 32% with major depression in the absence of dysthymia, were at risk for a recurrent episode of major depression.

Information on the course of cyclothymia is limited to studies investigating the offspring of bipolar patients; however, the reliability of these data are limited by the fact that in most of the reported studies the offspring were first interviewed during adulthood. Klein and colleagues (1985) found that the clinical course of bipolar offspring (ages 15 to 21) diagnosed with cyclothymia ($N = 9$) and bipolar II disorder ($N = 1$) is similar to the clinical course reported in previous studies of adult outpatient and nonclinical cyclothymia (Akiskal et al., 1977; Depue et al., 1981).

The age of onset of cyclothymia in Klein and colleagues' (1985) subjects ranged from 7 to 15, with an average onset age of 12.4 years. Hypomanic and depressive episodes developed within a year of each other. Other studies report that cyclothymia usually has its onset in the early or mid-teens (ages 12 to 14), and rarely occurs later than early adulthood (Akiskal et al., 1977; Depue et al., 1981; Klein et al., 1986).

In Klein and colleagues' (1985) cohort of patients with cyclothymia, periods of hypomania had an average duration of 1.8 days, and depressive phases had an average duration of 2.3 days. Twenty percent with cyclothymia or bipolar II disorder experienced less than 6 periods of depression a year, while the rest of the cohort reported experienced more than 12 periods of depression (Klein et al., 1985). The distribution of hypomanic episodes was identical to that of depressive episodes. Therefore, the oscillations between depression and hypomania were relatively rapid.

At present, no data are available on the probability of recovery and relapse in children with cyclothymia.

COMPLICATIONS

In the last three decades, there has been a dramatic increase in the rate of suicide in children and adolescents, and suicide is now the third leading cause of death among adolescents and young adults (Holinger, 1978, 1979, 1980). Identifying the clinical correlates of suicide attempts during childhood and adolescence would provide important information for primary prevention, early intervention, and treatment.

Friedman and colleagues (1982) report that 69% of their adolescent inpatients diagnosed with primary dysthymia attempted suicide. This is similar to the inpatients with major depression who attempted suicide (67%) and higher than those diagnosed with secondary dysthymia (50%).

Using the lethality of suicide attempt measures on the Schedule for Affective Disorders and Schizophrenia (SADS) (Endicott & Spitzer, 1978), Friedman and colleagues (1982) divided their patients according to minimal to mild attempt or severe to extremely lethal attempt. Seventy-five percent ($N = 3$ of 4) of the secondary dysthymics who attempted suicide and 72% ($N = 8$ of 11) of the primary dysthymics who attempted suicide made only minimal to mild suicide attempts. Fifty percent ($N = 5$ of 10) of the probands with major depression who attempted suicide made minimal to mildly lethal attempts, and 20% ($N = 2$ of 10) made attempts that were severe to extremely lethal. No proband with secondary dysthymia made a severe or extreme suicide attempt, and only 1 of the 11 primary dysthymics who attempted suicide made a severe or extreme attempt.

Another study (Robbins & Alessi, 1985) reports that of 9 adolescent patients diagnosed with dysthymia, 7 did not attempt suicide, 1 made two or more attempts, and 1 made a medically serious suicide attempt. Of the 4 cyclothymic adolescents, 2 made two or more suicide attempts.

EPIDEMIOLOGY

There are no published epidemiologic studies of the prevalence of dysthymia in children. The only work that approximates this was done by Kashani and colleagues (1983). They reported that the current point prevalence of RDC minor depression in 189 children 9 years old in New Zealand was 2.5%, and the cumulative lifetime incidence of minor depression was 9.7%. However, since they did not specify the duration of the minor depression, their data cannot be used to estimate the prevalence of dysthymia, since if the duration of the minor depression was less than 1 year, the episode would not meet criteria for dysthymia. We did not find any reports on the prevalence or incidence of childhood cyclothymia in the general population.

For psychiatrically referred populations, the New York Longitudinal Study followed 133 middle-and upper-middle-class individuals from early infancy to early adulthood after they were referred for behavioral problems. Three subjects (2.2%) were diagnosed with DSM-III dysthymic disorder (Chess, Thomas, & Hassibi, 1983).

Kovacs and colleagues' (1984a) prospective follow-up of 65 school-age children (selected if they had a depressive disorder of any type, or adjustment disorder with depressed mood) found that 19 children were diagnosed with dysthymic disorder and no major depression, and 9 had dysthymia and a concomitant major depression at study entry. Twenty-six children were diagnosed with major depression alone.

In a study of 100 adolescent substance users who were interviewed in a youth drop-in counseling center, 16 were diagnosed with concomitant major depressive and dysthymic episodes, 6 with a possible depression, 5 with only dysthymic disorder, and 7 with only major depressive disorder (Kashani, Keller, Solomon, Reid, & Mazzola, 1985).

In another study, 14% of 64 adolescent psychiatric inpatients were diagnosed with dysthymia, and 6% with cyclothymia (Robbins & Alessi, 1985). Friedman and colleagues (1982) report a high percentage (53%) of dysthymic patients in their affective disorder adolescents. One-third of this "dysthymic" cohort, however, are described as atypically depressed, having a dysthymia of less than 1 year's duration (with an average of 4.6 months). Fine, Moretti, Haley, and Marriage (1984) report that 53% of their children and adolescents with a diagnosis of affective disorder were dysthymic, which is 25% of the entire sample.

FAMILIAL PATTERN

In a study of 24 children with affectively ill biological parents, Beardslee, Keller, and Klerman (1985) report that 8% of the children were diagnosed with dysthymic disorder.

The 3 children diagnosed with dysthymia in the New York Longitudinal Study (Chess et al., 1983) had negative family histories for mental illness, but marked chronic stressful life situations and experiences predating the onset of the depression.

In their study of children (ages 15 to 21) of parents with bipolar I disorder, Klein and colleagues (1985, 1986) report that 27% of the offspring had some form of bipolar affective illness, primarily cyclothymia (24%). None of the children of the psychiatric control patients were diagnosed with any form of bipolar illness.

In a 3-year prospective follow-up of 68 referred juvenile offspring or siblings of bipolar patients, 18% were diagnosed dysthymic and 15% cyclothymic at study entry. After 3 years of follow-up, 2 of the 10 dysthymics developed hypomania (Akiskal et al., 1985).

DIFFERENTIAL DIAGNOSIS

The Relationship of Childhood Dysthymia to Major Depression

The DSM-III-R criteria for dysthymia are similar to the criteria for major depression except that the symptoms must persist for at least 1 year for a diagnosis of dysthymia, fewer symptoms are required, and the presence of psychotic features precludes the diagnosis of dysthymia. As in adults, whether childhood dysthymia is qualitatively or quantitatively different from major depression has yet to be established (Keller, Sessa, & Jones, in press).

Keller and Shapiro (1982) coined the term *double depression* to describe patients with a chronic low-grade depressive disorder whose course was punctuated by episodes of major depression superimposed on the underlying disorder that preceded the onset of the major depression by at least 2 years. Kovacs and colleagues (1984a, 1984b) have reported on the occurrence of double depression in their cohort of school-age children. Inclusion criteria for this study were that at intake, or within 2 months of intake, children had to meet DSM-III criteria for major depression (full or partially remitted episode, in either a unipolar or bipolar illness), dysthymia, or adjustment disorder with depressed mood. At study entry, 14% of this depressed cohort were diagnosed simultaneously with episodes of major depression and dysthymia. Major depressive disorder was the most common concomitant diagnosis of children presenting with dysthymia.

Another study (Kashani et al., 1985) reports that 16% of a sample of 100 adolescent substance users who were interviewed in a youth drop-in counseling center presented with double depression. Similar findings have been reported by investigators of adult dysthymic patients. In a study where patients were selected only if they had a major depressive disorder, Keller and Shapiro (1982) found that 26% of adults with a major depressive disorder also had an underlying chronic depression.

Although empirical data are not yet available to establish the relationship between dysthymia and major depression in children or adults, Kovacs and colleagues (1984b) use the following rationale to support their position that major depression and dysthymia in the children should be viewed as two separate entities. They reason that, because dysthymia tends to have an earlier onset than major depression and frequently precedes episodes of major depression, some investigators will suggest that dysthymia is a prodrome to major depression or a developmentally mediated stage in the development of major depression. However, Kovacs and colleagues

(1984b) are of the opinion that this view is challenged by the findings that dysthymia persists after the onset of major depression (Kovacs et al., 1984a) and that the chronic low-grade depression occurs for several years prior to the onset of a major depression. Additionally, although the majority of Kovacs and colleagues' dysthymic children develop a major depression, only 38% of the patients with major depression have an underlying dysthymia (Kovacs et al., 1984a, 1984b). Based on these data, Kovacs and colleagues conclude "that dysthymic disorder and major depressive disorders are related but separately diagnosable psychiatric entities in school-aged children and that dysthymia may 'weaken' the [child] and prepare the ground for major depression" (1984b, p. 648).

In summary, prospective longitudinal studies are needed to assess the reliability and validity of various diagnostic criteria for childhood dysthymia and to understand the relationship of dysthymia and major depression in children.

Dysthymia and Personality Disorders

We could not find any reports on the differential diagnosis of dysthymia and personality disorders in children. As previously discussed, there has been controversy in the adult literature about whether dysthymia is a personality variant or an affective disorder. In addition, because of their enduring problems with guilt, low self-esteem, and poor interpersonal skills, dysthymic adults often are diagnosed as having a concurrent DSM-III-R Axis II personality disorder (Keller et al., in press). Similarly, abnormal personality traits have been observed in children; however, since most systems of nomenclature preclude the diagnosis of a personality disorder in children before age 15, the relationship between early-onset dysthymia and most personality disorders remains speculative in children and adolescents.

Several studies of adolescent and adult dysthymic patients have reported a preponderance of coexisting borderline and antisocial personality disorders (Perry, 1985; Roy, Sutton, & Pickar, 1985). Friedman and colleagues (1982) reported rates of concurrent personality disorder in 24 hospitalized dysthymic adolescents. Although 8 of these 24 patients were chronically depressed for less than 1 year, these investigators did not differentiate between patients with dysthymia as defined in the DSM-III-R and those with a chronic depression of less than 1 year, averaging 4.6 months' duration. Therefore, when referring to their "dysthymic" cohort, Friedman and colleagues (1982) refer to dysthymic and atypically depressed adolescents. Sixteen of this dysthymic group of patients were considered primary dysthymics (patients in whom dysthymia was not preceded by any psychiatric illness other than an affective disorder) and 8 were considered secondary dysthymics (patients in whom dysthymia was preceded by a nonaffective psychiatric illness). Thirty-one percent ($N = 5$ of 16) of the primary dysthymics had a concurrent borderline personality disorder, compared to 25% ($N = 2$ of 8) of the secondary dysthymics who had a concurrent borderline personality disorder. Until data are available to prove otherwise, clinicians and researchers should be aware of the comorbidity of borderline and antisocial personality disorders with dysthymia in children and adolescents.

Comorbidity of Dysthymia with Nonaffective Disorders

Kovacs and colleagues (1984a, 1984b) have described the concurrent diagnoses of dysthymic disorder and nonaffective disorders in children. Ninety-three percent ($N = 26$ of 28) of the children diagnosed with dysthymic disorder also met DSM-III criteria for other conditions. The most common nonaffective disorder was anxiety disorder (36%), followed by attention deficit disorder (14%), and, finally, conduct disorder (11%). Children with major depression and dysthymia were equally likely to present with coexisting nonaffective clinical conditions, although children with adjustment disorder with depressed mood were far less likely to have concurrent disorders.

Because no other study reports on the comorbidity or differential diagnosis of childhood dysthymia, the generalizability of the high proportion of coexisting psychiatric disturbances reported by Kovacs and colleagues (1984a, 1984b) cannot be evaluated. However, with respect to major depression, other studies have reported on the preponderance of coexisting anxiety, attention deficit, and conduct disorders (Carlson & Cantwell, 1980; Puig-Antich, 1982; Puig-Antich, Blau, & Marx, 1978). The high proportion of children with a coexisting anxiety disorder in Kovacs and colleagues' study is similar to that in adult studies, which note a high frequency of anxiety in depressed patients (Roth, Gurney, & Garside, 1972; Woodruff, Guze, & Clayton, 1972).

Reporting on the comorbidity of alcohol and drug abuse in hospitalized adolescents, Friedman and colleagues (1982) found that 55% ($N = 6$ of 11) of patients with primary dysthymia and no concurrent borderline personality disorder had alcohol abuse and 36% ($N = 4$ of 11) had drug abuse, compared to 33% of the secondary dysthymics without a concurrent borderline personality disorder who had concomitant alcohol abuse and 37% who had drug abuse. Primary dysthymics who were concurrently diagnosed with borderline personality disorder showed a 20% rate of alcohol abuse and 40% rate of drug abuse. The two secondary dysthymics with concurrent borderline personality disorder did not show drug or alcohol abuse.

Fine, Moretti, Haley, and Marriage (1985) report that, although conduct and other psychiatric disorders share some depressive features with dysthymia, they "clearly demonstrate less severe depressive features than dysthymic disorder or major depression" (p. 176).

Cyclothymia

There are even fewer published data on the differential diagnosis of cyclothymia and its comorbidity with other disorders in children and adolescents. Given the controversy in the adult literature over whether cyclothymia is an independent diagnosis or a mild form of bipolar affective disorder (Keller, 1987), the paucity of data on the differential diagnosis of childhood cyclothymia is understandable. Furthermore, because of the clinical similarities between cyclothymia and bipolar I and bipolar II disorder, cyclothymia in children and adults remains a difficult differential diagnosis for clinicians.

Klein and colleagues (1985) report that 71% ($N = 5$ of 7) of bipolar patients' offspring who were diagnosed with a nonaffective disorder also received concomitant affective diagnoses (cyclothymia, $N = 3$; bipolar II disorder and dysthymia, $N = 2$). Thirty-six percent ($N = 5$ of 14) of the bipolar offspring with affective diagnoses also exhibited nonaffective disorders, and in all cases except one, the onset of the nonaffective condition preceded the affective disorder. The nonaffective diagnoses given included panic, phobic or generalized anxiety disorder, conduct disorder or antisocial personality, alcoholism, and drug abuse.

In Akiskal and colleagues' (1985) prospective follow-up of 68 bipolar offspring and siblings who were referred to the investigators' mood clinic because of the presence of psychopathologic manifestations, 11 adolescents with poly–substance abuse who did not meet criteria for an affective disorder at study entry were reclassified as having either cyclothymic or dysthymic disorder during follow-up. In this study, it is noteworthy that no patient met the criteria for anxiety neurosis or antisocial personality despite some patients' manifestation of anxiety symptoms and antisocial behaviors. Nearly half of the intake cases presented with mood fluctuations, personality disturbances, and substance abuse that did not meet the criteria for major affective disorder. In comparison to attention deficit disorder, these manifestations were phasic and did not respond to selected somatic treatment, and many subjects with these intermittent clinical features represented a cyclothymic level of affective disturbance (Akiskal et al., 1985).

CLINICAL MANAGEMENT

There have been no controlled, double-blind studies on the treatment of dysthymia and cyclothymia in children. However, there is descriptive information on the levels of psychotherapy and somatotherapy administered to children with dysthymia and cyclothymia in naturalistic studies.

Of Kovacs and colleagues' (1984a) cohort of children with major depression, dysthymia, or adjustment disorder with depressed mood, 63% received treatment during their index episode and 23% had only assessment contacts. Three children received somatic treatment: Two received a short course of imipramine hydrochloride after extended episodes of major depression, and one was prescribed diazepam during the course of dysthymic disorder. The rest of the treated patients received a heterogeneous mixture of psychosocial care with varying durations, frequency of contact, and type, which was administered during different intervals of the course of the disorder. Analyzing their treatment data in two categories, received or did not receive treatment, Kovacs and colleagues (1984a) found no significant differences in recovery rates between treated and untreated cases of dysthymia. However, since the treatments were not controlled this does not allow us to determine the efficacy of treatment.

In Klein and colleagues' (1985) study of the offspring of bipolar patients, 27% ($N = 10$ of 37) received some form of professional treatment. Of those offspring,

4 were diagnosed with cyclothymia and 1 with dysthymia, leading the authors to conclude that the treatment received by this high-risk group was brief and unsystematic.

In an uncontrolled trial of somatotherapy with the referred juvenile offspring and siblings of bipolar patients, Akiskal and colleagues (1985) report that the response to electroconvulsive therapy, tricyclic antidepressants, or lithium carbonate was comparable to the response of adult bipolar patients, although the actual rates of response were not cited. Adolescents receiving treatment in this trial were over 12 years old and had intermittent depressive symptoms or cyclothymic mood swings, with psychosis, suicidal behavior, or incapacitated functioning.

REFERENCES

Akiskal, H.S. (1983). Dysthymic and cyclothymic disorders: A paradigm for high-risk research in psychiatry. In J.M. Davis & J.W. Maas (Eds.), *The affective disorders*. Washington, DC: American Psychiatric Press.

Akiskal, H.S., Djenderedjian, A.M., Rosenthal, R.H., & Khani, M.K. (1977). Cyclothymic disorder: Validating criteria for inclusion in the bipolar affective group. *American Journal of Psychiatry, 134*, 1227–1233.

Akiskal, H.S., Downs, J., Jordan, P., Watson, S., Daugherty, D., & Pruitt, D.B. (1985). Affective disorders in referred children and younger siblings of manic-depressives. *Archives of General Psychiatry, 42*, 996–1003.

Akiskal, H.S., Rosenthal, T.L., Haykal, R.F., Lemmi, H., Rosenthal, R.H., & Scott-Strauss, A. (1980). Characterological depressions: Clinical and sleep EEG findings separating "subaffective dysthymias" from "character-spectrum disorders." *Archives of General Psychiatry, 37*, 777–783.

American Psychiatric Association. (1980). *Diagnostic and statistical manual of mental disorders* (3rd ed.). Washington, DC: Author.

American Psychiatric Association. (1987). *Diagnostic and statistical manual of mental disorders* (3rd ed., rev.). Washington, DC: Author.

Beardslee, W.R., Keller, M.B., & Klerman, G.L. (1985). Children of parents with affective disorder. *International Journal of Family Psychiatry, 6*, 283–299.

Carlson, G.A., & Cantwell, D.P. (1980). Unmasking masked depression in children and adolescents. *American Journal of Psychiatry, 137*, 445–449.

Chess, S., Thomas, A., & Hassibi, M. (1983). Depression in childhood and adolescence: A prospective study of six cases. *Journal of Nervous & Mental Disease, 171*, 411–420.

Cloninger, C.R., Reich, T., & Yokoyama, S. (1983). Genetic diversity, genome organization, and investigation of the etiology of psychiatric diseases. *Psychiatric Developments, 3*, 225–246.

Cytryn, L., McKnew, D.H., & Bunney, W.E. (1980). Diagnosis of depression in children: A reassessment. *American Journal of Psychiatry, 137*, 22–25.

Cytryn, L., McKnew, D.H., Zahn-Wexler, C., Radke-Yarrow, M., Gaensbauer, T.J., Harmon, R.J., & Lamour, M. (1984). A developmental view of affective disturbances in the children of affectively ill parents. *American Journal of Psychiatry, 141*, 219–222.

Depue, R.A., Slater, J.F., Wolfstetter-Kausch, H., Klein, D., Goplerud, E., & Farr, D. (1981). A behavioral paradigm for identifying persons at risk for bipolar depressive disorders:

A conceptual framework and five validation studies. *Journal of Abnormal Psychology*, *90*, 381–437.

Endicott, J., & Spitzer, R. (1978). A diagnostic interview: The schedule for affective disorders and schizophrenia. *Archives of General Psychiatry*, *35*, 837–844.

Fine, S., Moretti, M., Haley, G., & Marriage, K. (1984). Depressive disorder in children and adolescents: Dysthymic disorder and the use of self-rating scales in assessment. *Child Psychiatry & Human Development*, *14*, 223–229.

Fine, S., Moretti, M., Haley, G., & Marriage, K. (1985). Affective disorders in children and adolescents: The dysthymic disorder dilemma. *Canadian Journal of Psychiatry*, *30*, 173–177.

Friedman, R.C., Clarkin, J.F., Corn, R., Aronoff, M.S., Hurt, S.W., & Murphy, M.C. (1982). DSM-III and affective pathology in hospitalized adolescents. *Journal of Nervous & Mental Disease*, *170*, 511–521.

Holinger, P.C. (1978). Adolescent suicide: An experimental study of recent trends. *American Journal of Psychiatry*, *135*, 754–756.

Holinger, P.C. (1979). Violent deaths among the young: Recent trends in suicide, homicide, and accidents. *American Journal of Psychiatry*, *136*, 1144–1147.

Holinger, P.C. (1980). Violent deaths as a leading cause of mortality: An epidemiologic study of suicide, homicide, and accidents. *American Journal of Psychiatry*, *137*, 472–476.

Kashani, J.H., Keller, M.B., Solomon, N., Reid, J.C., & Mazzola, D. (1985). Double depression in adolescent substance users. *Journal of Affective Disorders*, *8*, 153–157.

Kashani, J.H., McGee, R.O., Clarkson, S.E., Anderson, J.C., Walton, L.A., Williams, S., Silva, P.A., Robins, A.J., Cytryn, L., & McKnew, D.H. (1983). Depression in a sample of 9-year-old children: Prevalence and associated characteristics. *Archives of General Psychiatry*, *40*, 1217–1223.

Keller, M.B. (1987). Differential diagnosis, natural course and epidemiology of bipolar disorder. In R.E. Hales & A.J. Frances (Eds.), *Psychiatry update: The American Psychiatric Association annual review* (Vol. 6). Washington, DC: American Psychiatric Press.

Keller, M.B., & Lavori, P.W. (1984). Double depression, major depression and dysthymia: Distinct entities or different phases of a single disorder? *Psychopharmacology Bulletin*, *20*, 399–402.

Keller, M.B., Sessa, F.M., & Jones, L.P. (in press). Chronic depressive disorders. In M.A. Thase, B.A. Edelstein, & M. Hersen (Eds.), *Handbook of outpatient treatment of adults*. New York: Plenum.

Keller, M.B., & Shapiro, R.W. (1982). Double depression: Superimposition of acute depressive episodes on chronic depressive disorders. *American Journal of Psychiatry*, *139*, 438–442.

Klein, D.N. (1974). Endogenomorphic depression: A conceptual and terminological revision. *Archives of General Psychiatry*, *31*, 447–454.

Klein, D.N., & Depue, R.A. (1984). Continued impairment in persons at risk for bipolar affective disorder: Results of a 19-month follow-up study. *Journal of Abnormal Psychology*, *93*, 345–347.

Klein, D.N., Depue, R.A., & Slater, J.F. (1985). Cyclothymia in the adolescent offspring of parents with bipolar affective disorder. *Journal of Abnormal Psychology*, *94*, 115–127.

Klein, D.N., Depue, R.A., & Slater, J.F. (1986). Inventory identification of cyclothymia: IX. Validation in offspring of bipolar I patients. *Archives of General Psychiatry, 43*, 441–445.

Kovacs, M., Feinberg, T.L., Crouse-Novak, M.A., Paulauskas, S.L., Pollock, M., & Finkelstein, R. (1984a). Depressive disorders in childhood: I. A longitudinal prospective study of characteristics and recovery. *Archives of General Psychiatry, 41*, 229–237.

Kovacs, M., Feinberg, T.L., Crouse-Novak, M.A., Paulauskas, S.L., Pollock, M., & Finkelstein, R. (1984b). Depressive disorders in childhood: II. A longitudinal study of the risk for a subsequent major depression. *Archives of General Psychiatry, 41*, 643–649.

Perry, J.C. (1985). Depression in borderline personality disorder: Lifetime prevalence at interview and longitudinal course of symptoms. *American Journal of Psychiatry, 142*, 15–21.

Peselow, E.D., Dunner, D.L., Fieve, R.R., & Lautin, A. (1982). Lithium prophylaxis of depression in unipolar, bipolar II, and cyclothymic patients. *American Journal of Psychiatry, 139*, 747–752.

Puig-Antich, J. (1982). Major depression and conduct disorder in prepuberty. *Journal of the American Academy of Child Psychiatry, 21*, 118–128.

Puig-Antich, J., Blau, S., & Marx, N. (1978). Prepubertal major depressive disorder: A pilot study. *Journal of the American Academy of Child Psychiatry, 17*, 695–707.

Robbins, D.R., & Alessi, N.E. (1985). Depressive symptoms and suicidal behavior in adolescents. *American Journal of Psychiatry, 142*, 588–592.

Roth, M., Gurney, C., & Garside, R.F. (1972). Studies in the classification of affective disorders: The relationship between anxiety states and depressive illness. *British Journal of Psychiatry, 121*, 147–161.

Rounsaville, B.J., Sholomskas, D., & Prusoff, B.A. (1980). Chronic mood disorders in depressed outpatients: Diagnosis and response to pharmacotherapy. *Journal of Affective Disorders, 2*, 73–88.

Roy, A.J., Sutton, M., & Pickar, D. (1985). Neuroendocrine and personality variables in dysthymic disorder. *American Journal of Psychiatry, 142*, 94–97.

Spitzer, R.L., Endicott, J., & Robins, E. (1985). *Research diagnostic criteria (RDC) for a selected group of functional disorders*. New York: New York State Psychiatric Institute.

Turner, W.J., & King, S. (1983). BPD$_2$, an autosomal dominant form of bipolar affective disorder. *Biological Psychiatry, 18*, 63–88.

Weissman, M.M., & Myers, J.K. (1978). Affective disorders in a U.S. urban community: The use of Research Diagnostic Criteria in an epidemiologic survey. *Archives of General Psychiatry, 35*, 1304–1311.

Woodruff, R.A., Guze, S.B., & Clayton, P.J. (1972). Anxiety neurosis among psychiatric outpatients. *Comprehensive Psychiatry, 13*, 165–170.

CHAPTER 17

Somatoform Disorders

JUDITH J. REGAN AND WILLIAM M. REGAN

DEFINITION

Hysteria is a term derived by Hippocrates from the Greek word meaning *"uterus."* It was hypothesized that the condition resulted from the migration of the uterus in widows and spinsters. The assumption of an organic cause continued to be in vogue until Mills wrote in 1890 that "hysteria in children has therefore no morbid anatomy that can be discriminated by either scalpel or microscope. The physical element must enter into the explanation of nearly all cases" (p. 967). Interest peaked in the late nineteenth century when hypnotism was noted to effect some drastic cures. Indeed, it was the painstaking analysis of a case of a hysterical neurosis that Freud employed as a basis for his theories of infantile sexuality.

Unfortunately, the concept of hysteria over time has had little consistency. Conflicting descriptions, observed manifestations, and theoretical approaches have provided little agreement about a consistent coherent entity with objective, well-defined criteria. In fact, the third edition of the *Diagnostic and Statistical Manual of Mental Disorders* (APA, 1980) abandoned the term completely amid significant controversy. Nevertheless, clinicians continue to refer to hysterical phenomena and personality traits.

The DSM-III approached the concept by dividing it into three separate parts representing the alterations in consciousness (dissociative disorders), physical symptomatology (somatoform disorders), and personality characteristics (histrionic) associated with this disorder. According to the DSM-III, somatoform disorders include the following: somatization disorder, conversion disorder, psychogenic pain disorder, and hypochondriasis.

HISTORICAL BACKGROUND

Modern concepts of somatoform disorders originated with Briquet, who thought that the disorder was a dysfunction of the central nervous system. He proposed that symptoms resulted from stressful environmental events that acted on the affective part of the brain in predisposed individuals. In his *Treatise on Hysteria* one of five cases was diagnosed before puberty. The children were noted to be fearful, timid, subject to intense emotional expressiveness, and extremely impressionable (see Mai & Marskey, 1980, 1981). In 1869, Reynolds reported cases in which the loss of function or pain was felt to be a result of an idea that the patient had about his or her own body. Charcot later linked the formulations in stating that the symptoms occurred in those individuals predisposed by heredity (Havens, 1966). He proposed that a traumatic event led to an idea that caused a functional lesion in the brain. Freud, working with Breuer, was the first to use the term *conversion* in a reference to the substitution of a somatic symptom for a repressed idea (Jones, 1953).

Diagnostic descriptions and terminology in regard to conversion disorders have changed markedly over the last 30 years. The original DSM (APA, 1952) described *conversion reactions* as functional symptoms in organs or parts of the body, usually those under voluntary control, due to "conversion" of the impulses causing anxiety. DSM-II (APA, 1968) changed the terminology to *hysterical neurosis, conversion type* and described the phenomenon as an involuntary psychogenic loss or disorder of function. Symbolism, secondary gain, and *la belle indifférence* were considered important elements of the clinical spectrum.

With publication of DSM-III (1980), diagnostic terms once again were changed. Conversion disorder consists primarily of pseudoneurologic symptoms; psychogenic pain disorder consists of a symptom-based disorder the diagnostic criteria for which are similar to those for conversion disorder; and somatization disorder is based on a history of multiple somatic complaints including prior conversion symptoms, sexual symptoms, and unexplained symptoms of pain.

Due to the lack of information and substantiated research of the other somatoform disorders in children and adolescence, our chapter will focus on the somatoform disorder most prominent in children and adolescence: conversion disorder.

While a number of etiologic theories abound regarding conversion disorders, there is a paucity of good studies addressing this issue.

The traditional psychodynamic explanation has been questioned by many authors. In this paradigm the symptom provides a solution to an unconscious conflict (A. Freud, 1976; Rangel, 1959). The conflict is most usually supposed to be between instinctual drives, such as aggression or sexuality, and prohibition by the superego of expression of these instincts. Symptoms expressed are believed to be symbolic of the conflict. Interpretations of conversion symptoms as a need to suffer or identification with a lost object are psychodynamic in origin (Engel, 1970). Looff (1970) found that children with conversion symptoms do have difficulty expressing feelings verbally.

Classical conditioning paradigms also provide a possible explanation for conversion symptomatology. Illness symptoms learned in childhood would be utilized as a coping mechanism (Barr & Abernathy, 1977; Kimball & Blindt, 1982). The use of physical symptoms to solve psychological problems may be transmitted within a family (Leybourne & Churchill, 1972). The importance of imitation and identification with significant persons in symptom formation has been discussed previously (Goodyer, 1980; Rock, 1971). Typically, the patient's symptoms are modeled after those of a physically ill family member. In addition, this mechanism often entails replication of symptoms of an illness the patient had earlier in life. For instance, a child with a seizure disorder may develop pseudo-seizures, and these may be difficult to distinguish from the original disorders. Psychodynamic theory emphasized somatic compliance. That is, the symptom choice was determined by a previous illness or constitutional inferiority of a particular organ function.

Of course, conversion disorders may be used as an acceptable means of reenacting the sick role. The individual can therefore avoid responsibilities and control or manipulate others (Celani, 1976; Haddock, 1967; Rabkin, 1964). Similarly, conversion symptoms may be used to express forbidden feelings or ideas when direct verbal communication for whatever reason is blocked. Hollender (1972) has suggested that the predominance of adult women with conversion disorders relates to the belief that directly expressing intense emotions is "not acting like a lady."

CLINICAL PICTURE

A common psychiatric disorder purported to be associated with conversion is that of the hysterical personality. However, even in adults, data in this regard are inconsistent. It now appears that a variety of personality types are associated, with the passive–dependent and passive–aggressive types being most frequent (Chodoff, 1958). Most authors reviewing conversion disorders in children and adolescents do not describe a typical pattern of histrionic personality traits. In addition, the high ratio of female to male patients does not seem to be borne out in this age group. This finding could be explained by the fact that prepubertal and early adolescent males are less concerned with dependency issues. Therefore, conflict over traditional sex roles may be less important in the development of conversion disorders in children than in adults.

The diagnosis is based on fulfillment of the diagnostic criteria as previously described. Lazare (1981) regards a number of traditional features previously associated with conversion as having no diagnostic value. These include symbolism of the symptom, secondary gain, hysterical personality, and *la belle indifférence*. These conclusions were drawn from a review of adult patients. In the child and adolescent population, variability of the symptoms over time and from one context to another, lack of organic pathology, presence of psychopathology either in the child or family members, identification of a major psychological stress, and susceptibility of the symptoms to suggestion all are reasonable to use in making the diagnosis of conversion. It is fairly clear that emotional unconcern (*la belle indifférence*) is not useful as a diagnostic criterion, per se, in children and in adolescents. Dubowitz and Hersov (1976) comment on its absence in each of their 5 cases. Rock (1971), however, considered it frequently present but felt that the children also demonstrated elements of depression such as low self-esteem and lack of confidence.

Differences in symptomatology in adults versus children and adolescents, while not well studied, are clearly present. Unilateral conversion symptoms in adults are more frequently found on the left side of the body (Galin, Diamond, & Braff, 1977; Stern, 1977), although there are some reports to the contrary (e.g., Fallik & Sigal,

1971). However, in a study of children and adolescents with unilateral conversion, 10 out of 11 children showed symptoms on the right side of the body. The single child with left-sided symptoms was left handed. As such, all of the patients lateralized in the direction of their handedness (Regan & LaBarbera, 1984). Explanations for the finding include Fallik and Sigal's (1971) proposal that conversion symptoms may be more likely to appear on the dominant side, since injuries more frequently occur on this side of the body. Alternatively, children and adolescents may "choose" the dominant limb because such disturbance is more incapacitating. Past clinical reports indicate that children and adolescents with conversion disorders appear to maximize their role as sick and physically disabled (Leybourne, 1972).

ASSOCIATED FEATURES

By present definitions, most conversions are suggestive of disorders of the nervous system, and therefore these patients often present to pediatric neurologists or pediatricians. Symptoms consisting of pain, although previously in the conversion category, are no longer considered to be conversion disorders by DSM-III criteria but remain a subtype of somatoform disorders. Symptoms involving a component of the autonomic nervous system (e.g., psychogenic urinary or fecal retention) have in the past been considered by some to be conversion disorders; however, most clinicians currently exclude these symptoms.

Ocular and neurologic symptoms are the more common presentations of conversion disorders in children and adolescents. Among neurologic symptoms, gait disturbance, weakness, limb malfunction, and pseudo-seizures predominate (Goodyer, 1980; Schneider & Rice, 1979). The range of disturbance can include anesthesias, paresthesias, hearing and visual defects, localized pain, vomiting, dermatographia, and other stigmata (Malmquist, 1971).

Although other psychiatric diagnoses or symptoms are frequently associated with conversion, a significant percentage do not have evidence of associated psychopathology. Folks, Ford, and Regan (1984) found that 44% of their adult conversion patients had no evidence of associated psychopathology. Absence of emotional problems therefore does not rule out the possibility of a conversion disorder.

Children typically are of normal or above-average intelligence (Rock, 1971). With adults, the more primitive and grossly nonphysiologic symptoms are observed in patients of rural background, while the symptoms of better educated population more closely simulate known disease (Ziegler, Imboden, & Meyer, 1960). In addition, adults are more likely to demonstrate poor insight and lower intelligence (Barnert, 1971).

COURSE AND PROGNOSIS

Organic disease is often difficult to distinguish from conversion disorder. Of Caplan's (1970) original sample, diagnosed as hysterical prior to psychiatric admission and investigation, 46% were found on discharge or follow-up to be suffering from an organic condition referable to the original complaint. Slater (1965) outlined the pitfalls of organic disease presenting as hysteria in adults, and Rivinus, Jamison, and Graham (1975) discussed the dangers of childhood neurological conditions being labeled psychiatric. Gatfield and Guze (1962) found neurologic disorder on follow-up in 17% of patients who were diagnosed as having conversion disorders. In another study, Rada, Armstrong, Meyer, and Krill (1973) found macular pathology in 3 of 18 children with visual conversion disorders followed for 1 year. Frequently, despite a typical clinical course during which the patient recovers after appropriate interventions, the possibility of later discovery of organic pathology remains. The initial presentation of the disorder may be identical to a conversion disorder without significant physical, laboratory, or X-ray findings. Adequate medical follow-up is essential to rule out such medical pathology over time. However, in terms of treatment, there is consensus that extensive and complex medical follow-up (with the associated lack of ruling out organic pathology) contributes to the consolidation and prolongation of the symptoms (Goodyer, 1980; Yates & Steward, 1976). Dubowitz and Hersov (1976) have examined the prolongation of symptoms by extensive physical investigation and reluctance to consider a psychiatric diagnosis and have advocated early collaboration between pediatrician and psychiatrist. Indeed, it appears that the participation of physicians and the family's tolerance of regression through illness provide further impetus to maintain the sick role and the associated secondary gains.

Children typically exhibit symptoms that are variable, fluctuate, and do not follow organic pathways. A traumatic event is likely to have occurred prior to the onset of symptomatology (Gross, 1979; Maloney, 1980; Rock, 1971). Spontaneous remission is more likely to occur in milder cases without severe psychological impairment or problem in affect, school performance, or peer relationships. Reassurance and medical suggestions alone commonly lead to rapid improvement. On the other hand, refractory cases are often described as depressed with impaired social relationships and overinvolvement with their families.

COMPLICATIONS

Clearly, a confounding problem in the treatment of conversion disorder is the presence of medical uncertainty. Rock (1971) noted that medical and nursing staff often exhibit considerable resistance to accepting the diagnosis. It is interesting how an ambivalent family is quick to pick up uncertainty in a particular medical staff person. An example is that of a 15-year-old girl with right upper extremity weakness whose family resisted a psychiatric diagnosis. A very well-meaning but overly involved family practitioner referred her for admission to a tertiary referral hospital. The family practitioner himself had been equivocal about the possibility of an organic disorder despite a very adequate workup, including CT, EEG, LP, EMG, and NCVs, all of which were within normal limits. After admission to a pediatric neurology service with a repeated extensive workup, the recommendation was for child psychiatric follow-up. After one outpatient visit the family failed to follow up with psychiatric treatment, returning instead to the family practitioner who at 3 months' follow-up again admitted the patient for diagnostic tests. Again, as Goodyer (1980) has stated, early intervention is indicated to prevent unnecessary physical investigation and symptom prolongation. Proctor's (1958) dismal follow-up results suggest early medical and psychological interventions are critical.

A complicating feature is a new, rarely reported form of child abuse, recently described by Woolcott, Aceto, Rutt, Bloom, and Glick (1982). This consists of an apparently well child being viewed as sick and prevented from functioning by the parent. Such cases are akin to the Munchausen's syndrome of the adult psychiatric community and are more commonly confused with unusual organic diseases than with conversion disorder.

EPIDEMIOLOGY

There is no consensus about the prevalence of conversion disorders in children, due to a number of factors. A wide variety of criteria as well as populations studied have made for an extreme in variance of these disorders. In the adult literature, attention has been paid to defining terminology and constructing an operational definition by which proper clinical studies can proceed (Chodoff, 1974; Guze, 1967; Stephens & Kamp, 1962). Child and adolescent studies are sparse by comparison and have suffered from a lack of clarity over what constitutes a conversion disorder. Various terms have been used throughout the past literature, including *hysteria* and *psychoneurosis*. Robins and O'Neal (1952), in a series of 41 patients followed up over 2 to 17 years, included cases of hypochondriasis and psychoneurosis. Proctor (1958) describes a clinical series of conversion and dissociative reactions that excludes hysterical character disorders but provides no criteria for the distinction. Rock (1971), in a study of 10 cases of "conversion hysteria," provides criteria for diagnosis. He required prominent symptoms (motor or sensory) with no apparent organic basis, onset or exacerbation with an emotionally significant event, and evidence of unconscious need on psychiatric examination.

Estimates of prevalence have varied with type of population studied and methods employed regarding definition. Thus Robins and O'Neal (1953) cite hysteria as being diagnosed in 8% of all psychiatric referrals and 0.08% of inpatients. Proctor (1958) and Forbis and Jones (1965) cite figures of 13% and 17%, respectively, of all cases referred to psychiatry. Caplan's (1970) study considers the overall incidence of hysteria to be less than 1% of inpatients, and Rutter, Graham, Chadwick, and Yule's (1976) epidemiological studies would suggest the diagnosis is rarer than clinicians have previously considered. More recently, the prevalence of conversion symptoms has varied from below 1% (Goodyer, 1981) to 8% (Regan & LaBarbera, 1984) to as high as 13% (Proctor, 1958) in an often quoted study of children referred to a psychiatry unit. Again, these differences can be attributed to the inclusion of dissociative reactions in addition to conversion, conversion alone, referral from a general hospital, psychiatrist referral, and so forth.

In general, there appears to be a higher reporting of conversion disorder from general pediatric, and neurologic samples than from the psychiatric population.

Rada, Meyer, and Kellner (1969) quote Eames as discovering tunnel vision in 9% of 193 schoolchildren, with three-fourths considered to be hysterical. Schneider and Rice (1979) describe conversion disorders in 2% of a pediatric neurology population from the ages of 6 to 19. Maloney (1980) reports an incidence of conversion disorders of 16.7% of pediatric inpatient child psychiatric evaluations. On the other hand, Lewis (1978) identified 5 diagnoses of conversion disorder in 129 requests for child psychiatric outpatient consultations. On inpatient units the incidence has ranged from 0.5% in Goodyer's (1980) sample to 13% in Proctor's (1958) study.

Part of such variability may be due to sociocultural factors. Proctor cites a fundamentalist "Bible Belt" population. Accordingly, Looff (1970) also found higher rates for Appalachian low- and middle-class children than for an urban group matched by age, sex, race, and socioeconomic class. It should be kept in mind, however, that "transient hysterical symptoms" occur normally in the course of development of many youngsters (Malmquist, 1971). Most studies suggest that age of onset is unlikely to be before 5 (Caplan, 1970; Rock, 1971; Stevens, 1969). There have been cases reported before this age, however (Caplan, 1970; A. Freud, 1926; Rock, 1971). Stephens and Kamp (1962) and Caplan (1970) report an equal sex distribution before puberty with an increase in girls in the pubescent and post-pubertal period. Proctor (1958) and Rock (1971) report an equal sex distribution regardless of age. The majority of recent reports indicate a predominance of females, with male predominance only occurring in young children (Goodyer, 1980; Turgay, 1980). A speculative explanation for this pattern holds that conversion symptoms involve the overplaying of passive–dependent and traditionally female personality characteristics (Celani, 1976). If so, female predominance should be less apparent among the elementary-school-age population, in which sex roles are less established than among adolescents.

It is not uncommon for children to develop conversion symptoms that either are transient or respond to pediatric intervention without psychiatric referral. A smaller proportion come to the attention of child psychiatrists in consultation with pediatric colleagues. An even smaller incidence seems to be those children requiring inpatient psychiatric treatment. As such, variability in incidence of reporting is related to severity and duration as well as sociocultural factors.

Both incidence and symptom choice appear related to cultural factors. Both the decline in the incidence of flamboyant symptomatology in the twentieth century and, for example, the high incidence reported by Proctor in the fundamentalist area of North Carolina suggest the large role that education and social class play in conversion symptomatology (Proctor, 1958).

FAMILIAL PATTERN

Family dynamics have been discussed in the pathogenesis of conversion disorders by several writers. Typical family patterns consist of a distant father and overprotective mother (Rock, 1971; Schneider & Rice, 1979; Yates & Steward, 1976). Maloney's

(1980) sample indicated a clinically depressed parent was involved in 85% of his cases as well as a major family crisis existing in 97% at the onset of the symptoms. Logically, considerable attention has been given to grief, object loss, dependency needs, and depression in families of conversion disorder patients.

Celani (1976) emphasizes the interpersonal environment fostering symptom formation. These families are characterized as reinforcing frailty, seductiveness, and passivity in their children. The interpersonal environment is structured to ensure attention and inhibit aggression, thereby fostering dependency and helplessness in the patient.

DIFFERENTIAL DIAGNOSIS

As previously mentioned, physical symptomatology without organic etiology is commonly associated with other psychiatric disorders. Symptoms associated with separation anxiety (headaches, stomachaches, etc.) are typically related to the current stressor and subside either after the separation is effected or when the pressure to separate is lessened. It is most unusual to see an actual loss of function physically in these children with separation anxiety. Likewise, the physical symptoms associated with overanxious disorder bear a direct relation to the anxiety present, and are part of an overall picture of fearfulness. The symptoms presented are usually concomitants of anxiety, such as nausea, tremulousness, and various pains. Depressive disorders in children and adolescents often present with a variety of physical complaints and little in the way of overt affective symptomatology. Lesse (1981), however, postulates the consideration of conversion symptoms as part of a masked depression. Pervasive developmental disorders or psychotic disorders may well present with conversion features. Unusual physical complaints in the absence of organic pathology should trigger a consideration of a psychotic process, necessitating further workup.

Regarding the subclasses of somatoform disorders in the DSM-III classification, the following applies to children and adolescents. Somatization disorder is a chronic, disabling, pervasive syndrome involving many organ systems and multiple medical or surgical interventions. The associated pathology is rare in children and adolescents if present at all. In addition, diagnosis of psychogenic pain disorder and hypochondriasis should also be avoided in childhood and adolescence except when it is a symptom of a conversion disorder. The literature does not support these diagnoses as distinct entities in children, and other diagnoses should be considered (Futterman, 1986). However, psychosomatic symptoms suggestive of somatoform disorders may be found in various other child and adolescent diagnoses. Common disorders that may feature these complaints include separation anxiety disorder, overanxious disorder, dysthymic disorders, and major depressive disorder. In general, it is preferable not to diagnose somatoform disorders in children if a more decisive diagnostic category is possible. For example, a child who develops headaches in anticipation of stressful events is likely to be suffering from an overanxious disorder. Children with separation anxiety disorder commonly will develop somatic symptoms (i.e., headaches, stomachaches) in relation to school attendance. Likewise, a child who develops somatic complaints following the illness or death of a close relative may be diagnosed as suffering an adjustment disorder: Preoccupation with an illness and death may be symptomatic of an affective disorder or overanxious disorder. On the other hand, the entity of true conversion disorder is more often clear and distinct. A conversion disorder should be readily diagnosed in any youngster with somatic symptoms for which there is not a discernible medical explanation (Futterman, 1986).

CLINICAL MANAGEMENT: RESEARCH FINDINGS

A wide variety of treatment techniques have been suggested for conversion disorders. However, an abundance of therapies usually suggests that no one treatment is very effective, and this is the case with conversion disorder. With conversion disorders each treatment approach appears to work to some degree in individual cases. Most authors recommend that the medical workup be limited and carried out as rapidly as possible, so as to avoid fostering secondary gain (Goodyer, 1980; Rock, 1971; Yates & Steward, 1976). A variety of measures have been recommended for symptom removal. Although it was previously held, there are no data indicating that symptom substitution will be a result of symptom removal. Among the therapies are psychotherapy: The cathartic treatment of Anna O. by Breuer was a major event in the development of psychoanalysis (Hollender, 1980). Many patients will have spontaneous remission of symptoms or demonstrate complete recovery after brief psychotherapy (Folks et al., 1984). Reassurance, suggestion, placebos, hypnosis, tranquilizers, biofeedback, reward management, relaxation techniques, behavior modification, faradic stimulation, and others have been reported as effective (Goodyer, 1980; Leybourne & Churchill, 1972; Rada et al., 1969; Schneider & Rice, 1979). The underlying similarity to the approaches just mentioned and a probable key to success is the belief of medical personnel that, in fact, there is no organic disorder. Thus, a tactful "escape" is made available, allowing the patient to give up the symptom after making the symptom unrewarding.

Individual and family therapy are often indicated, and after relief of symptomatology, an assessment needs to be made regarding the degree of psychopathology in the child and family members. Treatment plans should be based on mutually agreed-upon goals rather than necessarily on the previous symptomatology. In Proctor's (1958) series, 92% of the patients terminated treatment unilaterally against medical advice. Since efforts at psychiatric follow-up are rarely followed through, appropriate medical and psychological intervention in the acute phase are essential.

Neurophysiological Component

Early theories of conversion postulated by Briquet and Charcot emphasized biological bases. Psychoanalytic thought preempted the biological consideration until recently. A neurophysiologic component was proposed by Whitlock (1967) and Ludwig (1972) with corticifugal inhibition of afferent stimuli as a mechanism of explaining conversion. Neuropsychological testing of conversion patients demonstrates heightened suggestibility, increased field dependency, and impairment of recent memory and of vigilance and attention (Bendefeldt, Miller, & Ludwig, 1976). The idea that conversion phenomena may be concrete representations of ideas blocked from verbal expression was advanced by Flor-Henry, and associates based on empirical data obtained with the Halstead-Reitan battery of neuropsychological assessment. These data indicate impairment of both dominant and nondominant cerebral hemispheres with relatively greater impairment for the dominant hemisphere (Flor-Henry, Fromm-Auch, Tapper, & Schopflocher, 1981). However, these data are obtained from adult patients, and, while intriguing, they cannot be directly extrapolated to the child and adolescent population at this time due to the lack of similar studies in this age group. Further research needs to be addressed in the realm of biological bases for conversion disorders in children and adolescents.

DSM-III-R

With publication of the DSM-III-R (APA, 1987) the following changes have occurred in categories of somatoform disorders:

1. Body dysmorphic disorder has been added. This condition is described as beginning in adolescence through the third decade of life. This is a preoccupation with some imagined defect in appearance in a normally appearing person.
2. Psychogenic pain disorder has been changed to somatoform pain disorder. A duration of 6 months has been added to the criteria.
3. Atypical somatoform disorder has been changed to undifferentiated somatoform disorder.
4. Somatization disorder and hypochondriasis are listed with minor changes in the diagnostic criteria.

The addition of body dysmorphic disorder will open up areas for new research. It seems to occur early in life and may become a predominant somatoform disorder found in adolescents and children, similar to conversion disorders.

REFERENCES

American Psychiatric Association (1952). *Diagnostic and statistical manual of mental disorders*. Washington, DC: Author.

American Psychiatric Association (1968). *Diagnostic and statistical manual of mental disorders* (2nd ed.). Washington, DC: Author.

American Psychiatric Association (1980). *Diagnostic and statistical manual of mental disorders* (3rd ed.). Washington, DC: Author.

American Psychiatric Assocation (1987). *Diagnostic and statistical manual of mental disorders* (3rd ed., rev.). Washington, DC: Author.

Barnert, C. (1971). Conversion reactions and psychophysiologic disorder: A comparative study. *Psychiatric Medicine, 2,* 205–220.

Bendefeldt, F., Miller, L.L., & Ludwig, A.M. (1976). Cognitive performance in conversion hysteria. *Archives of General Psychiatry, 33,* 1250–1254.

Burr, R., & Abernathy, A. (1977). Conversion reaction—Differential diagnosis in the light of biofeedback research. *Journal of Nervous and Mental Disease, 164,* 287–292.

Caplan, H.L. (1970). *Hysterical conversion symptoms in childhood.* Unpublished dissertation, University of London.

Celani, D. (1976). An interpersonal approach to hysteria. *American Journal of Psychiatry, 133,* 1414–1418.

Chodoff, P. (1974). The diagnosis of hysteria: An overview. *American Journal of Psychiatry, 131,* 1073–1078.

Chodoff, P., & Lyons, H. (1958). Hysteria, the hysterical personality and "hysterical" conversion. *American Journal of Psychiatry, 114,* 734–740.

Dubowitz, V., & Hersov, L. (1976). Management of children with nonorganic (hysterical) disorders of motor function. *Developmental Medicine & Child Neurology, 18,* 358–368.

Engel, G.L. (1970). Conversion symptoms. In C.M. Macbryde (Ed.), *Signs and symptoms: Applied pathologic physiology and clinical interpretation.* Philadelphia: Lippincott.

Fallik, A., & Sigal, M. (1971). Hysteria: The choice of symptom site. *Psychotherapy & Psychosomatics, 19,* 310–318.

Flor-Henry, P., Fromm-Auch, D., Tapper, M., & Schopflocher, D. (1981). A neurophysiological study of the stable syndrome of hysteria. *Biological Psychiatry, 16,* 601–626.

Folks, D.G., Ford, C.V., & Regan, W.M. (1984). Conversion symptoms in a general hospital. *Psychosomatics, 25,* 285–295.

Forbis, O., & Jones, R. (1965). Hysteria in childhood. *Southern Medical Journal, 3,* 1221–1225.

Freud, S. (1958). Management of an analysis of a case of hysteria. In J. Strachey (Ed.), *Collected papers* (Vol. 3). New York: Basic.

Freud, S. (1959). The aetiology of hysteria. In J. Strachey (Ed.), *Collected papers* (Vol. 1). New York: Basic.

Freud, S. (1959). Early studies on the psychical mechanism of hysterical phenomena. In J. Strachey (Ed.), *Collected papers* (Vol. 5). New York: Basic.

Freud, A. (1976). An hysterical symptom in a child of 2 years and 3 months. *International Journal of Psycho-Analysis, 7,* 227–240.

Futterman, E.H. (1986). *Somatoform disorders in children and adolescents.* New York: Basic.

Galin, D., Diamond, R., & Braff, D. (1977). Lateralization of conversion symptoms: More frequent on the left. *American Journal of Psychiatry, 134,* 578–580.

Gatfield, P.D., & Guze, G.B. (1962). Prognosis and differential diagnosis of conversion reaction. *Disorders of the Nervous System, 23,* 623.

Goodyer, I. (1980). Hysterical reactions in childhood. *Journal of Child Pyschology & Psychiatry, 22,* 179.

Gross, M. (1979). Incestuous rape. A cause for hysterical seizures in four adolescent girls. *American Journal of Orthopsychiatry, 29,* 704.

Guze, S.B. (1967). Diagnosis and management of hysterical contracture in children. *American Journal of Psychiatry, 124*, 491–496.

Haddock, S.L. (1967). Hysterical personality traits. *Archives of General Psychiatry, 16*, 750–757.

Havens, L. (1966). Charcot and hysteria. *Journal of Nervous & Mental Disease, 141*, 505–516.

Hollender, M.H. (1972). Conversion hysteria (a post-Freudian reinterpretation of 19th century psychosocial data). *Archives of General Psychiatry, 26*, 311–314.

Hollender, M.H. (1980). The case of Anna O, a reformulation. *American Journal of Psychiatry, 137*, 797–800.

Jones, E. (Ed.). (1953). *The life and work of Sigmund Freud*. New York: Basic.

Kimball, C.P., & Blindt, K. (1982). Some thoughts on conversion. *Psychosomatics, 23*, 647–649.

Lazare, A. (1981). Current concepts in psychiatry: Conversion symptoms. *New England Journal of Medicine, 305*, 745–748.

Leybourne, P., & Churchill, S. (1972). Symptom discouragement in treating hysterical reactions of childhood. *International Journal of Child Psychotherapy, 1*, 111–114.

Lesse, S. (1981). Hypochondria and psychosomatic disorders masking depression in adolescents. *American Journal of Psychotherapy, 35*, 356.

Lewis, M. (1978). Child psychiatric consultation in pediatrics. *Pediatrics, 62*, 359.

Looff, D.H. (1970). Psychophysiologic and conversion reactions in children: Selective incidence in verbal and nonverbal families. *Journal of the American Academy of Child Psychiatry, 9*, 318.

Ludwig, A.M. (1972). Hysteria: A neurobiologic theory. *Archives of General Psychiatry, 27*, 771–777.

Mai, F.M., & Marskey, H. (1981). Briquet's concept of hysteria: An historical perspective. *Canadian Journal of Psychiatry, 26*, 57–63.

Mai, F.M., & Marskey, H. (1980). Briquet's treatise on hysteria: A synopsis and commentary. *Archives of General Psychiatry, 37*, 1401–1405.

Malmquist, C.P. (1971). Hysteria in childhood. *Postgraduate Medicine, 50*, 112.

Maloney, M.J. (1980). Diagnosing hysterical conversion reactions in childhood. *Journal of Pediatrics, 97*, 1016.

Mills, C.K. (1890). Hysteria. In J.D. Keating (Ed.), *Cyclopedia of the diseases of children—Medical and surgical*. Philadelphia: Lippincott.

Proctor, J.T. (1958). Hysteria in childhood. *American Journal of Orthopsychiatry, 28*, 394.

Rabkin, R. (1964). Conversion hysteria as a social maladaptation. *Psychiatry, 27*, 349–363.

Rada, R.T., Krill, A.E., Meyer, G.G., & Armstrong, D. (1973). Visual conversion reaction in children: II. Follow-up. *Psychosomatics, 14*, 271.

Rada, R.T., Meyer, G.G., & Kellner, R. (1969). Visual conversion reaction in children: I. Diagnosis. *Psychosomatics, 10*, 23.

Rangell, L. (1959). The nature of conversion. *Journal of the American Psychoanalytic Association, 7*, 632–662.

Regan, J., & LaBarbera, J.D. (1984). Lateralization of conversion symptoms in children and adolescents. *American Journal of Psychiatry, 141*, 1279–1280.

Reynolds, J.R. (1869). Remarks on paralysis and other disorders of motion and sensation, dependent on idea. *British Medical Journal, 2*, 483–485.

Rivinus, T.M., Jamison, L.L., & Graham, P.M. (1975). Childhood organic neurological disease presenting as psychiatric disorder. *Archives of Disturbed Children, 50*, 115–119.

Robins, E., & O'Neal, P. (1953). Clinical features of hysteria in children with a note on prognosis. *Nervous Children, 10*, 246–271.

Rock, N.L. (1971). Conversion reactions in childhood. A clinical study of childhood neurosis. *Journal of the American Academy of Child Psychiatry, 101*, 65–78.

Rutter, M., Graham, P., Chadwick, O., & Yule, W. (1976). Adolescent turmoil: Fact or fiction. *Journal of Child Psychology & Psychiatry & Applied Disciplines, 17*, 35–36.

Schneider, S., & Rice, D. (1979). Neurologic manifestations of childhood hysteria. *Journal of Pediatrics, 94*, 153.

Slater, E. (1965). Diagnosis of hysteria. *British Medical Journal, 1*, 1395–1399.

Stephens, J.H., & Kamp, M. (1962). On some aspects of hysteria. *Journal of Nervous & Mental Disease, 134*, 305–309.

Stern, D.B. (1977). Handedness and the lateral distribution of conversion reactions. *Journal of Nervous & Mental Disease, 164*, 122–128.

Stevens, H. (1969). Conversion hysteria revisited by the pediatric neurologist. *Clinical Proceedings of Childrens Hospital, 25*, 27–32.

Turgay, A. (1980). Conversion reactions in children. *Psychiatric Journal of the University of Ottawa, 5*, 287–294.

Whitlock, F. (1967). The aetiology of hysteria. *Acta Psychiatrica Scandinavica, 43*, 144–162.

Woollcott, P., Aceto, T., Rutt, C., Bloom, M., & Glick, R. (1982). Doctor shopping with the child as proxy patient: A variant of child abuse. *Journal of Pediatrics, 101*, 297.

Yates, A., & Steward, M. (1976). Conversion hysteria in childhood, a case report and a reminder. *Clinical Pediatrics, 15*, 379.

Ziegler, F., Imboden, J., & Meyer, E. (1960). Contemporary conversion reaction: A clinical study. *American Journal of Psychiatry, 116*, 901–909.

CHAPTER 18

Substance Use Disorders

M. JEROME FIALKOV

DEFINITION

Diagnosis and classification of substance use disorders reflect prevailing cultural attitudes and theoretical biases. In recent times, these disorders have been recognized as independent and discrete diagnostic entities separate from other psychiatric conditions. In the third edition of the *Diagnostic and Statistical Manual of Mental Disorders* (DSM-III) (APA, 1980) nine separate classes of substances are listed as causes of substance use disorders: (1) alcohol; (2) barbiturates or similarly acting sedatives or hypnotics; (3) amphetamines or similarly acting sympathomimetics; (4) opioids; (5) cannabis; (6) cocaine; (7) phencyclidine (PCP) or similarly acting arylcyclohexylamines; (8) hallucinogens; and (9) tobacco. Each class of substances is designated as producing abuse, dependence, or both.

The substance use disorders are distinguished from the substance-induced organic mental disorders. The term *substance use disorders* refers to the maladaptive behavior associated with more or less regular use of the substances, while the substance-induced organic mental disorders describe the direct acute or chronic effects of these substances on the central nervous system, be they behavioral, cognitive, motor, or physiological (e.g., intoxication or withdrawal). However, the distinction between the substance-induced organic mental disorders and substance use disorders is, in practice, rather blurred.

For most classes of substances, but by no means all, pathological use results in both abuse and dependence. According to DSM-III, substance abuse is the pattern of pathological use for at least 1 month that causes impairment in social or occupational functioning. To distinguish substance abuse from nonpathological use, a pattern of pathological use must be demonstrated by the user's maladaptive behavior relative to the substance used. Criteria established to determine pathological use include the user's inability to diminish or stop use; intoxication throughout the day; repeated but unsuccessful efforts to control use through periods of temporary abstinence or by restriction of substance ingestion to certain times of the day; continued substance

The author acknowledges Maureen Fialkov for her unwavering support and secretarial assistance and William Suvak for the bibliography.

use despite serious physical disability known by the subject to be exacerbated by use of the substance; and need of the substance for adequate functioning or complications resulting directly from excessive substance use (e.g., alcoholic blackouts, opioid overdose).

For substance dependence to be diagnosed, evidence of tolerance or withdrawal must be present. Almost invariably a pattern of pathological use precedes the diagnosis of substance dependence and causes impairment in social or occupational functioning, although, less frequently, the disorder can be limited to a physiological dependence (as in the neonatal withdrawal syndrome). *Tolerance* refers to the markedly increased quantity of the substance required to achieve the desired effect or, conversely, the markedly diminished effect resulting from the regular use of the same quantity. There is considerable individual variability in the amount of the substance required to achieve the desired effect. For this reason, the determining feature of tolerance is the individual's report of marked increase in quantity of the substance consumed over time to achieve intoxication. *Withdrawal* results from discontinuation of or reduction in intake of a substance previously regularly used by the individual to induce a physiological state of intoxication. *Physical dependence* is the altered physiological state produced by the repeated administration of a substance to prevent the appearance of a syndrome characteristic for each substance—the withdrawal or abstinence syndrome. These are general phenomenological syndromes that can be further subclassified according to etiology, in this case by the substance involved.

Because most children and younger adolescents use substances relatively rarely, physical dependence and associated chronic syndromes are infrequent occurrences. Adolescents exhibit evidence of pathological use but often do not meet the DSM-III criteria for abuse, although they often show impairment in academic (occupational) and, to a lesser extent, social functioning. Intoxication is the most frequent substance-induced disorder occurring among adolescent drug users. Recurrent bouts of intoxication of sufficient severity, frequency, and intensity are evidence of substance abuse and the harbinger of dependence. It is this type of ambiguity that creates confusion in diagnosis and early treatment of adolescent drug users.

HISTORY

Alcohol is the oldest documented compound of abuse. Records discussing its disabling effects and its control date back to Egypt and Mesopotamia. Widespread drinking occurred in early Greece and Rome, prompting considerable efforts to enforce moderation. The ancient world does not seem to have experienced any other significant drug use problem (see Austin, 1979, for details).

Beginning in the sixteenth century, however, psychoactive substance use began to rise and so did concern over abuse. This was the era of exploration and colonization that brought contact with new peoples who used new substances: tobacco, coca, cocoa, and cassina from the New World; coffee from Arabia and Turkey; the kola nut from Africa; and tea from China. Western explorers and travelers in their turn carried both old and new substances to the rest of the world. Technological developments in alcohol distillation and coffee bean roasting further helped by making these substances more readily available and pleasant to consume and less expensive. Advances in distillation made it possible to increase the potency of alcoholic beverages 400 to 500% (from 14% to 50% or more in alcoholic content), making it easier to get drunk, liberating humanity from dependency on viticulture and from the difficult transportation of wine and beer. As illustrated by the London gin epidemic and the widespread use of spirits in the American west, readily available cheap spirits under certain sociocultural conditions could have disastrous results.

While relatively little information is available on youth drug abuse prior to the 1950s and 1960s, the political upheaval and social crises of that era brought the drug problem to the awareness of U.S. society at large. In the 1950s marijuana use was popularized by "beat generation" author Jack Kerouac. In the 1960s it gained widespread popularity among college and high school students. Since the 1970s the use of marijuana has transcended all social strata and all age groups—the estimated number of regular users of marijuana in the United States in the 1980s ranges from 16 to 30 million.

The late 1950s and 1960s also saw a rash of fad drugs whose popularity quickly waned. In 1959, there was a craze for glue sniffing among young people, particularly boys in the age range of 13 to 15. LSD, used as an adjunct to psychotherapy in the 1950s, was popularized in the 1960s particularly as a result of proselytizing by Dr. Timothy Leary. Phencyclidine started out as an anesthetic but soon became popular with adolescents as PCP or "angel dust." Methaqualone or Quaalude came into general use as a "downer" but has since been withdrawn from the market. Amyl nitrite became popular among homosexual groups, where it was used to postpone and enhance orgasm during sexual intercourse.

Amateur and professional athletics were plagued by drug abuse to the extent that in 1976 the Olympic Games authorities required urinalysis of medal winners and other selected entrants. By 1983 there were mass disqualifications at the Pan American Games for the use of anabolic steroids, a synthesized form of the male hormone testosterone.

At the end of World War II, the new United Nations adopted a protocol that brought drug control under the jurisdiction of the World Health Organization (WHO), still the most important international agency in the field. From 1948 to 1964 the agency spearheaded a series of agreements that severely limited international trade in opium and restricted legal trade in cocaine and marijuana to supplies necessary for medical and scientific usage. Today, WHO continues to collect the most reliable worldwide statistics on drug abuse, including alcoholism.

Over the past 100 years, the terminology used to describe the substance use disorders has been repeatedly revised as concepts about the nature of chronic substance-using behavior have evolved. In 1964 the World Health Organization (WHO) Expert Committee on Addiction-Producing Drugs recommended substitution of the term *drug dependence* for the terms *addiction* and *habituation*. The WHO formulation made it necessary to define dependence on each variety of drug separately and implied an important distinction between psychic and physical dependence. This terminology was in common use until publication in 1980 of DSM-III, which divided substance use disorders into two major categories: abuse and dependence.

The WHO memorandum on nomenclature and classification of drug- and alcohol-related problems (Edwards, Arif, & Hodgson, 1981) defined drug dependence as a syndrome manifested by a behavioral pattern in which the use of a given psychoactive drug, or class of drugs, is given much higher priority than other behaviors that once had higher value. The dependence syndrome, however, should be regarded not as a discrete entity but as occurring along a continuum. The WHO Task Force suggested a syndromal approach to diagnosis based on operational criteria of a cognitive, behavioral, and physiological nature, which need not all be present at the same time nor with the same intensity. This model followed a provisional description provided by Edwards and Gross (1976) for the alcohol dependence syndrome consisting of seven essential elements involving both biologic process and learning. These key elements were incorporated into the proposed criteria for DSM-III-R (Rounsaville, Spitzer, & Williams, 1986).

Little if any research has addressed the relevance of this concept of the dependence syndrome for adolescents and children. Adolescents who meet these criteria are likely to be in an advanced stage of the dependence syndrome. Preadolescents and adolescents at risk for substance abuse need to be identified early in the course of the syndrome. However, the relationship of susceptibility to the onset of substance use disorders in this age group remains unclear and was not incorporated into the DSM-III criteria.

CLINICAL PICTURE

All psychoactive substances are capable of causing intoxication, each induces a psychological dependence, and all are self-administered to attain an optimal state of well-being (Jaffee, 1980). Clinical presentation of psychoactive substance use can be reduced to the following responses: intoxication, toxic reactions, panic reactions, flashback phenomena, psychotic reactions, organic mental disorder, and withdrawal (or abstinence) syndrome (Lipowski, 1975; Schuckit, 1985). While researchers tend to focus on individual psychoactive substances in their study of drug effect, clinicians have noted that most reactions in clinical practice follow multiple substance use (Clayton, 1986; Cohen, 1981).

Intoxication is the most common clinical presentation of substance use (Cohen, 1986a). Two kinds of intoxication can be identified. The most common form includes the cerebellar signs of gait ataxia, slurred speech, poor coordination, and nystagmus. The central nervous system (CNS) depressants such as alcohol and the sedative hypnotics, phencyclidine, and the volatile solvents are mostly responsible for this type of intoxication. A second kind of intoxication involves the sympathomimetic-type drugs such as the amphetamines and cocaine, hallucinogens, and cannabis, in which the cerebellar signs are minimal but the alterations in perception, cognition, and emotion are evident. Opiate intoxication is somewhere between the two types in terms of symptomatology. Behavioral manifestations of substance-induced intoxication are reflected in loquacity, psychomotor retardation, irritability, poor memory, short attention span, restlessness, increased physical and sexual aggression, poor judgment, and impulsivity.

Intoxication lies along a continuum extending from sober consciousness to intoxication of varying intensity, including delirium, convulsions or coma, and possibly death. *Toxic reactions* are really overdoses occurring when the individual has taken excessive amounts of the drug so that the body support systems no longer function adequately (Schuckit, 1985). Clinically, the individual will present with unstable vital signs. Life-threatening overdoses are most often associated with the CNS depressants, opioids, phencyclidines, and some inhalable solvents.

Alcohol idiosyncratic intoxication, formerly called pathological intoxication, is a variant of the alcohol intoxication state. This condition manifests itself as a maladaptive behavioral response, often in the form of assaultive behavior following ingestion of an amount of alcohol insufficient to induce intoxication in most people. There is usually a subsequent amnesia for the period of intoxication. The behavior is said to be atypical for the individual. Some individuals with this disorder are said to have abnormal electroencephalograms (EEG) associated with a past history of head trauma or encephalitis. The medicolegal aspect of crimes committed during an incident of idiosyncratic intoxication is usually viewed with some skepticism by the courts, since evasion of responsibility may be suspected with claims that alcohol precipitated the seizurelike episode.

Panic reactions usually occur in naive users who have typically taken marijuana, hallucinogen, or a stimulant for the first time. Shortly after ingestion of the drug and with onset of the drug effect the individual develops an acute fear of losing control, of having done physical harm to himself or herself, or of going "crazy." Physical findings reflect fear, anxiety, and sympathetic nervous system overactivity, manifesting as tachycardia, increased respiratory rate, elevated blood pressure, slightly dilated pupils, and excessive perspiration.

The *flashback* phenomenon is the unwanted recurrence of drug effects usually as a result of cannabis or hallucinogen use. Other related drugs with the potential include Ketamine (a hallucinatory anesthetic resembling PCP), morning glory seeds, and large amounts of amphetamines (Cohen, 1977). Flashbacks occur suddenly and unexpectedly with full intensity. They usually last for only a few minutes but may persist several hours.

Patients may experience flashbacks after a single ingestion, but usually there is a history of many ingestions. They may recur occasionally or as frequently as several times per day. Shick and Smith (1970) divided flashbacks into three categories: perceptual flashbacks; somatic flashbacks; and emotional flashbacks. The perceptual flashbacks are the most common, with the somatic and emotional flashbacks the most distressing. They are almost always accompanied by an acute panic reaction. The perceptual flashbacks are most often visual, although any sensory modality may be affected. Visual phenomena include intensification of colors, visual illusions such as halo effects, shimmering, pseudo-hallucinations (the appearance of geometric forms and figures that the patient realizes are not there), and occasionally true hallucinations of insects or animals. Patients may experience frequent spontaneous visual imagery. The somatic flashbacks consist of feelings of depersonalization in which the patient's body or body parts feel unnatural, unreal, or foreign and may be accompanied by numbness, paresthesia, or pain. Emotional flashbacks are often the most upsetting and consist of a recreation of very distressing emotions associated with the original hallucinogenic experience. These emotions include loneliness, panic, or depression, and may be so intense that the patient becomes suicidal. The individual may also complain of a mild altered time sense similar to the slowing of the perception of time under the influence of the hallucinogen.

With *psychotic reactions,* the drug user loses contact with reality and experiences hallucinations and/or delusions in the midst of a clear sensorium with stable vital signs and no evidence of withdrawal symptoms or signs. Although these symptoms are quite dramatic, they usually are self-limiting and tend to disappear over the course of several days or weeks (Wilford, 1982). Drug-induced psychotic reactions are usually seen in individuals who have repeatedly consumed CNS depressants, stimulants, hallucinogens, phencyclidines, and cannabinoids. Most of these drug-induced states last for a day to a week at most and are usually totally reversible (with the exception of psychoses induced by phencyclidine and STP). The hallucinations tend to be auditory rather than visual and are often accusatory in nature. In the case of stimulant (amphetamine) psychosis there may also be haptic (tactile) hallucinations in which the individual feels things crawling on him or her (formication). These are also experienced in cocaine and alcohol withdrawal states. Paranoid states of jealousy, suspiciousness, and ideas of reference are also frequently observed. The existence of a cannabis psychosis is controversial in the United States, although a common reason for referral to mental hospitals in countries such as Morocco and India (Chopra & Smith, 1974; Thacore, 1973).

Large doses of almost any psychoactive drug can cause an *organic state* marked by confusion, disorientation, and an overall decrease in mental functioning along with stable vital signs but the absence of signs of withdrawal. At very high levels, the physical signs and symptoms of a toxic overdose predominate. The drugs most often associated with this condition are the CNS depressants, stimulants, solvents, and phencyclidines (Schuckit, 1985). The organic brain syndrome in the case of the CNS depressants, including alcohol and barbiturates, can occur as part of intoxication or overdose or during withdrawal. Adolescents on barbiturates for epilepsy may have insufficient medication and go into a withdrawal state or, if suicidal, may take an overdose. Alcohol, on the other hand, the most frequently used drug by adolescents, can have both acute and chronic effects, causing mental confusion and clouding of consciousness through its direct effect as in intoxication and indirect consequences of alcohol intake, such as trauma (e.g., subdural hematoma) or metabolic disturbances (e.g., hypoglycemia).

The *withdrawal or abstinence syndrome* consists of the development of physiological and psychological symptoms when psychoactive substances are discontinued too quickly. Four types of withdrawal (or abstinence) phenomena are identified according to etiology (Cohen, 1986b): CNS depressants; opiates; stimulants; and a miscellaneous group that includes cannabis, nicotine, and certain other psychoactive agents. Adolescents rarely develop physical dependence or withdrawal symptoms.

The fetus of the pregnant woman who uses narcotics, sedative hypnotics, or psychotomimetic or stimulant drugs is inevitably exposed to these drugs in utero and thus to the possibility of their toxic or addicting effects. Birth of the child of an addicted mother can precipitate a withdrawal state (Finnegan, 1979). In the late 1950s the great majority of cases were due to heroin. More recently, methadone has come into widespread use and has become the predominant drug responsible for withdrawal symptoms in neonates.

The most commonly observed signs and symptoms of neonatal narcotic withdrawal are tremors, high-pitched cry, hyperactivity, irritability, sneezing, increased muscle tone, frantic sucking of the fists, and regurgitation. The onset of the symptoms in the large majority of cases is between 4 and 24 hours of age and is unusual after 72 hours. Methadone withdrawal appears within the first 2 or 3 days of life, although there have been reported cases of onset delayed as long as 2 weeks or more. It is possible that other substances such as barbiturates or diazepam may also be involved. Chronic heavy alcohol use by the mother, in addition to causing possible teratogenic effects, may result in a neonatal abstinence syndrome (Nichols, 1967; Pierog, Chandavasu, & Wexler, 1977; Schaefer, 1962). Hingson and colleagues (1982) found that marijuana users were more likely than nonusers to have offspring with withdrawallike symptoms (tremors and high-pitched cry) that were attributable to maternal marijuana use rather than nicotine or alcohol. The changes disappear after a month. Thus if used during pregnancy marijuana constitutes a serious health hazard.

ASSOCIATED FEATURES

The associations between psychoactive substance use disorders and psychiatric conditions in adolescence and young adulthood are complex and variable. Psychiatric disorders may cause substance use, result from substance use, or be a chance association—a temporal association between substance use and the onset of a psychiatric disorder does not imply any cause–effect relationship. Substance use may precipitate an independent psychiatric disorder such as schizophrenia, paranoid state, or affective disorder in a predisposed individual or be the result of a psychiatric illness with attempts at self-medication with alcohol or amphetamines (Khantzian, 1985).

There is a strong relationship between illicit psychoactive substance use and psychiatric disorder in adolescents. At age 16 years, 59% of girls and 44% of boys referred to psychiatric clinics were reported by their parents to use drugs or alcohol as compared to only about 10% of demographically matched, nonreferred 16-year-olds (Achenbach & Edelbrock, 1981). Factor analysis of behavior problems for the referred group showed that alcohol and drug use was correlated primarily with the syndrome of delinquent behavior (conduct disorder) (Achenbach, 1978; Achenbach & Edelbrock, 1979). Other epidemiological studies have confirmed this association between delinquency and substance use (Clayton, 1981; Elliott, Huizinga, & Ageton, 1985; Kandel, Davies, Karus, & Yamaguchi, 1986).

Substance abuse (including alcohol abuse) is common among incarcerated delinquents, most of whom have conduct disorder as a primary or secondary diagnosis (Fialkov, 1984; McManus, Alessi, Grapentine, & Brickman, 1984). In a retrospective study of 41 consecutively admitted adolescent outpatients not initially diagnosed as suffering from substance use disorders, 59% had associated conduct disorder (Roehrich & Gold, 1986). In a study of adolescent alcohol abusers attending an emergency room, 30% of males and 18% of the females were diagnosed as having conduct disorder (Reichler, Clement, & Dunner, 1983). Conduct disorder and behavioral disturbances in childhood precede the initiation of drug use in adolescence and are often associated with learning problems in school, low self-esteem, depressive mood, and rebelliousness (Kandel, 1982; Kaplan, 1980; Paton, Kessler, & Kandel, 1977).

Studies carried out among adults have shown that alcohol and psychoactive substances are used to cope with affective disorder (Mirin & Weiss, 1986). In an adolescent psychiatric population receiving inpatient intervention, one-third were assigned a diagnosis of major affective disorder (Semlitz & Gold, in press). Depression was most commonly associated with alcohol abuse on an emergency service (Reichler et al., 1983). One-third of the substance abusers attending a youth counseling center included significantly more depressed individuals than the general population (Kashani, Keller, Solomon, Reid, & Mazzola, 1985). Sixteen percent suffered from a "double depression," with a chronic type of depression persisting more than a year superimposed on a major depression. These depressed adolescents may also suffer from an underlying conduct disorder (primary or secondary) associated with substance use. Treatment with an antidepressant of this subgroup of individuals may be of relevance (Puig-Antich, 1982).

It has been suggested that the coexistence of hyperactivity, attentional deficits, and impulsivity is characteristic of individuals at high risk for alcoholism (Alterman & Tarter, 1983; Wood, Wender, & Reimherr, 1983). Hyperactive adolescents have been shown to consume alcohol more frequently than controls (Blouin, Bornstein, & Trites, 1978; Mendelson, Johnson, & Stewart, 1971), although other studies of somewhat larger samples appear to contradict those findings (Feldman, Denhoff, & Denhoff, 1979; Loney, Kramer, & Milich, 1981). Nevertheless, other investigations suggest that, in general, hyperactives and controls are comparable in their drug and alcohol use and hyperactivity (attention deficit disorder) per se does not lead to increased risk for alcoholism in adulthood (Alterman & Tarter, 1986; Weiss & Hechtman, 1986), nor does stimulant treatment in childhood predispose these individuals to greater substance use in adulthood (Laufer, 1971; Milman, 1979; Weiss & Hechtman, 1986). However, hyperactivity coupled with aggression appears to be a powerful predictor of future substance use (Eyre, Rounsaville, & Kleber, 1982; Loney, 1980) and of a poor outcome to treatment for the condition in adulthood (Gittelman, Mannuzza, Shenker, & Bonagura, 1985).

COURSE AND PROGNOSIS

For most individuals, initial experimentation and subsequent, more regular patterns of use typically develop during early adolescence. This occurs in a relatively ordered fashion: first experimentation with coffee and tea, followed sequentially by wine or beer, tobacco and/or hard liquor, marijuana, and other illicit drugs (hallucinogens, stimulants, depressants, and narcotics) (Hamburg, Kraemer, & Jahnke, 1975; Kandel, 1975). Adolescents rarely proceed directly from the "gateway drugs" (tobacco, beer, and wine) to illicit drugs such as heroin and cocaine without the intermediate steps of using hard liquor and marijuana (Donovan & Jessor, 1983; Kandel, 1975). This is not absolute; in some communities inhalants may be the first substances abused by children.

The usual range for initiating and using drugs is between the ages of 14 and 21, peaking at about 18 years and then declining sharply. The pattern of cocaine use is different, showing later initiation of use, which continues to rise in young adulthood (Johnston, O'Malley, & Bachman, 1986; Kandel & Yamaguchi, 1985). The rates for initiation for prescribed and nonmedical use of psychoactive substances (the minor tranquilizers, sedatives, and stimulants) also tend to increase in young adulthood.

The years of intensive use of alcohol and illicit drugs correspond to the period in which most individuals prepare for their adult roles in life by completing their education, obtaining employment, and entering into marriage and parenthood (Kandel, Davies, Karus, & Yamaguchi, 1986). Among both men and women, use of marijuana and other illicit drugs in adolescence correlates with subsequent job instability, instability of marriage, resulting in an increased rate of divorce or separation, and participation in at least one type of delinquency in the preceding 12 months. An adolescent drug use pattern also predicted a negative health outcome (being ill in bed within the previous year). Adolescent drug use also has an effect on psychological functioning in young adulthood, with an increased rate of depressive mood and psychosomatic symptoms. This suggests that in adulthood increased use of prescribed psychotropic medication may be related to psychological distress (Kandel & Yamaguchi, 1985).

In summary, youth who initiate substance use before age 15 are at increased risk for drug disorders in young adulthood. Antisocial and alcoholic relatives in association with personal alcohol problems, heavy tobacco use, antisocial behavior, depression, and anxiety increase the risk of substance use disorders, particularly if they were present before age 15. Nevertheless, it is difficult to predict which drug users are likely to progress from use to problem use (Robins & Przybeck, 1985).

IMPAIRMENT

Chronic ingestion of heavy doses of alcohol is associated with a number of organic changes, some of which can be irreversible. These physical and neurological consequences generally occur in young and middle adulthood (Tarter & Van Thiel, 1985).

Prolonged use of stimulants may lead to cerebrovascular changes, and investigators have reported cerebral hemorrhages, subarachnoid bleeding, subdural hematomas, and vascular lesions resembling periarteritis nodosa (Connell, 1958). There is also some anecdotal evidence of decreased intellectual ability and concentration due to chronic stimulant use (Grant, Mohns, Miller, & Reitan, 1976; Grant et al., 1978).

Numerous clinical reports from several countries have described heavy, chronic cannabis users who exhibit behaviors that some observers have labeled *amotivational syndrome* (Kolansky & Moore, 1972; McGlothlin & West, 1968). Included in the various descriptions of this syndrome are the following characteristics: apathy; reduced drive and ambition; impaired ability to carry out complex tasks; failure to pursue long-term plans; reduced tolerance to frustration; diminished communication skills; neglect of personal appearance; and sluggish mental responses. The syndrome takes several weeks to clear after the termination of drug administration, suggesting that the symptoms are due to CNS changes rather than the continued presence of cannabis. Other psychoactive substances such as alcohol, sedative-hypnotics, and opiates are thought to be responsible for causing a similar amotivational state, essentially due to chronic intoxication. Few definitive studies have been conducted to determine whether chronic substance use affects educational attainment or motivation in college or career training (Mellinger, Somers, Davidson, & Manheimer, 1976). Reduction in college aspirations tends to precede rather than to follow the initiation into illicit drugs other than marijuana (Kandel, 1981).

Whether consistent marijuana use produces microscopic or macroscopic alterations in brain structure has been variably answered. Animal studies have revealed long-lasting impairment of learning ability after a period of chronic cannabis treatment (Negrete, 1982), in addition to structural changes such as cerebral atrophy after long-term oral administration of cannabis (McGahan, Dubin, & Sassenrath, 1984). This raises the possibility of residual cerebral damage in human chronic cannabis users. One recent controlled study revealed decreased, regional cerebral blood flow in male chronic cannabis users, which returned to normal levels after an extended period of abstinence (Tunving, Thulin, Risberg, & Warkentin, 1986). With the more potent marijuana currently available, it is possible that serious physical consequences of chronic cannabis use will become more prevalent.

Volatile solvents have particular relevance for youth; they may be the initial drug abused by grammar school and junior high school students. Frequently individuals abusing solvents present with a rapid onset of confusion and disorientation. Electroencephalographic findings were similar (Christiansson & Karlsson, 1957) to the stage 2–stage 3 electroencephalographic changes of delirium as originally reported by Romano and Engel (1944). Only a minority of youth using volatile solvents on a long-term basis display neurological symptoms. In the majority they are quickly reversible and are likely to be due to transient rather than permanent brain changes. Persistent effects have been reported in some cases of volatile substance abuse. Cerebellar signs, such as nystagmus, titubating gait, ataxia, and tremor of the limbs, have been caused by chronic toluene abuse. The cerebellar signs were significantly correlated with the width of cerebellar sulci and superior cerebellar cisterns on CT scan (Fornazzari, Wilkinson, Kapur, & Carlen, 1983). Permanent neuropsychological deficits have not been convincingly confirmed by available research (Ron, 1986).

COMPLICATIONS

Adolescents predisposed to become dependent on psychoactive substances often suffer with psychiatric disturbances and painful affect states. The psychoactive substance use serves a "prosthetic" function, helping them to regulate and modulate feelings of self-esteem, relationships, and behavior (Weider & Kaplan, 1969; Wurmser, 1974). Their substance use results in withdrawal from family, friends, school, work, and recreational pursuits. They tend to experience low self-esteem and overwhelming feelings of despair, rage, or shame. Illegal activities pursued in support of their drug habit may result in promiscuous sexual activity, with concomitant increased risk of premature pregnancy, venereal disease, malnutrition, or physical abuse. These adolescents may drop out of school and become involved increasingly in delinquent activities and the associated deviant peer relationships that reinforce escalating use of more potent psychoactive substances (Niven, 1986).

Physical complications include trauma, overdose, withdrawal syndromes, and the complications of parenteral drug use. Trauma and overdose are by far the most common in adolescents. Trauma is a consequence of accidents, suicide attempts, or assaults related to drug abuse. All psychoactive substances impair psychomotor performance for complex tasks and have special implications for driving accidents. In a study of males, 15 to 34 years, who died in motor vehicle accidents, one or more drugs were found in the blood of 81% of the victims. Alcohol was detected in 70%, cannabinoids in 37%, and cocaine in 11%. Cannabinoids were found in combination with alcohol in 81% of the cases (Williams, 1985).

Overdose of psychoactive substances, both intentional and accidental, frequently involves ingestion of more than one substance. Accidental overdose occurs when a user ingests drugs of unknown concentration or an already intoxicated user continues to ingest drugs. Young children or naive adolescents who have been experimenting with alcohol, tobacco, marijuana, or solvents for the first time may unintentionally overdose.

Withdrawal typically occurs infrequently in adolescent substance abusers. In those instances when it does occur it is generally due to narcotics (Niven, 1986). Seizures, delirium, and death are the most serious consequences of withdrawal.

The majority of adolescents do not use drugs parenterally. Virtually all severe complications of parenteral drug use are related to infections or the injection of adulterants (Dimijian, 1976). More recently, acquired immune deficiency syndrome (AIDS) has become a potentially hazardous complication for intravenous drug users (Friedland et al., 1985).

Depression, with and without suicidal ideation, is the most frequent psychiatric complication of psychoactive substance abuse or dependence. The depression is related to several factors: the pharmacological effects of the drugs, the preexisting personality of the user, and the psychosocial problems that develop as the user moves farther and farther into an addictive life-style. Users of any kind of psychoactive substance may experience severe depression and attempt suicide, the drug most commonly used being one of the central nervous system depressants.

The relationship between suicide, completed or attempted, depression, and psychoactive substance use needs to be clarified. It appears that the important factor associated with suicidal ideation is not depression per se but the feeling of hopelessness (Kazdin, French, Unis, Esveldt-Dawson, & Sherick, 1983), a finding consistent with studies of adult suicide attempters (Beck, Kovacs, & Weissman, 1975). However, suicidal behavior in young people can occur in the absence of depression but may be associated with high rates of serious alcohol and drug abuse (Headlam, Goldsmith, Hanenson, & Rauh, 1979; Garfinkel & Golombek, 1983), although this may vary according to region and country (Hawton, 1986).

Those adolescents who successfully complete suicide tend to be older adolescent males, who are clinically depressed and abusers of drugs and alcohol (Brent, 1987; Husain & Vandiver, 1984). Many fatal motor vehicle accidents involving adolescents are thought to represent suicidal equivalents (Finch & Poznanski, 1971). Many of these victims (16 to 19 years old) have been found to have a blood alcohol content (BAC) above 0.10%. Marijuana is often used in combination with alcohol, aggravating already impaired psychomotor functioning.

Drug-induced psychoses are usually seen in individuals who have repeatedly consumed stimulants, hallucinogens, and CNS depressants (Tsuang, Simpson, & Kronfol, 1982). The onset of the drug-induced psychosis is generally in late adolescence, with age of first admission to hospital on average 2 to 3 years later. The large majority of drug-induced psychosis sufferers experience a relatively brief course with fewer symptoms and signs, which tend to be more in the nature of confusion, disorientation, or severe memory deficit and visual hallucinations. These individuals are hospitalized on average less than a month. In those individuals in whom the psychotic symptoms are more persistent, only a small proportion are thought to develop chronic schizophrenia (Bowers, 1977; Erard, Luisada, & Peale, 1980). A family history of schizophrenia or affective disorder and a premorbid personality disorder are predictive of a more prolonged schizophrenialike state (Tsuang et al., 1982).

Violent behavior is more likely to occur among the adolescent and young adult population group than among older substance users. Alcohol, barbiturates, stimulants, and phencyclidine are most frequently associated with violence. There is less chance of violent aggressive behavior in heroin addicts than in other substance users because of its tendency to diminish aggression. Alcohol is most likely to be associated with violence in adolescence because of the frequency and quantities consumed per drinking session. Alcohol is one of the major drugs involved in criminal assaults by adolescents (Tinklenberg et al., 1974), often in association with marijuana and barbiturates. Substance use produces false feelings and ideas of suspicion and persecution, and feelings of omnipotence and bravado. These paranoid thought disorders can lead to bursts of violence and hyperactivity, which in turn can lead to criminal behavior. Ordinarily only moderate doses of the substance lead to violence and criminality. Small doses do not generally lead to aggressiveness, and large doses are usually incapacitating (Connell, 1958; Fauman & Fauman, 1979; Linder, Lerner, & Burns, 1981).

EPIDEMIOLOGY

Because of the existence of a number of cross-sectional surveys of particular populations and a small number of high-quality longitudinal and cohort-sequential studies, it is now possible to chart trends in use. However, the alcohol field, in contrast to the drug abuse field, has far more consistency across studies in the ways the ingestion of the substance is measured. This is facilitated by the fact that alcohol is regulated, it comes in a form that can be precisely measured, and there is a long history of concern about alcohol and the abuse of it. It is generally agreed that one must measure the frequency and quantity of intake within binge occasions and the contexts and consequences of use and abuse. In the drug abuse field, measurement becomes a more formidable task because of the lack of regulation, the wide variety of drugs available to users, and the generally low prevalence rates for most of these substances.

Clayton and Ritter (1985) question whether the focus of attention should be on the specific pharmacological class of drugs being used most frequently or on drug combinations. Most adolescent substance users are quite likely to have used or abused a number of illicit substances in addition to their contemporaneous use of both cigarettes and alcohol (Clayton, 1986; Farley, Santo, & Speck, 1979; Kovach & Glickman, 1986).

The National Institute on Drug Abuse (NIDA) supports a number of epidemiological studies including a periodic national survey of drug use in the household population (the National Survey on Drug Abuse) (Miller et al., 1983) and an annual nationwide survey of drug use among high school seniors (the Monitoring the Future Survey) (Johnston et al., 1986). In 1982 a parallel survey was conducted of about 2400 high school seniors, dependents of military personnel who attended 33 overseas schools administered by the Department of Defense (Johnston, O'Malley, & Davis-Sacks, 1983). In 1980 and again in 1982 surveys were conducted with a worldwide random sample of U.S. military personnel (Bray et al., 1983; Burt & Biegel, 1980). In 1974 and again in 1978, Rachal, Maisto, Guess, and Hubbard (1982) conducted a study of alcohol and drug use among students in the seventh through twelfth grades. Barnes (1984), in her New York State survey, used the same frequency and quantity questions on 27,000 students in seventh through twelfth grades in the survey sponsored by the National Institute on Alcohol Abuse and Alcoholism.

The National Survey of Drug Abuse sample is divided into three segments: youth 12 to 17 years old; young adults 18 to 25 years old; and adults 26 years or older. In this study the percentage of youths 12 to 17 years old who had ever tried marijuana rose during the 1970s from 14% in 1972 to 31% in 1979 (Fishburne, Abelson, & Cisin, 1980). In 1982, the lifetime prevalence of marijuana use among youth was slightly lower at 27%. The downturn observed for use of marijuana between 1979 and 1982 occurred in the use of other drugs such as the hallucinogens (e.g., LSD, peyote, PCP). Stimulants, sedatives, tranquilizers, and analgesics usually obtained via prescription for legitimate medical purposes also showed a slight increase in their nonmedical use. Cocaine use was high but relatively stable. At the time of this survey (1982) it was difficult to predict which direction cocaine use would take.

For the first time in 1986, data were available from the Monitoring the Future Survey on the prevalence and trends in drug use among young adults who had completed high school in 1975. The period of young adulthood (late teens and early to mid-twenties) is particularly important because this tends to be a time of peak levels of use for many drugs. The findings and trends in drug use from these studies were remarkably consistent with those obtained from the National Survey of Drug Abuse. Eleven separate classes of drugs are distinguished in this report: marijuana (including hashish), inhalants, hallucinogens, cocaine, heroin, natural and synthetic opiates other than heroin, stimulants (more specifically, amphetamines), sedatives, tranquilizers, alcohol, and cigarettes. Separate statistics are presented for several subclasses of drugs: PCP and LSD, barbiturates and methaqualone, and the amyl and butyl nitrites. This study contains data from only those seniors present on the day the survey was administered. The approximately 20% of each birth cohort who become school dropouts and those who are chronically absent are not adequately represented in these surveys.

Over the 10-year period from 1975 to 1985, the years 1978 and 1979 marked the crest of a long and dramatic rise in marijuana use among American high school students. The steady decline since 1979 halted in 1985. Lifetime, annual, monthly, and daily use prevalences now stand at 54%, 41%, 26%, and 4.96%, respectively. This halt was also observed among college students and the full young adult sample. As in the National Survey of Drug Abuse, there was a decline in the use of tranquilizers, barbiturates, stimulants (the second most widely used class after marijuana), and methaqualone. Use of LSD, opiates other than heroin, and inhalants has remained relatively stable. Concurrent with this decline in overall involvement with illicit drugs came the disturbing finding that cocaine use increased among seniors in 1985. Current use (i.e., use in the prior 30 days) rose from 4.9% in 1983 to 6.7% in 1985. Some 17% of seniors in 1985 had tried it. The lifetime prevalence and active use rose dramatically with age as people passed into their mid-twenties. Among 27-year-olds in the follow-up study, roughly 40%—4 in every 10 of these young adults—reported trying cocaine, in contrast to 10% who had used cocaine as seniors in 1976. Despite the widely publicized dangers associated with cocaine use, no dramatic changes are noted in perceived harmfulness (Johnston et al., 1986).

Regarding alcohol use, since 1980, the monthly prevalence of alcohol use among seniors gradually declined from 72% in 1980 to 66% in 1985. The sex difference has diminished gradually since the study began a decade ago. College students reported an increase in the occasions for heavy drinking, rising from 52% in 1982 to 57% in 1985. Cigarettes comprise the most frequent class of substance used on a daily basis among high school students. In summary, Johnston and his colleagues concluded that the overall picture of drug use improved considerably. Nevertheless, this nation's high school students and other young adults showed a level of involvement with illicit drugs that is greater than can be found in any other industrialized nation in the world.

In 1982, Johnston and colleagues conducted a study of about 2400 high school seniors selected randomly from 33 schools overseas that educate dependents of military personnel. Comparison with their civilian counterparts reveals exactly the same proportion that have tried illicit drugs. Lifetime prevalence rates in the two populations were nearly identical for certain drugs (marijuana, hallucinogens, sedatives). Rates of use for cocaine, stimulants, the amyl and butyl nitrites, and methaqualone were lower than for seniors stateside. Daily use of marijuana was lower among the overseas seniors while daily drinking and cigarette smoking were higher abroad. The similarities between the two groups of seniors regarding levels of drug use are far more striking than the differences.

In 1980 and again in 1982 surveys were conducted with a worldwide random sample of U.S. military personnel. The general prevalence rates for use during the previous 30 days had decreased for all drugs. These findings for all of the drug classes other than alcohol compared quite favorably in 1982 with the rates observed for the same period in the class of 1982 Monitoring the Future sample. Alcohol was the exception. In 1982, some 83% of the E1–E5 military personnel had used alcohol in some form during the preceding 30 days. Among high school seniors in 1982, 70% had used alcohol during the preceding 30 days. This points to alcohol as a source of difficulty in the military.

In 1974, Rachal and colleagues conducted a study of alcohol and drug use among more than 13,000 students who were part of a national sample of seventh and eighth, ninth and tenth, and eleventh and twelfth graders. In 1978 they conducted another cross-sectional survey, this time among 4918 students representative of those in the tenth through the twelfth grades (Rachal et al., 1982). Barnes (1984), using the same frequency and quantity questions, measured the current alcohol consumption of a representative sample of more than 27,000 students in seventh through twelfth grades throughout New York State. Using the same drinking classification, their findings were quite similar and comparable to the alcohol use data from the Monitoring the Future studies and the National Survey on Drug Abuse data. By age 15 or 16, about 3 of 4 youths, on average, have used alcoholic beverages during the previous year. Using the frequency–quantity measures to create a typology of alcohol users ranging from abstainers to heavier drinkers, Rachal and colleagues found that 27.4% of students in tenth, eleventh, and twelfth grades in 1978 drank once a week or more often. Despite the time difference, the findings were quite similar to those of the more recent New York State study. Among students in tenth through twelfth grades, the proportions of drinkers and heavier drinkers are greater than among the samples of students in seventh through twelfth grades. For example, in the Rachal study in 1974, 28.8% of students in tenth through twelfth grades are drinkers, and 29% of the students in this group are either moderate to heavy or heavy drinkers. In New York State, 40% were in the two heavier drinking categories, figures somewhat higher than for the United States as a whole. From the epidemiological point of view, alcohol use appears to have leveled out among youth, albeit at a high rate. This also applies to young adults who graduated from high school 10 years ago (class of 1976), confirming the ceiling effect.

The age at which alcohol use is most likely to begin is 13, followed by the year before and after, that is, ages 12 and 14 (Barnes & Welte, 1986; Blane & Hewitt, 1977). The probability of starting illicit substance use peaks at the ages of 14 and 15. By the age of 15, the typical student has a 58% probability of having had one or more experiences with illicit substances, particularly marijuana (Frank et al., 1985). Beginning drug use before age 15 years is predictive of increased risk of drug disorders in young adulthood, regardless of sex, race, and education (Robins

& Murphy, 1967; Robins & Przybeck, 1985). However, initiation into drug use of cigarettes, alcohol, and marijuana tends to increase through 18 years of age and then declines sharply. Cocaine is the only illicit drug that shows continuing increases in the risk of initiation, probably reflecting historical trends (Johnston et al., 1986; Kandel & Yamaguchi, 1985).

A number of investigators have examined the "stepping-stone" theory of substance use. The theory evolved in the mid-1960s with the widely publicized notion that marijuana use was a dangerous first step to eventual heroin addiction. However, epidemiological data did not support this contention. Nevertheless, a clear finding has emerged with progression from use of alcohol to marijuana to other substance use. Alcohol is the "gateway" drug for all other drug use (Donovan & Jessor, 1983; Welte & Barnes, 1985). In other words, unless alcohol is used first, there is very little use of any other drugs, including marijuana. Similarly, adolescents are unlikely to go on to use hard drugs such as cocaine or heroin unless they have used marijuana first.

Of particular concern is the combined use of alcohol and other illicit substances (or polydrug abuse). Alcohol and marijuana is the most widespread combination among secondary school students, followed by alcohol and cocaine (Clayton, 1986; Farley et al., 1979; Frank et al., 1985). Not only are alcohol and illicit drug abuse strongly linked, but these substance abuse behaviors are both strongly correlated with other adolescent problem behaviors such as delinquency, school problems, and family conflict, and other interpersonal problems (Braucht, 1982; Jessor, Graves, Hanson, & Jessor, 1968). Moreover, they are predictive in adulthood of alcoholism and antisocial personality in males and depression and phobias in females (Robins & Przybeck, 1985).

FAMILIAL PATTERN

Information supporting familial influence in abuse of substances other than alcohol is scarce, and available results are inconsistent. Most of the studies compare families of alcoholics with those of nonalcoholics.

Alcoholics have been found to be six times more likely than nonpsychiatric patients and more than two times more likely than psychiatric patients to report parental alcoholism (Cotton, 1979). The risk appears to increase with the number of alcoholic relatives and the closeness of the genetic relationship. Thus the lifetime expectancy rate for becoming alcoholic in the population at large is estimated to be about 3 to 5% among men and 0.1 to 1% among women. Rate of alcoholism in sons of alcoholic parents may reach between 20 and 50% and in daughters of alcoholics between 3 and 8%. Since most individuals are reared by their natural parents, other approaches have been utilized to determine the relative contributions of environmental and hereditary influence. For example, twin studies have demonstrated a concordance rate of 60% or higher for the identical twin of an alcoholic while the risk for fraternal twins is 30% or less (Kaij, 1960; Partanen, Brunn, & Markkanen, 1966). However, the most impressive evidence supporting genetic influences on familial transmission of alcoholism comes from adoption-type studies. Half-sibling and adoption studies document a fourfold increased risk for alcoholism in the adopted-out sons and daughters of alcoholics separated from their biological parents in infancy and raised without knowledge of their parents' drinking problem (Bohman, Sigvardsson, & Cloninger, 1981; Cloninger, Bohman, & Sigvardsson, 1981; Goodwin et al., 1974; Schuckit, Goodwin, & Winokur, 1972). Being raised by an alcoholic adoptive parent but with no alcoholic biological parents does not appear to increase the risk for the problem.

Human genetics studies of familial transmission of substance abuse other than alcoholism are relatively rare. Family studies have revealed a trend for preference of similar types of drugs within families; monozygotic twins show greater similarity for drug preference or response than dizygotic pairs (Liston, Simpson, Jarvik, & Guthrie, 1981; Pederson, 1981; Tennant, 1976).

Alcohol abuse and other forms of substance abuse are not considered homogeneous, discrete clinical disorders. This is thought to be due to the influence of both familial and sociocultural factors, which change from one generation to the next (Cloninger, Sigvardsson, Reich, & Bohman, 1986). Three types of alcohol abusers with distinct clinical features and different genetic and environmental backgrounds can be distinguished (Bohman, Cloninger, Von Knorring, & Sigvardsson, 1984). These types have been called milieu-limited alcoholism, male-limited alcoholism, and antisocial behavior disorder with alcohol abuse. Milieu-limited alcoholism affects both males and females of alcoholic natural parents and is usually mild, with no history of criminality. Male-limited alcoholism is a hereditary form of alcoholism passed from natural father to son regardless of the son's adoptive environment at a rate nine times more frequent than in the general population. The women in the families of male-limited alcoholics have no excess of alcohol abuse but are somatizers, characterized by recurrent complaining of headache, backache, and vague abdominal problems from an early age (Cloninger, Sigvardsson, Von Knorring, & Bohman, 1984; Sigvardsson, Von Knorring, Bohman, & Cloninger, 1984). The third type of alcohol abuser is characterized by prominent violent criminal behavior and multiple registrations for alcohol abuse, seldom requiring medical or psychiatric treatment (Bohman et al., 1984).

Substance abuse with alcohol in particular is often associated with dysfunctional interactional patterns that reflect the change in role definition (Jackson, 1954), poor communication skills (Gorad, 1971; Kennedy, 1976), and repetitive, pathological interactions that maintain the alcoholic's drinking, sometimes paradoxically, with adaptive, homeostatic, and meaningful consequences for the dynamics of the family system (Davis, Berenson, Steinglass, & Davis, 1974). Alcoholic families tend to perceive high levels of conflict in their environment (Moos & Moos, 1976) and tend to be more rigid and less flexible in adjusting to changing expectations (Kennedy, 1976). They increase the rate and amount of verbal output while drinking (Moos, Bromet, Tsu, & Moos, 1979) as well as their assertive or aggressive responses. The drinking response to the conflict distinguishes these marriages from others. However, the family can also play a protective role in preventing the intergenerational transmission of alcoholism. Families with an alcoholic member who indulge in certain rituals marking major developmental transitions such as births, graduations, and marriages tend to have a better prognosis (Wolin, Bennett, Noonan, & Teitelbaum, 1980).

The role of substance use in family violence has received some attention. Alcohol use appears to be an important causal factor in family violence, including spouse beating and child abuse (Gelles & Straus, 1970). Children under 18 years of alcohol- and opiate-addicted families are more likely to have experienced physical or sexual abuse and to have been seriously neglected (Black & Mayer, 1980).

DIFFERENTIAL DIAGNOSIS

With acute intoxication and toxic reactions, the patient has ingested appreciably more than the customary or therapeutic amount of a psychoactive substance and presents with unstable vital signs. The condition may be accompanied by a psychotic reaction or organic brain syndrome. There are no major psychiatric disorders that mimic overdose, with the possible exception of a catatoniclike stupor seen in severe depression. However, physical disorders that can cause comalike hypoglycemia or severe electrolyte abnormalities must be considered. Also, adolescents and young adults may have sustained head injuries or taken combinations of drugs that adversely affect functioning. Seizures may occur as a direct result of intoxication with codeine, propoxyphene, amphetamines, cocaine, or LSD. They may also be secondary to CNS anoxia after overdose of depressant drugs or be unrelated to drug ingestion but nevertheless present with the symptoms of an acute confusional state.

Panic reactions tend to persist for the duration of the drug's action, for example, up to 12 hours for LSD and closer to 2 to 4 hours for mescaline and peyote. Acute panic reactions may be distinguished from the acute toxic reactions that result from an overdose of hallucinogens. Acute toxic reactions present with varying combinations of somatic symptoms, perceptual changes, confusion and disorientation, anxiety and depression, paranoid thinking, and suspiciousness. Acute panic reactions also tend to present with varying combinations of those symptoms, but anxiety predominates and is out of proportion to the other effects (Ungerleider & Frank, 1976). The hallucinogens must also be differentiated from reactions to amphetamines, belladonna derivatives, and schizophrenia.

Not all prolonged adverse reactions to a hallucinogen are flashbacks. Paranoid or anxiety reactions should be distinguished because of a different approach to their management. Certain temporal lobe epilepsies may present as momentarily altered states during which colorful visual displays are seen. Depersonalization, derealization, déjà vu, and fugue experiences may occur in association with partial seizures. Hypnagogic and hypnopompic imagery experienced while falling asleep or waking up are similar to flashback hallucinatory episodes. Flashbacks need to be differentiated from drug-induced psychoses, schizophrenic reactions, and organic brain syndromes. Drug-induced psychoses tend to be prolonged and continuous with the original hallucinogenic experience. Neither the onset nor the cessation of symptoms occurs suddenly as in the case of flashbacks.

Any psychiatric disorder capable of producing a psychotic reaction (schizophrenia, mania, organic mental disorder, or depression) must be considered. If the psychosis is determined to be drug related, identification of the drug involved is helpful in predicting recovery time (Schuckit, 1985). Depressant drugs can produce a temporary psychosis characterized by acute onset of symptoms, a clear sensorium, auditory hallucinations, and paranoid delusions. Stimulant psychosis mimics acute schizophrenia or mania. Hallucinogen-induced psychoses usually clear within a few weeks. Persistence beyond that time suggests a preexisting psychiatric problem exacerbated by drug use. Prolonged psychotic reaction following phencyclidine use has been reported (Yesavage & Freman, 1978) and seems to be related to the amount of the substance ingested. The existence of cannabinoid-induced psychoses has been in question. The temporary paranoid state accompanied by visual hallucinations is probably a reaction to excessive doses of the drug (Smart & Adlaf, 1982). Frankly psychotic states that do not dissipate within hours to days are thought to reflect a prior psychiatric disorder rather than a condition sui generis (Negrete, 1982). However, in some cases the onset of psychotic symptoms is directly related to an increase in cannabis consumption without any evidence of a premorbid abnormal personality. Symptoms in these cases last 1 to 6 weeks but may last as long as a year. Relapse into psychosis is common with resumption of cannabis use (Bernardson & Gunne, 1972; Palsson, Thulin, & Tunving, 1982).

CLINICAL MANAGEMENT: RESEARCH FINDINGS

Illicit drug use may occur in the home, the emergency room, physician's office, school, or any other space where youth tend to congregate. It may affect the fetus in utero, neonates, preschoolers, children of elementary school age, adolescents, and young adults of both sexes, all ethnic backgrounds, religious persuasions, and socioeconomic strata.

In the emergency situation, life-threatening problems are the first priority. A complete history from the patient and family members, physical examination, and comprehensive laboratory testing for drugs of abuse are the sine qua non of accurate diagnosis of substance use (Gold, Verebey, & Dackis, 1985; Verebey, Martin, & Gold, in press). The youth may be intoxicated, experiencing a panic state, flashbacks, withdrawal from one or more drugs, or an exacerbation of a concurrent illness and/ or injury or combinations of symptoms. Few adolescents require a formal medical detoxification with the exception of severe alcohol, benzodiazepine, barbiturate, and opiate abusers. Nonetheless, every adolescent deserves a full medical and psychiatric evaluation. Medical evaluation must include a physical and neurological examination, nutritional assessment, thyroid function tests, CBC and SMA, and evaluation for venereal disease and/or pregnancy. Serum and urine samples for drug analysis are a necessary component (Semlitz & Gold, in press). Neuroendocrine testing (dexamethasone suppression test and TRH) are helpful in deciding on diagnoses of affective disorder. Family assessment is also essential. Based on this information, obtained during the initial assessment process, a decision is made as to the most appropriate treatment setting.

A comprehensive approach to treatment services allows the development of several strategies to meet the needs of a variety of youth (Kusnetz, 1985). Little information is available about the effectiveness of treatment modalities and programs for adolescent substance abusers. Such treatment programs tend to operate independently and rarely have the resources or inclination to evaluate how effective they are in dealing with adolescent clients (Smith, Levy, & Striar, 1979). They also fail to follow up on clients, particularly early dropouts, so that outcome of intervention (or lack of it) is generally based on hearsay.

Many different types of adolescent drug treatment resources have been devised and include such settings as therapeutic communities, halfway houses, outpatient programs, and specialized counseling programs in family services units, often associated with city- or county-run clinics (Filstead & Anderson, 1983; Kusnetz, 1985). Although remarkably little is known of the effectiveness of treatment and long-term outcome, a few studies have addressed these issues systematically and in depth. Three of the largest studies were those of the Drug Abuse Reporting Program (DARP) (Sells & Simpson, 1979), the Treatment Outcome Prospective Study (TOPS) (Hubbard, Cavanaugh, Craddock, & Rachal, 1985), and the study of predicted treatment outcomes for juvenile and young adult clients in the Pennsylvania Substance Abuse System (Rush, 1979). All of these involve descriptive rather than controlled studies and must be viewed with caution. Most adolescents are admitted to drug-free outpatient programs (DFOP) with a minority entering residential programs. Few of these residential programs are specifically designed for adolescents, who are likely to receive treatment similar to that of the adult clients. Day-care or alternative school programs serve a small proportion of adolescent substance users and provide more comprehensive services than outpatient programs. Substance abusers with serious psychological problems are treated in programs located in licensed hospitals or other medical and psychiatric settings. However, cost of inpatient hospitalization tends to preclude long-term treatment. Long-term follow-up (after 4 to 6 years) revealed that adolescents generally had a favorable outcome, including significant reductions in the use of "hard" drugs such as opiates but that marijuana and alcohol use was not influenced. In addition, there was a reduction in criminal activities (Sells & Simpson, 1979). In the Treatment Outcome Prospective Study (TOPS), the residential program respondents fared better than those who were attending drug-free outpatient programs. Indeed, in the drug-free outpatient programs there were continuing high levels of alcohol and marijuana use (as in the DARP study), suggesting that treatment had a limited effect on the adolescents' substance use (Hubbard, Cavanaugh, Rachal, Schlenger, & Ginzburg, 1983). Hubbard and colleagues (1983) concluded that early treatment can give a youth a better chance for rehabilitation or, at the least, interrupt the development of more serious drug careers.

Youth most likely to have a successful treatment outcome were, according to Rush (1979), enrolled in an educational program, nonopiate abusers, white, and older at initial use of the drug. Negatively correlated with successful treatment outcome was being a multiple drug abuser. Duration of time in residential treatment was positively related to eventual productivity, with the reverse true for adolescent clients in outpatient drug-free programs. Juveniles who had the best potential for being productive needed to be in the program for relatively short periods.

In an analysis of 30 drug-free outpatient programs for adolescents, program variables that predicted successful outcome included treatment of a large number of adolescent clients, having a special school for school dropouts, a relatively large budget (presumably to attract better staff), employment of experienced counselors or therapists, provision of special services such as vocational counseling, recreational services, and birth control services, use of therapeutic techniques incorporating crisis intervention, gestalt therapy, music and art therapy, and group confrontation in addition to allowing and encouraging free expression and spontaneous action by clients (Friedman & Glickman, 1986). In a vocational program serving drug-abusing male delinquents, improvement occurred in a number of problem areas of behavior, adjustment, and attitude, but there was no significant reduction in illicit drug use (Friedman, Utada, & Glickman, 1986). An off-campus supportive life skills program was even less effective than the vocational training and job placement program within the context of a structured school milieu.

A prevention strategy is particularly important with young people who have a family member with an alcohol or drug problem. They can be helped to cope with this reality through individual therapy or through group therapy with other youths in a similar situation. Family therapy or assistance in getting help may be obtained from Alcoholics Anonymous, Al-Anon, family counseling centers, or other human service agencies.

In 1984, the National Institute on Drug Abuse identified several basic approaches to substance abuse prevention programs (Bell & Battjes, 1985): drug abuse education and affective education as educational modes; alternative programs; psychosocial approaches (resistance strategies referred to as "social inoculation") and personal and social skills training; and cognitive–developmental training, which focuses on physiological reactions to smoking experimentation and user perceptions. These prevention programs were conducted primarily in junior high schools and focused on the use of tobacco but are applicable to alcohol and other substance use.

Drug abuse prevention programs initiated in the late 1960s and early 1970s focused almost exclusively on providing youth with information on drugs and their effects. These information dissemination programs used "fear-arousal" messages designed to scare individuals enough to deter them from smoking, drinking, or using drugs. The moralistic overtones lacked credibility, and results indicated increased levels of drug use by program participants.

Affective educational programs attempt to enrich the personal and social development of students and to train them in decision-making skills. The foci of these programs are values clarification and decision making, improvement of interpersonal skills through activities such as communication training, peer counseling, and assertiveness training, and increasing students' abilities to meet their needs through social institutions (Moskowitz, 1983). Most of these interventions were largely ineffective in preventing substance use or abuse and did not contain adequate evaluation components to assess their impact on substance use behaviors (Schaps, DiBartolo, Moskowitz, Palley, & Churgin, 1981). They relied too much on an experiential approach with too little emphasis on the acquisition of the necessary skills to increase personal and social competence, particularly in resisting peer pressures to begin using one or more substances.

The same fate was met by alternative programs that focused not on drugs per se but on community projects intended to reduce alienation and to provide young people with opportunities for recreation, socialization, and informal education. Recent findings from community programs for heart disease prevention may provide some valuable insights into this form of intervention (Johnson & Solis, 1983).

The psychosocial approach to intervention is based on social learning theory (Bandura, 1977) and problem behavior theory (Jessor & Jessor, 1977). Some approaches place primary emphasis on increasing students' awareness of pro-substance-use social pressures (referred to as psychological inoculation) and on teaching specific techniques for resisting such pressures; others emphasize the development of more general coping skills and focus on the most significant underlying determinants of tobacco, alcohol, and drug use through personal and social skills training. Such generalized programming may be delivered in the context of comprehensive school health programs. This has been demonstrated to be an effective intervention for cessation of adolescent cigarette smoking (Evans, 1976) and has been elaborated on by other investigators to include the use of older peers as primary change agents and role playing to enhance pressure resistance skills (McAlister, Perry, & Maccoby, 1979). In addition to providing students with general life skills, this prevention strategy applies the skills specifically to the problem of substance abuse. Throughout the program, direct connections are made between the use of general life skills and the issues of smoking, drinking, and drug taking. For example, in addition to general assertive skills such as the use of "no" statements, requests, and the assertive expression of rights, students are taught how to use these skills to resist direct interpersonal pressure to smoke, drink, or use drugs. Both prevention strategies have demonstrated a reduction in cigarette smoking over a 6-month period (Schinke & Gilchrist, 1983), teenage pregnancy (Schinke, Blythe, Gilchrist, & Burt, 1981), and smoking and alcohol and marijuana use (Botvin, Baker, Renick, Filazzola, & Botvin, 1984).

These promising results notwithstanding, it is unclear how effective such preventions are when implemented under less than optimal conditions and populations other than white middle-class junior high school students. Whether these approaches will prevent substance abuse in other more vulnerable populations remains to be demonstrated.

DSM-III-R

Revisions in DSM-III-R (APA, 1987) for the substance use disorder category (Rounsaville et al., 1986; Williams, 1986) are, in part, based on a WHO memorandum on nomenclature and classification of drug- and alcohol-related problems (Edwards et al., 1981). In DSM-III-R the term *substance* has been replaced with *psychoactive substance* and the diagnostic class changed to *psychoactive substance use disorders*. Several new categories have been added to cover dependence on cocaine, phencyclidine, and related drugs (hallucinogens and inhalants). In addition, *barbiturate and similarly acting sedative hypnotic* use has been changed to *sedative, hypnotic, or anxiolytic* use.

Polysubstance dependence refers to the use of at least three categories of psychoactive substance (not including nicotine and caffeine) over at least a 6-month period with no single psychoactive substance predominating.

Since the distinction between abuse and dependence is difficult to make, the definition of *dependence* was broadened to include clinically significant behaviors, cognitions, and symptoms that indicate a substantial degree of involvement with a psychoactive substance and risk of impairment in physical, social, and occupational functioning. Thus most instances of DSM-III abuse are subsumed under the DSM-III-R (APA, 1987) category of dependence. However, those cases that do not meet the criteria for dependence, even though their substance use is maladaptive, are now assigned to a residual category (psychoactive substance abuse).

DSM-III-R requires the presence of at least three clinically significant behaviors, cognitions, or symptoms to reflect a substantial degree of psychoactive substance use, as well as risk of impairment in physical, social, and occupational functioning. Examples include frequent preoccupation with seeking or taking the substance; taking the substance in larger amounts or over a longer period than intended; tolerance to or withdrawal from the substance; and continued use of the substance despite persistent social, occupational, psychological, or physical problems caused or exacerbated by the substance. Severity criteria indicate whether the dependence is mild, moderate, severe, in partial remission, or in full remission. The disturbance caused by the substance should have persisted for at least a month or have occurred repeatedly over a longer period of time.

Psychoactive substance abuse becomes a residual category, defined as a condition that does not meet the criteria for dependence. Nevertheless, the maladaptive pattern of substance use is indicated by either one of the following (in contrast to the three behaviors for dependence):

1. Continued use despite a persistent social, occupational, psychological, or physical problem caused or exacerbated by use of the substance
2. Recurrent use in situations when use is hazardous (e.g., driving while intoxicated)

(Symptoms of the disturbance should have persisted for at least 1 month or have occurred repeatedly over a longer period of time, but with the individual not meeting the criteria for psychoactive substance dependence for the specific substance.)

REFERENCES

Achenbach, T.M. (1978). Psychopathology of childhood: Research problems and issues. *Journal of Consulting & Clinical Psychology, 46,* 759–776.

Achenbach, T.M., & Edelbrock, C.S. (1979). The Child Behavior Profile: II. Boys aged 12–16 and girls aged 6–11 and 12–16. *Journal of Consulting & Clinical Psychology, 47*, 223–233.

Achenbach, T.M., & Edelbrock, C.S. (1981). Behavioral problems and competencies reported by parents of normal and disturbed children aged 4 through 16. *Monographs of the Society for Research in Child Development, 46*, Serial No. 188.

Alterman, A.I., & Tarter, R.E. (1983). The transmission of psychological vulnerability: Implications for alcoholism etiology. *Journal of Nervous & Mental Disease, 171*, 147–154.

American Psychiatric Association. (1980). *Diagnostic and statistical manual of mental disorders* (3rd ed.). Washington, DC: Author.

American Psychiatric Association. (1987). *Diagnostic and statistical manual of mental disorders* (3rd ed., rev.). Washington, DC: Author.

Austin, G.A. (1979). *Perspectives on the history of psychoactive substance use* (DHEW Publication No. (ADM) 79-810). Washington, DC: U.S. Government Printing Office.

Bandura, A. (1977). *Social learning theory*. Englewood Cliffs, NJ: Prentice-Hall.

Barnes, G.M. (1984). *Alcohol use among secondary school students in New York State*. Buffalo: Research Institute on Alcoholism.

Barnes, G.M., & Welte, J.W. (1986). Patterns and predictors of alcohol use among 7–12th grade students in New York State. *Journal of Studies on Alcohol, 47*, 53–62.

Beck, A.T., Kovacs, M., & Weissman, A. (1975). Hopelessness and suicidal behavior: An overview. *Journal of the American Medical Association, 234*, 1146–1149.

Bell, C.S., & Battjes, R. (Eds.). (1985). *Prevention research: Deterring drug abuse among children and adolescents. NIDA Research Monograph 63* (DHHS Publication No. (ADM) 85-1334). Washington, DC: U.S. Government Printing Office.

Bernardson, G., & Gunne, L.M. (1972). Forty-six cases of psychosis in cannabis abusers. *International Journal of the Addictions, 7*, 9–16.

Black, R., & Mayer, J. (1980). Parents with special problems: Alcoholism and opiate addiction. In C.H. Kempe & R.E. Helfer (Eds.), *The battered child* (3rd ed.) (pp. 104–113). Chicago: University of Chicago Press.

Blane, H.T., & Hewitt, L.E. (1977). *Alcohol and youth: An analysis of the literature, 1960–1975*. Prepared for the National Institute on Alcohol Abuse and Alcoholism (Publication No. PB-268-698). Springfield, VA: National Technical Information Service.

Blouin, A.G.A., Bornstein, R.D., & Trites, R. (1978). Teenage alcohol use among hyperactive children: A 5-year followup study. *Journal of Pediatric Psychology, 3*, 188–194.

Bohman, M., Cloninger, C.R., Von Knorring, A.L., & Sigvardsson, S. (1984). An adoption study of somatoform disorders: III. Crossfostering analysis and genetic relationship to alcoholism and criminality. *Archives of General Psychiatry, 41*, 872–878.

Bohman, M., Sigvardsson, S., & Cloninger, C.R. (1981). Maternal inheritance of alcohol abuse: Crossfostering analysis of adopted women. *Archives of General Psychiatry, 38*, 965–969.

Botvin, G.J., Baker, E., Renick, N., Filazzola, A.D., & Botvin, E.M. (1984). A cognitive–behavioral approach to substance abuse prevention. *Addictive Behaviors, 9*, 137–147.

Bowers, M.B., Jr. (1972). Acute psychosis induced by psychotomimetic drug abuse: I Clinical findings. *Archives of General Psychiatry, 34*, 832–835.

Braucht, G.N. (1982). Problem drinking among adolescents: A review and analysis of psychosocial research. In *Alcohol and health, Monograph no. 4. Special populations issues* (Publ. No. (ADM) 82-1193). Washington, DC: U.S. Government Printing Office.

Bray, R.M., Guess, L.L., Mason, R.E., Hubbard, R.L., Smith, D.G., Marsden, M.E., & Rachal, J.V. (1983). *Highlights of the 1982 worldwide survey of alcohol and nonmedical drug use among military personnel.* Research Triangle, NC: Research Triangle Institute.

Brent, D.A. (1987). Correlates of the medical lethality of suicide attempts in children and adolescents. *Journal of the American Academy of Child & Adolescent Psychiatry, 26,* 87–91.

Burt, M.R., & Biegel, M.M. (1980). *Worldwide survey of nonmedical drug use and alcohol use among military personnel: 1980.* Bethesda, MD: Burt Associates.

Chopra, G.S., & Smith, J.W. (1974). Psychotic reactions following cannabis use in East Indians. *Archives of General Psychiatry, 30,* 24–27.

Christiansson, G., & Karlsson, B. (1957). Sniffing: A means of intoxication among children. *Svenska Lakartidningen, 54,* 33–44.

Clayton, R.R. (1981). The delinquency and drug use relationship among adolescents: A critical review. In D.J. Lettieri & J.P. Ludford (Eds.), *Drug abuse and the American adolescent. NIDA Research Monograph 38* (DHHS Publication No. (ADM) 81-1166). Washington, DC: U.S. Government Printing Office.

Clayton, R.R. (1986). Multiple drug use: Epidemiology, correlates, and consequences. In Galanter, M. (Ed.), *Recent developments in alcoholism* (Vol. 4). New York: Plenum.

Clayton, R.R., & Ritter, C. (1985). The epidemiology of alcohol and drug abuse among adolescents. *Advances in Alcohol & Substance Abuse, 4 (4/4),* 41–67.

Cloninger, C.R., Bohman, M., & Sigvardsson, S. (1981). Inheritance of alcohol abuse: Cross fostering analysis of adopted men. *Archives of General Psychiatry, 38,* 861–868.

Cloninger, C.R., Sigvardsson, S., Reich, T., & Bohman, M. (1986). Inheritance of risk to develop alcoholism. In M.C. Braude & J.M. Chao (Eds.), *Genetic and biological markers in drug abuse and alcoholism, NIDA Research Monograph 66* (DHHS Publication No. (ADM) 86-1444). Washington, DC: U.S. Government Printing Office.

Cloninger, C.R., Sigvardsson, S., Von Knorring A.L., & Bohman, M. (1984). An adoption study of somatoform disorders: II. Identification of two discrete somatoform disorders. *Archives of General Psychiatry, 41,* 863–871.

Cohen, S. (1977). Flashbacks. *Drug Abuse & Alcoholism Newsletter, 6,* 1–3.

Cohen, S. (1981). The effects of combined alcohol/drug abuse on human behavior. In S.E. Gardner (Ed.), *Drug and alcohol abuse: Implications for treatment* (DHHS Publication No. (ADM) 85-958). Washington, DC: U.S. Government Printing Office.

Cohen, S. (1986a). Intoxication. *Drug Abuse and Alcoholism Newsletter, 15(7)* .

Cohen, S. (1986b). Withdrawal. *Drug Abuse and Alcoholism Newsletter, 15(8).*

Connell, P.H. (1958). *Amphetamine psychosis. Maudsley Monographs No. 5.* London: Oxford University Press.

Cotton, N.S. (1979). The familial incidence of alcoholism: A review. *Journal of Studies in Alcoholism, 40,* 89–116.

Davis, D.I., Berenson, D., Steinglass, P., & Davis, S. (1974). The adaptive consequences of drinking. *Psychiatry, 37,* 309–315.

Dimijian, G.G. (1976). Differential diagnosis of emergency drug reactions. In P.G. Bourne

(Ed.), *A treatment manual for acute drug abuse emergencies* (DHEW Publication No. (ADM) 76-230). Washington, DC: U.S. Government Printing Office.

Donovan, J.E., & Jessor, R. (1983). Problem drinking and the dimension of involvement with drugs: A Guttman scalogram analysis of adolescent drug use. *American Journal of Public Health, 73,* 543–552.

Edwards, G., Arif, A., & Hodgson, R. (1981). Nomenclature and classifications of drug and alcohol related problems. *Bulletin of the World Health Organization, 59,* 225–242.

Edwards, G., & Gross, M.M. (1976). Alcohol dependence: Provisional description of a clinical syndrome. *British Medical Journal, 1,* 1058–1061.

Elliott, D.S., & Ageton, A.L. (1976). The relationship between drug use and crime among adolescents. In Research Triangle Institute, *Appendix to drug use and crime: Report of the Panel on Drug Use and Criminal Behavior* (NTIS No. PB 259 167). Springfield, VA: National Technical Information Service.

Elliott, D.S., Huizinga, D., & Ageton, S.S. (1985). *Explaining delinquency and drug use.* Beverly Hills: Sage.

Erard, R., Luisada, P.V., & Peale, R. (1980). The PCP psychosis: Prolonged intoxication or drug induced functional illness? *Journal of Psychedelic Drugs, 12,* 235–251.

Evans, R.I. (1976). Smoking in children: Developing a social psychological strategy of deterrence. *Preventive Medicine, 5,* 122–127.

Eyre, S.L., Rounsaville, B.J., & Kleber, H. (1982). History of childhood hyperactivity in a clinical population of opiate addicts. *Journal of Nervous & Mental Disorders, 170,* 522–529.

Farley, E.C., Santo, Y., & Speck, D.W. (1979). Multiple drug abuse patterns of youths in treatment. In G.M. Beschner & A.S. Friedman (Eds.), *Youth drug abuse problems, issues and treatment.* Lexington, MA: Lexington Books.

Fauman, M.A., & Fauman, B.J. (1979). Violence associated with phencyclidine abuse. *American Journal of Psychiatry, 135,* 1584–1586.

Feldman, S., Denhoff, E., & Denhoff, J. (1979). The attention disorders and related syndromes: Outcome in adolescence and young adult life. In L. Stern & E. Denhoff (Eds.), *Minimal brain dysfunction: A developmental approach.* New York: Masson.

Fialkov, M.J. (1984). *Final report of the service project to provide mental health services to mentally ill juvenile offenders committed to the Youth Development Center at Waynesburg.* Unpublished manuscript, University of Pittsburgh, Office of Education and Regional Programming.

Filstead, W.J., & Anderson, C.H. (1983). Conceptual clinical issues in the treatment of adolescent alcohol and substance misusers. *Child & Youth Services, 6 (1/2),* 103–116.

Finch, S.M., & Poznanski, E.O. (1971). *Adolescent suicide.* Springfield IL: Charles C. Thomas.

Finnegan, L.P. (Ed.). (1979). *Drug dependence in pregnancy: Clinical management of mother and child* (DHEW Publication No. (ADM) 79-678). Washington, DC: U.S. Government Printing Office.

Fishburne, P.M., Abelson, H.I., & Cisin, I. (1980). *National survey on drug abuse: Main findings: 1979* (DHHS Publication No. (ADM) 80-976). Washington, DC: U.S. Government Printing Office.

Fornazzari, L., Wilkinson, D.A., Kapur, B.M., & Carlen, P.L. (1983). Cerebellar cortical and functional impairment in toluene abusers. *Acta Neurologica Scandinavica, 67,* 319–329.

Frank, B., Lipton, D., Marel, R., Schmeidler, J., Barnes, G., & Welte, J. (1985). *A double danger: Relationship between alcohol use and substance use among secondary school students in New York State*. Buffalo: Research Institute in Alcoholism.

Friedland, G.H., Harris, C., Burkus-Small, C., Shine, D., Moll, B., Darrow, W., & Klein, R.S. (1985). Intravenous drug abusers and the acquired immunodeficiency syndrome (AIDS). Demographic, drug use and needle-sharing patterns. *Archives of Internal Medicine, 145*, 1413–1417.

Friedman, A.S., & Glickman, N.W. (1986). Program characteristics for successful treatment of adolescent drug abuse. *Journal of Nervous & Mental Diseases, 174*, 669–679.

Friedman, A.S., Utada, A., & Glickman, N.W. (1986). Outcome for court-referred drug-abusing male adolescents of an alternative activity treatment program in a vocational high school setting. *Journal of Nervous & Mental Diseases, 174*, 680–688.

Garfinkel, B.D., & Golombek, H. (1983). Suicidal behavior in adolescence. In H. Golombek & B.D. Garfinkel (Eds.), *The adolescent and mood disturbance*. New York: International University Press.

Gelles, R.J., & Straus, M.A. (1979). Violence in the American family. *Journal of Social Issues, 35*, 15–39.

Gittelman, R., Mannuzza, S., Shenker, R., & Bonagura, N. (1985). Hyperactive boys almost grown up: Psychiatric status. *Archives of General Psychiatry, 42*, 937–947.

Gold, M.S., Verebey, K., & Dackis, C.A. (1985). Diagnosis of drug abuse, drug intoxication and withdrawal states. *Fair Oaks Hospital Psychiatry Letter, 3*, 23–34.

Goodwin, D.W., Schulsinger, F., Moller, N., Hermansen L., Winokur, G., & Guze, S.B. (1974). Drinking problems in adopted and nonadopted sons of alcoholics. *Archives of General Psychiatry, 3*, 164–169.

Gorad, S.L. (1971). Communication styles and interaction of alcoholics and their wives. *Family Process, 10*, 475–489.

Grant, I., Adams, K.M., Carlin, A.S., Rennick, P.M., Judd, L.L., & Schoof, K. (1978). The collaborative neuropsychological study of polydrug users. *Archives of General Psychiatry, 35*, 1063–1074.

Grant, I., Mohns, L., Miller, M., & Reitan, R.M. (1976). A neuropsychological study of polydrug users. *Archives of General Psychiatry, 33*, 973–978.

Hamburg, B.A., Kraemer, H.C., & Jahnke, W. (1975). A hierarchy of drug use in adolescence: Behavioral and attitudinal correlates of substantial drug use. *American Journal of Psychiatry, 132*, 1155–1163.

Hawkins, J.D., Lishner, D., & Catalano, R.F. (1985). Childhood predictors and the prevention of adolescent substance abuse. In C.L. Jones & R.J. Battjes (Eds.), *Etiology of drug abuse: Implications for prevention. NIDA Research Monograph No. 56* (DHHS Publication No. (ADM) 85-1335). Washington, DC: U.S. Government Printing Office.

Hawton, K. (1986). *Suicidal behavior in children and adolescents*. Beverly Hills: Sage.

Headlam, H.K., Goldsmith, J., Hanenson, I.B., & Rauh, J.L. (1979). Demographic characteristics of adolescents with self poisoning. A survey of 235 instances in Cincinnati, Ohio. *Clinical Pediatrics, 18*, 147–154.

Hingson, R., Alpert, J.J., Day, N., Dooling, E., Kayne, H., Morelock, S., Oppenheimer, E., & Zuckerman, B. (1982). Effects of maternal drinking and marijuana use on fetal growth and development. *Pediatrics, 70*, 539–546.

Hubbard, R.L., Cavanaugh, E.R., Craddock, S.G., & Rachol, J.V. (1985). Characteristics, behaviors, and outcomes for youth in the TOPS. In A.S. Friedmand and G.M. Beschner

(Eds.), *Treatment services for adolescent substance abusers. NIDA Treatment Research Monograph Series* (DHHS Publication No. (ADM)85-1342) Washington, DC: U.S. Government Printing Office.

Hubbard, R.L., Cavanaugh, E.R., Rachal, J.V., Schlenger, W.E., & Ginzburg, H.M. (1983). Alcohol use and problems among adolescent clients in drug treatment programs. *Alcohol Health & Research World, 7(4)*, 10–18.

Husain, S.A., & Vandiver, T. (1984). *Suicide in children and adolescents.* New York: SP Medical and Scientific Books.

Jackson, J.K. (1954). The adjustment of the family to the crisis of alcoholism. *Quarterly Journal of Studies on Alcohol, 15*, 562–586.

Jaffe, J.H. (1980). Drug addiction and drug abuse. In A.G. Gilman, L.S. Goodman, & A. Gilman (Eds.), *The pharmacological basis of therapeutics* (6th ed.). New York: Macmillan.

Jessor, R., Graves, T.D., Hanson, R.C., & Jessor, S.L. (1968). *Society, personality and deviant behavior: A study of a triethnic community.* New York: Holt, Rinehart & Winston.

Jessor, R., & Jessor, S.L. (1977). *Problem behavior and psychosocial development: A longitudinal study of youth.* New York: Academic.

Johnson, C.A., & Solis, J. (1983). Comprehensive community program for drug abuse prevention: Implications of the community heart disease prevention programs for future research. In T.J. Glynn, C.G. Leukefeld, & J.P. Ludford (Eds.), *Preventing adolescent drug abuse: Intervention strategies. NIDA Research Monograph 47* (DHHS Publication No. (ADM) 83-1280). Washington, DC: U.S. Government Printing Office.

Johnston, L.D., O'Malley, P.M., & Bachman, J.G. (1986). *Drug use among American high school students, college students, and other young adults. National trends through 1985* (DHHS Publication No. (ADM) 86-1450). Washington, DC: U.S. Government Printing Office.

Johnston, L.D., O'Malley, P.M., & Davis-Sacks, M.L. (1983). *A worldwide survey of seniors in the Department of Defense dependent schools: Drug use and related factors, 1982.* Ann Arbor, MI: Institute for Social Research.

Kaij, L. (1960). *Studies on the etiology and sequelae of abuse of alcohol.* Lund, Sweden: Department of Psychiatry, University of Lund.

Kandel, D.B. (1975). Stages in adolescent involvement in drug use. *Science, 190*, 912–914.

Kandel, D.B. (1981). Drug use by youth: An overview. In D.J. Lettieri & J.P. Ludford (Eds.), *Drug abuse and the American adolescent. NIDA Research Monograph 38* (DHHS Pub. No. (ADM) 81-1166). Rockville, MD: NIDA.

Kandel, D.B. (1982). Epidemiological and psychosocial perspectives on adolescent drug use. *Journal of the American Academy of Child Psychiatry, 21*, 328–347.

Kandel, D.B., Davies, M., Karus, D., & Yamaguchi, K. (1986). The consequences in young adulthood of adolescent drug involvement. *Archives of General Psychiatry, 43*, 746–754.

Kandel, D.B., & Yamaguchi, K. (1985). Developmental patterns of the use of legal, illegal and medically prescribed psychotropic drugs from adolescence to young adulthood. In C.L. Jones & R.J. Battjes (Eds.), *Etiology of drug abuse: Implications for prevention. NIDA Research Monograph 56* (DHHS Publication No. (ADM) 85-1335). Washington, DC: U.S. Government Printing Office.

Kaplan, H.B. (1980). *Deviant behavior in defense of self.* New York: Academic.

Kashani, J.H., Keller, J.B., Solomon, N., Reid, J.C., & Mazzola, D. (1985). Double depression in adolescent substance users. *Journal of Affective Disorders, 8*, 153–157.

Kazdin, A.E., French, N.H., Unis, A.S., Esveldt-Dawson, K., & Sherick, R. B. (1983). Hopelessness, depression and suicidal intent among psychiatrically disturbed inpatient children. *Journal of Consulting & Clinical Psychology, 51*, 504–510.

Kennedy, D.L. (1976). Behavior of alcoholics and spouses in a simulation game situation. *Journal of Nervous & Mental Diseases, 162*, 23–24.

Khantzian, E.J. (1985). On the psychological predisposition for opiate and stimulant dependence. *Fair Oaks Hospital Psychiatry Letter, 3*(1), 1–4.

Kolansky, H., & Moore, W.T. (1972). Clinical effects of marijuana on the young. *International Journal of Psychiatry, 10*, 55–67.

Kovach, J.A., & Glickman, N.W. (1986). Levels and psychosocial correlates of adolescent drug use. *Journal of Youth & Adolescence, 15*, 61–77.

Kusnetz, S. (1985). An overview of selected adolescent substance abuse treatment programs. In A.S. Friedman & G.M. Beschner (Eds.), *Treatment services for adolescent substance abusers* (DHHS Publication No. (ADM) 35-1342). Washington, DC: U.S. Government Printing Office.

Laufer, M.W. (1971). Longterm management and some follow-up findings on the use of drugs with minimal cerebral syndrome. *Journal of Learning Disabilities, 4*, 55–58.

Linder, R.L., Lerner, S.E., & Burns, R.S. (1981). *PCP: The devil's dust*. Belmont, CA: Wadsworth.

Lipowski, Z.J. (1975). Organic brain syndromes: Overview and classification. In D.F. Benson & D. Blumer (Eds.), *Psychiatric aspects of neurologic disease*. New York: Grune & Stratton.

Liston, E.H., Simpson, J., Jarvik, L., & Guthrie, D. (1981). Morphine and experimental pain in identical twins. In L. Gedda, P. Parisi, & W.E. Nance (Eds.), *Twin research. Epidemiological and clinical studies* (Vol. 3). New York: Alan R. Liss.

Loney, J. (1980). The Iowa theory of substance abuse among hyperactive adolescents. In D.J. Lettieri, M. Sayers, & T.W. Pearson (Eds.), *Theories on drug abuse. National Institute on Drug Abuse Research Monograph 30* (DHHS Publication No. (ADM) 80-967). Washington, DC: U.S. Government Printing Office.

Loney, J., Kramer, J., & Milich, R. (1981). The hyperactive child grows up: Predictors of symptoms, delinquency and achievement at follow-up. In K.D. Gadow & J. Loney (Eds.), *Psychosocial aspects of drug treatment for hyperactivity*. Boulder, CO.: Westview.

McAlister, A., Perry, C., & Maccoby, N. (1979). Adolescent smoking: Onset and prevention. *Pediatrics, 63*, 650–658.

McGahan, J.P., Dubin, A.B., & Sassenrath, E. (1984). Longterm delta-9-tetrahydrocannabinol treatment: Computed tomography of the brains of rhesus monkeys. *American Journal of Diseases of Children, 138*, 1109–1112.

McGlothlin, W.H., & West, L.J. (1968). The marijuana problem: An overview. *American Journal of Psychiatry, 125*, 126–134.

McManus, M., Alessi, N.E., Grapentine, W.L., & Brickman, A. (1984). Psychiatric disturbance in serious delinquents. *Journal of the American Academy of Child Psychiatry, 23*, 602–615.

Mellinger, G.D., Somers, R.H., Davidson, S.T., & Manheimer, D.I. (1976). The amotivational syndrome and the college student. In R.L. Dornbush, A.M. Freedman, & M. Fink (Eds.), Chronic cannabis use. *Annals of the New York Academy of Sciences, 282*, 37–55.

Mendelson, W.B., Johnson, N.E., & Stewart, M.A. (1971). Hyperactive children as teenagers: A follow-up study. *Journal of Nervous & Mental Disease, 153*, 273–279.

Miller, J.D., Cisin, I.H., Gardner-Keaton, H., Harrell, A.V., Wirtz, P.W., Abelson, H.I., & Fishburne, P.M. (1983). *National survey on drug abuse: Main findings 1982* (DHHS Publication No. (ADM) 83-1263). Washington, DC: U.S. Government Printing Office.

Milman, D.H. (1979). Minimal brain dysfunction in childhood: Outcome in late adolescence and early adult years. *Journal of Clinical Psychiatry, 40,* 371–380.

Mirin, S.M., & Weiss, R.D. (1986). Affective illness in substance abusers. *Psychiatric Clinics of North America, 9,* 503–514.

Moos, R., Bromet, E., Tsu, V., & Moos, B. (1979). Family characteristics and the outcome of treatment for alcoholism. *Journal of Studies on Alcohol, 40,* 78–88.

Moos, R., & Moos, B. (1976). A typology of family social environments. *Family Process, 15,* 357–372.

Moskowitz, J.M. (1983). Preventing adolescent substance abuse through drug education. In T.J. Glynn, C.G. Leukefeld, & J.P. Ludford (Eds.), *Preventing adolescent drug abuse: Intervention strategies. NIDA Research Monograph 47* (DHHS Publication No. (ADM) 83-1280). Washington, DC: U.S. Government Printing Office.

Negrete, J.C. (1982). Psychiatric effects of cannabis use. In K.O. Fehr & H. Kalant (Eds.), *Adverse health and behavioral consequences of cannabis use. Working papers for the ARF/WHO scientific meeting, Toronto, 1981.* Toronto: Addiction Research Foundation.

Nichols, M.M. (1967). Acute alcohol withdrawal syndrome in a newborn. *American Journal of Diseases of Children, 113,* 714–715.

Niven, R.G. (1986). Adolescent drug abuse. *Hospital & Community Psychiatry, 37,* 596–607.

Palsson A., Thulin, S.O., & Tunving, K. (1982). Cannabis psychoses in South Sweden. *Acta Psychiatrica Scandinavica, 66,* 311–321.

Partanen, J., Brunn, K., & Markkanen, T. (1966). *Inheritance of drinking behavior.* New Brunswick, NJ: Rutgers University Center of Alcohol Studies.

Paton, S., Kessler, R., & Kandel, D.B. (1977). Depressive mood and illegal drug use: A longitudinal analysis. *Journal of Genetic Psychology, 131,* 267–289.

Pederson, N. (1981). Twin similarity for usage of common drugs. In L. Gedda, P. Parisi, & W.E. Nance (Eds.), *Twin research 3: Epidemiological and clinical studies.* New York: Alan R. Liss.

Pierog, S., Chandavasu, O., & Wexler, I. (1977). Withdrawal syndrome in infants with the fetal alcohol syndrome. *Journal of Pediatrics, 90,* 630–633.

Puig-Antich, J. (1982). Major depression and conduct disorder in prepuberty. *Journal of American Academy of Child Psychiatry, 21,* 118–128.

Rachal, J.V., Maisto, S.A., Guess, L.L., & Hubbard, R.L. (1982). Alcohol use among youth. In *Alcohol consumption and related problems (Alcohol and Health Monograph No. 1)* (DHHS Pub. No. (ADM) 82-1190). Washington, DC: U.S. Government Printing Office.

Reichler, B.D., Clement, J.L., & Dunner, D.L. (1983). Chart review of alcohol problems in adolescent psychiatric patients in an emergency room. *Journal of Clinical Psychiatry, 44,* 338–339.

Robins, L., & Murphy, G.E. (1967). Drug use in a normal population of young Negro men. *American Journal of Public Health, 57,* 1580–1596.

Robins, L.N., & Przybeck, T.R. (1985). Age of onset of drug use as a factor in drug and other disorders. In C.L. Jones & R.J. Battjes (Eds.), *Etiology of drug abuse: Implications for prevention. NIDA Research Monograph 56* (DHHS Publication No. (ADM) 85-1335). Washington, DC: U.S. Government Printing Office.

Roerich, H., & Gold, M.S. (1986). Diagnosis of substance abuse in an adolescent psychiatric population. *International Journal of Psychiatry in Medicine, 16*, 137–143.

Romano, J., & Engel, G.L. (1944). Delirium: I. Electroencephalographic data. *Archives of Neurology & Psychiatry, 51*, 356–377.

Ron, M.A. (1986). Volatile substance abuse: A review of possible long-term neurological, intellectual and psychiatric sequelae. *British Journal of Psychiatry, 148*, 235–246.

Rounsaville, B.J., Spitzer, R.L., & Williams, J.B.W. (1986). Proposed changes in DSM-III substance use disorders: Description and rationale. *American Journal of Psychiatry, 143*, 463–468.

Rush, T.V. (1979). Predicting treatment outcomes for juvenile and young adult clients in the Pennsylvania substance abuse system. In G.M. Beschner & A.S. Friedman (Eds.), *Youth drug abuse: Problems, issues and treatment*. Lexington, MA: Lexington Books.

Schaefer, O. (1962). Alcohol withdrawal syndrome in a newborn infant of a Yukon Indian mother. *Canadian Medical Association Journal, 87*, 1333–1334.

Schaps, E., Dibartolo, R., Moskowitz, J., Palley, C., & Churgin, S. (1981). Primary prevention evaluation research: A review of 127 impact studies. *Journal of Drug Issues, 11*, 17–43.

Schinke, S.P., Blythe, B.J., Gilchrist, L.D., & Burt, G.A. (1981). Primary prevention of adolescent pregnancy. *Social Work Groups, 4*, 121–135.

Schinke, S.P., & Gilchrist, L.D. (1983). Primary prevention of tobacco smoking. *Journal of School Health, 53*, 416–419.

Schuckit, M.A. (1985). *Drug and alcohol abuse* (2nd ed.). New York: Plenum.

Schuckit, M.A., Goodwin, D.A., & Winokur, G.A. (1972). Study of alcoholism in half siblings. *American Journal of Psychiatry, 128*, 1132–1136.

Sells, S.B., & Simpson, D.D. (1979). Evaluation of treatment outcome for youths in the drug abuse reporting program (DARP): A followup study. In G.M. Beschner & A.S. Friedman (Eds.), *Youth drug abuse: Problems, issues and treatment*. Lexington, MA: Lexington Books.

Semlitz, L., & Gold, M.S. (in press). Diagnosis and treatment of adolescent substance abuse. In R.C. Hall (Ed.), *Psychiatry and medicine*.

Shick, J.F., & Smith, D.E. (1970). Analysis of the LSD flashback. *Journal of Psychedelic Drugs, 3*, 13–19.

Sigvardsson, S., von Knorring, A.L., Bohman, M., & Cloninger, C. R. (1984). An adoption study of somatoform disorders: 1. The relationship of somatization to psychiatric disability. *Archives of General Psychiatry, 41*, 853–862.

Smart, R.G., & Adlaf, E.M. (1982). Adverse reactions and seeking medical treatment among student cannabis users. *Drug & Alcohol Dependence, 9*, 201–211.

Smith, D., Levy, S., & Striar, D. (1979). Treatment services for youthful drug users. In B.M. Beschner & A.S. Friedman (Eds.), *Youth drug abuse: Problems, issues and treatment*. Lexington, MA: Lexington Books.

Tarter, R.E., & Van Thiel (Eds.). (1985). *Alcohol and the brain: Chronic effects*. New York: Plenum.

Tennant, F.S. (1976). Dependency traits among parents of drug abusers. *Journal of Drug Education, 6*, 83–88.

Thacore, V.R. (1973). Bhang psychosis. *British Journal of Psychiatry, 123*, 225–229.

Tinklenberg, J.R., Murphy, P.L., Murphy, P., Darley, C.F., Roth, W.T., & Kopell, B.S. (1974). Drug involvement in criminal assaults by adolescents. *Archives of General Psychiatry, 30*, 685–689.

Tsuang, M.T., Simpson, J.C., & Kronfol, Z. (1982). Subtypes of drug abuse with psychosis: Demographic characteristics, clinical features and family history. *Archives of General Psychiatry, 39*, 141–147.

Tunving, K., Thulin, S.O., Risberg, J., & Warkentin, S. (1986). Regional cerebral blood flow in longterm heavy cannabis use: Preliminary communication. *Psychiatry Research, 17*, 15–21.

Turanski, J.J. (1983). Reaching and treating youth with alcohol related problems: A comprehensive approach. *Alcohol Health and Research World, 7(4)*, (4) 3–9.

Ungerleider, J.T., & Frank, I.M. (1976). Management of acute panic reactions and flashbacks resulting from LSD ingestion. In P.G. Bourne (Ed.), *A treatment manual for acute drug abuse emergencies* (DHEW Pub. No. (ADM) 76-230). Rockville, MD: National Clearinghouse for Drug Abuse Information.

Verebey,K., Martin, D., & Gold, M.S. (in press). Interpretation of drug abuse testing: Strengths and limitations of current methodology. In R.C. Hall (Ed.), *Psychiatry and medicine*.

Weider, H., & Kaplan, E. (1969). Drug use in adolescents. *Psychoanalytic Study of the Child, 24*, 399–431.

Weiss, G., & Hechtman, L.T. (1986). *Hyperactive children grown up*. New York: Guilford.

Welte, J.W., & Barnes, G.M. (1985). Alcohol: The gateway to other drug use among secondary school students. *Journal of Youth & Adolescence, 14*, 487–498.

Wilford, B.B. (1982). *Drug abuse: A guide for the primary care physician*. Chicago: American Medical Association.

Williams, A.F., Peat, M.A., Crouch, D.J., Wells, J.F., & Finkle, B.S. (1985). Drugs in fatally injured young male drivers. *Public Health Reports, 100*, 19–25.

Williams, J.B.W. (1986). DSM-III-R preview: A look at organic mental and substance use disorders. *Hospital & Community Psychiatry, 37*, 995–996.

Wolin, S.J., Bennett, L.A., Noonan, D.L., & Teitlebaum, M.A. (1980). Disrupted family rituals: A factor in the intergenerational transmission of alcoholism. *Journal of Studies in Alcohol, 41*, 199–214.

Wood, D., Wender, P.H., & Reimherr, F. W. (1983). The prevalence of attention deficit disorder, residual type, or minimal brain dysfunction in a population of male alcoholic patients. *American Journal of Psychiatry, 38*, 95–98.

Wurmser, L. (1974). Psychoanalytic considerations of the etiology of compulsive drug use. *Journal of the American Psychoanalytic Association, 22*, 820–843.

Yesavage, J.A., & Freman, A.M. (1978). Acute PCP intoxication. *Journal of Clinical Psychiatry, 39*, 664–666.

CHAPTER 19

Gender Identity Disorders

KENNETH J. ZUCKER

DEFINITION

Gender identity, one's basic sense of self as a male or a female, constitutes a core aspect of personality. Normative research has shown that the first behavioral signs of gender development can be observed at least as early as the second or third year of life (e.g., Fagot & Leinbach, 1985; Huston, 1985). Because gender identity is such a fundamental aspect of the self, most persons do not consciously attend to it; just as most persons do not consciously attend to certain physiological states, such as breathing. At a broader level, Cucchiari (1981) notes that a "genderless" sociocultural system has never been observed or discovered by ethnographers, which has tempted some anthropologists and others to speculate on the nature of culture without gender.

Clinicians, perhaps with less expansive goals, have focused on understanding the development of persons whose gender identity departs radically from the norm. Such persons become preoccupied with gender, much as someone with emphysema becomes preoccupied with respiration. In DSM-III (APA, 1980) the new diagnoses of gender identity disorder of childhood and transsexualism reflected the fruits of many years of work with such persons.

Table 19.1 shows the DSM-III criteria for gender identity disorder of childhood. For both boys and girls, the A criterion reflects the child's sense of discomfort with his or her assigned sex. The B criteria reflect the apparent correlates of such discontent in relation to various components of sex-typed behavior, although it can be seen that the specifics differ between the sexes. The merits of these differences are addressed in the section on differential diagnosis.

HISTORICAL BACKGROUND

The systematic study of gender identity disorders in children, mainly boys, began with a number of clinical reports in the early 1960s (Bakwin, 1960; Green & Money, 1960, 1961a, 1961b; Zuger, 1966). At least three lines of influence seem to have sparked clinical and research interest in these children. Prior to 1960, Money and

TABLE 19.1.   DSM-III Diagnostic Criteria for Gender Identity Disorder of Childhood

For males:

A. Strongly and persistently stated desire to be a girl, or insistence that he is a girl.
B. Either (1) or (2):
   (1) persistent repudiation of male anatomic structures, as manifested by at least one of the following repeated assertions:
       (a) that he will grow up to become a woman (not merely in role)
       (b) that his penis or testes are disgusting or will disappear
       (c) that it would be better not to have a penis or testes
   (2) preoccupation with female stereotypical activities as manifested by a preference for either cross-dressing or simulating female attire, or by a compelling desire to participate in the games and pastimes of girls
C. Onset of the disturbance before puberty

For females:

A. Strongly and persistently stated desire to be a boy, or insistence that she is a boy (not merely a desire for any perceived cultural advantage from being a boy).
B. Persistent repudiation of female anatomic structures, as manifested by at least one of the following repeated assertions:
   (1) that she will grow up to become a man (not merely in role)
   (2) that she is biologically unable to become pregnant
   (3) that she will not develop breasts
   (4) that she has no vagina
   (5) that she has, or will grow, a penis
C. Onset of the disturbance before puberty.

Reprinted with permission from the *Diagnostic and Statistical Manual of Mental Disorders* (3rd ed.). © 1980 American Psychiatric Association.

his colleagues had published a number of papers on gender development in children with hermaphroditism (e.g., Money, Hampson, & Hampson, 1955, 1957). Despite an anomalous sexual biology, gender development in these children was apparently normal and without conflict, as long as the "sex of rearing" was consistent and without ambivalence. When gender conflict occurred, it was held that parental and professional indecision regarding the child's sex, often due to the ambiguous appearance of the genitalia, was the responsible factor. Given this context, boys with an apparently normal sexual biology who displayed extreme cross-gender behavior must have provided an interesting contrast group.

A second line of influence was the awareness that extreme childhood cross-gender behavior was associated with adult "perversions," such as homosexuality and transvestism, a correlation also noted by some of the nineteenth-century European "first-generation" scholars of sexology. Green and Money (1961a) pointed out that despite these previous observations "many persons . . . would 'pooh-pooh' the idea that adult effeminacy, including homosexuality and transvestism, has antecedent signs which can be recognized . . . in childhood" (p. 286).

The third line of influence was the increasing recognition of persons, without detectable physical abnormality, who suffered from a basic sense of discontent with their gender identity. Erotic attraction to same-sex partners was not experienced as "homosexual" by such persons because of their strong identification with the sex-typed characteristics of the opposite sex. Ferenczi (1914/1980), for example, used the term *subject homoerotics* to describe men who felt and behaved like women. Other terms capturing the same basic phenomenology were introduced, among them Cauldwell's (1949) *psychopathia transsexualis*. With publication of the Christine Jorgensen case (see Hamburger, 1953) and Benjamin's (1954, 1966) work, the phenomenon of transsexualism began to interest clinicians and researchers. As numerous retrospective studies have shown, transsexuals recall an extensive childhood cross-gender history, thus providing the basis for speculation that children "at risk" for transsexualism could be identified and studied *in statu nascendi* (Green, 1968; Stoller, 1968).

CLINICAL PICTURE

Over the years, a reasonably coherent picture has emerged of the behavioral signs that characterize the gender identity disorder of childhood. In a boy, one might observe the following: verbal statements that he is, or would like to be, a girl; cross-dressing in girls' or women's clothing; a preference for culturally stereotypic feminine toys and activities; emulation of females in fantasy play; admiration of females; a preference for girls as playmates; display of feminine or effeminate motoric movements; a high-pitched or effeminate voice; expression of dislike of his sexual anatomy (e.g., hiding his penis, sitting to urinate); and an aversion to rough-and-tumble play and group sports. In a girl, the inverse is essentially observed: verbal statements that she is, or would like to be, a boy; a preference for masculine clothing co-occurring with an aversion to culturally stereotypic girls' clothing (e.g., dresses); a preference for culturally stereotypic masculine toys and activities; emulation of males in fantasy play; admiration of males; a preference for boys as playmates; display of exaggerated masculine motoric movements; attempts to speak in a "deep" or gruff voice; expression of dislike of her sexual anatomy (e.g., wanting to have a penis, standing to urinate); and an interest in rough-and-tumble play and group sports (with boys). When all of these behaviors are present, one is probably dealing with the most severe form of childhood cross-gender identification.

There is some evidence that the complete DSM-III diagnostic criteria are more likely to be met in younger children. In a study by Zucker, Finegan, Doering, and Bradley (1984), the mean age of 21 gender-referred children (16 boys, 5 girls) who met the DSM-III criteria was 6.6 years, whereas the mean age of the 15 gender-referred children (all boys) who did not was 9.7 years ($p < .001$). In a second cohort of 36 gender-referred children, the mean age of the 18 children (15 boys, 3 girls) who met the criteria was 6.5 years, whereas the mean age of the 18 children (16 boys, 2 girls) who did not was 8.9 years ($p < .001$). In Zucker and colleagues' (1984) study, the children who met the criteria showed more extreme patterns of cross-gender behavior than their non–DSM-III counterparts, as judged by parent report and behavioral tests. By and large, the differences in gender role behavior remained significant, even after the disparity in age was taken into account. Thus there appeared to be some evidence for the concurrent validity of the DSM-III criteria.

Although much of the basic phenomenology is now clear, the nature of the disturbance in "identity" still requires clarification. In a small series of extremely feminine boys, Stoller (1968) claimed that they "not only wish at times that they were girls . . . [but also] maintain . . . they are . . . females" (p. 200). His observations suggested that the children virtually misclassify their gender identity.

Subsequent studies have shown that most cross-gender-identified children do not misclassify their assigned sex, although they usually wish to be of the opposite sex (e.g., Coates, 1985; Zucker, Doering, Bradley, & Finegan, 1980). Stoller would not be surprised by this finding, as he would argue that misclassification would be expected only in the most extreme cases; in my own experience, however, it has rarely been found even in the most extreme cases. When misclassification occurs, it is in very young children, suggesting an age-related phenomenon, rather than something etiologically unique, as Stoller has hypothesized (for further discussion, see Coates & Zucker, 1988; Zucker, 1982, 1985).

Somewhere between the belief that one is and the wish to be the opposite sex is the clinical claim that these children are gender "confused" (e.g., Bradley, 1985). This notion seems to have arisen in part from the inability to observe the misclassification described by Stoller (1968). In what sense, however, are these children confused? They do not appear to suffer from simple cognitive gender confusion, since on tests of gender constancy (e.g., Slaby & Frey, 1975) the vast majority of gender-disturbed children answer correctly the question "Are you a girl or a boy?" and its negation (Zucker et al., 1980). Tuber and Coates (1985) examined the Rorschach responses of 14 feminine boys and reported that overt gender confusion (e.g., transformation of gender in single percepts of people) was a characteristic response. They concluded that such responses reflected "the fluidity, permeability, and confusion of boundaries between male and female identifications" (p. 261). Unfortunately, detailed quantitative information was not provided and a subsequent study (Lozinski, 1988) did not find much evidence for gender confusion as defined by Tuber and Coates, although there was a significant asymmetry in sex-typed representations of persons and objects. But confusion may refer to other behavioral phenomena. It may reflect the child's ambivalence about whether it is better to be a boy or a girl (for whatever reason), it may refer to the blurring of gender identity during intense fantasy play, and so on. Further research will have to operationalize more clearly what is meant by the term *gender confusion*. At present, it might be best to conceptualize the disturbance in identity as resting on a spectrum, with wishing to be of the opposite sex, confusion, and misclassification representing degrees of severity.

ASSOCIATED FEATURES

The general psychosocial functioning of gender-disturbed children has been a contentious issue, particularly from a theoretical perspective. In DSM-III, little attention was paid to the matter: "Some of these children, particularly girls, show no other signs of psychopathology. Others may display serious signs of disturbance, such as phobias or persistent nightmares" (pp. 264–265).

A number of research studies, almost exclusively with boys, have attempted to assess the general psychological functioning of these children. Diverse approaches to measurement have been utilized, including standardized behavior problem questionnaires (e.g., Bates, Bentler, & Thompson, 1973; Coates & Person, 1985; Zucker, 1985), ratings of social behavior in structured situations (Bates, Bentler, & Thompson, 1979), projective tests (e.g., Ipp, 1986; Kolers, 1986), and ascertainment of other psychiatric disorders (Coates & Person, 1985). On average, these studies show that clinic-referred boys with gender identity problems display levels of general psychopathology commensurate with those of matched psychiatric controls and greater than those of normal controls. Overcontrolled behavioral psychopathology has been the most common finding, which is interesting, given that this pattern is more commonly found in girls than in boys (Achenbach, 1966; Silvern & Katz, 1986).

The conceptual question concerns the nature of the relation between the general and the gender psychopathology:

1. Is the general psychopathology secondary and simply the result of social ostracism, as implied in the DSM-III?
2. Is the gender identity disorder secondary to a more basic disturbance in personality development, as some psychoanalytic theoreticians suggest?
3. Are the two types of psychopathology orthogonal, that is, unrelated and determined by independent processes?
4. Is some type of reciprocal influence involved, dependent on specific characteristics of the child and family?
5. Finally, is it possible that the answer varies from case to case, so that the clinician must decide which possibility is most plausible (and the researcher must decide which possibility is most common across a group of cases)?

At present, the answer to the conceptual question is far from clear. The clinician, therefore, needs to give careful consideration to the significance of these associated features in the development of a treatment plan.

COURSE AND PROGNOSIS

Age at Onset

The clinical and research literature shows that the first behavioral signs of childhood gender disturbance usually appear during the preschool years. In Green's (1976) study of feminine boys, for example, the peak year of onset of cross-dressing was between the second and third birthday, and 94% of the boys had begun to cross-dress by age 6. In most cases, it appears that all of the cross-gender behaviors that have been discussed emerge during the preschool years, much as do the signs of more typical gender identification.

From a conceptual standpoint, this similarity would suggest that the underlying mechanisms for both patterns may be the same, albeit mirror images of each other (cf. Cicchetti, 1984). From a practical perspective, at least two points can be made. First, the tendency among professionals to minimize the significance of extensive early cross-gender behavior as "only a phase" is probably an error. Normative and clinical studies show quite clearly the importance of the preschool years for the development of gender identity. One might even go so far as to suggest that the establishment of a stable and secure sense of gender identity is an important "developmental task" of this age period. Second, cases in which there is an abrupt appearance of cross-gender behavior in middle or late childhood are probably due to different, or unusual, etiological variables.

Stability

Information regarding the course of cross-gender identification within childhood itself has been studied from both cross-sectional and longitudinal perspectives. To date, there is evidence for both stability and change. Based on clinical observations, Zuger (1978) noted "a kind of 'decay' or burning out of . . . symptoms, completely in some, partially in others, and not at all in a few" (p. 368). Cross-sectional studies employing objective measures have also found a reduction in cross-gender behavior with age (e.g., Bates, Skilbeck, Smith, & Bentler, 1974), and, as noted earlier, the likelihood of making a DSM-III diagnosis of gender identity disorder of childhood lessens with age (Zucker et al., 1984).

Longitudinal 1-year follow-up data on 44 of 55 gender-disturbed children were provided by Zucker, Bradley, Doering, and Lozinski (1985). Based on multiple measures of sex-typed behavior, they found that cross-gender behavior, on average, did not increase over the 1-year period; rather, it either remained stable or declined. In some respects, these data may underestimate stability, because most of the parents were concerned about their child's behavior, and degree of behavioral change correlated positively with a number of therapeutic variables. This latter finding suggests that individual differences in stability may be more than random variation (cf. Zuger, 1978). Whether such differences have predictive utility for gender identity, sexual orientation, and general psychiatric adjustment in the adolescent years and beyond is not yet known.

Follow-Up

A number of prospective studies of cross-gender-identified boys have reached a point where it is possible to provide some information on postpubertal gender identity and sexual orientation. Green's (1987) study is the most comprehensive, and can be used as a frame of reference for the other studies (e.g., Davenport, 1986; Lebovitz, 1972; Money & Russo, 1979; Zuger, 1984). Available follow-up data on case reports have been discussed by Zucker (1985, pp. 143–153).

Less than 10% of children followed prospectively have persisted in their cross-gender identification to the extent of requesting sex reassignment surgery (Zucker, 1985). Green (1987), for example, reported that only 1 of 44 boys appeared to be transsexual (or at least strongly gender dysphoric). Zuger (1984) reported that 1 of

39 boys was transsexual, but this youngster committed suicide before he received surgery. Follow-up data are less clear with regard to how many boys remain gender dysphoric, but not to the extent of wanting to proceed with sex-change surgery.

The most common atypical outcome reported so far concerns sexual orientation. At a follow-up mean age of 19.0 years (range 14 to 24), Green (1987, Ch. 4) reported that 33 of 44 boys were either bisexual or homosexual in fantasy (Kinsey ratings of 2 to 6); the remaining 11 boys were heterosexual or primarily heterosexual in fantasy (Kinsey ratings of 0 to 1). Of the 30 boys who reported overt behavior, 24 were bisexual or homosexual and 6 were heterosexual. These data may underestimate the prevalence of a bisexual or homosexual outcome, since at the time of follow-up the boys who were heterosexual in fantasy were significantly younger than the boys who were bisexual or homosexual in fantasy (16.8 vs. 19.7 years, respectively). A similar age difference was present for those who had also engaged in overt sexual behavior. Green (1987), however, does provide some external evidence supporting the validity of the sexual orientation outcome data.

These follow-up outcome data provide some of the strongest evidence that cross-gender identification in childhood constitutes a discrete syndrome (cf. Rutter, 1978). Of course, this does not mean that the linkage between patterns of gender behavior in childhood and postpubertal sexual orientation is understood. The data simply provide more evidence of the importance of understanding the nature of this relation.

The relatively low percentage of transsexual outcomes also requires explanation. Perhaps it is due to a base rate problem, as Weinrich (1985) suggests. Alternatively, it is possible that evaluation in childhood somehow interrupts the "natural history" of transsexualism, given that so much attention is paid to the variable of gender identity during therapy. Other explanations are also likely, including poor measurement of "true" gender dysphoria in childhood (see the section on clinical picture). Clearly, more work is needed to understand the determinants of outcome for individual children.

IMPAIRMENT

In DSM-III, poor same-sex peer relations constituted the only noted impairment. The presence of impairment was attributed almost exclusively to the negative reaction of peers to the child's cross-gender behavior.

Clinical studies also point to impaired relations with the same-sex parent, particularly when that parent is concerned about the child's behavior. Once the behavior has become dystonic for the family as a whole, its continuation can lead to increased strain in both mother–child and father–child relations.

As noted in the section on associated features, the presence, on average, of overcontrolled general psychopathology also has relevance to the child's functioning. Clinical experience suggests that the range of impairment is broad, with some children functioning quite well and others showing severe problems in many spheres of development.

COMPLICATIONS

In DSM-III, the sole complication listed was transsexualism. As noted in the section on course and prognosis, the prospective studies of boys showed that a small minority do seem to remain severely gender disturbed after puberty. It is not clear, however, whether transsexualism is a complication as this term is used in medicine or simply a continuation of the same primary disorder.

Because homosexuality is no longer considered a mental illness, it is not included in DSM-III as a complication of the gender identity disorder of childhood. This should not, however, distract the clinician from attending to the unique problems posed by being a member of a minority group.

Little is known about the long-term psychological well-being of gender-disturbed children, including their capacity to form meaningful interpersonal relationships. It is also not known whether there are differences in the general functioning of those who develop a homosexual as opposed to a heterosexual orientation. It is hoped that some of the prospective studies will be able to address these matters.

EPIDEMIOLOGY

No formal prevalence and incidence studies that identify "cases" of childhood gender disturbance have been conducted. There are, however, a number of studies in which the prevalence of specific cross-gender behaviors has been assessed. These studies, coupled with clinical experience, allow us to draw some conclusions with regard to the prevalence of childhood cross-gender identification.

Perhaps the most general statement that can be made is that childhood gender disturbance is a rare phenomenon. In this respect, it is like other uncommon child psychiatric syndromes, such as autism. For example, if one relied on prevalence estimates for adult transsexualism, then 1 in 24,000 to 37,000 boys and 1 in 103,000 to 150,000 girls would be expected to have the gender identity disorder of childhood (see Meyer-Bahlburg, 1985). This is, however, probably a lower-bound estimate, since many gender-disturbed children do not develop transsexualism in later life (see section on course and prognosis).

Upper-bound estimates can be gauged from two sources: studies that report the prevalence of a cross-gender history in adult homosexuals, and studies of children in which the prevalence of specific cross-gender behaviors has been assessed. With regard to the former, one must first establish the prevalence of exclusive or near-exclusive preferential homosexuality. The best data on this score suggest, at least among men, a prevalence rate of 2 to 6% (for a recent review, see Whitam & Mathy, 1986). Given that about 50% of adult homosexual men recall a childhood cross-gender history, a prevalence rate of about 1 to 3% can be inferred for boys. A similar conclusion can probably be drawn for girls.

Studies of specific cross-gender behaviors in children also provide data relevant to epidemiological issues. Achenbach and Edelbrock's (1981) Child Behavior Checklist

(CBCL), for example, includes two items pertaining to cross-gender identification: "behaves like opposite sex" and "wishes to be of opposite sex." Among nonreferred boys (N = approximately 500) aged 4 to 13 grouped at 2-year intervals, the percentage of mothers who endorsed the first item ranged from 0.7% in boys aged 12 to 13 to 6.0% in boys aged 4 to 5. Endorsement of the second item ranged from 0 to 2.3%. Among nonreferred girls (N = approximately 500) maternal endorsement was higher: For the first item, the range was 9.6 to 12.9%; for the second item, the range was 1.9 to 5.0%.

Studies that have assessed patterns of actual cross-gender behavior are of even greater interest. Fagot (1977), for example, found that among 207 preschoolers, 7 boys (6.6%) and 5 girls (4.9%) displayed moderate cross-gender free-play preferences, as defined by statistical criteria. This type of study probably best identifies the upper-bound prevalence of childhood cross-gender identification, at least within the age range under consideration.

It is not clear whether psychiatric status per se increases the risk for gender disturbance. The two CBCL items pertaining to cross-gender identification occurred in a greater percentage of referred than nonreferred boys and girls, although the amount of variance accounted for by clinical status was small (see Achenbach & Edelbrock, 1981, p. 36). In a study of 100 boys aged 6 to 12 referred to the only child psychiatry clinic in Newfoundland, Sreenivasan (1985) reported that none met the DSM-III criteria for gender identity disorder of childhood. Based on a 26-item weighted "effeminacy" index, however, there was evidence for considerable individual variation in cross-gender behavior. Trisection of the range for the total score at equidistant points resulted in a classification of 15% of the sample as "high" in effeminacy. Whether this type of distribution would be found in a normal control group is an open question. Moreover, assessment studies in which specific gender role behaviors have been measured have not found that atypical gender role behavior is associated with psychiatric status per se (e.g., Bates et al., 1979; Zucker, Doering, Bradley, & Finegan, 1982).

Although the true prevalence of childhood gender disturbance remains a matter of debate, it is apparent that actual referrals for assessment are more common for boys than for girls. In the author's clinic, the male:female sex ratio has been 8.6:1 (N = 112). Rekers (1985) has reported a much larger sex ratio, 30:1. There are probably two factors that account for this strong sex difference in referral rates. First, it may well be that boys are more vulnerable to gender disturbance than girls, much as they are to a variety of other child psychiatric conditions (Eme, 1979). Second, cultural factors appear to be related to a more negative or worried response to cross-gender behavior in boys than in girls. For example, same-sex peers are much less likely to want to be friends with an exclusively feminine boy than with an exclusively masculine girl (Zucker, Wilson, & Stern, 1985), and adults are more likely to have long-term worries (e.g., homosexuality) about a feminine boy than about a masculine girl (Antill, 1987; Martin, 1985). Because there is greater tolerance for girlhood masculinity (cf. Feinman, 1981), it may be that some girls with a true gender disorder go unnoticed until adolescence, when expectations for sociosexual interaction increase. In my clinic, the male:female sex ratio for transsexualism during adolescence is 2:1 ($N = 30$). In the Clarke Institute's Gender Identity Clinic for adults, the male:female sex ratio for transsexualism is even smaller, approaching parity (Blanchard, Clemmensen, & Steiner, 1987). Thus the true sex ratio for childhood gender disturbance is probably somewhat smaller than has been reported so far.

Over the past 20 years, much has been written about changing gender roles. Has this had any impact on the incidence of childhood gender disturbance? Lothstein (1983) reports having received

> a number of calls from mothers who had intentionally tried to "masculinize" their 1-year-old girls (or "feminize" their 1-year-old boys) in order to prepare their children for what they viewed as radically new social roles. To their dismay, their experiments were failing. As their children reached age 4, instead of exhibiting an androgynous sex role, they were evidencing a stereotypical cross-gender role which was frightening to their parents. (p. 248)

Unfortunately, there are no hard epidemiological data with regard to incidence. Zucker (1985) has noted that there is little evidence that patterns of gender role behavior in children have changed substantially, although experiments have shown how one might reduce sex-stereotyped behavior, at least in the short term (see Katz, 1986). In the author's clinic, there has been no significant change in the number of referrals per year over an 8-year period (1978–1986).

FAMILIAL PATTERN

DSM-III states that there is "no information" with regard to familial pattern. One question that can be asked is whether there is any evidence that disorders of gender identity "run in families." To date, formal studies employing the family history method have not been conducted, so the answer remains sketchy.

In a small study of extremely feminine boys, Stoller (1969) reported that their mothers were gender dysphoric in childhood and only grudgingly relinquished their masculinity in adolescence. In a larger-scale study, Green, Williams, and Goodman (1985) reported a trend for the mothers of feminine boys to have been more "tomboyish" in childhood than the mothers of control boys, although the adolescent sociosexual experience of both groups of mothers was similar. No systematic data have been reported with regard to gender development in the fathers of feminine boys.

Based on parent report and behavioral measures, the preadolescent siblings of gender-disturbed children have been found to display conventional patterns of sex-typed behavior (e.g., Zucker et al., 1985). At the time the proband was assessed, no siblings in the family appeared to have a gender identity disorder. Case reports of both identical (Chazan, in press; Green & Stoller, 1971) and fraternal twins (Esman, 1970; Zucker, Bradley, & Hughes, 1987) have also yielded discordance with regard to gender identity disorder.

Data on gender development in the offspring of homosexual and transsexual parents are also relevant to the question of familiality. Studies of children reared by a homosexual parent have generally found them to display conventional patterns of gender role behavior (e.g., Golombok, Spencer, & Rutter, 1983; Green, Mandel, Hotvedt, Gray, & Smith, 1986; Hoeffer, 1981; Kirkpatrick, Smith, & Roy, 1981), although none of these studies have followed the children long enough to assess their sexual orientation. Green (1978) reported similar findings in 16 children reared at least for a time by a transsexual mother or a transsexual father, although Rekers, Mead, Rosen, and Brigham (1983) found that 1 of 46 gender-disturbed boys had a mother intent on having sex reassignment surgery.

The literature on transsexualism is too patchy to draw any firm conclusions with regard to familiality (Hoenig, 1985). A recent study of homosexual men, however, suggests that they are more likely to have a bisexual or homosexual brother than are unmarried heterosexual men, 22% versus 4% (Pillard & Weinrich, 1986; see also Pillard, Poumadere, & Carretta, 1981). Further research is clearly needed to assess the extent of convergence and divergence between the literature on children and the literature on adults with regard to the question of familiality.

DIFFERENTIAL DIAGNOSIS

It is not difficult to recognize and diagnose gender identity disorder when a child presents with the "full-blown" syndrome. As Meyer-Bahlburg (1985) points out, however, there is as yet some unmarked "zone of transition between clinically significant cross-gender behavior and mere statistical deviations from the gender norm" (p. 682). From a diagnostic standpoint, this is probably the most common issue that the clinician will confront. One example might be boys whose gender role behavior is conventionally masculine, except that they eschew competitive group sports (e.g., football) and rough-and-tumble play. In my own clinical experience, I have not been referred many such boys, but a general practitioner might well be asked whether or not such a child has a gender identity problem. If the other signs of cross-gender identification are not present, then it is highly unlikely that such a problem exists.

In my experience, a more common diagnostic problem involves children who manifest multiple signs of cross-gender identification but do not verbalize the desire to be of the opposite sex. Since the A criterion is not met (see Table 19.1), the DSM-III diagnosis cannot be given. Typically, these children are over the age of 8 at the time of assessment and a developmental history often reveals the presence of cross-sex wishes at an earlier age. Despite the denial of wanting to be of the opposite sex, the clinical picture suggests a strong identification with the opposite sex and a devaluation of one's own sex. Rosen, Rekers, and Friar (1977) suggested that such children could be diagnosed as having a gender role disturbance. In DSM-III the residual diagnosis of atypical gender identity disorder could be given, but it is not really clear in what sense such children are "atypical," for example, with respect to etiology and natural history.

Another problem of differential diagnosis concerns boys who cross-dress but do not manifest other signs of cross-gender identification; in fact, they appear to be conventionally masculine. The cross-dressing itself also appears to differ from those cases in which it is part of a more extensive disturbance in gender identity. Typically, it involves the use of maternal underclothing, which is concealed under the boy's own clothing. The texture of the clothing is often important, as soft and silky items are preferred. The putative motivation does not seem to be to enhance the fantasy of being a girl. Retrospective data from adolescents and adults suggest that such boys may be at risk for subsequent transvestism in which erotic arousal is associated with wearing female clothing (see Coates & Zucker, 1988; Stoller, 1985). In DSM-III, the residual diagnosis of atypical gender identity disorder can be given in such cases.

Diagnostic issues for girls revolve around the B criteria. It can be seen in Table 19.1 that these criteria differ from the criteria for boys in two ways. First, for girls, as is not the case for boys, feelings of aversion for one's sexual anatomy are not included in the evidence for anatomic dysphoria. Statements that essentially deny the reality, or future reality, of the girl's anatomic status or biological capabilities are the only evidence considered valid. Second, DSM-III does not include a criterion comparable to the boy's preoccupation with female stereotypical activities.

Clinical experience suggests that the criteria for B prevent the clinician from making a positive diagnosis of gender identity disorder, even though the clinical evidence suggests the presence of disturbance. As argued elsewhere (Zucker, 1982), it is unrealistic to expect a literal denial of female anatomy, although misgivings regarding it can be documented in much the same way as those of the gender-disturbed boy regarding his male anatomy.

Part of the rationale for omitting from B a reference to culturally stereotypic masculine behavior is the concern that such behavior would not differentiate gender-disturbed girls from other girls who have strong masculine gender role preferences, such as "tomboys," but who are not gender dysphoric. Unfortunately, the precise ways in which these two groups of girls differ from each other is not clear. Zucker (1985) suggested that a strong aversion toward female clothing and cosmetics might be one characteristic differentiating the two groups, and it is likely that the intensity of the cross-sex wish and the presence of anatomic dysphoria are two other behaviors that would aid in the process of differential diagnosis. Continued study of both referred and nonreferred samples of masculine girls (e.g., Green, Williams, & Goodman, 1982) will perhaps clarify these and other issues.

CLINICAL MANAGEMENT: RESEARCH FINDINGS

Treatment of cross-gender-identified children has spanned the armamentaria available to the clinician, including behavior therapy, psychoanalytically oriented therapy, group therapy, family therapy, and eclectic combinations of these approaches. A detailed review of these various strategies is available elsewhere (Zucker, 1985; Zucker & Green, in press).

Rekers (1977, 1985) and his colleagues have provided the largest data base of single-case reports with regard to behavior therapy. The most common forms of intervention have been differential social attention, self-regulation, and the token economy. These interventions have been directed at various targets, including toy and dress-up play, peer affiliation, and mannerisms; interestingly, none of the interventions has focused specifically on the child's verbal statements or fantasies about wanting to be of the opposite sex. Typically, treatment has been conducted in the clinic or in the home.

In general, Rekers and his colleagues have reported success either in reducing cross-sex behaviors or in increasing same-sex behaviors. Both stimulus and response specificity have, however, been common limitations of the treatment interventions, which has led other clinicians to search for strategies that are more effective in promoting generalization (e.g., Hay, Barlow, & Hay, 1981). Despite these problems, short-term follow-ups within childhood provide evidence for durability of treatment effects (see Zucker, 1985).

To date, only limited postpubertal follow-up data have been provided by Rekers and his group. For example, Rekers (1985) reported that more than 50 children had been comprehensively treated and that follow-up results suggested permanent changes in gender identity. By this, one presumes that there is an absence of gender dysphoria or the continuation of the childhood request to become a member of the opposite sex. As yet, Rekers has not provided any information with regard to postpubertal sexual orientation. Green (1987, p. 261), however, reported that two boys treated by Rekers were bisexual at follow-up (the researchers worked at the same university).

There have been no formal studies evaluating the effectiveness of psychotherapy with cross-gender-identified children, although some of the case reports are exceptionally detailed (e.g., Schultz, 1979). The focus of treatment in these reports varies, but it often involves the child's sense of self as a boy or a girl, interpersonal relations with family members and peers, and general issues pertaining to ego functioning. Many of these reports indicate changes in gender identity and gender role behavior by the end of treatment.

Psychodynamic approaches have stressed parental factors as central to the genesis and maintenance of childhood cross-gender identification; accordingly, parents have often been involved in treatment. In fact, some therapists have argued that the role of the parents is essential in the overall treatment process (see Coates & Zucker, 1988). The more eclectic approach discussed by Green, Newman, and Stoller (1972; see also Newman, 1976) has also emphasized the importance of the parents' role in the treatment plan. Zucker, Bradley, Doering, & Lozinski (1985) provided some empirical evidence of the merit in working with parents, finding that the number of parent therapy sessions correlated more strongly than the number of child therapy sessions with reductions in cross-gender behavior between assessment and a 1-year follow-up in a sample of 44 gender-disturbed children.

At present, there is not enough information to evaluate the long-term effects of these treatment approaches, although the short-term results seem similar to what has been achieved with behavioral approaches. Formal comparative therapy studies

TABLE 19.2. **DSM-III-R Diagnostic Criteria for Gender Identity Disorder of Childhood**

For males:

A. Persistent and intense distress about being a boy and an intense desire to be a girl, or more rarely, insistence that he is a girl.

B. Either (1) or (2):

   (1) preoccupation with female stereotypical activities, as shown by a preference for either cross-dressing or simulating female attire, or by an intense desire to participate in games and pastimes of girls and rejection of male stereotypical toys, games, and activities

   (2) persistent repudiation of male anatomic structures, as indicated by at least one of the following repeated assertions:

     (a) that he will grow up to become a woman (not merely in role)

     (b) that his penis or testes are disgusting or will disappear

     (c) that it would be better not to have a penis or testes

C. The boy has not yet reached puberty.

For females:

A. Persistent and intense distress about being a girl, and a stated desire to be a boy (not merely a desire for any perceived cultural advantages from being a boy), or insistence that she is a boy.

B. Either (1) or (2):

   (1) persistent marked aversion to normative feminine clothing and insistence on wearing stereotypical masculine clothing, e.g., boys' underwear and other accessories

   (2) persistent repudiation of female anatomic structures, as evidenced by at least one of the following:

     (a) an assertion that she has, or will grow, a penis

     (b) rejection of urinating in a sitting position

     (c) assertion that she does not want to grow breasts or menstruate

C. The girl has not yet reached puberty.

Reprinted with permission from the *Diagnostic and Statistical Manual of Mental Disorders* (3rd ed. rev.). © 1987 American Psychiatric Association.

are also not available, so the most effective way to work with gender-disturbed children remains unclear.

DSM-III-R

Table 19.2 shows the DSM-III-R (APA, 1987) diagnostic criteria for gender identity disorder of childhood. It can be seen that the criteria for boys have remained much the same, with only some rewording of both the A and B criteria. The B criteria for girls, however, have changed in two ways. First, they now include statements that reflect negative feelings about one's sexual anatomy (instead of just statements that deny their reality), as one critique suggested (Zucker, 1982). Second, they include a new subcategory that reflects the gender-disturbed girl's marked aversion to culturally stereotypic feminine clothing. These changes should reduce the probability of "false negatives" in the diagnostic process.

REFERENCES

Achenbach, T.M. (1966). The classification of children's psychiatric symptoms: A factor analytic study. *Psychological Monographs*, *80* (7, Whole No. 615).

Achenbach, T.M., & Edelbrock, C.S. (1981). Behavioral problems and competencies reported by parents of normal and disturbed children aged four through sixteen. *Monographs of the Society for Research in Child Development*, *46*(1), Serial No. 188.

American Psychiatric Association. (1980). *Diagnostic and statistical manual of mental disorders* (3rd ed.). Washington, DC: Author.

American Psychiatric Association. (1987). *Diagnostic and statistical manual of mental disorders* (3rd ed., rev.). Washington, DC: Author.

Antill, J.K. (1987). Parents' beliefs and values about sex roles, sex differences, and sexuality: Their sources and implications. In P. Shaver & C. Hendrick (Eds.), *Sex and gender*. Newbury Park, CA: Sage.

Bakwin, H. (1960). Transvestism in children. *Journal of Pediatrics*, *56*, 294–298.

Bates, J.E., Bentler, P.M., & Thompson, S.K. (1973). Measurement of deviant gender development in boys. *Child Development*, *44*, 591–598.

Bates, J.E., Bentler, P.M., & Thompson, S.K. (1979). Gender-deviant boys compared with normal and clinical control boys. *Journal of Abnormal Child Psychology*, *7*, 243–259.

Bates, J.E., Skilbeck, W.M., Smith, K.V.R., & Bentler, P.M. (1974). Gender role abnormalities in boys: An analysis of clinical ratings. *Journal of Abnormal Child Psychology*, *2*, 1–16.

Benjamin, H. (1954). Transsexualism and transvestism as psychosomatic somato-psychic syndromes. *American Journal of Psychotherapy*, *8*, 219–230.

Benjamin, H. (1966). *The transsexual phenomenon*. New York: Julian.

Blanchard, R., Clemmensen, L.H., & Steiner, B.W. (1987). Heterosexual and homosexual gender dysphoria. *Archives of Sexual Behavior*, *16*, 139–152.

Bradley, S.J. (1985). Gender disorders in childhood: A formulation. In B.W. Steiner (Ed.), *Gender dysphoria: Development, research, management*. New York: Plenum.

Cauldwell, D. (1949). Psychopathia transsexualis. *Sexology*, *16*, 274–280.

Chazan, S.E. (in press). Paired opposites: Mirror gender identity in a case of identical twins. *Current Issues in Psychoanalytic Practice*.

Cicchetti, D. (1984). The emergence of developmental psychopathology. *Child Development*, *55*, 1–7.

Coates, S. (1985). Extreme boyhood femininity: Overview and new research findings. In Z. DeFries, R.C. Friedman, & R. Corn (Eds.), *Sexuality: New perspectives*. Westport, CT: Greenwood Press.

Coates, S., & Person, E.S. (1985). Extreme boyhood femininity: Isolated behavior or pervasive disorder? *Journal of the American Academy of Child Psychiatry*, *24*, 702–709.

Coates, S., & Zucker, K.J. (1988). Gender identity disorders in children. In C.J. Kestenbaum & D.T. Williams (Eds.), *Handbook of clinical assessment of children and adolescents* (vol. II). New York: New York University Press.

Cucchiari, S. (1981). The gender revolution and the transition from the bisexual horde to patrilocal band: The origins of gender hierarchy. In S.B. Ortner & H. Whitehead (Eds.), *Sexual meanings: The cultural construction of gender and sexuality*. Cambridge: Cambridge University Press.

Davenport, C.W. (1986). A follow-up study of 10 feminine boys. *Archives of Sexual Behavior*, *15*, 511–517.

Eme, R.F. (1979). Sex differences in childhood psychopathology: A review. *Psychological Bulletin, 86*, 574–595.

Esman, A.H. (1970). Transsexual identification in a three-year-old twin: A brief communication. *Psychosocial Process, 1*, 77–79.

Fagot, B.I. (1977). Consequences of moderate cross-gender behavior in preschool children. *Child Development, 48*, 902–907.

Fagot, B.I., & Leinbach, M.D. (1985). Gender identity: Some thoughts on an old concept. *Journal of the American Academy of Child Psychiatry, 24*, 684–688.

Feinman, S. (1981). Why is cross-sex-role behavior more approved for girls than for boys? A status characteristic approach. *Sex Roles, 7*, 289–300.

Ferenczi, S. (1980). The nosology of male homosexuality (homoerotism). In S. Ferenczi, *First contributions to psychoanalysis*. New York: Brunner/Mazel. (Original work published 1914.)

Golombok, S., Spencer, A., & Rutter, M. (1983). Children of lesbian and single-parent households. *Journal of Child Psychology & Psychiatry, 24*, 551–572.

Green, R. (1968). Childhood cross-gender identification. *Journal of Nervous & Mental Disease, 147*, 500–509.

Green, R. (1974). *Sexual identity conflict in children and adults*. New York: Basic.

Green, R. (1976). One-hundred ten feminine and masculine boys: Behavioral contrasts and demographic similarities. *Archives of Sexual Behavior, 5*, 425–446.

Green, R. (1978). Sexual identity of 37 children raised by homosexual or transsexual parents. *American Journal of Psychiatry, 135*, 692–697.

Green, R. (1987). *The "sissy boy syndrome" and the development of homosexuality*. New Haven: Yale University Press.

Green, R., Mandel, J.B., Hotvedt, M.E., Gray, J., & Smith, L. (1986). Lesbian mothers and their children: A comparison with solo parent heterosexual mothers and their children. *Archives of Sexual Behavior, 15*, 167–184.

Green, R., & Money, J. (1960). Incongruous gender role: Nongenital manifestations in prepubertal boys. *Journal of Nervous & Mental Disease, 131*, 160–168.

Green, R., & Money, J. (1961a). Effeminacy in prepubertal boys: Summary of 11 cases. *Pediatrics, 27*, 286–291.

Green, R., & Money, J. (1961b). "Tomboys" and "sissies." *Sexology, 28*, 2–5.

Green, R., Newman, L.E., & Stoller, R.J. (1972). Treatment of boyhood "transsexualism." An interim report of four years' experience. *Archives of General Psychiatry, 26*, 213–217.

Green, R., & Stoller, R.J. (1971). Two monozygotic (identical) twin pairs discordant for gender identity. *Archives of Sexual Behavior, 1*, 321–327.

Green, R., Williams, K., & Goodman, M. (1982). Ninety-nine "tomboys" and "non-tomboys": Behavioral contrasts and demographic similarities. *Archives of Sexual Behavior, 11*, 247–266.

Green, R., Williams, K., & Goodman, M. (1985). Masculine or feminine gender identity in boys: Developmental differences between two diverse family groups. *Sex Roles, 12*, 1155–1162.

Hamburger, C. (1953). The desire for change of sex as shown by personal letters from 465 men and women. *Acta Endocrinologica, 14*, 361–375.

Hay, W.M., Barlow, D.H., & Hay, L.R. (1981). Treatment of stereotypic cross-gender motor behavior using covert modeling in a boy with gender identity confusion. *Journal of Consulting & Clinical Psychology, 49,* 388–394.

Hoeffer, B. (1981). Children's acquisition of sex-role behavior in lesbian-mother families. *American Journal of Orthopsychiatry, 51,* 536–544.

Hoenig, J. (1985). Etiology of transsexualism. In B.W. Steiner (Ed.), *Gender dysphoria: Development, research, management.* New York: Plenum.

Huston, A. (1985). The development of sex typing: Themes from recent research. *Developmental Review, 5,* 1–17.

Ipp, H.R. (1986). *Object relations of feminine boys: A Rorschach assessment.* Unpublished doctoral dissertation, York University, Downsview, Ontario.

Katz, P.A. (1986). Modification of children's gender-stereotyped behavior: General issues and research considerations. *Sex Roles, 14,* 591–602.

Kirkpatrick, M., Smith, K., & Roy, R. (1981). Lesbian mothers and their children: A comparative study. *American Journal of Orthopsychiatry, 51,* 545–551.

Kolers, N. (1986). *Some ego functions in boys with gender identity disturbance.* Unpublished doctoral dissertation, York University, Downsview, Ontario.

Lebovitz, P.S. (1972). Feminine behavior in boys: Aspects of its outcome. *American Journal of Psychiatry, 128,* 1283–1289.

Lothstein, L.M. (1983). *Female-to-male transsexualism: Historical, clinical, and theoretical issues.* Boston: Routledge & Kegan Paul.

Lozinski, J.A. (1988). *Sex-typed responses in the Rorschach protocols of cross-gender-identified children.* Unpublished master's thesis, University of Toronto, Toronto, Ontario.

Martin, C.L. (1985, August). *Why are tomboys and sissies evaluated differently?* Paper presented at the meeting of the American Psychological Association, Los Angeles.

Meyer-Bahlburg, H.F.L. (1985). Gender identity disorder of childhood: Introduction. *Journal of the American Academy of Child Psychiatry, 24,* 681–683.

Money, J., Hampson, J.G., & Hampson, J.L. (1955). Hermaphroditism: Recommendations concerning assignment of sex, change of sex and psychologic management. *Bulletin of the Johns Hopkins Hospital, 97,* 284–300.

Money, J., Hampson, J.G., & Hampson, J.L. (1957). Imprinting and the establishment of gender role. *Archives of Neurology & Psychiatry, 77,* 333–336.

Money, J., & Russo, A.J. (1979). Homosexual outcome of discordant gender identity/role: Longitudinal follow-up. *Journal of Pediatric Psychology, 4,* 29–41.

Newman, L.E. (1976). Treatment for the parents of feminine boys. *American Journal of Psychiatry, 133,* 683–687.

Pillard, R.C., Poumadere, J., & Carretta, R.A. (1981). Is homosexuality familial? A review, some data, and a suggestion. *Archives of Sexual Behavior, 10,* 465–475.

Pillard, R.C., & Weinrich, J.D. (1986). Evidence of familial nature of male homosexuality. *Archives of General Psychiatry, 43,* 808–812.

Rekers, G.A. (1977). Assessment and treatment of childhood gender problems. In B.B. Lahey & A.E. Kazdin (Eds.), *Advances in clinical child psychology* (Vol. 1). New York: Plenum.

Rekers, G.A. (1985). Gender identity problems. In P.A. Bornstein & A.E. Kazdin (Eds.), *Handbook of clinical behavior therapy with children.* Homewood, IL: Dorsey.

Rekers, G.A., Mead, S., Rosen, A.C., & Brigham, S.L. (1983). Family correlates of male childhood gender disturbances. *Journal of Genetic Psychology*, *142*, 31–42.

Rosen, A.C., Rekers, G.A., & Friar, L.R. (1977). Theoretical and diagnostic issues in child gender disturbances. *Journal of Sex Research*, *13*, 89–103.

Rutter, M. (1978). Diagnostic validity in child psychiatry. *Advances in Biological Psychiatry*, *2*, 2–22.

Schultz, N.M. (1979). *Severe gender identity confusion in an eight-year-old boy*. Unpublished doctoral dissertation, Yeshiva University.

Silvern, L.E., & Katz, P.A. (1986). Gender roles and adjustment in elementary-school children: A multidimensional approach. *Sex Roles*, *14*, 181–202.

Slaby, R.G., & Frey, K.S. (1975). Development of gender constancy and selective attention to same-sex models. *Child Development*, *46*, 849–856.

Sreenivasan, U. (1985). Effeminate boys in a child psychiatric clinic: Prevalence and associated factors. *Journal of the American Academy of Child Psychiatry*, *24*, 689–694.

Stoller, R.J. (1968). Male childhood transsexualism. *Journal of the American Academy of Child Psychiatry*, *7*, 193–209.

Stoller, R.J. (1969). Parental influences in male transsexualism. In R. Green & J. Money (Eds.), *Transsexualism and sex reassignment*. Baltimore: Johns Hopkins University Press.

Stoller, R.J. (1985). Maternal influences in creating fetishism in a two-year-old boy. In E.J. Anthony & G.H. Pollock (Eds.), *Parental influences in health and disease*. Boston: Little, Brown.

Tuber, S., & Coates, S. (1985). Interpersonal phenomena in the Rorschachs of extremely feminine boys. *Psychoanalytic Psychology*, *2*, 251–265.

Weinrich, J.D. (1985). Transsexuals, homosexuals, and sissy boys: On the mathematics of follow-up studies. *Journal of Sex Research*, *21*, 322–328.

Whitam, F.L., & Mathy, R.M. (1986). *Male homosexuality in four societies: Brazil, Guatemala, the Philippines, and the United States*. New York: Praeger.

Zucker, K.J. (1982). Childhood gender disturbance: Diagnostic issues. *Journal of the American Academy of Child Psychiatry*, *21*, 274–280.

Zucker, K.J. (1985). Cross-gender-identified children. In B.W. Steiner (Ed.), *Gender dysphoria: Development, research, management*. New York: Plenum.

Zucker, K.J., Bradley, S.J., Doering, R.W., & Lozinski, J.A. (1985). Sex-typed behavior in cross-gender-identified children: Stability and change at a one-year follow-up. *Journal of the American Academy of Child Psychiatry*, *24*, 710–719.

Zucker, K.J., Bradley, S.J., & Hughes, H.E. (1987). Gender dysphoria in a child with true hermaphroditism. *Canadian Journal of Psychiatry*, *32*, 602–609.

Zucker, K.J., Doering, R.W., Bradley, S.J., & Finegan, J.K. (1980, March). *Gender constancy judgments in gender-disturbed children: A comparison to sibling and psychiatric controls*. Paper presented at Child Psychiatry Day, Hospital for Sick Children, Toronto.

Zucker, K.J., Doering, R.W., Bradley, S.J., & Finegan, J.K. (1982). Sex-typed play in gender-disturbed children: A comparison to sibling and psychiatric controls. *Archives of Sexual Behavior*, *11*, 309–321.

Zucker, K.J., Finegan, J.K., Doering, R.W., & Bradley, S.J. (1984). Two subgroups of gender-problem children. *Archives of Sexual Behavior*, *13*, 27–39.

Zucker, K.J., & Green, R. (in press). Gender identity disorder of childhood. In T.B. Karasu (Ed.), *Treatment of psychiatric disorders*. Washington, DC: American Psychiatric Association.

Zucker, K.J., Wilson, D.N., & Stern, A. (1985, April). *Children's appraisals of sex-typed behavior in their peers*. Paper presented at the meeting of the Society for Research in Child Development, Toronto.

Zuger, B. (1966). Effeminate behavior present in boys from early childhood: I. The clinical syndrome and follow-up studies. *Journal of Pediatrics, 69*, 1098–1107.

Zuger, B. (1978). Effeminate behavior present in boys from childhood: Ten additional years of follow-up. *Comprehensive Psychiatry, 19*, 363–369.

Zuger, B. (1984). Early effeminate behavior in boys: Outcome and significance for homosexuality. *Journal of Nervous & Mental Disease, 172*, 90–97.

CHAPTER 20

Anorexia Nervosa and Bulimia Nervosa

DAVID S. GOLDBLOOM AND PAUL E. GARFINKEL

DEFINITION

Anorexia nervosa (AN) is an eating disorder characterized by self-imposed starvation due to relentless pursuit of thinness and morbid fear of fatness; this leads to varying degrees of emaciation and significant medical and psychiatric complications. Its name is itself a misnomer that gives rise to common misconceptions about the nature of the disorder; there is no true loss of appetite in AN until the more severe stage of the illness is reached. Rather, a determined battle is waged against sensations of hunger to achieve an illusory mastery.

Various diagnostic criteria have been proposed in the last two decades to characterize rigorously a disorder that has been described clinically for hundreds of years; these largely similar sets of criteria are described elsewhere (Garfinkel & Kaplan, 1986). The DSM-III (APA, 1980), and more recent DSM-III-R (APA, 1987), criteria for AN (see Table 20.1) provided a clinically useful, inclusive definition that has met with broad acceptance. Modifications to these criteria are discussed. Definitions and diagnoses impose at times arbitrary boundaries on the manifestations of psychiatric disorders that do not always make clinical sense. This has generated the less than satisfactory diagnoses of a *partial syndrome of AN* (Szmukler, 1983), *subclinical AN* (Button & Whitehouse, 1981), and *atypical eating disorder* (Mitchell, Pyle, Hatsukami, & Eckert, 1986). These categories reflect both an ambiguity inherent in psychiatric diagnosis and an attitudinal overlap between AN and culturally sanctioned beliefs. Nevertheless, the serious medical and psychiatric manifestations of AN and characteristic psychological features (Garner, Olmsted, & Garfinkel, 1983) argue for definition of AN as a distinct psychiatric disorder and not a mere exaggeration of Western social values.

The definition of bulimia is complicated by its multiple meanings as a symptom, as a subtype of AN, and as an autonomous disorder. As a symptom, it describes the phenomenon of binge eating, that is, the rapid ingestion of a large amount of

Dr. Goldbloom gratefully acknowledges the support of a Centennial fellowship from the Medical Research Council of Canada during the preparation of this chapter. Dr. Garfinkel is the recipient of a grant from the Ontario Mental Health Foundation and the Medical Research Council of Canada for works described in this chapter.

TABLE 20.1.   DSM-III and DSM-III-R Diagnostic Criteria for Anorexia Nervosa

DSM-III	DSM-III-R
A. Intense fear of becoming obese, which does not diminish as weight loss progresses	A. Refusal to maintain body weight over a minimal normal weight for age and height, e.g., weight loss leading to maintenance of body weight 15% below expected; or failure to make expected weight gain during period of growth, leading to body weight 15% below expected
B. Disturbance of body image, e.g., claiming to "feel fat" even when emaciated	B. Intense fear of becoming obese, even though underweight
C. Weight loss of at least 25% of original body weight or, if under 18 years of age, weight loss from original body weight plus projected weight gain expected from growth charts may be combined to make the 25%	C. Disturbance in the way in which one's body weight, size, or shape is experienced, e.g., claiming to "feel fat" even when emaciated, belief that one area of the body is "too fat" even when obviously underweight
D. Refusal to maintain body weight over a minimal normal weight for age and height	D. In females, absence of at least 3 consecutive menstrual cycles when otherwise expected to occur (primary or secondary amenorrhea)
E. No known physical illness that would account for the weight loss	

Source: Reprinted with permission from the *Diagnostic and Statistical Manual of Mental Disorders* (3rd ed. and 3rd ed., rev.). © 1980, 1987 American Psychiatric Association.

food in a discrete period of time. There are definitional difficulties here with arbitrary determination of food quantity and duration of eating to qualify as a binge; at a clinical level, however, patients are usually able to distinguish between a normal meal and a bulimic episode. Purely as a symptom, bulimia may occur in a variety of medical disorders from Parkinson's disease to the Prader-Willi syndrome. As a subtype of AN, it alternates with the intense dietary restriction of the disorder and may be present in about 50% of cases of AN (Casper, Eckert, Halmi, Goldberg, & Davis, 1980; Garfinkel, Moldofsky, & Garner, 1980). Here, the definition of bulimia extends beyond the binge-eating symptom to accommodate the context of AN; it is associated with a loss of control, post-binge self-deprecation, and usually the wish to purge the ingested calories. Finally, bulimia exists as an autonomous syndrome in individuals who are neither emaciated nor bulimic secondary to medical illness. The recognition of this syndrome is relatively recent, and its definition continues to evolve. The DSM-III (APA, 1980) criteria for bulimia (see Table 20.2) have been criticized for being overinclusive in not specifying any symptom severity, and inadequate in not requiring a core psychological feature in the form of a morbid fear of fatness. An alternative is the syndrome of bulimia nervosa (BN), which includes the loss of control over eating, a repertoire of behaviors to control body weight, and characteristic intense preoccupation with weight and shape (Fairburn & Garner, 1986) as originally defined and revised by Gerald Russell (1979, 1983) and now incorporated into DSM-III-R (APA, 1987). Russell's diagnostic criteria for BN are presented in Table 20.3. BN represents a more restrictive and usually

TABLE 20.2. DSM-III Diagnostic Criteria for Bulimia and DSM-III-R Diagnostic Criteria for Bulimia Nervosa

Bulimia, DSM-III	Bulimia Nervosa, DSM-III-R
A. Recurrent episodes of binge eating (Rapid consumption of a large amount of food in a discrete period of time, usually less than 2 hours)	A. As per DSM-III
B. At least 3 of the following: I) Consumption of high-caloric, easily-ingested food during a binge II) Inconspicuous eating during a binge III) Termination of such eating episodes by abdominal pain, sleep, social interruption, or self-induced vomiting IV) Repeated attempts to lose weight by severely restrictive diets, self-induced vomiting, or use of cathartics and/or diuretics V) Frequent weight fluctuations greater than 10 pounds due to alternating binges and fasts	B. During the eating binges there is a feeling of a lack of control over the eating behavior
C. Awareness that the eating pattern is abnormal and fear of not being able to stop voluntarily	C. The individual regularly engages in either self-induced vomiting, use of laxatives or diuretics, strict dieting or fasting, or vigorous exercise, in order to prevent weight gain
D. Depressed mood and self-deprecating thoughts following eating binges	D. A minimum average of two binge-eating episodes per week for at least 3 months
E. The bulimic episodes are not due to anorexia nervosa or any known physical disorder	E. Persistent overconcern with body shape and weight

Source: Reprinted with permission from the *Diagnostic and Statistical Manual of Mental Disorders* (3rd ed. and 3rd ed., rev.). © 1980, 1987 American Psychiatric Association.

TABLE 20.3. Russell's Diagnostic Criteria for Bulimia Nervosa

Bulimia nervosa—original criteria (Russell, 1979)
1. The patients suffer from powerful and intractable urges to overeat.
2. They seek to avoid the "fattening" effects of food by inducing vomiting or abusing purgatives or both.
3. They have a morbid fear of becoming fat.

Bulimia nervosa—revised criteria (Russell, 1983)
1. The patients have preoccupations with food, irresistible cravings for food, and repeated episodes of overeating.
2. They employ devices aimed at counteracting the "fattening" effects of food.
3. They have a psychopathology resembling that of classical anorexia nervosa.
4. They have had a previous overt or cryptic episode of anorexia nervosa.

more clinically severe definition of the syndrome of bulimia; the term BN has now met with broad acceptance and is used hereafter. The latest revisions to the diagnostic criteria are discussed at the end of this chapter. Other names for bulimic disorders such as *bulimarexia* (Boskind-Lodahl, 1976) and the *dietary chaos syndrome* (Palmer, 1979) are no longer needed.

HISTORICAL BACKGROUND

Current Western cultural preoccupations with thinness and fitness have led some people to misconstrue eating disorders as mere epiphenomena of modern social mores. While today's prevailing attitudes may have heightened awareness of and even made desirable eating disorders, AN and BN have well-documented historical descriptions extending back over centuries.

While various accounts of asceticism, starvation, and emaciation in young women date from as early as the Middle Ages (Bell, 1985), the description of two cases of "nervous consumption" by Richard Morton in 1694 is widely acknowledged as the earliest of classical AN. He noted this disease to be chronic and difficult to treat unless intervention occurs shortly after onset. He also described the initial ego-syntonic nature of AN, that "at first it flatters and deceives the patient, for which reason it happens for the most part that the physician is consulted too late" (p. 11). He recognized associated affective disturbance in the form of depression and anxiety as well as the edema of starvation and the importance of therapeutic refeeding.

In the nineteenth century, more complete descriptions by Gull (1874) and Lasegue (1873) also generated the name AN as well as synonyms of apepsia hysterica and anorexia hysterica. Gull noted that AN was a disease of adolescent and young adult females that occasionally occurred in males. He observed secondary amenorrhea, bradycardia, hyperactivity, and bulimia as clinical features. Lasegue recognized the difference between the food avoidance in AN and the true anorexia of depression or carcinoma, as well as the denial of illness by patients and the development of unusual food preferences. Gull emphasized the primacy of food and nursing care in treatment and cautioned against medications. He warned of the risk of death from starvation. Virtually all of these careful observations and recommendations are valid today.

In this century, thinking about AN has evolved in parallel with dominant conceptual trends in psychiatry. In the context of neuropsychiatry and renewed interest in the central nervous system in the early 1900s, a pathologist noted an association between cachexia and adenohypophyseal destruction in a patient (Simmonds, 1914). This misleading association spawned a variety of biological treatments for AN for two decades. Then the ascendant influence of psychoanalytic thinking overtook the biological model and flourished through the 1940s and 1950s. AN was formulated as a defense against guilt-ridden oral impregnation fantasies (Waller, Kaufman, & Deutsch, 1940). The progression of psychological theories evolved beyond drive theory to include the importance of object relations, cognitive psychology, and family interactions (Garfinkel & Garner, 1982). Important contributors have included

Hilde Bruch, who emphasized both faulty interactional patterns between the infant and the mother in AN and resultant perceptual and conceptual disturbances (Bruch, 1973). In particular, she identified disturbances in body image, interoceptive disturbances, and an overwhelming sense of personal ineffectiveness. Empirical psychometric research has validated much of her theory and observation. The significance of ongoing as well as remote patterns of familial interaction has been recognized and has led to enhanced therapeutic modalities (Minuchin, 1978). Finally, the renaissance of biological psychiatry in the last two decades has led to a flurry of investigations into the biological derangements in AN and a belated appreciation of the work of Ancel Keys (1950) in recognizing the biology and psychology of human starvation. The danger of a theoretical pendulum swing back to the reductionism of earlier times has been averted by the general acceptance of a multidetermined model of AN (Andersen, 1985; Garfinkel & Garner, 1982).

The history of BN is less well celebrated, likely due to its relatively recent recognition as a clinical entity and its potential to escape medical detection. The symptom of binge eating, called *boolmot* in Hebrew and *bulimy* in Greek, was described in the Babylonian Talmud (Kaplan & Garfinkel, 1984). The modern history of BN has been well summarized by Casper (1983). Many classic descriptions of AN included observation of the bulimic aspects of this disorder. In 1944, a detailed history of BN in the context of a past history of AN chronicled many of the attitudes and behaviors seen in BN patients today (Binswanger, 1944). A definitive description of 30 patients with BN by Gerald Russell (1979) ushered in current awareness of this distinct disorder.

CLINICAL PICTURE

The central feature of AN is the individual's marked pursuit of thinness with the associated conviction that her body is too large (Garfinkel & Garner, 1982). The enduring existence of AN over centuries suggests that this reflects more than an enhancement of current social preoccupations with weight and shape. Rather, its origins are more complex and varied. It may emanate from a past history of obesity that was associated with taunting and social failure; it may reflect a symbolic focus in a search for personal mastery that in turn betrays a sense of ineffectiveness. It may also provide a retreat from the maturing process of adolescence, as expressed by development of secondary sexual characteristics (Crisp, 1980).

Its initial manifestation is deceptively benign; AN may often begin with a diet. Despite the ubiquity of dieting, the beginnings of clinical AN differ from usual dieting in important ways. Typical dieting features a fixed target weight, variably successful restraint, an enhancement of social interaction, a relinquishing of prohibitions once the target is reached, and usually a gradual return to prediet weight. In AN, an early warning sign in dieting is the occurrence of shifting weight goals and an escalating sense of being overweight as weight loss occurs. The desired weight keeps dropping, and abstention from high-calorie foods becomes a more global food aversion. Social contacts diminish. At this point, despite an evolving emaciation that may alarm the family, the patient typically denies being thin or ill and is uninterested in professional help to reverse her weight loss. Rather, she sees her health as being further enhanced by losing more weight.

The disturbance in body image that accompanies the drive for thinness and underlies the denial of emaciation lies somewhere between an overvalued idea and a true delusion. This distinction is largely semantic, as it responds neither to logical argument nor to antipsychotic medication. Well described clinically by Bruch (1973), this disturbance has been confirmed empirically with body size estimation via calipers (Slade & Russell, 1973) and a distorting photograph (Freeman, Thomas, Solyom, & Koopman, 1985; Garner, Garfinkel, Stancer, & Moldofsky, 1976). It is a typical but not universal feature of AN. What creates this disturbance is unknown. Hypotheses include a fixation at a concrete operational stage of Piagetian development, regression from the maturational meaning of menarche, and the linkage of self-worth with body fat in an inversely proportional relationship.

The intensity of the drive for thinness generates a repertoire of eating behaviors familiar to families of patients and to clinicians. Food is avoided, toyed with rather than eaten, or secretly disposed of. A variety of excuses and evasions for missed meals appears. An often complex set of rules regarding foods and their manner of consumption develops, with a seemingly encyclopedic awareness of caloric content and magical beliefs about different food groups. There is usually a long list of forbidden foods.

For those AN patients of the bulimic subtype, the forbidden foods are typically those consumed in a binge—namely, high-calorie, carbohydrate-rich items. This is followed by efforts to counteract the ingestion of calories by vomiting, laxative or diuretic abuse, severe food restriction, or intensive exercising. Physical fitness becomes a means to avoid fatness.

Diminishing consumption of food is paralleled by an increasing preoccupation with it. Patients may collect recipes and work in food-related jobs. This intensifies the fear of yielding to the impulse to eat and further heightens the prohibitions against it. Characteristic thinking styles emerge, including a black-and-white pattern of reasoning called dichotomous thinking (Garner & Bemis, 1982); a pound gained is perceived as an ineluctable trajectory toward obesity. This pattern extends importantly beyond food to intrapsychic and interpersonal beliefs. Coupled with such an attitude is a profound sense of self-mistrust, whether it relates to biological signals of hunger and satiety or to more purely emotional states.

Because of the initially ego-syntonic nature of the disorder, patients rarely present to physicians complaining of weight loss. Rather, they may request assistance for dieting in the absence of obesity or may seek help for the secondary features of their AN. Included are constipation with a request for laxatives, bloating or frank edema with a request for diuretics, hypokalemia due to vomiting, secondary amenorrhea, or depression. If vomiting is a regular feature of the disorder, erosion of tooth enamel may lead to a dental diagnosis of AN.

The clinical picture of BN has been delineated only recently in a systematic fashion (Fairburn & Cooper, 1984). A morbid fear of fatness is the overriding psychological preoccupation, and this is coupled with a past history of unequivocal AN in 25% of an English sample. Psychometric assessment of eating attitudes paralleled the results obtained in AN samples. A past personal history and family history of obesity and depression are common. American studies of DSM-III bulimia indicate a significant coexistence of alcohol and drug abuse (Mitchell, Hatsukami, Eckert, & Pyle, 1985).

When the prevalence and importance of bulimia in the context of AN were recognized (Casper et al., 1980; Garfinkel et al., 1980), distinguishing clinical features of this subgroup were noted. These included a wide variety of impulsive behaviors, including stealing, self-mutilation, suicide attempts, and substance abuse. Compared to restricting AN, this subgroup tended to be more socially and sexually active.

In terms of psychopathology, current empirical research indicates little difference between patients with BN and those with the bulimic subtype of AN (Garner, Olmsted, & Garfinkel, 1985). Weight alone fails to distinguish bulimic groups in terms of attitudes and beliefs about food, weight, and shape.

The bulimic patient may binge up to several times per day, and often reports cognitive preoccupation with foods, social isolation, and impaired professional functioning because of the demands of the bulimia. There is less contentment with the disorder than is seen in AN, and patients are more likely to seek treatment. Binges may be triggered by any strong unpleasant feelings (anxiety, depression, anger, loneliness) or may occur at times as a habit. Patients frequently report a sense of frenzy, loss of control, or frank dissociation during the binge, which can last from minutes to hours. Binges are usually terminated by running out of food, physical fullness, abdominal pain, sleepiness, or social interruption; a psychological sense of satiety is notably absent. There is wide variability in the personal experience of the binge itself in terms of effect on anxiety or dysphoria, but guilt and self-deprecation are common afterward.

The binge is usually followed by efforts to counteract dreaded calories. The commonest sequela is vomiting, often induced with a finger or by manual pressure on the abdomen; many patients report an eventual ability to vomit spontaneously by bending over. Some use syrup of ipecac to induce vomiting; the toxicity of this practice is discussed later. Laxative, diuretic, or diet pill abuse is an alternative or adjunct to emesis.

As in AN, the patient may not openly acknowledge the disorder—although in BN in women at normal weight, this may reflect more the shame and self-loathing associated with bulimic behaviors. Again, it may be the observation of sequelae of the disorder that leads to diagnosis.

ASSOCIATED FEATURES

Physiological

Effects of Starvation

Virtually every body system is affected by starvation; the physiological changes seen in AN reflect not only caloric deprivation but also homeostatic mechanisms that conserve energy. These manifest themselves through a variety of symptoms. Secondary amenorrhea is almost inevitable in postpubertal AN, and in a minority of cases may precede significant weight loss (Fries, 1977). Evidence suggests a hypothalamic disturbance in gonadotropin function underlying this feature (Garfinkel & Garner, 1982). Other starvation effects commonly seen clinically include sinus bradycardia, hypothermia, abdominal bloating, constipation, dry skin and the development of lanugo body hair, and edema (Mitchell, 1986). Recent research has revealed much of the underlying neurohormonal and neurotransmitter changes that produce these features, but these are reviewed in detail elsewhere (Kennedy & Garfinkel, 1987). Simmonds's preoccupation with the pituitary of 70 years ago has been superseded by hypotheses about the hypothalamus in AN patients (Gold et al., 1986) using sophisticated measures. Advances in imaging techniques have yielded evidence of structural brain changes in terms of ventricular enlargement in AN patients (Artmann, Grau, Adelmann, & Schlieffer, 1985; Datlof, Coleman, Forbes, & Kriepe, 1986). Structural and functional changes may give rise to symptoms of impaired concentration, depression, and irritability, and signs of impaired cognitive functioning (Strupp, Weingartner, Kaye, & Gwirtsman, 1986). Similarly, nuclear medicine studies have defined a delay in gastric emptying that likely partially accounts for the bloating commonly described by such AN patients (McCallum et al., 1985).

Other neuroendocrine features of starvation include elevation of plasma growth hormone levels, reduced serum triiodothyronine levels (T3) accompanied by elevated reverse T3 levels, and altered cortisol metabolism with failure of dexamethasone suppression (Garfinkel & Garner, 1982).

Effects of Bingeing and Purging

Both the means used to carry out the behaviors and the consequences provide a variety of signs and symptoms; some of these are evident instantly on clinical contact. Marked bilateral parotid gland enlargement is characteristic, and may be accompanied by elevations in plasma amylase of pancreatic or salivary origin (Kaplan, 1987; Levin, Falko, Dixon, Gallup, & Saunders, 1980). Erosions on the dorsum of the hand (Russell, 1979) arise from friction against the teeth during digital induction of vomiting (Williams, Friedman, & Steiner, 1986); they may be a clue to covert BN. Depletion of potassium through vomiting and diuretic abuse can lead to cardiac complications and reflects a broader disturbance in the form of hypokalemic, hypochloremic metabolic alkalosis. Abuse of laxatives results in both intermittent diarrhea and chronic constipation. Dental enamel erosions and caries can result from the acidity of vomitus in over one-third of a clinical population (Simmons, Grayden, & Mitchell, 1986).

There are no primary or trait-dependent physiological features known at this time of patients with eating disorders. Thus virtually all known physiological disturbances seen in AN and BN are secondary to starvation or the means of calorie avoidance. They are listed more fully later in the chapter as complications.

Psychological

Affective Disorder

While clinicians have long recognized an association between affective symptoms and eating disorders, its precise nature still awaits elucidation. In one study of AN patients, more than one-third met research criteria for a diagnosis of a major depressive episode (Piran, Kennedy, Garfinkel, & Owens, 1985). However, starvation itself induces many of the classic vegetative symptoms of depression as well as neuroendocrine disturbances similar to those seen in affective disorders (Halmi, 1985). While response to antidepressant drugs in BN has led some to perceive eating disorders as a variant of affective disorders, there is reason for considerable caution (Altshuler & Weiner, 1985) in both diagnosis and treatment. The intimate relationship between mood and food still awaits clarification.

Anxiety Disorder

Half of a sample of 47 AN patients met research criteria for a lifetime diagnosis of panic disorder and one-third also showed evidence of social phobia (Piran et al., 1985). Again, the confound of significant nutritional disturbance and the affects elicited by threats to the pursuit of thinness provide an important context for the prevalence of anxiety disorders in this population. Research studies have not adequately addressed the relationship between eating and anxiety disorders.

Personality Disorder

Clinical experience has placed restricting AN in the arena of compulsive, passive–aggressive, avoidant, and dependent personality traits, with both bulimic AN and BN falling into the spectrum of borderline, histrionic, narcissistic, and antisocial features. Whether these traits precede the eating disorder or are awakened from a subclinical level by the eating disorder is unknown. There is a paucity of research in this area. A recent study of 68 patients with AN or BN, using both clinical and psychometric evaluation, confirmed a high prevalence of avoidant personality disorder (60%) in restricting AN, and an equally significant prevalence of borderline personality disorder (55%) in the bulimic group (Piran, Lerner, Garfinkel, Kennedy, & Brouillette, in press).

COURSE AND PROGNOSIS

AN and BN are usually gradual in onset, secretive in nature, and often chronic in course. Research on course and prognosis has been hampered by methodological problems, including sampling bias, diagnostic vagaries, variable outcome criteria, loss of patients to follow-up, and duration of follow-up (Theander, 1985). Nevertheless, Theander's follow-up of 94 Swedish eating-disordered patients for a minimum of 24 years showed that less than one-third recovered within 3 years and that more than one-third were ill for greater than 6 years. Of his sample, 13% had died of

AN at follow-up and a further 4% had committed suicide. While these data may reflect earlier, less successful treatments of AN and BN, they also underscore the significant mortality associated with these disorders over time.

In addition to mortality, there is a significant psychiatric morbidity associated with AN; adequate follow-up of BN has not yet been done. Detailed follow-up of 60 Canadian women with AN 5 to 14 years after initial presentation revealed significant psychopathology (Toner, Garfinkel, & Garner, 1986) in comparison with a control group. Both restricting and bulimic AN patients had markedly elevated lifetime prevalence of affective disorder, chiefly major depression, compared to controls. The same held true for anxiety disorders. Subtype of AN did not distinguish outcome except in the case of substance abuse disorders, where the prevalence was significantly greater in the bulimic subtype. Short-term follow-up (1 to 3 years) of patients treated for BN with a behavioral approach showed good improvement in eating behavior for fewer than half the sample and "persistent dysphoria" in more than half the sample, but the data suffer from methodological limitations (Hsu & Holder, 1986).

Mortality in eating disorders may emanate from starvation itself, the means to induce it, the methods to treat it, and suicide. The use of ipecac to induce vomiting can lead to myocardial toxicity, and the depletion of potassium may lead to arrhythmias. This state, when coupled with overaggressive refeeding, can lead to sudden cardiac death (Isner, Roberts, Heymsfield, & Yager, 1985; Powers, 1982).

COMPLICATIONS

A multisystem panoply of complications accompanies eating disorders. These are summarized in Table 20.4 and reviewed in detail elsewhere (Jacobs & Schneider, 1985; Mitchell, 1986).

EPIDEMIOLOGY

The same methodological problems seen in outcome studies plague those of incidence and prevalence. AN and BN are predominantly disorders of the female—at least 90% of cases. Studies of age of onset show bimodal peaks at 14 and 18 years (Halmi, Casper, Eckert, Goldberg, & Davis, 1979). A significant number of women develop the disorder in young adulthood. While AN was originally described and is now caricatured as a disease of the upper classes, research indicates a downward social drift in the last decade in its epidemiology (Garfinkel et al., 1980).

Current accepted prevalence rates among Western adolescent and young adult women are 1% for AN and 2 to 4% for BN. Semantic and diagnostic confusion over the term *bulimia* has led to gross overestimates of its prevalence that have limited clinical significance. Nevertheless, eating disorders may be occult (Kutcher, Whitehouse, & Freeman, 1985) or may be more prevalent in high-risk groups (Garfinkel, Garner, & Goldbloom, 1987).

FAMILIAL PATTERN

While recognition of the importance of the family in eating disorders began more than a century ago, little systematic research has explored this, and none has been prospective or controlled in design. Stereotypes of a domineering, intrusive mother and an absent, passive father do not always apply clinically and do not always appear in psychometric evaluations. Nevertheless, some studies have distinguished the bulimic's intrafamiliar environment from that of the restrictor as being more chaotic, conflictual, and openly hostile (Strober & Humphrey, 1987).

Genetic implications exist in the increased prevalence of AN among siblings of AN probands, which may range from 3 to 10%—well in excess of that expected for the general population. A number of twin studies show a concordance rate of 38 to 50% from monozygotic twins as opposed to 11% for dizygotic twins (Garfinkel & Garner, 1982). This may reflect a heightened psychological struggle for identity in the context of biological duplication as much as a genetic diathesis. These disorders do not "breed true." Evidence points to an increased familial prevalence of other, possibly related, psychiatric disorders, such as depression and alcoholism, particularly among families of bulimic probands (Strober, Salkin, Burroughs, & Morrell, 1982), which may have implications for both biological predisposition and treatment.

DIFFERENTIAL DIAGNOSIS

Psychiatric

Increased awareness of eating disorders may lead to overdiagnosis based on inadequate consideration of their distinctive features (Garfinkel, Garner, Kaplan, Rodin, & Kennedy, 1983). Other psychiatric disorders that may ostensibly mimic AN include conversion disorder, schizophrenia, and depression. Distinguishing features of these disorders are summarized in Table 20.5. Vomiting to counteract caloric ingestion in BN must be distinguished from intensely symbolic vomiting as seen in conversion disorder (Garfinkel, Kaplan, Garner, & Darby, 1983).

Medical

The major somatic causes of weight loss are easily distinguished from AN by psychiatric interview and physical examination. Gastrointestinal disturbances such as malabsorption, regional enteritis, and ulcers do not feature the core psychological preoccupations of AN. Neoplasias of the pituitary and periphery may also superficially mimic AN. Tuberculosis similarly induces weight loss, as do endocrine disturbances such as Addison's disease, diabetes mellitus, hypopitutarism, and hyperthyroidism.

The symptom of binge eating, typically in the absence of a morbid fear of fatness or associated purging behaviors, occurs in a variety of medical disorders. These may include Parkinson's disease, the Prader-Willi syndrome, Huntington's chorea,

TABLE 20.4. Complications of Eating Disorders

Complications	Frequency	Cause	Treatment
Cardiovascular System			
Bradycardia	Common	Starvation	Responds to weight restoration
Hypotension	Common	Starvation	Responds to weight restoration
Arrhythmias	Infrequent	Starvation, fluid depletion usually provoked by exercise in starvation; may be due to hypokalemia	Responds to weight restoration or potassium supplements
Cardiomyopathy	Rare	Emetine toxicity from ipecac	Stop the ipecac
Central Nervous System			
Nonspecific EEG changes	Common	Starvation	Weight restoration
Reversible cortical atrophy	Uncommon	Starvation	Weight restoration
Renal/Electrolytes			
Hypokalemia	Common	Loss of potassium from multiple routes (vomiting, diarrhea, and diuretics)	Prevent purging; may need a potassium supplement
		Salt restriction and water intoxication (to meet weight goals)	Well-balanced diet with appropriate amount of fluids
Increased BUN	Uncommon	Dehydration	Rehydration
Metabolic alkalosis	Common	Purging	Prevent purging
Edema	Common	Not clearly understood	Elevate feet for 1 hour t.i.d.; avoid salt; do not use diuretic

Gastrointestinal system			
Parotitis	Common	Mechanical trauma; starvation	No specific treatments; stop binges and vomiting
Early satiety	Common	Delayed gastric emptying	Domperidone 20 mg t.i.d.
Gastric dilatation	Rare	Rapid refeeding	Avoid oral feeding; use IV feeding
Constipation	Common	Starvation; reliance on laxative	Use diet—emphasis on dietary bulk, fruits, vegetables and try to avoid laxatives
Dental caries	Common	Acidic nature of vomitus	Dental consult
Hyperamylasemia	Common in bulimia	Unknown	Prevent purging
Gastric rupture	Rare	Bingeing	Surgery
Superior mesenteric artery syndrome	Rare	Weight loss	Weight restoration
Musculoskeletal system			
Myopathy	Uncommon	Starvation; hypokalemia; emetine myotoxicity of ipecac	Weight restoration; stop ipecac abuse
Osteoporosis	Rare	Starvation	Weight restoration
Thyroid			
Decreased serum T3 and increased reverse T3	Common	Starvation	Weight restoration
Persistent amenorrhea	Infrequent	Low weight; emotional stress	Restore weight to 90% of average
Hematological changes			
Anemia	Infrequent	Bone marrow hypoplasia due to starvation	Weight restoration; may need iron
Thrombocytopenia	Rare	Starvation	Weight restoration
Hypercholesterolemia	Common	Unknown	Balanced diet
Hypercarotenemia	Infrequent	Ingestion of high carotene foods	Balanced diet

TABLE 20.5. Clinical Features of Anorexia Nervosa, Conversion Disorders, Schizophrenia, and Depression

Feature	Anorexia Nervosa	Conversion Disorder	Schizophrenia	Depression
Intense drive for thinness	Marked	None	None	None
Self-imposed starvation	Marked (due to fear of body size)	None	Marked (due to delusions about food)	None
Disturbance in body image	Present (lack of awareness of change in body size and lack of satisfaction or pleasure in the body)	None	None	None
Appetite	Maintained (but with fear of giving in to impulse)	Variable	Maintained	True anorexia
Satiety	Usually bloating, nausea, early satiety	Variable	Variable	Variable
Avoidance of specific foods	Present (for carbohydrates or foods presumed to be high in "calories")	None	Present (of foods that are thought to be poisoned)	Loss of interest in all food
Bulimia	Present in 30 to 50%	May occur	Rare	Rare
Vomiting	Present (to prevent weight gain)	Present (expresses some symbolic meaning)	Rare (to prevent undesirable effects on the body)	None
Laxative abuse	Present (to prevent weight gain)	Infrequently present (expresses some symbolic meaning)	None	None
Activity level	Increased	Reduced or no change	No change	Reduced
Amenorrhea	Present	Present	Present	Present

Source: P.E. Garfinkel, D.M. Garner, A.S. Kaplan, G. Rodin, & S. Kennedy, 1983, "Differential Diagnosis of Emotional Disorders That Cause Weight Loss," *Canadian Medical Association Journal, 129*, pp. 939–945. Reprinted with permission.

Klein-Levin syndrome, and increased intracranial pressure. No known medical illness simulates the larger picture of BN.

CLINICAL MANAGEMENT: RESEARCH FINDINGS

Rigorous outcome data on treatment of eating disorders are limited; every form of psychiatric and psychological therapy has been described (Garner & Garfinkel, 1985; Garfinkel & Garner, 1987) in relation to AN and BN.

Psychological Treatment

Controlled psychosocial treatment studies of AN have recently been reported in the literature (Russell, Szmukler, Dare, & Eisler, 1987) ; the difficulties of psychotherapy research in general are compounded by the presence of a life-threatening disorder in a young population. There is a widespread clinical consensus that the traditional psychoanalytic approach is relatively ineffective and that a cognitive–behavioral approach coupled with an explicit goal of weight restoration and a trusting relationship is more helpful (Hsu, 1986). A clinical trial comparing cognitive–behavioral and psychodynamic psychotherapy in AN and BN is in progress (Garner, personal communication, 1987).

For BN, a number of studies have indicated a role for cognitive–behavioral therapy in symptom reduction (Garner, Fairburn, & Davis, 1987). Whether these treatments provide an enduring change in underlying attitudes and beliefs awaits confirmation.

Biological Treatment

All available evidence indicates that for AN food remains the drug of choice. Despite clinical popularity of the use of chlorpromazine or a benzodiazepine for sedation or control of premeal anxiety, controlled studies in AN have failed to yield clinically significant benefits from amitriptyline, cyproheptadine, pimozide, sulpiride, and lithium. While these medications may play an adjunctive role in individual cases, no data support their widespread or routine use.

The last few decades have witnessed burgeoning research evidence on the role of medications in the treatment of BN. Imipramine, desipramine, and phenelzine have demonstrated efficacy against BN in double-blind placebo-controlled trials. Similar trials of amitriptyline and mianserin have failed to yield benefit greater than placebo (Pope & Hudson, 1986). Research on drug agonists of central serotonergic activity, such as fluoxetine and fenfluramine, as well as antagonists of central opioid activity, such as naltrexone, holds promise.

The next decade of treatment research in eating disorders should include comparative trials of different psychotherapies as well as of pharmacotherapy versus psychotherapy. It is likely that, as in depression, clinical management will continue to require an artful blend of a number of treatment modalities.

DSM-III-R

The revised diagnostic criteria for AN and BN are presented in Tables 20.1 and 20.2. While necessarily arbitrary, they reflect a significant improvement over DSM-III. For AN, the proportion of weight loss required has decreased from 25 to 15% below expected weight, and amenorrhea has been added as a criterion. This allows for diagnosis of the significant number of subjects who develop amenorrhea prior to substantial weight loss.

For BN, the revisions have become more stringent in setting a minimum frequency for binge-eating episodes and more realistic in dropping coincident AN as an exclusion criterion. Further, the name change to bulimia nervosa and the addition of the psychological criterion of a persistent overconcern with body weight and shape decrease semantic and phenomenologic confusion. BN is less widespread than DSM-III bulimia, and the greater precision of the BN criteria will be useful in evaluating research and treatment.

REFERENCES

Altshuler, K.A., & Weiner, M.F. (1985). Anorexia nervosa and depression: A dissenting view. *American Journal of Psychiatry*, *142*, 328–332.

American Psychiatric Association. (1980). *Diagnostic and statistical manual of mental disorders* (3rd ed.). Washington, DC: Author.

American Psychiatric Association. (1987). *Diagnostic and statistical manual of mental disorders* (3rd ed., rev.). Washington, DC: Author.

Andersen, A.E. (1985). *Practical comprehensive treatment of anorexia nervosa and bulimia*. Baltimore: Johns Hopkins University Press.

Artmann, M., Grau, H. Adelmann, M., & Schlieffer, R. (1985). Reversible and non-reversible enlargement of cerebrospinal fluid spaces in anorexia nervosa. *Neuroradiology*, *27*, 304–312.

Bell, R.M. (1985). *Holy anorexia*. Chicago: University of Chicago Press.

Binswanger, L. (1944). Der fall Ellen West. *Schweizer Archiv für Neurologie und Psychiatrie*. Translated in R. May, E. Angel, & H. Ellenberger (Eds.), *Existence*. New York: Basic (1957).

Boskind-Lodahl, M. (1976). Cinderella's stepsisters: A feminist perspective on anorexia nervosa and bulimia. *Signs: Journal of Women in Culture & Society*, *2*, 342–356.

Bruch, M. (1973). *Eating disorders: Obesity, anorexia nervosa, and the person within*. New York: Basic.

Button, E.J., & Whitehouse, A. (1981). Subclinical anorexia nervosa. *Psychological Medicine*, *11*, 509–516.

Casper, R.C. (1983). On the emergence of bulimia nervosa as a syndrome: A historical view. *International Journal of Eating Disorders*, *2*, 3–16.

Casper, R.C., Eckert, E.D., Halmi, K.A., Goldberg, S.C., & Davis, J.M. (1980). Bulimia: Its incidence and clinical importance in patients with anorexia nervosa. *Archives of General Psychiatry*, *37*, 1030–1035.

Crisp, A.H. (1980). *Anorexia nervosa: Let me be*. London: Academic.

Datlof, S., Coleman, P.D., Forbes, G.B., & Kriepe, R.E. (1986). Ventricular dilatation on CAT scans of patients with anorexia nervosa. *American Journal of Psychiatry, 143*, 96–98.

Fairburn, C.G., & Cooper, P.J. (1984). The clinical features of bulimia nervosa. *British Journal of Psychiatry, 144*, 238–246.

Fairburn, C.G., & Garner, D.M. (1986). The diagnosis of bulimia nervosa. *International Journal of Eating Disorders, 5*, 403–419.

Freeman, R.J., Thomas, C.D., Solyom, L., & Koopman, R.F. (1985). Clinical and personality correlates of body size overestimation in anorexia nervosa and bulimia nervosa. *International Journal of Eating Disorders, 4*, 439–456.

Fries, H. (1977). Studies on second amenorrhea, anorectic behaviour, and body-image perception: Importance for the early recognition of anorexia nervosa. In R. Vigersky (Ed.), *Anorexia nervosa*. New York: Raven.

Garfinkel, P.E., & Garner, D.M. (1982). *Anorexia nervosa: A multidimensional perspective*. New York: Brunner/Mazel.

Garfinkel, P.E., & Garner, D.M. (Eds.). (1987). *The role of drug therapies for the eating disorders*. New York: Brunner/Mazel.

Garfinkel, P.E., Garner, D.M., & Goldbloom, D.S. (1987). Eating disorders: Implications for the 1990's. *Canadian Journal of Psychiatry, 32*, 624–631.

Garfinkel, P.E., Garner, D.M., Kaplan, A.S., Rodin, G., & Kennedy, S. (1983). Differential diagnosis of emotional disorders that cause weight loss. *Canadian Medical Association Journal, 129*, 939–945.

Garfinkel, P.E., & Kaplan, A.S. (1986). Anorexia nervosa: Diagnostic conceptualizations. In K.D. Brownell & J.P. Foreyt (Eds.), *Handbook of eating disorders*. New York: Basic.

Garfinkel, P.E., Kaplan, A.S., Garner, D.M., & Darby, P.L. (1983). The differentiation of vomiting/weight loss as a conversion disorder from anorexia nervosa. *American Journal of Psychiatry, 140*, 1019–1022.

Garfinkel, P.E., Moldofsky, M., & Garner, D.M. (1980). The heterogeneity of anorexia nervosa: Bulimia as a distinct subgroup. *Archives of General Psychiatry, 37*, 1036–1040.

Garner, D.M., & Bemis, K.M. (1982). A cognitive behavioural approach to anorexia nervosa. *Cognitive Research and Therapy, 6*, 1–27.

Garner, D.M., Fairburn, C., & Davis, R. (1987). Cognitive behavioural treatment of bulimia nervosa: A critical appraisal. *Behaviour Modification, 11*, 398–431.

Garner, D.M., & Garfinkel, P.E. (Eds.). (1985). *Handbook of psychotherapy for anorexia nervosa and bulimia*. New York: Guilford.

Garner, D.M., Garfinkel, P.E., Stancer, H.C., & Moldofsky, H. (1976). Body image disturbances in anorexia nervosa and obesity. *Psychosomatic Medicine, 38*, 227–336.

Garner, D.M., Olmsted, M.P., & Garfinkel, P.E. (1983). Does anorexia nervosa occur on a continuum? Subgroups of weight-preoccupied women and their relationship to anorexia nervosa. *International Journal of Eating Disorders, 2*, 11–19.

Garner, D.M., Olmsted, M.P., & Garfinkel, P.E. (1985). Similarities among bulimic groups selected by different weights and weight histories. *Journal of Psychiatric Research, 19*, 129–134.

Gold, P.W., Gwirtsman, H., Avgerinos, P.C., Nieman, L.K., Gallucci, W.T., Kaye, W., Jimerson, D., Ebert, M., Rittmaster, R., Loriaux, D.L., & Chrousos, G.P. (1986). Abnormal hypothalamic-pituitary-adrenal function in anorexia nervosa. *New England Journal of Medicine*, *314*, 1335–1342.

Gull, W.W. (1874). Anorexia nervosa (apepsia hysterica, anorexia hysterica). *Transactions of the Clinical Society of London*, 7, 22–28.

Halmi, K.A. (1985). Relationship of the eating disorders to depression: Biological similarities and differences. *International Journal of Eating Disorders*, 4, 667–680.

Halmi, K.A., Casper, R.C., Eckert, E.D., Goldberg, S.C., & Davis, J.M. (1979). Unique features associated with age of onset of anorexia nervosa. *Psychiatry Research*, *1*, 209–215.

Hsu, L.K.G. (1986). The treatment of anorexia nervosa. *American Journal of Psychiatry*, *143*, 573–581.

Hsu, L.K.G., & Holder, D. (1986). Bulimia nervosa: Treatment and short-term outcome. *Psychological Medicine*, *16*, 65–70.

Isner, J.M., Roberts, W.C., Heymsfield, S.B., & Yager, J. (1985). Anorexia nervosa and sudden death. *Annals of Internal Medicine*, *102*, 49–52.

Jacobs, M.B., & Schneider, J.A. (1985). Medical complications of bulimia: A prospective evaluation. *Quarterly Journal of Medicine*, *214*, 177–182.

Kaplan, A.S. (1987). Hyperamylasemia and bulimia: A clinical review. *International Journal of Eating Disorders*, *6*, 537–543.

Kaplan, A.S., & Garfinkel, P.E. (1984). Bulimia in the Talmud. *American Journal of Psychiatry*, *141*, 721.

Kennedy, S.M., & Garfinkel, P.E. (1987). Neuroendocrine function in anorexia nervosa and bulimia. In C.B. Nemeroff & P.T. Loosen (Eds.), *Handbook of clinical psychoneuroendocrinology*. New York: Guilford.

Keys, A., Brozek, J., Henschel, A., Mickelson, O., & Taylor, H.L. (1950). *The biology of human starvation*. Minneapolis: University of Minnesota Press.

Kutcher, S.P., Whitehouse, A.M., & Freeman, C.P.L. (1985). "Hidden" eating disorders in Scottish psychiatric inpatients. *American Journal of Psychiatry*, *142*, 1475–1478.

Lasegue, C. (1873). On hysterical anorexia. *Medical Times & Gazette*, 2, 265–266, 367–369.

Levin, P.A., Falko, J.M., Dixon, K., Gallup, E.M., & Saunders, W. (1980). Benign parotid enlargement in bulimia. *Annals of Internal Medicine*, *93*, 827–829.

McCallum, R.W., Grill, B.B., Lange, R., Planky, M., Glass, E.E., & Greenfield, D.G. (1985). Definition of a gastric emptying abnormality in patients with anorexia nervosa. *Digestive Diseases & Sciences*, *30*, 713–722.

Minuchin, S., Rosman, B.L., & Baker, L. (1978). *Psychosomatic families: Anorexia nervosa in context*. Cambridge, MA: Harvard University Press.

Mitchell, J.E. (1986). Anorexia nervosa: Medical and physiological aspects. In K.D. Brownell & J.P. Foreyt (Eds.), *Handbook of eating disorders*. New York: Basic.

Mitchell, J.E., Hatsukami, D., Eckert, E.D., & Pyle, R.L. (1985). Characteristics of 275 patients with bulimia. *American Journal of Psychiatry*, *142*, 482–485.

Mitchell, J.E., Pyle, R.L., Hatsukami, D., & Eckert, E.D. (1986). What are atypical eating disorders? *Psychosomatics*, *27*, 21–28.

Morton, R. (1694). *Phthisiologica: or, a treatise of consumptions*. London: Smith & Walford.

Palmer, R.L. (1979). The dietary chaos syndrome: A useful new term? *British Journal of Medical Psychology*, *52*, 187–190.

Piran, N., Kennedy, S., Garfinkel, P.E., & Owens, M. (1985). Affective disturbance in eating disorders. *Journal of Nervous & Mental Diseases*, *173*, 395–400.

Piran, N., Lerner, P., Garfinkel, P.E., Kennedy, S.M., & Brouillette, C. (in press). Personality disorders in restricting and bulimic forms of anorexia nervosa. *International Journal of Eating Disorders*.

Pope, H.G., & Hudson, J.I. (1986). Antidepressant therapy for bulimia: Current status. *Journal of Clinical Psychiatry*, *47*, 339–345.

Powers, P.S. (1982). Heart failure during treatment of anorexia nervosa. *American Journal of Psychiatry*, *139*, 1167–1170.

Russell, G.F.M. (1979). Bulimia nervosa: An ominous variant of anorexia nervosa. *Psychological Medicine*, *9*, 429–448.

Russell, G.F.M. (1983). Anorexia nervosa and bulimia nervosa. In G.F.M. Russell & L. Hersov (Eds.), *Handbook of psychiatry: Vol. 4. The neuroses and personality disorders*. Cambridge: Cambridge University Press.

Russell, G.F.M., Szmukler, G.I., Dare, C., & Eisler, I. (1987). An evaluation of family therapy in anorexia nervosa and bulimia nervosa. *Archives of General Psychiatry*, *44*, 1047–1056.

Simmonds, M. (1914). Ueber embolische prozesse in der hypophysis. *Archives of Pathology and Anatomy*, *217*, 226–239.

Simmons, M.S., Grayden, S.K., & Mitchell, J.E. (1986). The need for psychiatric–dental liaison in the treatment of bulimia. *American Journal of Psychiatry*, *143*, 783–784.

Slade, P.D., & Russell, G.F.M. (1973). Experimental investigations of bodily perception in anorexia nervosa and obesity. *Psychotherapy & Psychosomatics*, *22*, 259–363.

Strober, M., & Humphrey, L. (1987). Familial contributions to the etiology and course of anorexia nervosa and bulimia. *Journal of Consulting and Clinical Psychology*, *5*, 654–659.

Strober, M., Salkin, B., Burroughs J., Morrell, W. (1982). Validity of the bulimia–restricter distinction in anorexia nervosa. *Journal of Nervous & Mental Disease*, *170*, 345–351.

Strupp, B.J., Weingartner, H., Kaye, W., & Gwirtsman, H. (1986). Cognitive processing in anorexia nervosa: A disturbance in automatic information processing. *Neuropsychobiology*, *15*, 89–94.

Szmukler, G.I. (1983). Weight and food preoccupation in a population of English schoolgirls. In *Understanding anorexia nervosa and bulimia*. Columbus, OH: Ross Laboratories.

Theander, S. (1985). Outcome and prognosis in anorexia nervosa and bulimia: Some results of previous investigations, compared with those of a Swedish long-term study. *Journal of Psychiatric Research*, *19*, 493–508.

Toner, B.B., Garfinkel, P.E., & Garner, D.M. (1986). Long-term follow-up of anorexia nervosa. *Psychosomatic Medicine, 48,* 520–529.

Waller, J.V., Kaufman, M.R., & Deutsch, F. (1940). Anorexia nervosa: Psychosomatic entity. *Psychosomatic Medicine, 2,* 3–16.

Williams, J.F., Friedman, I.M., & Steiner, H. (1986). Hand lesions characteristic of bulimia. *American Journal of Diseases of Children, 140,* 28–29.

CHAPTER 21

Functional Enuresis and Encopresis

DANIEL M. DOLEYS

FUNCTIONAL ENURESIS

Definition

DSM-III-R defines functional enuresis as "repeated involuntary or intentional voiding of urine during the day or night into bed or clothes, after an age at which continence is expected" (APA, 1987, p. 84). Episodes must occur at least twice per month for children 5 to 6 years old and once per month for older children. Chronological age must be at least 5 and mental age 4. The enuresis cannot be attributable to physical causes.

There are about 90 different types of urinary incontinence (Lund, 1963), but more than 90% fall into the functional category. The two basic subtypes are primary (continuous) and secondary (discontinuous). Primary enuretics have never been continent, whereas the secondary enuretic has had at least a year of continence. Approximately 80% of enuretics are primary. Enuresis can be further subdivided into diurnal (daytime), nocturnal (nighttime), or both.

Surprisingly, little is known about daytime enuresis. There appears to be no commonly accepted definition. Some have proposed a single wet day per month (Hallgren, 1956; Oppel, Harper, & Rider, 1968). Others have also included frequency and urgency in the definition.

Historical Background

The term *enuresis* is derived from Greek terminology and means "to make water." Enuresis was first recognized as a medical problem in 1550 B.C. (Glicklich, 1951). It was included as a disease in the first English pediatric text.

Treatment of enuresis has frequently been rather inhumane. Parents have been known to beat their children, set them with their wet clothes on hot radiators, shame and ridicule them, display wet clothing and/or bedding, and tie off the penis. Surprisingly, punishment, especially in the form of embarrassment, was done with professional approval. Even though Mowrer and Mowrer described the urine alarm as a treatment for nocturnal enuresis as early as 1938, abusive types of treatments can still be heard of, and unenlightened professionals still tell parents, "Don't worry, your child will grow out of it."

Some present-day therapies make no more theoretical sense, given the available data, than did ground hedgehog or viscera of pigs and urine from spayed swine used in the fifteenth and sixteenth centuries. Even as recently as the nineteenth century, steel spikes in the mattress, cauterization of the urethra with silver nitrate, and inflated rubber bags in the vagina to compress the bladder neck were used.

Today the treatment of nocturnal enuresis is both more humane and more commercial. Several mail-order catalogs sell urine alarms, with the instructions "rubber stamped." Fortunately, no assembly is required, but often batteries are not included. There are even "in the home" treatment companies. Some demonstrate their credibility by boasting approval by certain magazines and lay groups. Treatment of enuresis has indeed become "big business."

Unfortunately, the unsuspecting parent is unaware of the large body of literature dealing with assessment, treatment, and devices available. While certain procedures, such as the urine alarm, are easily implemented and in fact work with perhaps the majority of enuretics, the lack of knowledgeable individual attending to the problem may well increase the rate of relapse. Also, there is good reason to believe that each failed treatment renders the problem more resistant to subsequent attempts.

Clinical Picture

The pattern of wetting for these children may vary considerably. Differences can be found in the frequency, magnitude, and timing of the episodes. Some may go extended periods without incontinence. The nocturnal enuretic may wet more than once per month. Some awaken immediately after wetting; others do not. Most will avoid the wet spot and may move to the floor for the rest of the night. Many parents complain of their children being "deep sleepers" and very hard to awaken. Arousal conditioning may be important, as it is generally easier for the child to become continent by learning to awaken to bladder distention at night rather than trying to sleep through the night.

Frequently, daytime enuretics do feel the urge to void but report that it is "too late." Urinary frequency and urgency are not uncommon. A few nocturnal enuretics report dreams of water, but this is not common. Nocturnal enuresis may occur in any stage of sleep.

Most children are embarrassed by the problem and reluctant to seek help. When behavioral problems coexist, they are likely to be a result rather than a cause of the enuresis and improve as the enuresis does. Parental attitude and compliance are highly correlated with successful treatment. Too often children present for treatment in late childhood or early teen years because some professional has suggested that the child wait.

When diurnal and nocturnal enuresis coexist, there is no indication that elimination of one problem affects the other. However, the author has found diurnal enuresis somewhat easier to treat. Success with daytime wetting may improve compliance and motivation for treatment of nighttime wetting, which can take considerably longer.

Associated Features

While it is commonly assumed that the majority of enuretic children have a higher incidence of behavioral and emotional disorders than nonenuretics, this has not been demonstrated. The incidence of behavioral problems among enuretics does appear greater than for nonenuretics (Rutter, Tizard, & Whitmore, 1970; Werry & Cohrssen, 1967), especially for girls, but the majority of enuretics have no additional problems. Secondary enuretics appear to have a higher rate of associated behavioral problems than do primary enuretics (Rutter et al., 1970). When associated pathology is observed, it is more likely to be a result rather than a cause of the enuresis and improves when continence is achieved.

An often ignored consequence of enuresis is urinary tract infection. The risk of infection is greater for females. If left untreated, infection can give rise to reduced functional capacity, progressive damage, and renal insufficiency.

The effect of enuresis on parental attitudes and attributions has become a recent concern (Butler, Brewin, & Forsythe, 1986; Morgan & Young, 1975), especially in light of the fact that enuresis has been associated with child abuse (Kempe & Helfer, 1972). Maternal intolerance is higher in lower socioeconomic groups and correlates with dropout from treatment and with an overly punitive approach by parents to the problem.

Course and Prognosis

The fact that 20% of children 5 years old and only about 2% of children 12 to 14 years old wet frequently enough to be considered enuretic suggests a high rate of spontaneous remission. Fifty percent of older children compared to 80% of younger children are of the continuous type. This suggests: (1) that children tend to relapse after they become continent; and/or (2) that some children begin to wet after they have had a period of continence. While it is true that, left untreated, the majority of enuretics appear to become continent, our understanding of this process is poor. It is fair to assume that many of these children are exposed to "home remedies" that may be very punitive, and at least untested. Ridicule by peers, social isolation, and reduced self-esteem and confidence are likely to be consequences of untreated enuresis. Some support for this is obtained from data showing children who are successfully treated often appear much better adjusted, happier, and more content (Baker, 1969; Dische, 1971; Werry & Cohrssen, 1965).

Impairment

The amount of impairment caused by daytime and nighttime enuresis is primarily related to child self-esteem and social behavior. In the very young, continence is often required to gain admission to certain school programs. Mostly, however, fear of detection limits the child's activities, especially being away from home overnight. With girls there is a higher likelihood of urinary tract infection.

Parental attitudes and attribution can impair normal parent–child relationships. Response can vary from total ambivalence to abuse. The effect on the child appears temporary, as improvement and measures of self-esteem are correlated with remission of enuresis.

Epidemiology

The prevalence rates of enuresis vary with age. It is estimated that about 15 to 20% of children 5 years old, 5% of children 10 years old, and 2 to 3% of children 12 to 14 years old are nocturnal enuretics (Rutter, Yule, & Graham, 1973). This disorder occurs about twice as often in boys as in girls. Enuresis is more common in lower socioeconomic groups and in fractured family situations (i.e., divorce, separation, death) and institutional settings.

A variety of factors have been implicated as being of etiological importance. Enuresis has been seen as an arousal disorder. EEG recordings note that children do wet in each of the four stages of sleep but rarely in REM (rapid eye movement). However, investigations have failed to differentiate between the depth of sleep, as measured by EEG, and arousability, a behavioral measure of how easily a child can be aroused. Recent data have not been supportive of enuresis being an arousal disorder (Mikkelsen et al., 1980), and studies comparing enuretics and nonenuretics on the dimension of arousability yield conflicting data (Bostack, 1958; Boyd, 1960; Braithwaithe, 1956; Kaffman & Elizur, 1977).

Genetic predisposition is considered based on the high concordance rates found among monozygotic versus dizygotic twins (Bakwin, 1973). Gerrard and his colleagues (Esperance & Gerrard, 1969; Zaleski, Gerrard, & Shokeir, 1973) have suggested that enuretics have smaller functional bladder capacity secondary to inadequate cortical inhibitions or allergic reactions. Overlap between functional bladder capacities of enuretics and nonenuretics has called this explanation into question (Rutter, 1973). In addition, increasing bladder capacity does not appear to be associated with decreased nocturnal enuresis, although there is some suggestion that it is correlated with daytime wetting.

Learning theory approaches enuresis as a habit deficiency resulting from inadequate or inappropriate learning experiences and/or reinforcement contingencies (Atthowe, 1973; Lovibond & Coote, 1970). Certainly, the conditioning-based treatments generated by this approach have been the most effective treatments. Psychodynamic approaches conceptualize enuresis as a symptom of some underlying conflict or emotional state (Pierce, 1952; Sperling, 1957). In fact, most enuretics do not appear to have emotional or behavioral disturbances. Symptom substitution, as predicted by this model, has not been documented, and psychodynamic therapies have proven to be inefficient or ineffective.

Prevalence figures for daytime enuresis are lower than for nighttime and range around 1% of 5-year-olds. It is slightly more common in girls and declines with age. About 30% of nocturnal enuretics also have diurnal problems. More than 75% of diurnal enuretics are continuous. Diurnal enuretics show a higher incidence of urinary frequency and urgency.

There is some suggestion that diurnal and nocturnal enuresis are governed by different mechanisms (Fiedling, 1980). The response patterns to treatment differ and there are higher rates of emotional and behavioral problems as well as encopresis in the diurnal enuretic.

Reduced bladder capacity, bladder instability, urinary infections, and psychological disturbances have been implicated as etiologically important. The "urge syndrome" or nonneurogenic bladder is found in girls who have diurnal and nocturnal wetting. These urges are accompanied by uninhibited bladder contractions and voiding. *Detrusor sphincter dyssynergia* refers to a lack of coordinated action between the internal and external urinary sphincters found in some diurnal enuretics (Fielding, 1982).

The lazy bladder syndrome is associated with low frequency and high functional bladder capacity and is found more frequently in boys. Chronic inhibition of voiding in the presence of the urge can give rise to overdistention of the bladder and bladder decompensation. These various diurnal patterns may be related to encouraging the child to void at the first sign of an urge or forced inhibition. A working model of diurnal bladder functioning has been proposed by Fielding (1982).

Familial Pattern

Familial pattern appears strong. It is estimated that nearly 75% of first-degree relatives of enuretics have also been enuretic. In addition, the concordance rates for monozygotic twins is nearly twice that for dizygotic twins: 68% versus 36% (Bakwin, 1971). However, this relationship is stronger for males than for females.

Differential Diagnosis

The main diagnostic groupings are related to duration of the problem and presence or absence of organic pathology. If a child has never been continent, he or she is described as a primary or continuous enuretic and he or she is described as secondary or discontinuous if continence has been achieved for a year or more. Small functional bladder capacities can be determined by use of the water-loading test or monitoring of voiding patterns. Urinary tract infections are present in about 10% of females and are detected by characteristics of the urinary stream and urinalysis. A general physical examination and urine culture can rule out most renal pathology. Voiding cystourethrogram, cystoscopy, and excretory urogram are invasive but useful diagnostic procedures for assessing organic pathology. These procedures should be reserved for those children recalcitrant to treatment or who display symptoms suggestive of neurogenic problems. Appropriate assessment is necessary and can yield many benefits (Fielding & Doleys, in press).

Clinical Management: Research Findings

The clinical management of nocturnal enuresis has fallen into four categories: drugs, bladder expansion, dry bed training, and urine alarm. A variety of stimulants, anticholinergics, tranquilizers, and antidepressants have been used. Imipramine hydrocholoride has emerged as having the greatest efficacy. However, total continence is realized in only 30% of cases, and relapse following withdrawal of the drug is as high as 95% (Stewart, 1975).

Bladder expansion exercises are directed at increasing functional bladder capacity, thereby allowing the child to retain during the night or until the distention cues are sufficiently strong to awaken him or her. Introduced and studied in the late 1960s and 1970s, the technique has not been proven superior to the urine alarm. However, it is frequently combined with the urine alarm and used as a component of dry bed training.

Dry bed training is a multifaceted program incorporating positive practice, positive reinforcement, retention control training, nighttime awakening, negative reinforcement, and full cleanliness training. Introduced by Azrin, Sneed, and Foxx (1973, 1974), it initially produced remarkable results and was seen as an alternative to the urine alarm. Replications have yielded inconsistent results. A series of well-controlled studies by Bollard (Bollard, 1982; Bollard & Nettelbeck, 1981; Bollard, Nettelbeck, & Roxbee, 1982; Bollard & Woodroofe, 1977) showed that dry bed training was about as effective as the urine alarm procedure and that its effect was diminished if the urine alarm was not used as part of the procedure.

The urine alarm has been the most popular of enuresis treatments. A urine-sensing device is placed on the bed or attached to the child's clothes. A bell or buzzer of sufficient intensity to awaken the child is triggered by voiding. A review of the studies from 1960 to 1975 showed 75% of children successfully treated, with treatment duration ranging from 5 to 12 weeks. Rate of relapse was approximately 40%, with nearly 70% of these successfully retreated (Doleys, 1977). Relapse continues to be a major issue. Various modifications in treatment, such as scheduling of the alarm, overlearning, extending treatment duration, and combining the urine alarm with drugs, have been explored as mechanisms to reduce relapse. Patient motivation, parental attitude and compliance, type of device, and proper assessment of the problem have been linked to outcome.

The treatment of daytime wetting has not received as much attention as the treatment of nighttime wetting. Retention control training combined with full cleanliness training has been used with success. Several detection devices (Dixon & Smith, 1976) are available allowing for a form of urine alarm training to be carried out. Scheduled visits to the bathroom, training and cue discrimination regarding bladder fullness, and systematic toilet training with reinforcement of appropriate behavior have also been employed depending upon the particular deficiency noted during assessment.

The use of EMG biofeedback therapy is seen with great regularity in treating dysfunctional bladder syndromes associated with diurnal enuresis (Maizels, King, & Firlit, 1979; Wear, Wear, & Cleeland, 1979). Treatment focuses on retraining the child to produce coordinated movements between the internal and external sphincters in response to increased bladder fullness. Some success has also been realized with cases of neurogenic bladders (Nergardh, van Hedenberg, Hellstrom, & Ericsson, 1974). This work is summarized in a chapter by Doleys (1983).

DSM-III-R

There have been a number of changes from DSM-III to DSM-III-R (APA, 1987). (1) The new definition specifies that wetting may be into clothes or bed. (2) A chronological age of 5 and mental age of 4 is included in the criteria. (3) Primary and secondary types are differentiated. (4) DSM-III indicated urinary tract infections as a complication, especially in girls, but this is omitted in the revision.

Except for number 4, the changes seem appropriate. There are enough data to correlate infection with enuresis that the author believes it should have remained. It is to be hoped that future editions will specifically include dysfunctional bladder syndromes, as several of these disorders are linked to toileting practices and correctable by behavioral procedures. This would seem to fit what most consider to be a functional versus organic problem.

FUNCTIONAL ENCOPRESIS

Definition

Functional encopresis has been defined as the "repeated involuntary (or, much more rarely, intentional) passage of feces into places not appropriate for that purpose (e.g., clothing or floor)" (APA, 1987, p. 82). There is some disagreement as to the age at which a child can be considered encopretic. It is sometimes difficult to differentiate the child who is encopretic from one who has never been toilet-trained. Information regarding the individual's general developmental rate, prior attempts at toilet training, and presence of bladder control is important in formulating the diagnosis. Most workers in this area, however, agree that socialized children in this society should be bowel-trained by the age of 4.

Functional encopresis is further differentiated as either primary (continuous) or secondary (discontinuous). The primary encopretic is one who has not achieved total fecal continence for the prior year. The secondary encopretic has demonstrated a period of fecal continence of at least a year. Children should also be differentiated according to the presence or absence of retention or constipation. This can vary in degree from 2 to 14 or more days. Retention may be secondary to "pot refusal syndrome" (Berg & Jones, 1964), where the encopretic child is being noncompliant. In other children, the retention or constipation may be secondary to avoidance behavior stimulated by fear of toileting and/or painful defecation (Doleys, 1979).

Historical Background

The term *encopresis* appears to have been established as the fecal equivalent of enuresis. It began to appear in the literature around the 1920s. For reasons that are unclear, encopresis seems to have fallen more into the medical–organic realm than enuresis. Enuresis is further differentiated in the *Merck Manual* as being organic or functional. It is interesting that the diagnostic term *encopresis* does not appear in the *Merck Manual*, but the condition is listed as *fecal incontinence*. The brief two-paragraph discussion relates only to those cases where organic pathology is evident and leaves the reader with the impression that all fecal incontinence is associated with organic pathology. Schaefer (1979) suggests that the first case of psychogenic or emotionally based fecal incontinence may have been reported by Fowler (1882). He also speculates that the term *encopresis* first appeared in the literature in a paper by Weissenberg (1926). Perhaps, as Schaeffer (1979) has suggested, Anthony (1957) best accounted for the relative paucity of literature on encopresis compared to enuresis by noting: "Clinicians on the whole, perhaps out of disgust, prefer neither to treat them (encopretics) nor to write about them" (p. 157).

Clinical Picture

The estimates of the incidence of functional encopresis vary from 1.5 to 7.5% of children. Newson and Newson (1968) reported that 2.8% of males 7 to 8 years of age and 0.7% of females of the same age were encopretic. It appears that boys generally outnumber girls 6 to 1. One detailed study performed by Levine (1975) examined 102 encopretics. Eighty-five percent were male, and 50% of the total sample were incontinent during the day and night. Most of the children denied the ability to detect the urge to defecate and complained of abdominal pains, poor appetite, and lethargy. Fecal impactions were found to one degree or another in approximately 75%; 40% were diagnosed as continuous encopretics. Familial, marital, and behavioral pathologies were not major contributing factors.

Many of these children are of average intellectual capacity and have undergone a variety of examinations for the problem. Parents present either ambivalent or thoroughly disgusted with the situation, including inadequate response on the part of the child to a variety of treatment attempts. Use of purgatives, regular toileting, restriction of privileges, shaming, and diet manipulation have usually been attempted with minimal or no results.

Associated Symptoms

A family disruption resulting from attempts to treat or control encopresis is not uncommon. The encopretic child may withdraw from social contact and indeed may be isolated from peers. Changes in school performance, both behaviorally and academically, may be present. The child may be subjected to ridicule by siblings and attempt to cover up the problem by discarding or hiding soiled underwear. Some become so desensitized to the presence of soiled underwear that they do not change their clothes until prompted to do so. Many will deny the problem upon initial interview, even when they are aware of the reason for being brought to treatment. Parental frustration may accelerate to the point of stimulating discipline that can border on abuse. Parents seem to have a much lower tolerance for encopresis than they do for enuresis. In some cases, the problem behavior is considered willful disobedience on the part of the child. The uneducated professional, unfortunately, does little to rectify this misconception, especially when all medical diagnostic studies are normal. Nocturnal encopresis is relatively rare and often is associated with the presence of organic pathology. The prognosis in such cases is considered poor to guarded.

Course and Prognosis

Incidence figures show that 1.2% of males and 0.3% of females are encopretic at 10 to 12 years of age (Rutter et al., 1970), which is about one-half the number noted for children 7 to 8 years of age. Spontaneous remission has been estimated at 13.5% of children 7.5 to 12 years of age, and 14 to 16% of children 5 to 19 years of age (Forsythe & Redmond, 1974). Longitudinal data noting the course of encopresis over time for a specified group and extending into the teenage years or beyond are not available. Figures are likely to differ for the continuous and discontinuous encopretics. As the incidence of encopresis in adulthood appears unknown, it would be tempting to assume that the vast majority, if not all, functionally encopretic children become continent eventually. This assumption, however, cannot be substantiated and does not take into account the trials and tribulations suffered by the parent(s) and children.

Research data and treatment outcome are rather promising. Comprehensive programs such as Doleys (1982), Wright (1973, 1975), and Levine (Levine & Bakow, 1976) report success rates of up to 100%. Follow-up duration varies from 3 to 36 months. Continuous encopretics respond more slowly than discontinuous and retentive slower than nonretentive in general.

Therefore, left untreated it is very likely that the encopretic child will become continent, but the psychological cost may be high. The prognosis for improvement in well-managed therapy is good, making it hard to justify nontreatment of these children.

Complications

The major complication of encopresis is megacolon. This condition arises secondary to excessive retention. Sustained distention of the colon stretches the muscles used to propel fecal material. Stretch receptors used to cue the presence of fecal mass become desensitized, thus resulting in more prolonged retention. In some instances, fecal retention has been associated with increased urinary frequency and decreased emptying, which can lead to bladder infection.

Impairment

The impairment to children with encopresis can be significant. Many become socially isolated for fear of detection by peers. When discovered, they are often exposed to ridicule. Self-esteem declines. Acting out may be present. Some lie about their problem, and others cover it up by hiding their underwear. Detection, however, appears inevitable. Family activities are orchestrated around the problem. For example, camps and overnight outings are avoided. Some children begin to retain as a mechanism of control, only to complicate the encopresis. Others learn that decreased activity may reduce frequency of bowel activity.

Encopretic children are often accused of being lazy and lacking in discipline and motivation. Few believe the children are often unable to detect the need to defecate. Parents and extended family try all sorts of "home remedies" before presenting the child for treatment, only to enhance the frustration. Iatrogenic factors enter in when the unsuspecting parent or child becomes exposed to any ill-prepared and uninformed professional.

Epidemiology

Estimates of the incidence of encopresis vary from 1.5 to 7.5% of children. Levine (1982) reported that 1.5% of second graders were encopretic. Bellman (1966) noted about 8% of 3-year-olds and 2.4% of 4-year-olds to be encopretic, with a decrease of 0.3% each year from 4 to 7 years of age. In another study, Newson and Newson (1968) found 2.3% of males and 0.7% of females 7 to 8 years of age to be encopretic. The problem occurs about six times more often in males than in females. About 0.5% of encopretics also have enuresis.

Levine (1975) examined 102 encopretics. Eighty-seven were between the ages of 4 and 13 years; 85% were male and 50% were incontinent during the day and night. Forty percent were continuous, and 75% had impactions. Familial, marital, and behavioral pathologies were not major contributing factors. Quality of parental interaction, coerciveness during toilet training, and ambivalence of parents have been cited as significant etiological factors (Anthony, 1957; Pinkerton, 1958). Constitutional predisposition, circumstances of the environment, and critical life events are also described (Levine, 1982).

Familial Pattern

Little is known regarding familial pattern in encopresis. Bellman (1966) did note that 15% of fathers of encopretics reported having encopresis at some time in their own lives.

Differential Diagnosis

Functional encopresis must be differentiated from disorders involving sensory or structural abnormalities. Constipation, especially early in life, may be associated with congenital hypothyroidism, anorectal anomalies (Hendren, 1978; Leape & Ramenofsky, 1978) or Hirschsprung's disease (aganglionic megacolon) (Ravitch, 1958). Crohn's disease resulting from thrombosis or scarring of inflamed bowel, malnutrition, cerebral palsy, and infectious polynephritis are all possibilities to be ruled out (Levine, 1982).

A physical examination and comprehensive history will rule out many of the disorders just named. X-ray films may be needed. Anorectal manometry (Engel,

1978; Schuster, 1968) is being used with increased frequency to assess internal and external anal sphincter activity. Some have indicated its use in differentiating functional from organic encopresis (Molnar, Taitz, Urwin, & Wales, 1983; Shaw, Bosher, & Blair, 1980). Paradoxical diarrhea is found in some children with megacolon and large impactions (Davidson, 1958). Differential diagnosis is required to ensure proper treatment. Biopsy and barium enema are seldom required.

Clinical Management: Research Findings

The research literature has been reviewed extensively elsewhere (Doleys, 1978, 1979, 1985; Parker & Whitehead, 1982; Schaefer, 1979; Walker, 1978). There are many procedures that have been implemented and shown to be successful, albeit with small numbers of subjects and without the appropriate controls. Inadequate description of the problem and subject, absence of long-term follow-up, and lack of the relationship between treatment success and subject characteristics have also plagued this area. However, several treatment programs have emerged as being successful and appear to have some common characteristics.

Adequate assessment and description of the problem are paramount. Appropriate subtyping and differential diagnosis are needed. Multiple features of the problem must be monitored in treatment. This was very nicely demonstrated in a recent article by O'Brien, Ross, and Christophersen (1986) where appropriate and inappropriate toileting and independent toileting were monitored, along with frequency of cathartics. Behavioral data are collected for a baseline (assessment), treatment, and follow-up. In clinical practice, there is an unfortunate tendency to initiate treatment without adequate baseline data. Frequent contact with the parents (who need to be thoroughly educated regarding the problem, the treatment, and the plan to ensure compliance) is necessary.

Most programs utilize frequent pants checks and regular toileting. Parents control the availability of underwear so that the child cannot cover up accidents by hiding soiled clothes. Bowel movements are prompted by use of cathartics and/or increased dietary fiber. Provisions are made for the management of retention or constipation. This may require occasional use of enemas and must be carefully monitored to avoid abuse. Doleys (1987) recommended that they be administered by medical personnel as opposed to the family. Some mechanism for fading the cathartics, enemas, and so forth should be in place.

Accidents are usually consequented by some form of full cleanliness training (Foxx & Azrin, 1973) or restriction of privileges. These procedures must be severe enough to have an impact on the behavior, but their application must be carefully monitored by the therapist. Parents are instructed on how to control their "emotional" reaction to accidents. Appropriate toileting is adequately reinforced. Tokens, star charts, praise, trips, increased privileges, and the like have all been used. Care is given to select and maintain use of meaningful reinforcers. Too often parents and the therapist issue what they think the child should like, rather than what the child in fact enjoys.

Independent toileting is the major focus of therapy, not just the reduction of accidents. Iatrogenic retention is watched for, as is the development of any other concomitant aberrant behavior. Frequent follow-up contact is maintained for at least a year post-treatment, and criteria for reimplementing treatment are established.

There are many variations on the program just outlined, but the essential components are present. Single-factor or modality therapy may work with specific cases, but it cannot be considered the "treatment of choice." Hospitalization may be required in the most recalcitrant or noncompliant cases, but as a rule it is not needed. Psychotherapy, and especially psychodynamically oriented therapy, has not proven effective in the treatment of childhood encopresis.

DSM-III-R

There are three changes in the diagnostic criteria from DSM-III to DSM-III-R. First, DSM-III-R requires "at least one such event a month for at least six months" (APA, p. 84), where no frequency requirement had previously been imposed. Second, the phrase in DSM-III, "in the individual's own socio-cultural setting" (APA, 1980, p. 82), has been omitted. Third, DSM-III-R specifies that the child must have a chronological and mental age of at least 4 years.

REFERENCES

American Psychiatric Association. (1980). *Diagnostic and statistical manual of mental disorders* (3rd ed.). Washington, DC: Author.

American Psychiatric Association. (1987). *Diagnostic and statistical manual of mental disorders* (3rd ed., rev.). Washington, DC: Author.

Anthony, E.G. (1957). An experimental approach to the psychopathology of childhood encopresis. *British Journal of Medical Psychology, 30,* 146–175.

Atthowe, J.M. (1973). Nocturnal enuresis and behavior therapy: A functional analysis. In R.B. Rubin, J. Henderson, H. Fensterheim, & L.P. Ullmann (Eds.), *Advances in behavior therapy* (Vol. 4). New York: Academic.

Azrin, N.H., & Foxx, R.M. (1974). *Toilet training in less than a day.* New York: Simon & Schuster.

Azrin, N.H., Sneed, T.J., & Foxx, R.M. (1973). Dry bed: A rapid method of eliminating bedwetting (enuresis) of the retarded. *Behaviour Research & Therapy, 11,* 427–434.

Azrin, N.H., Sneed, T.J., & Foxx, R.M. (1974). Dry bed: Rapid elimination of childhood enuresis. *Behaviour Research & Therapy, 12,* 147–156.

Baker, B.L. (1969). Symptom treatment and symptom substitution in enuresis. *Journal of Abnormal Psychology, 74,* 42–49.

Bakwin, H. (1971). Enuresis in twins. *American Journal of Diseases of Children, 58,* 806–809.

Bakwin, H. (1973). The genetics of enuresis. *Clinics in Developmental Medicine, 48,* 73–77.

Bellman, M. (1966). Studies on encopresis. *Acta Paediatrica Scandinavica* (Suppl. 70).

Berg, L., & Jones, K.V. (1964). Functional fecal incontinence in children. *Archives of Disease in Childhood, 39,* 465–472.

Bollard, J.A. (1982). *A systematic modification of dry-bed training for the treatment of nocturnal enuresis.* Doctoral dissertation, University of Adelaide, South Australia.

Bollard, J.A., & Nettlebeck, T. (1981). A comparison of dry-bed training and standard urine alarm conditioning—Treatment of childhood bedwetting. *Behaviour Research & Therapy, 19,* 215–226.

Bollard, J.A., Nettelbeck, T., & Roxbee, L. (1982). Dry-bed training for childhood bedwetting: A comparison of group with individually administered parent instruction. *Behavior Research & Therapy, 20,* 209–217.

Bollard, R.J., & Woodroffe, P. (1977). The effect of parent-administered dry-bed training on nocturnal enuresis in children. *Behaviour Research & Therapy, 15,* 159–165.

Bostack, J. (1958). Exterior gestation, primitive sleep, enuresis and asthma: A study in aetiology. *Medical Journal of Australia, 149,* 185–192.

Boyd, M.M. (1960). The depth of sleep in enuretic school children and in non-enuretic controls. *Journal of Psychosomatic Research, 4,* 274–281.

Braithwaithe, J.V. (1956). Some problems associated with enuresis. *Proceedings of the Royal Society of Medicine, 49,* 33–39.

Butler, R.J., Brewin, C.R., & Forsythe, W.T. (1986). Maternal attributions and tolerance for nocturnal enuresis. *Behaviour Research and Therapy, 24,* 307–312.

Davidson, M.D. (1958). Constipation and fecal incontinence. In E.H. Bakwin (Ed.), *Pediatric clinics of North America.* Philadelphia: Saunders.

Dische, S. (1971). Management of enuresis. *British Medical Journal, 2,* 22–36.

Dixon, J., & Smith, P.S. (1976). The use of pants alarm in daytime toilet training. *British Journal of Mental Subnormality, 22,* 20–25.

Doleys, D.M. (1977). Behavioral treatments for nocturnal enuresis in children: A review of the recent literature. *Psychological Bulletin, 84,* 30–54.

Doleys, D.M. (1978). Assessment and treatment of enuresis and encopresis in children. In M. Hersen, R.M. Eisler, & P.M. Miller (Eds.), *Progress in behavior modification* (Vol. 6). New York: Academic.

Doleys, D.M. (1979). Assessment and treatment of childhood encopresis. In A.J. Finch & P.O. Kendall (Eds.), *Treatment and research in child psychopathology.* New York: Spectrum.

Doleys, D.M. (1983). Enuresis and encopresis. In T. Ollendick & M. Hersen (Eds.), *Handbook of child psychopathology.* New York: Plenum.

Doleys, D.M. (1985). Enuresis and encopresis. In P. Bernstein & A.E. Kazdin (Eds.), *Handbook of clinical behavior therapy with children.* New York: Dorsey.

Doleys, D.M. (in press). Encopresis. In M. Hersen & C.G. Last (Eds.), *Child behavior therapy casebook.* New York: Plenum.

Engel, B.T. (1978). The treatment of fecal incontinence by operant conditioning. *Auto-Medica, 2,* 101–108.

Esperanca, M., & Gerrard, J.W. (1969). Nocturnal enuresis: Comparison of the effect of imipramine and dietary restriction of bladder capacity. *The Canadian Medical Association Journal, 101,* 721–724.

Fielding, D. (1980). The response of day and night wetting children and children who wet only at night to retention control training and the enuresis alarm. *Behaviour Research & Therapy, 18*, 305–317.

Fielding, D.M. (1982). An analysis of the behaviour of day and night wetting children: Towards a model of micturition control. *Behaviour Research & Therapy, 20*, 49–60.

Fielding, D.M., & Doleys, D.M. (in press). Elimination problems: Enuresis and encopresis. In E.J. Mach & L.J. Terdal (Eds.), *Behavioral assessment of childhood disorders* (2nd ed.). New York: Guilford.

Forsythe, W.I., & Redmond, A. (1974). Enuresis and spontaneous cure rate: Study of 1124 enuretics. *Archives of Diseases in Childhood, 49*, 259–263.

Fowler, G.B. (1882). Incontinence of feces in children. *American Journal of Obstetrics & Disorders of Women & Children, 15*, 985–988.

Foxx, R.M., & Azrin, N.N. (1973). *Toilet training the retarded*. Champaign, IL: Research Press.

Glicklich, L.B. (1951). A historical account of enuresis. *Pediatrics, 8*, 859–876.

Hallgren, B. (1956). Enuresis: I. A study with reference to the morbidity of risk and symptomatology. *Neurologica Scandinavica, 31*, 379–404.

Hendren, W.H. (1978). Constipation caused by anterior location of the anus and its surgical correction. *Journal of Pediatric Surgery, 13*, 505–512.

Kaffman, M., & Elizur, E. (1977). Infants who become enuretic: A longitudinal study of 161 kibbutz children. *Child Development Monographs, 42*.

Kempe, C.H., & Helfer, R.E. (1972). *Helping the battered child and his family*. Oxford, England: Lippincott.

Leape, L.L., & Ramenofsky, M.L. (1978). Anterior ectopic anus: A common cause of constipation in children. *Journal of Pediatric Surgery, 13*, 627–630.

Levine, M.D. (1975). Children with encopresis: A descriptive analysis. *Pediatrics, 56*, 412–416.

Levine, M.D. (1982). Encopresis: Its potentiation, evaluation and alleviation. *Pediatric Clinics of North America, 29*, 315–330.

Levine, M.D., & Bakow, H. (1976). Children with encopresis: A study of treatment outcome. *Pediatrics, 58*, 845–852.

Lovibond, S.H., & Coote, M.A. (1970). Enuresis. In C.G. Costello (Ed.), *Symptoms of psychopathology*. New York: Wiley.

Lund, C.J. (1963). Types of urinary incontinence. In C.J. Lund (Ed.), *Clinical obstetrics and gynecology*. New York: Harper & Row.

Maizels, M., King, L.R., & Firlit, C.F. (1979). Urodynamic feedback: A new approach to treat vesicle sphincter dyssynergia. *Journal of Urology, 122*, 205–209.

Mikkelsen, E.J., Rapoport, J.L., Nee, L., Greunau, C., Mendelsen, W., & Gillin, C. (1980). Childhood enuresis: I. Sleep patterns and psychopathology. *Archives of General Psychiatry, 37*, 1139–1144.

Molnar, D., Tartz, L.S., Erin, O.M., & Wales, J. (1983). Anorectal manometry results in defecation disorders. *Archives of Diseases in Childhood, 58*, 257–261.

Morgan, R.T.T., & Young, G.C. (1975). Parental attitudes and the conditioning treatment of childhood enuresis. *Behaviour Research & Therapy, 13*, 197–199.

Nergardh, A., von Hedenberg, C., Hellstrom, B., & Ericsson, N. (1974). Continence training of children with neurogenic bladder dysfunction. *Developmental Medicine & Child Neurology, 16,* 47–52.

Newson, J., & Newson, E. (1968). *Four-year-old in the urban community.* London: Allen & Unwin.

O'Brien, S., Ross, L.V., & Christophersen, E.R. (1986). Primary encopresis: Evaluation and treatment. *Journal of Applied Behavioral Analysis, 19,* 137–145.

Oppel, W.C., Harper, P.A., & Rider, R.V. (1968). The age of attaining bladder control. *Pediatrics, 42,* 614–626.

Parker, L., & Whitehead, W. (1982). Treatment of urinary and fecal incontinence in children. In D.C. Russo & J.W. Varni (Eds.), *Behavioral pediatrics: Research and practice.* New York: Plenum.

Pierce, C.M. (1972). Enuresis. In A.M. Freedman & H.I. Kaplan (Eds.), *The child: His psychological and cultural development.* New York: Atheneum.

Pierce, C.M. (1975). Enuresis and encopresis. In A.M. Friedman, H.I. Kaplan, & B.J. Sadock (Eds.), *Comprehensive textbook of psychiatry* (Vol. 2). Baltimore: Williams & Wilkins.

Pinkerton, P. (1958). Psychogenic megacolon in children: The implications of bowel negativism. *Archives of Diseases in Childhood, 33,* 371–380.

Ravitch, M.M. (1958). Pseudo Hirschsprung's disease. *Annals of Surgery, 148,* 781–795.

Rutter, M. (1973). Indication for research. In I. Kolvin, E.C. MacKeith, & S.R. Meadow (Eds.), *Bladder control and enuresis.* Philadelphia: Lippincott.

Rutter, M., Tizard, J., & Whitmore, K. (Eds.) (1970). *Education, health and behavior.* London: Longman.

Rutter, M., Yule, W., & Graham, P. (1973). Enuresis and behavioural deviance: Some epidemiological considerations. In I. Kolvin, R.C. MacKeith, & S.R. Meadows (Eds.), *Bladder control and enuresis.* London: Heinman.

Schaefer, C.R. (1979). *Childhood encopresis and enuresis: Causes and therapy.* New York: Van Nostrand Reinhold.

Schuster, M.M. (1968). Motor action of rectum and anal sphincter in continence and defecation. In C.F. Code (Ed.), *Handbook of physiology: Alimentary canal IV.* Washington, DC: American Physiological Society.

Shaw, A., Bosher, P., & Blair, K. (1980). Anorectal manometry for evaluating defecation disorders. *Virginia Medical Journal, 107,* 366–370.

Sperling, M. (1965). Dynamic considerations and treatment of enuresis. *Journal of the American Academy of Child Psychiatry, 4,* 19–31.

Stewart, M.A. (1975). Treatment of bedwetting. *Journal of the American Medical Association, 232,* 281–283.

Walker, C.E. (1978). Toilet training, enuresis, encopresis. In P.R. Magrad (Ed.), *Psychological management of pediatric problems* (Vol. I). Baltimore: University Park Press.

Wear, J.B., Wear, R.B., & Cleeland, C. (1979). Biofeedback in urology and urodynamics: Preliminary observations. *Journal of Urology, 119,* 464–468.

Weissenberg, S. (1926). Uber enkopresis. *Z. Kinderheilk, 40,* 674–677.

Werry, J.S., & Cohrssen, J. (1965). Enuresis: An etiologic and therapeutic study. *Journal of Pediatrics, 67,* 423–431.

Wright, L. (1973). Handling the encopretic child. *Professional Psychology*, *4*, 137–144.

Wright, L. (1975). Outcome of a standardized program for treating psychogenic encopresis. *Professional Psychology*, *6*, 453–456.

Zaleski, A., Shokeir, M.H.K., & Gerrard, J.W. (1972). Enuresis: Familial incidents and relationships to allergic disorders. *Canadian Medical Association Journal*, *106*, 30–31.

Zaleski, A., Gerrard, J.W., & Shokeir, M.H.K. (1973). Nocturnal enuresis: The importance of a small bladder capacity. In I.Kolvin, R.C. MacKeith, & S.R. Meadow (Eds.), *Bladder control and enuresis*. Philadelphia: Saunders.

CHAPTER 22

Fire Setting and Pyromania

DAVID J. KOLKO

From a legal perspective, arson is today the fastest growing crime in the United States, and it is the most costly as well (Wooden & Berkey, 1984). Of the nearly three million fires reported across the country, almost one in five is committed by a juvenile. Recent Uniform Crime Reports indicate that juveniles account for 40% of arson arrests and convictions (U.S. Federal Bureau of Investigation, 1987). The diagnosis of pyromania has been reserved for those severely disturbed individuals whose fire setting appears to reflect some idiosyncratic impulse or need. Before evaluating its historical background and contemporary utility, the criteria for pyromania as stated in the third edition of the *Diagnostic and Statistical Manual of Mental Disorders* (DSM-III) (APA, 1980) will be presented. Revised diagnostic criteria in DSM-III-R (APA, 1987) will be examined throughout the chapter and in the final section.

DEFINITION

DSM-III defines pyromania as a psychiatric disorder that involves the following criteria: (1) recurrent failure to resist impulses to set fires; (2) an increasing sense of tension before setting fires; (3) an experience of intense pleasure, gratification, or release at the time of committing the act; (4) a lack of motivation such as monetary gain or sociopolitical ideology for setting fires; and (5) the absence of an organic mental disorder, schizophrenia, antisocial personality, or conduct disorder (APA, 1980). Thus psychiatric nosology regards pyromania as a disorder of impulse control.

HISTORICAL BACKGROUND

While the term *pyromania* often has been used interchangeably with other related terms, such as *fire setting* and *arson*, the diagnostic entity of pyromania has had a long history in the psychiatric literature. A brief overview and evaluation of this

Completion of this chapter was supported in part by NIMH grant #39976.

tradition will be presented prior to a review of significant diagnostic and assessment characteristics in the clinical picture.

Interest in the diagnosis of pyromania has continued for more than a century, with the earliest accounts published representing fire setting as a form of moral insanity (Prichard, 1822, 1837) or moral mania (Ray, 1838). It was Ray (1844) who first used the term *pyromania* to refer to a distinct form of insanity for which the offender was not responsible. Pyromania was later treated as a form of mental disorder or illness (Dunglison, 1874; Ogston, 1878), before being rejected altogether by practitioners adopting the scientific approach (Everts, 1887; Pilgrim, 1885). Nevertheless, reference to pyromania as a mental disorder continued in psychoanalytic formulations and case reports, and later accounts based on impulse theory (Magee, 1933; Stekel, 1924). In the first *Diagnostic and Statistical Manual of Mental Disorders*, pyromania was described as an obsessive–compulsive reaction (APA, 1952), but it was deleted from the second edition (APA, 1968).

Clinical and experimental reports offer little support for the diagnostic integrity of pyromania. While some investigators have reported estimates as high as 40% in selected adult samples (Mavromatis & Lion, 1977), many have argued that pyromania is extremely rare (Macdonald, 1977; Zeegers, 1984). Case-controlled and clinical–descriptive studies have reported that few adult patients exhibiting arson have received the diagnosis of pyromania (Bradford, 1982; Geller, 1984; Geller & Bertsch, 1985; Hill et al., 1982; Koson & Dvoskin, 1982; Yesavage, Benezech, Ceccaldi, Bourgeois, & Addad, 1983). Pyromania in children was originally reported in Lewis and Yarnell's (1951) classic treatise on the topic. With continued juvenile involvement in arson, there has been greater interest in applying this diagnosis to children and adolescents. However, as in the case of adults, few juvenile fire setters have actually received this diagnosis (Kuhnley, Hendren, & Quinlan, 1982). Instead, such children are often diagnosed with conduct disorder (Kazdin & Kolko, 1986; Kolko, Kazdin, & Meyer, 1985; Kuhnley et al. 1982; Stewart & Culver, 1982).

Difficulty in rendering the diagnosis of pyromania may be influenced by several factors. First, since many children, and perhaps adults, are referred to a clinic after setting one fire, the primary diagnostic criterion (recurrent failure to resist the impulse) listed in DSM-III often was not fulfilled (see Kolko, 1985), despite the fact that many of these children might set fires at a later date. Indeed, in DSM-III-R *recurrent* is now replaced by *on more than one occasion*. Second, some children may plan a fire in advance or may exhibit adequate self-control, thus reducing the likelihood that the incident is perceived as impulsive. Third, the diagnosis according to DSM-III could not be made when fire setting was due to conduct disorder (APA, 1980, pp. 46–47). By contrast, DSM-III-R no longer disqualifies the diagnosis of pyromania when fire setting is due to conduct disorder, although there still are some implicit reservations. Finally, the diagnosis of pyromania has traditionally been associated with psychodynamic formulations and assigned to adult patients (see Heath, Gayton, & Hardesty, 1976). As noted by Wooden and Berkey (1984), the diagnosis of pyromania appears to be reserved for those juveniles who engage in severe fire setting, however defined. Given the fact that serious fire setting has been noted frequently, the following represent assessment and diagnostic considerations likely to prove useful in evaluating the nature and severity of the child's fire-setting behavior. Where appropriate, special reference will be made to the diagnosis of pyromania.

CLINICAL PICTURE

The clinical and empirical literature on juvenile fire setting is essentially still in its infancy. Recent research findings have begun to suggest certain sociodemographic and clinical characteristics in an attempt to articulate a clinical picture, although it bears repeating that such findings represent trends or patterns rather than definitive conclusions at this point.

As noted earlier, an essential feature of pyromania is its "purposeful" setting "on more than one occasion." Indeed, many children have been found to engage in this behavior repeatedly. This is particularly apparent in the case of older children. Certain adolescents have been referred primarily for repeated fire setting that is often regarded as dangerous and deliberate (Jacobson, 1985b; Lewis & Yarnell, 1951; Stewart & Culver, 1982). Lewis and Yarnell (1951) observed that a sizable subgroup of adolescents was responsible for numerous fires, with many of them setting more than five fires. Repeated fire setting has also been noted by more recent, large-scale studies of psychiatric patients (Bumpass, Fagelman, & Brix, 1983; Kolko & Kazdin, 1988, in press; Kuhnley et al., 1982). In contrast, most younger children have been found to set a single fire in the home. Many of these children may cease this activity upon swift parental consequation or prompt referral. Unfortunately, the absence of prospective studies makes it difficult to determine who and how many of these children will set another fire. For some psychiatrically disturbed fire-setting children, both child and parent reports confirm at least a 2-year history of the behavior, supporting the notion of historical continuity for this activity (Kolko & Kazdin, in press). Repetitive fire setting has been likewise documented for adult arsonists (Koson & Dvoskin, 1982).

The nature of the fire setter's reasons or motives for engaging in this activity is also of primary importance in understanding the clinical picture. DSM-III-R posits "tension or affective arousal before the act" (p. 326) and fascination with fire as criteria for pyromania. The implicit tension- or affective-reduction model, as noted earlier, is difficult to apply to children, much less adults. However, a common motive among children entails some form of curiosity in, attraction to, or interest in fire (Kolko, 1985). The most prevalent reason given among one large sample of children was that they liked the fire, the excitement it engendered, and the fire engines (Lewis & Yarnell, 1951). Though such children represent a small percentage of fire setters among disturbed children (Wooden & Berkey, 1984), the majority of children who have set accidental fires that come to the attention of fire service officials have simply been playing with matches. These children are reported by parents to "perk up their ears" when hearing or seeing fires and firetrucks, to prefer toys that resemble fire-related equipment, and to talk about fire in conversation.

One recent study of inpatients found that fire setters were significantly more interested in various fire-related events and activities than non–fire setters (Kolko & Kazdin, in press). Thus some children make attempts at experimentation and exploration with fire that get out of control and destroy property.

At the other extreme fall those fire setters who set fires to mediate a motive of revenge or retaliation, aggression, or intimidation. The use of fire as a weapon or as some form of counterattack has been frequently described. Many children have sought revenge against adults (Gruber, Heck, & Mintzer, 1981; Lewis & Yarnell, 1951; Macht & Mack, 1968). The one general motive ascribed to these children implicates their need for "power enhancement," whereby they resort to fire setting as an expression of hostility and aggression in response to feeling a lack of control (Wooden & Berkey, 1984, p. 35). When fire setting has been committed in schools, the motivation has usually been revenge or spite (Karchmer, 1983). Fires resulting from these motives are often set after an experience of failure, frustration, or rejection. The prominence of anger following interpersonal conflict has been determined for adults as well (Jordan, 1985). Interestingly, a lack of motivation is a diagnostic criterion for pyromania. Although deliberate fire setting of this type was specifically excluded in the DSM-III, it is conceivable that the older child's or adolescent's deliberate act of fire setting might provide an experience consistent with the tension-reduction component found in pyromania. Regardless of its relationship to pyromania, the motive of aggression is prominent among fire setters and often accounts for the clinical concern regarding this behavior.

A related characteristic of the fire setter that has received only scant attention is limited social effectiveness and skill, often manifested by emotional expressiveness difficulties. Fire setters have often been characterized as extremely passive, withdrawn, and restricted affectively (Kolko & Kazdin, 1986). Problems in the expression of anger have been reported (Awad & Harrison, 1976; Siegelman & Folkman, 1971). Among the behavioral correlates of fire setting that have been evaluated in the literature, social maladjustment or isolation is one of the most significant (Kolko, 1985). Studies and clinical reports have suggested that fire setters experience difficulties establishing and maintaining relationships (Jacobson, 1985; Kaufman, Heins, & Reiser, 1961; Nurcombe, 1964; Vandersall & Wiener, 1970) and handling interpersonal conflict (Sakheim, Vigdor, Gordon, & Helprin, 1985). For example, fire setters have been described as being more easily led by peers and likely to play alone than non–fire setters (Wooden & Berkey, 1984). They also engage in fewer social activities or events than non–fire setters (Heath, Hardesty, Goldfine, & Walker, 1983).

It is plausible that interpersonal limitations of this nature may be due to deficiencies in basic social or expressiveness skills. One recent study found that fire setters were perceived by their parents to be more socially unskilled than non–fire setters (Kolko et al., 1985). Impairments in social judgment and the capacity to form positive attachments to people have also been noted (Sakheim et al., 1985). Such findings are consistent with data based on adult samples indicating that arsonists have been found to be less assertive than other offenders (Rice & Chaplain, 1979), generally passive (Mavromatis & Lion, 1977), and interpersonally limited or inept (Prins, 1978; Vreeland & Waller, 1980). Some arsonists have been described as passive–aggressive, suggesting an inability to express anger directly (Hill et al., 1982). Consequently, it is argued that arsonists may use fire to achieve interpersonal outcomes in a concealed or nonconfrontive manner, without the need for direct expression of their motives to the victim. When used in this way, fire becomes a dramatic method of influencing others that requires little effort and no direct communication, but produces a sizable and immediate effect.

Since most studies of fire setters have been directed toward patient populations, it is not surprising that individual psychiatric disorders have been found associated with this activity. Early studies noted the presence of psychotic or schizophrenic symptomatology (Bender, 1959; Kaufman et al., 1961; Vandersall & Wiener, 1970). Only recently, however, have controlled studies been conducted using DSM-III criteria. (At the time of writing, none is available that follows DSM-III-R criteria.) Fire-setting children have generally received the diagnosis of conduct disorder (Heath et al., 1983; Kazdin & Kolko, 1986; Kolko et al., 1985; Sakheim et al., 1985; Stewart & Culver, 1982). A recent examination of the distribution of diagnoses in fire-setting and control groups from an outpatient population indicated a significant relationship between fire setting and conduct disorder (Heath, Hardesty, Goldfine, & Walker, 1985). In that study, only 2 of 32 fire setters were diagnosed with pyromania. Fire setters have also been diagnosed more often with attention deficit disorder than non–fire setters (Kuhnley et al., 1982).

Children who set fires appear to evince a cluster of conduct problems and/or antisocial behaviors likely to qualify for the diagnosis of conduct disorder. In accord with this diagnostic picture, such children have been found to exhibit more individual antisocial and delinquent acts, such as stealing, lying, running away, truancy, property destruction (Jacobson, 1985a; Kolko, 1985; Kolko & Kazdin, 1986; Kuhnley et al., 1982; Wooden & Berkey, 1984), and, to a lesser extent, aggression (Kolko et al., 1985), than non–fire setters. Recent findings indicating that these activities appear to cluster together in antisocial and delinquent youth have suggested that fire setting may be conceptualized as a "covert" or concealed behavior (Loeber & Schmaling, 1985). Although the specific meaning of this description awaits clarification and validation, it seems useful to conceive of disturbed fire setters as generally exhibiting antisocial behaviors that are often committed on a concealed basis and without direct confrontation of a victim.

In terms of general demographic features, fire setters have been found consistently among the entire age range. The majority are approximately 8 years of age, with a second group of children around 13 years of age. This early age is significantly younger than the modal age (13) of conduct-disordered children (Jacobson, 1985a). The bimodal age distribution of fire setters is consistent with the previous discussion of motives that distinguishes between young children who exhibit curiosity but few other problems on the one hand and older disturbed adolescents who use fire as a weapon on the other (see Fineman, 1980; Karchmer, 1983; Kolko, 1985). Recent empirical evidence also supports the existence of subgroups of fire setters divided into a younger group whose primary referral reason is fire setting at home and an older group exhibiting various antisocial behaviors that include fire setting (Jacobson, 1985b). Indeed, one recent analysis found significant differences in the behavioral patterns evinced by fire setters in three different age groups (Wooden & Berkey, 1984). The older children in that sample were noted to exhibit more diverse and complicated problems.

Juvenile fire setting occurs most often in males. In fact, the behavior is approximately 10 times more common in males than in females (see Kolko, 1985), although the incidence is somewhat common among female psychiatric patients (Kolko et al., 1985). More males have been found among fire-setting than among conduct-disordered samples (Jacobson, 1985a). In contrast to early findings suggesting a relationship between fire setting and intellectual retardation, most fire setters are of average intellectual functioning. Only a few fire setters from recent case studies have been described with some form of mental retardation, with one study noting specific reading retardation (Jacobson, 1985a).

The family environments of fire-setting children have been rarely articulated in an empirical, rather than impressionistic, fashion. In the majority of cases involving young children who are curious about fire, no discernible pathology has been identified. Thus these children generally reside in families containing both parent figures who provide a supportive, consistent, and affectionate environment (Wooden & Berkey, 1984). Conversely, seriously disturbed fire setters, particularly those referred to psychiatric clinics, have been reared in families characterized by isolation or prolonged absences from parents, especially fathers (Fine & Louie, 1979; Gruber et al., 1981; Stewart & Culver, 1982). A higher proportion of fire setters in some samples were placed in residential settings (Ritvo, Shanok, & Lewis, 1982) or adopted as children (Kuhnley et al., 1982) than non–fire setters.

Relatedly, family relationship disturbances have been described in the form of excessively harsh disciplinary practices, most significantly, physical abuse (Gruber et al., 1981; Jayaprakash, Jung, & Panitch, 1984; Ritvo et al., 1982). Fire setters have also acknowledged greater use of excessive corporal punishment by their parents than non–fire setters (Sakheim et al., 1985; Wooden & Berkey, 1984). The troubled families from which many disturbed fire setters come are often unaffectionate, distant, negative, and conflictual (Siegelman & Folkman, 1971; Vandersall & Wiener, 1970). Concomitantly, parental limitations in providing adequate care for the overall emotional and behavioral needs of the child have been described. The parents of nonreferred fire-setting children have been characterized as rejecting and punitive (Kafry, 1980), and difficulties in setting firm limits at home have been noted among the parents of troubled fire setters. More serious psychiatric and psychological disturbances also have been reported. The specific forms of dysfunction have been diverse, including schizophrenic or psychotic disorders, depression, and antisocial behavior (Bumpass et al., 1983; Fine & Louie, 1979; Lewis & Yarnell, 1951; Stewart & Culver, 1982). Such characteristics are likely further to exacerbate already weak parent–child relations and perhaps may contribute to or accelerate the conditions under which a fire is committed.

ASSOCIATED FEATURES

Those characteristics regarded as associated features are probably so characterized due to their relative neglect in empirical studies or findings suggesting an inconsistent relationship to fire setting. One such variable pertains to limited academic achievement and learning ability. Poor school performance was originally noted for nearly one-half (Yarnell, 1940) and three-quarters (Nurcombe, 1964) of two early samples, and in other studies as well (see Fineman, 1980; Kaufman et al., 1961). A recent comparative study found that fire setters received higher ratings of truancy, behavioral problems in school, and learning problems than non–fire setters (Wooden & Berkey, 1984). Adult arsonists have also been found to experience academic problems (Bradford, 1982).

Recent attention has been paid to the presence of hyperactivity in fire setters. Many of these children have been described as overactive (Gruber et al., 1981; Kaufman et al., 1961; Nurcombe, 1964; Vandersall & Wiener, 1970). In addition to receiving this diagnosis more often than non–fire setters (Kuhnley et al., 1982), fire setters have been rated as more impulsive and overactive on clinical measures (Jacobson, 1985a; Wooden & Berkey, 1984). The child's overactivity has been linked to other impulse control difficulties, such as increased risk taking, mischievousness, and defiance (Kafry, 1980).

While much has been written about the role of enuresis and cruelty to animals, there is little empirical evidence to support this association. Most studies and case reports acknowledge little relationship, if any, between fire setting and enuresis (Heath et al., 1976; Jacobson, 1985b; Nurcombe, 1964; Sakheim et al., 1985; Wooden & Berkey, 1984; Yarnell, 1940). The relationship between fire setting and cruelty to animals is mixed (Heath et al., 1983; Wooden & Berkey, 1984).

Although generally neglected in empirical studies, mention must be made of the potential impact of stressful precipitating life events. The significance of specific stressors is generally more evident in the case of the older fire-setting child. Previously reported events have included sudden alterations in family relationships due to separation, divorce, or death (Fineman, 1980; Strachan, 1981; Vandersall & Wiener, 1970). In the large-scale study conducted by Wooden and Berkey (1984), parents of fire setters acknowledged more than twice the number of current family disruptions. These parents also reported that fire setters had experienced more severe stress in the 6 months that preceded the fire-setting episode, which included an experience of punishment in some cases. Reports of adolescents who have initiated fire setting during inpatient hospitalization have also highlighted the role of idiosyncratic situations or events as antecedents (Boling & Brotman, 1975; Rosenstock, Holland, & Jones, 1980). The suggestion that disturbed fire setters are reacting to some form of personal loss or frustration deserves further consideration (Karchmer, 1983).

The relationship between fire setting and sexual arousal or conflict has been frequently discussed in various formulations (Gold, 1962; Lewis & Yarnell, 1951). Yarnell (1940), for example, reported that nearly all of the children in her sample exhibited sexual conflict, with many having been involved in alternative sexual experiences. Some recent studies have obtained evidence suggesting that fire setters evince a higher level of sexual arousal or fantasy excitement, as well as greater sexual conflicts and gender identity confusion than non–fire setters (Sakheim et al., 1985). Fire setters have also received higher ratings of sexual misbehavior than non–fire setters (Jacobson, 1985a). While the sexual preoccupation of adult arsonists has been reported (McKerracher & Dacre, 1966; Scott, 1974; Tennent, McQuaid, Loughnane, & Hands, 1974), other studies provide mixed evidence for this particular relationship among juveniles (Kolko, 1985; Lewis & Yarnell, 1951) and adults (Hurley & Monahan, 1969; Soothill & Pope, 1973). Most of these studies, however, have been flawed by limited and impressionistic assessment information, often being limited to case reports that describe the child's sexual activities (Wooden & Berkey, 1984). With more recent attention being paid to the role of sexual abuse among fire setters, especially females (Wooden & Berkey, 1984), the relationship between sexual preoccupation or mistreatment and fire setting may be more adequately examined.

One final correlate of fire setting is the presence of a cluster of additional behaviors dealing with fire. Both DSM-III and DSM-III-R note that individuals with pyromania may engage in activities that maintain exposure to fire, such as observing neighborhood fires, setting fire alarms, and showing an interest in fire equipment. Though few studies have assessed such activities, some seriously disturbed fire-setting juveniles have also exhibited what may be described as a fire-setting syndrome. The components of this syndrome have included playing with matches and firecrackers, waiting for the firemen to arrive, putting their fires out, and an interest in becoming a firefighter (Wooden & Berkey, 1984). Such characteristics are consistent with early descriptions of fire "buffs" or "bugs" (Lewis & Yarnell, 1951). It still remains to be determined whether these behaviors are more commonly observed in fire setters, whether disturbed or not.

COURSE AND PROGNOSIS

Little information has been disseminated regarding the likelihood of recidivism among and the follow-up status of fire setters. For fire setters referred for inpatient treatment, the rate of recidivism has been 23% (Stewart & Culver, 1982). Other studies have noted recidivism but no specific rates (Kuhnley et al., 1982; Parrish et al., 1985; Siegelman & Folkman, 1971; Wooden & Berkey, 1984).

Mixed evidence exists regarding prognosis. The clinical import of fire setting has been supported in one study of inpatients that found that repeaters were more antisocial and symptomatic and less compliant, and resided in families with more psychiatrically disturbed parents (Stewart & Culver, 1982). There have also been findings suggesting more psychological, social, and family adjustment difficulties among nonpatient recidivists (Siegelman & Folkman, 1971).

The prognostic significance of juvenile fire setting in terms of subsequent arson and criminality has also been examined. No studies have documented the developmental course of fire setting to suggest its continuity into adulthood. The only study of arson recidivism followed 67 of 79 adult offenders charged with arson for a 20-year period (Soothill & Pope, 1973). Only 3 men were reconvicted for the offense, each of whom had been convicted earlier for stealing as well. Subsequent convictions among the sample were for larceny, breaking and entering, and property damage. While impressive for its length, the study's findings are subject to qualification since 40% were imprisoned for arson and 32% were placed on probation or committed to a psychiatric hospital, and since juveniles received different dispositional sentences than adults. Studies of adult arsonists have revealed both individual and familial characteristics that are similar to those previously described for juveniles, including recidivism, motives of revenge and pleasure, parental absences and pathology, school underachievement, and antisocial behaviors (Bradford, 1982; Hill et al., 1982; Koson & Dvoskin, 1982; Yesavage et al., 1983).

An alternative source of information documenting clinical course comes from studies evaluating the relationship between juvenile fire setting and later criminal behavior. Following a psychiatric examination covering behavior problems in childhood, Hellman and Blackman (1966) found that 74% of aggressive prisoners had the triad of enuresis, cruelty to animals, and fire setting, compared to 28% of nonaggressive prisoners ($p < .001$). There were also significant group differences in the presence of each of these symptoms. Twice as many prisoners in the aggressive as in the nonaggressive group (16 vs. 8) had a history of fire setting. A similar study of institutionalized delinquents documented the triad in 13% of the cases (Wax & Haddox, 1974). In contrast, the results of a third study found virtually no reference to either of these three behaviors in an evaluation of the predictors of violence based on the published literature, and interviews with both professionals and convicts (Justice, Justice, & Kraft, 1974).

With few predictive studies of fire setting, the relationship between adult antisocial behavior and other manifestations of conduct disorder is pertinent to understanding the impact of fire setting (Lefkowitz, Eron, Walder, & Huesmann, 1977; Loeber, 1982; Loeber & Dishion, 1983; Loeber & Schmaling, 1985; Patterson, 1982; Robins, 1978). The general findings based on this literature suggest that: (1) adult and childhood antisocial behaviors are interconnected; (2) the variety of childhood antisocial behavior is a good predictor of adult criminality; (3) family circumstances such as large size, parental separation, and limited child-rearing skills are useful in predicting recidivism; and (4) overt behaviors such as aggression and disobedience decline between the ages of 10 and 16 years, and are replaced by more covert behaviors such as lying and stealing.

Such findings bear implications for the fire-setting child. First, the diverse clinical pictures noted earlier implicate a variety of dysfunctions that may heighten the risk for subsequent criminal behavior (Robins, 1978), especially given the stability of antisocial behavior (Loeber, 1982). Second, the emergence of covert behaviors after age 10 suggests that fire setting may be just one of several salient acts associated with offenses committed against property whose frequency increases during adolescence. The presence of covert behaviors has been noted to increase the likelihood of recidivism (Loeber, 1982). Third, many of the family characteristics predictive of delinquency and recidivism have been reported for fire setters. The fact that fire setting was the second most powerful predictor of persistent conduct disorder among male clinic patients from a total of 10 variables provides recent support for these relationships (Kelso & Stewart, 1986). Additional predictive studies are now needed to replicate these findings and further clarify the type and extent of continued fire setting among different child populations.

IMPAIRMENT

The degree of impairment generally varies from mild to severe as a function of the presence and severity of associated clinical features. In the majority of cases, impairment is only minimal, as the child can be maintained adequately in an ordinary academic and home situation. However, some fire-setting children have been described as dangerous. Jacobson (1985b), for example, found that one-fifth of his sample (104) were classified as dangerous, due to such features as primary referral for fire setting, perpetration of serious damage, early age of onset of fire setting, and parental dysfunction. Related characteristics believed to be associated with increased impairment include the presence of aggression and impulsivity, severe defiance, anger arousal, single-parent family, and school problems (cf. Gaynor, 1985; Karchmer, 1983). Of course, the impact of these and other characteristics on individual impairment should be documented in longitudinal studies.

COMPLICATIONS

Complications that arise from acts of fire setting have rarely been discussed. Most often, the complications stem from legal consequences that may ensue in cases that come to the attention of fire service or police officials. Some fire setters, especially those over the age of 10, are referred to juvenile authorities for sentencing and disposition (Strachan, 1981). Children whose fires result in major property damages are especially likely to experience complications as part of the sequelae of a fire-setting incident. Such fires may have several serious and direct economic, medical, disciplinary, social, and familial consequences. However, it is difficult to determine how many and which juveniles have appeared in juvenile court or were formally convicted of arson, and what, if any, specific consequences were imposed.

An additional complication includes the possibility of legal charges or juvenile justice system contact for involvement in other antisocial activities. Theft, vandalism, and truancy may be correlates of fire setting that may bolster the case for prosecution. Nevertheless, many children so charged are diverted away from legal involvement through referral to community mental health or social service agencies for therapeutic intervention.

EPIDEMIOLOGY

Empirical data documenting the prevalence of fire setting in children and adolescents are virtually nonexistent. Achenbach and Edelbrock (1981) provide relevant prevalence information from a large-scale study ($N = 1300$) of parent reports using the Child Behavior Checklist (CBCL). Fire setting was ascribed to up to 3% of nonreferred boys and girls. Fire setting was reported for up to 7% of referred girls between the ages of 8 and 9 years, and 10 and 13 years. For referred boys, rates of fire setting ranged from 6% to 20%, with boys between the ages of 8 and 12 years showing the highest rates.

Two additional studies provide sample prevalence rates of fire setting. One study of 860 outpatients reported that only 20 (2.3%) were noted to set fires (Vandersall & Wiener, 1970). In contrast, a study of 544 children referred to residential treatment found that 90 (16.5%) children had set fires (Gruber et al., 1981). Although the representativeness of these two studies is certainly in question, it is possible that such estimates underestimate the incidence of fire setting due to limitations in the assessment of this behavior. When fire-setting interest and activity are surveyed through direct interviews with young normal children, the percentages reported for these two behaviors are as high as 80 and 45%, respectively (Kafry, 1980). Other surveys of both patient and nonpatient populations are needed to reflect more accurately the extent of fire-setting behavior.

FAMILIAL PATTERN

As noted earlier, a few studies have documented the presence of various psychiatric disorders in the parents of fire setters, though none provide a comparison with parents of non–fire setters. In the only comparison study examining parental characteristics, Kazdin and Kolko (1986) found that parents of inpatient fire setters tended to show a higher incidence of current and past mental disorder using a structured interview than parents of inpatient non–fire setters, but the differences were nonsignificant. However, parents of fire setters were found to be more depressed and to acknowledge a greater range of psychiatric symptoms. The possibility that parents of fire setters are also more likely to have a history of fire setting or arson has been discussed (Wooden & Berkey, 1984), but cannot be determined at this time.

DIFFERENTIAL DIAGNOSIS

Although children who set fires receive the diagnosis of conduct disorder more often than other diagnoses, certain evidence points to the presence of additional diagnoses in such children. As noted in previous studies (Heath et al., 1976; Wooden

& Berkey, 1984), fire setting has occasionally been associated with psychotic syndromes and schizophrenia. In these cases, fire setting may occur in response to hallucinations involving themes of persecution, self-abuse, and control. Alternatively, fire setting in children may reflect an involvement in dyssocial activities, with motives such as crime concealment and arson for pay (Karchmer, 1983). Of course, some children who set fires receive multiple diagnoses (Nurcombe, 1964; Vandersall & Wiener, 1970). However, many of these children have not received an adequate diagnostic assessment (Kolko, 1985). Since most studies of fire setters are directed toward hospitalized or disturbed groups, it remains to be determined which and how many formal psychiatric diagnoses appear related to fire setting among other child populations.

CLINICAL MANAGEMENT

Strategies found effective in the management and treatment of childhood fire setters have been described in a few sources (see Fineman, 1980; Kolko, 1985; Kolko & Ammerman, 1988). Community-based programs sponsored by the fire service have been utilized extensively in curtailing the fire setting of young children deemed at low risk for recidivism (Federal Emergency Management Agency, 1979, 1983; National Fire Protection Association, 1979; Gaynor, McLaughlin, & Hatcher, 1984). Such programs teach children basic fire safety concepts and activities in the context of an educational curriculum, and may include a volunteer "companion" to serve as an appropriate role model. When regarded as necessary, some of these programs make referrals to mental health clinics (see Kolko, in press).

Children who are seen through the mental health system have, in general, been exposed to procedures that are primarily based on the social learning model, as has been described in recent clinical case studies. What limited evidence is available suggests that an array of cognitive–behavioral techniques have been associated with reduced fire setting and, at times, improvements in adjustment in selected areas. For example, practitioners have employed satiation or supervised practice fires to extinguish the child's interest in fire play and teach proper control over the behavior (Jones, 1981; Welsh, 1971; Wolff, 1984). Certain programs have included satiation as well as token reinforcement for appropriate alternative behaviors (Kolko, 1983) or response cost for involvement with fire (Holland, 1969). Specific skills-training procedures have also been incorporated into multicomponent interventions, such as self-instruction to control fire-setting urges (MacDonald & Brazier, 1982) and negative imagery to reduce the appeal of fire (Stawar, 1976). A related technique, graphing, which consists of a visual representation of the child's fire-setting behavior, precipitating events, and mediating emotional reactions, has been used to increase the child's awareness of specific cycles likely to elicit fire setting and responsibility for initiating the incident (Bumpass et al., 1983).

In a few cases, diverse interventions were directed toward multiple target behaviors. One program incorporated social skills training to alter interpersonal deficits, overcorrection to satiate fire play, covert sensitization to reduce the appeal of fire play, and training in specific fire safety skills (McGrath, Marshall, & Prior, 1979). This noteworthy intervention was associated with improvements in both fire setting and desired social activities. An extension of this program to which three additional components were added (relaxation training, response cost for fire setting, visit to a burn unit) was also found to reduce fire setting (Koles & Jensen, 1985). While these clinical reports convey optimism in the treatment of fire-setting activity, improvements are needed to rectify both technical and methodological limitations in the literature, most notably, inadequate functional analysis, weak methodologies, and poorly articulated treatment descriptions. Likewise, large-scale treatment studies are needed to facilitate treatment planning for different children.

DSM-III-R

The newer DSM-III-R diagnostic criteria (APA, 1987) bear implications for conduct disorder and pyromania, both of which make reference to fire setting. A more comprehensive list of diagnostic criteria appears for conduct disorder, though this list continues to include fire setting as an associated symptom. The diagnosis of pyromania still reflects a repeated failure (i.e., more than once) to resist impulses to set fires, but differs from the previous definition by including the following: (1) a reference to persistent fascination with fire; (2) an expansion in the degree of involvement in fires (i.e., fire setting, witnessing fires, participating in its aftermath); and (3) exclusionary conditions implicating the individual's motives (e.g., monetary gain, ideology, criminal behavior, response to hallucinations). The empirical basis for these criteria is still unclear, however. Only through further application of these criteria will the clinical pictures of fire-setting youth be meaningfully represented.

REFERENCES

Achenbach, T.M., & Edelbrock, C.S. (1981). Behavioral problems and competencies reported by parents of normal and disturbed children aged four through sixteen. *Monographs of the Society for Research in Child Development*. Chicago: Society for Research in Child Development.

American Psychiatric Association (1952). *Diagnosis and statistical manual of mental disorders*. Washington,DC: Author.

American Psychiatric Association (1968). *Diagnostic and statistical manual of mental disorders* (2nd ed.). Washington, DC: Author.

American Psychiatric Association (1980). *Diagnostic and statistical manual of mental disorders* (3rd ed.). Washington, DC: Author.

American Psychiatric Association (1987). *Diagnostic and statistical manual of mental disorders* (3rd ed., rev.). Washington, DC: Author.

Awad, G., & Harrison, S. (1976). A female firesetter: A case report. *Journal of Nervous & Mental Disease, 163*, 432–437.

Bender, L. (1959). Children and adolescents who have killed. *American Journal of Psychiatry*, *116*, 510–513.

Boling, L., & Brotman, C. (1975). A firesetting epidemic in a state mental health care center. *American Journal of Psychiatry*, *132*, 946–950.

Bradford, J.M.W. (1982). Arson: A clinical study. *Canadian Journal of Psychiatry*, *27*, 188–196.

Bumpass, E.R., Fagelman, F.D., & Brix, R.J. (1983). Intervention with children who set fires. *American Journal of Psychotherapy*, *37*, 328–345.

Dunglison, R. (1874). *Medical lexicon: A dictionary of medical science* (new ed.). Philadelphia: Henry C. Lea.

Everts, O. (1887). Are dipsomania, kleptomania, pyromania, etc., valid forms of mental disease? *American Journal of Insanity*, *44*, 52–59.

Federal Emergency Management Agency. (1979). *Interviewing and counseling juvenile firesetters*. Washington, DC: U.S. Fire Administration

Federal Emergency Management Agency. (1983). *Juvenile firesetters handbook: Dealing with children ages 7–14*. Washington, DC: U.S. Fire Administration

Fine, S., & Louie, D. (1979). Juvenile firesetters: Do the agencies help? *American Journal of Psychiatry*, *136*, 433–435.

Fineman, K.R. (1980). Firesetting in childhood and adolescence. *Psychiatric Clinics of North America*, *3*, 483–500.

Gaynor, J. (1985). Child and adolescent fire setting: Detection and intervention. *Feelings and Their Medical Significance*, *27*, 1–10. Columbus, OH: Ross Laboratories.

Gaynor, J., McLaughlin, P.M., & Hatcher, C. (1984). *The Firehawk-children's program: A working manual*. San Francisco: National Firehawk Foundation.

Geller, J. (1984). Arson: An unforeseen sequela of deinstitutionalization. *American Journal of Psychiatry*, *141*, 504–508.

Geller, J.L., & Bertsch, G. (1985). Fire-setting behavior in the histories of a state hospital population. *American Journal of Psychiatry*, *142*, 464–468.

Gold, L.H. (1962). Psychiatric profile of the fire-setter. *Journal of Forensic Sciences*, *7*, 404–417.

Gruber, A.R., Heck, E.T., & Mintzer, E. (1981). Children who set fires: Some background and behavioral characteristics. *American Journal of Orthopsychiatry*, *51*, 484–488.

Heath, G.A., Gayton, W.F., & Hardesty, V.A. (1976). Childhood firesetting. *Canadian Psychiatric Association Journal*, *21*, 229–237.

Heath, G.A., Hardesty, V.A., Goldfine, P.E., & Walker, A.M. (1983). Childhood firesetting: An empirical study. *Journal of the American Academy of Child Psychiatry*, *22*, 370–374.

Heath, G.A., Hardesty, V.A., Goldfine, P.E., & Walker, A.M. (1985). Diagnosis and childhood firesetting. *Journal of Clinical Psychology*, *41*, 571–575.

Hellman, D.S., & Blackman, N. (1966). Enuresis, fire-setting and cruelty to animals: A triad predictive of adult crime. *American Journal of Psychiatry*, *122*, 1431–1435.

Hill, R.W., Langevin, R., Paitich, D., Handy, L., Russon, M.A., & Wilkinson, L. (1982). Is arson an aggressive act or a property offense? A controlled study of psychiatric referrals. *Canadian Journal of Psychiatry*, *27*, 648–654.

Holland, C.J. (1969). Elimination by the parents of firesetting behaviour in a 7-year-old boy. *Behaviour Research & Therapy*, *7*, 135–137.

Hurley, W., & Monahan, T.M. (1969). Arson: The criminal and the crime. *British Journal of Criminology, 9*, 4–21.

Jacobson, R.R. (1985a). Child firesetters: A clinical investigation. *Journal of Child Psychology & Psychiatry, 26*, 759–768.

Jacobson, R.R. (1985b). The subclassification of child firesetters. *Journal of Child Psychology & Psychiatry, 26*, 769–775.

Jayaprakash, S., Jung, J., & Panitch, D. (1984). Multifactorial assessment of hospitalized children who set fires. *Child Welfare, 63*, 74–78.

Jones, F.D.E. (1981). Therapy for firesetters. *American Journal of Psychiatry, 138*, 261–262.

Jordan, N. (1985). Arson as weapon of choice. *Psychology Today*, May, p. 67.

Justice, B., Justice, R., & Kraft, I. (1974). Early-warning signs of violence: Is a triad enough? *American Journal of Psychiatry, 131*, 457–459.

Kafry, D. (1980). Playing with matches: Children and fire. In D. Canter (Ed.), *Fires and human behaviour*. Chichester, England: Wiley.

Karchmer, C.L. (1983). *Juvenile firesetter and school arson prevention programs*. Hartford, CT: Aetna Life Insurance Company.

Kaufman, I., Heins, L., & Reiser, D. (1961). A re-evaluation of the psychodynamics of firesetting. *American Journal of Orthopsychiatry, 31*, 123–136.

Kazdin, A.E., & Kolko, D.J. (1986). Parent psychopathology and functioning among childhood firesetters. *Journal of Abnormal Child Psychology, 14*, 315–329.

Kelso, J., & Stewart, M.A. (1986). Factors which predict the persistence of aggressive conduct disorder. *Journal of Child Psychology & Psychiatry, 27*, 77–86.

Koles, M.R., & Jenson, W.R. (1985). Comprehensive treatment of chronic fire setting in a severely disordered boy. *Journal of Behavior Therapy & Experimental Psychiatry, 16*, 81–85.

Kolko, D.J. (1983). Multicomponent parental treatment of firesetting in a developmentally disabled boy. *Journal of Behavior Therapy & Experimental Psychiatry, 14*, 349–353.

Kolko, D.J. (1985). Juvenile firesetting: A review and critique. *Clinical Psychology Review, 5*, 345–376.

Kolko, D.J., & Ammerman, R.T. (1988). Firesetting. In M. Hersen & C. Last (Eds.), *Child behavior therapy casebook*. New York: Plenum Press.

Kolko, D.J. (in press). Community interventions for juvenile firesetters: A survey of two national programs. *Hospital and Community Psychiatry*.

Kolko, D.J., & Kazdin, A.E. (1986). A conceptualization of firesetting in children and adolescents. *Journal of Abnormal Child Psychology, 14*, 49–62.

Kolko, D.J., & Kazdin, A.E. (1988). Parent-child correspondence in identification of fire setting among child psychiatric patients. *Journal of Child Psychology and Psychiatry, 29*, 175–184.

Kolko, D.J., & Kazdin, A.E. (in press). Prevalence of fire setting and related behaviors among child psychiatric patients. *Journal of Consulting and Clinical Psychology*.

Kolko, D.J., Kazdin, A.E., & Meyer, E.C. (1985). Aggression and psychopathology in childhood firesetters: Parent and child reports. *Journal of Consulting & Clinical Psychology, 53*, 377–385.

Koson, D.F., & Dvoskin, J. (1982). Arson: A diagnostic study. *Bulletin of the American Academy of Psychiatry & Law, 10*, 39–49.

Kuhnley, E.J., Hendren, R.L., & Quinlan, D.M. (1982). Firesetting by children. *Journal of the American Academy of Child Psychiatry, 21*, 560–563.

Lefkowitz, M.M., Eron, L.D., Walder, L.O., & Huesmann, L.R. (1977). *Growing up to be violent: A longitudinal study of the development of aggression*. New York: Pergamon.

Lewis, N.O.C., & Yarnell, H. (1951). Pathological firesetting (pyromania). *Nervous & Mental Disease, Monograph No. 82*. Nicholasville, KY: Coolidge Foundation.

Loeber, R. (1982). The stability of antisocial and delinquent child behavior: A review. *Child Development, 53*, 1431–1446.

Loeber, R., & Dishion, T. (1983). Early predictors of male delinquency: A review. *Psychological Bulletin, 94*, 68–99.

Loeber, R., & Schmaling, K.B. (1985). Empirical evidence for overt and covert patterns of antisocial conduct problems: A meta-anlysis. *Journal of Abnormal Child Psychology, 13*, 337–352.

Macht, L.B., & Mack, J.E. (1968). The firesetter syndrome. *Psychiatry, 31*, 277–288.

Macdonald, J.M. (1977). *Bombers and fire-setters*. Springfield, IL: Charles C. Thomas.

MacDonald, L., & Brazier, B. (1982). Eliminating the firesetting behavior of a mentally retarded adolescent. *Journal of Practical Approaches to Developmental Handicap, 6*, 10–12.

Magee, J.H. (1933). Pathological arson. *Scientific Monthly, 37*, 358–361.

Mavromatis, M., & Lion, J.R. (1977). A primer on pyromania. *Diseases of the Nervous System, 38*, 954–955.

McGrath, P., Marshall, P.T., & Prior, K. (1979). A comprehensive treatment program for a firesetting child. *Journal of Behavior Therapy & Experimental Psychiatry, 10*, 69–72.

McKerracher, D.W., & Dacre, J.I. (1966). A study of arsonists in a special security hospital. *British Journal of Psychiatry, 112*, 1151–1154.

National Fire Protection Association. (1979). *Learn not to burn*. Quincy, MA: National Fire Protection Association.

Nurcombe, B. (1964). Children who set fires. *Medical Journal of Australia, 1*, 579–584.

Ogston, F. (1878). *Lectures on medical jurisprudence*. Philadelphia: Lindsay & Blakiston.

Parrish, J.M., Capriotti, R.M., Warzak, W.J., Handen, B.L., Wells, T.J., Phillipson, S.J., & Porter, C.A. (1985). *Multivariate analysis of juvenile firesetting*. Paper presented at the Annual Meeting of the Association for the Advancement of Behavior Therapy, Houston.

Patterson, G.R. (1982). *A social learning approach: Vol. 3. Coercive family process*. Eugene, OR: Castalia.

Pilgrim, C.W. (1885). Pyromania (so-called), with report of a case. *American Journal of Insanity, 41*, 456–465.

Prins, H.A. (1978). "Their candles are all out" (Macbeth) . . . or are they. *Royal Society of Health Journal, 98*, 191–195.

Ray, I. (1838). *A treatise on the medical jurisprudence of insanity*. Boston: Charles C. Thomas & James Brown.

Ray, I. (1844). *A treatise on the medical jurispurdence of insanity* (2nd ed.). Boston: William D. Tickner & Co.

Rice, M.E., & Chaplin, T.C. (1979). Social skills training for hospitalized male arsonists. *Journal of Behavior Therapy and Experimental Psychiatry, 10*, 105–108.

Ritvo, E. Shanok, S.S., & Lewis, D.O. (1982). Firesetting and nonfiresetting delinquents: A comparison of neuropsychiatric, psychoeducational, experiential, and behavioral characteristics. *Child Psychiatry & Human Development, 13*, 259–267.

Robins, L.N. (1978). Sturdy childhood predictors of child antisocial behaviour: Replications from longitudinal studies. *Psychological Medicine, 8*, 611–622.

Rosenstock, H.A., Holland, A., & Jones, P.H. (1980). Firesetting on an adolescent inpatient unit: An analysis. *Journal of Clinical Psychiatry, 41*, 20–22.

Sakheim, G.A., Vigdor, M.G., Gordon, M., & Helprin, L.M. (1985). A psychological profile of juvenile firesetters in residential treatment. *Child Welfare, 64*, 453–476.

Scott, D. (1974). *The psychology of fire.* New York: Charles Scribner's Sons.

Siegelman, E.Y., & Folkman, W.S. (1971). *Youthful firesetters: An exploratory study in personality and background.* Springfield, VA: U.S.D.A. Forest Service.

Soothill, K.L., & Pope, P.J. (1973). Arson: A twenty-year cohort study. *Medicine, Science & the Law, 13*, 127–138.

Stawar, T.L. (1976). Fable mod: Operantly structured fantasies as an adjunct in the modification of firesetting behavior. *Journal of Behavior Therapy & Experimental Psychiatry, 7*, 285–287.

Stekel, W.C. (1924). *Peculiarities of behavior.* New York: Boni & Liveright.

Stewart, M.A., & Culver, K.W. (1982). Children who set fires: The clinical picture and a follow-up. *British Journal of Psychiatry, 140*, 357–363.

Strachan, J.C. (1981). Conspicuous firesetting in children. *British Journal of Psychiatry, 138*, 26–29.

Tennent, T.G., McQuaid, A., Loughnane, T., & Hands, N.J. (1971). Female arsonists. *British Journal of Psychiatry, 119*, 497–502.

U.S. Federal Bureau of Investigation. (1987). *Crime in the United States,* Washington, DC: U.S. Government Printing Office.

Vandersall, J.A., & Wiener, J.M. (1970). Children who set fires. *Archives of General Psychiatry, 22*, 63–71.

Vreeland, R.G., & Waller, M.B. (1980, September). *Social interactions in families of firesetting children.* Presented at the Annual Meeting of the American Psychological Association, Montreal.

Wax, D.E., & Haddox, V.G. (1974). Enuresis, fire-setting and animal cruelty: A triad predictive of violent behavior. *Journal of Psychiatry & the Law, 2*, 45–71.

Welsh, R.S. (1971). The use of stimulus satiation in the elimination of juvenile firesetting behavior. In A.M. Graziano (Ed.), *Behavior therapy with children.* Chicago: Aldine.

Wolff, R. (1984). Satiation in the treatment of inappropriate firesetting. *Journal of Behavior Therapy & Experimental Psychiatry, 15*, 337–340.

Wooden, W.S., & Berkey, M.L. (1984). *Children and arson: America's middle class nightmare.* New York: Plenum.

Yarnell, H. (1940). Firesetting in children. *American Journal of Orthopsychiatry, 10*, 272–286.

Yesavage, J.A., Benezech, M., Ceccaldi, P., Bourgeois, M., & Addad, M. (1983). Arson in mentally ill and criminal populations. *Journal of Clinical Psychiatry, 44*, 128–130.

Zeegers, M. (1984). Criminal fire-setting: A review and some case studies. *Medicine & Law, 3*, 171–176.

PART 3

Special Topics

CHAPTER 23

Developmental Issues

LIZETTE PETERSON, DANIEL J. BURBACH, AND JOHN CHANEY

Developmental aspects of child psychiatric diagnosis were rarely considered even a decade ago. Recently, however, numerous investigators have persuasively argued that knowledge of child development is essential to effective diagnosis of child psychopathology (e.g., Achenbach, 1982; Cicchetti, 1984; Garber, 1984; Gelfand & Peterson, 1985; Greenspan & Lourie, 1981; Tanguay, 1984). In this chapter, our goal is to describe how an understanding of development can contribute to the diagnosis of child psychopathology. To accomplish this goal, we address not only the continuities and discontinuities of child and adult psychopathology but also the shortcomings of some traditional psychiatric nomenclatures that fail to address the role of development in the etiology, course, and outcome of psychiatric disorders. In addition, we consider the rapidly emerging field of developmental psychopathology, especially as it pertains to the diagnosis of child dysfunction. Next, a variety of innovative, developmentally appropriate methods of assessment are considered, with an emphasis on procedures used to diagnose psychopathology during infancy and early childhood. Finally, the potential of developmentally based classification systems is briefly explored.

CONTINUITY AND DISCONTINUITY IN PSYCHOPATHOLOGY

Childhood

Proponents of developmentally based diagnostic frameworks do not deny that there are some continuities in psychopathology during childhood. Some disturbances such as delinquency (Loeber, 1982) and Type A behavior (Matthews & Angulo, 1980) seem to remain stable throughout childhood. In other cases, one type of early maladaptive behavior predicts a very different kind of problem in later childhood. For example, avoidance of the caretaker as infants predicts preschoolers' later excessive dependency on the teacher (Sroufe, Fox, & Pancake, 1983), and initial negative reactions to maternal separation during hospitalization predict learning disabilities in adolescents (Douglas, 1975). However, there is no compelling evidence that dysfunction at one point in childhood *definitively* predicts pathology later in childhood (Garber, 1984). Stability of pathology in childhood seems to be the exception rather than the rule.

Later Life

The absence of compelling continuities in psychopathology across the life span seems to be particularly at odds with the conceptualization many have entertained of childhood disorders as precursors to adult psychopathology. It was not uncommon in the past to evaluate the merit of a child diagnostic category in terms of its ability to predict future disturbance (Garber, 1984). It is true that several severe disorders, such as childhood schizophrenia (Robins, 1966), and marked deficits, such as inadequate peer relationships (John, Mednick, & Schulsinger, 1982; Roff & Ricks, 1970), appear strongly related to adult psychopathology. It is also true that disturbance of one form in childhood can present as a different form of pathological dysfunction in later life. For instance, institutional rearing may lead to later social difficulties (Rutter, Quinton, & Liddle, 1983); poor coping strategy development in childhood may leave an individual unable to adapt effectively to later stressful life events (Rutter, 1986); and childhood impulsiveness and aggressiveness rather than isolated, withdrawn behavior during childhood may predict adult schizophrenia (Robins, 1966).

However, most children with emotional problems become essentially normal adults (Garber, 1984). Many studies indicate that problems such as shyness (Masterson, 1967; Victor & Halverson, 1976), anxious, fearful, or phobic behavior (Agras, Chapin, & Oliveau, 1972; Rutter & Garmezy, 1983), and sleep disturbances (Robins, 1978) appear to be transient in nature, and are not carried over to adulthood. Most forms of behavioral disorder can be observed intermittently in normal children who evidence no subsequent disturbance (Rutter, Tizard, Yule, Graham, & Whitmore, 1976; Wenar, 1982). In other cases, disorders brought on by maladaptive responses to environmental stressors at a given point in development can be expected to resolve with further development or changes in the environment (Lefkowitz & Burton, 1978; Thomas & Chess, 1972). Thus early disorders are not necessarily pathognomonic of later dysfunction.

ADULTOMORPHIC CLASSIFICATION

The lack of continuity between child and adult psychopathology suggests the inappropriateness for child diagnosis of most traditional nomenclatures that are based on the study of adult psychopathology. (We exclude the more recent empirically evolved classification schemes that have focused specifically on children.) Most traditional systems of diagnosis merely employ downward extrapolations of adult symptomatology and terminology. The erroneous assumption that these adult-based categories can be effectively altered accurately to reflect disorders in childhood without independent validation with children has been termed *adultomorphism* (Phillips, Draguns, & Bartlett, 1975).

Gelfand and Peterson (1985) argued that it is generally inappropriate to apply diagnostic procedures developed for one group to another group, whether the application cuts across cultural, socioeconomic, gender, or age parameters. First, there is no guarantee that child and adult forms of a disturbance will be manifest in the same fashion. Thus when adult-based classification schemes are used, signs specific to children can be missed (Carlson & Garber, 1986). Second, the adult-based criteria for various disorders may be overinclusive, particularly for very young children. For example, Crowther, Bond, and Rolf (1981) noted that several behaviors thought to represent pathological functioning in adults were exhibited by more than one-fifth of the preschoolers in their sample, yet these children were not viewed as maladapting by their parents and teachers. Thus these behaviors were not found to be pathological either in statistical frequency or in their impact on the child's psychosocial functioning. In still other instances, classification systems based on adult dysfunction identify distinct categories of disturbance that often present in children as a single disorder. This is a particular problem when it is precisely the co-occurrence of the presumably separate disorders that is predictive of later dysfunction. Rescorla (1986), for example, reported a close relationship between seemingly disparate categories (aggressive–destructive behavior and anxiety, sadness, and emotional insecurity) in preschool children, and he noted that children who have both constellations of behaviors differed from children with either category alone. Finally, pathology is typically defined by a syndrome or a pattern of behaviors. It is possible that many constellations of problem behaviors in children may differ from those seen in adults, due in part to the wider range and variety of normal behaviors available to children in comparison with adults (Achenbach, 1980).

Temporal specifications are also a problem. Some classification systems, such as DSM-III, specify temporal stability on some dimensions (e.g., Axis 2—developmental disorders), although this kind of stability is not often seen in childhood (Rutter & Shaffer, 1980). Other cases using temporal parameters (e.g., Axis 5—highest level of adaptive functioning *in the last year*) have very different implications for a rapidly developing child than for an adult. Similarly, diagnostic criteria for many syndromes include a duration requirement for certain symptoms. Because the specified time period is usually equivalent for children and adults, most nomenclatures are necessarily more stringent for younger children. That is, a year in the life of a 10-year-old represents a significantly greater proportion of time than a year in the life of a 40-year-old, and thus a 1-year criterion has different meaning across the life span.

Some classifications appear to postulate etiologies that have been demonstrated in adults but not in children. For instance, DSM-III (APA, 1980) substitutes *dementia* for the previously used diagnosis *disintegrative psychosis*. This change occurred despite findings suggesting that the clinical features of disintegrative psychosis differ greatly in children and adults, and that children do not typically show the neurological abnormalities (Evans-Jones & Rosenbloom, 1978) necessary for the diagnosis of dementia.

Finally, and most importantly, because the proponents of adultomorphic classification systems regard psychopathology as homologous in children and adults, they often fail to recognize that pathology is usually relative to the age of the individual in question. Whether pathology is defined as statistically rare behavior or as maladaptive psychological functioning, the age of the individual in question usually determines the degree to which the behavior is considered pathological. To illustrate this point, Wenar (1982) began his text on psychopathology with three stories. In the first, a boy responds suddenly with violent physical aggression. In the second, a son announces to his father that he intends to be a girl when he grows up. In the third, a mother worries that her child is "going crazy" because she believes she can cause automobile accidents by wishing them and fears crablike monsters under her bed. In all three stories, the most relevant question to ask is: "How old is the child?" Physical aggression, incomplete gender identification, and fears of fantasy creatures are all aspects of normal development, anticipated in the majority of preschool children. Only at older ages do such behaviors signify psychopathology. It thus becomes necessary to view psychopathology in reference to the continuum of normal development. This premise has led to renewed interest in the relationship between development and psychopathology, and is responsible for the emergence of a new area of study in childhood disorders, known as *developmental psychopathology*.

DEVELOPMENTAL PSYCHOPATHOLOGY AND DIAGNOSIS

Achenbach (1974) used the term *developmental psychopathology* as the title for a text that began, "This is a book about a field that hardly exists yet." Ten years later, Cicchetti (1984) in a special issue of *Child Development* described developmental psychopathology as a now existent field. Cicchetti discussed the theoretical convergence of classical developmental psychology and clinical psychology in the introduction to a series of papers addressing different aspects of developmental psychopathology. Gelfand and Peterson (1985) similarly considered the interface of these two historically separate areas, and described some of the reasons behind the historical schism between developmental and clinical child psychology. Developmental psychology, with its traditional emphasis on nomothetic approaches and description of normal development, has historically avoided the idiographic and clinical aspects of diagnosis (Elkind, 1982; Gelfand & Peterson, 1985). In turn, clinical child psychologists have avoided obtaining a background in normal development and have drawn many of their conceptualizations of psychopathology from theoreticians, such as S. Freud (1905), Abraham (1927), Adler (1916), and Hartmann (1939), who based their conceptualizations of pathology on adult renditions of childhood experiences but never really studied children at all (Tyson, 1986).

Partially because of the historical rift between developmental and clinical child psychology and partially because of the nature of developmental theory, there are a variety of different attitudes toward classification within developmental psychopathology. Some developmentalists believe that classification is antithetical to the basic tenets of developmental psychology (Santostefano, 1971). These authors suggest that "diagnosis" implies that behavior is static and that individuals cannot be classified on the basis of stable personality traits. That is, the developmental view focuses on fluid behavioral traits and change rather than stability. Of course, some would argue that disorders and not stable personality traits of children themselves should be classified (Cantwell, 1980; Rutter, 1965). Even within such a viewpoint, however, there remains much controversy concerning which aspects of the child's functioning are best viewed as units of a disorder (Garber, 1984). Further, it is unclear what impact diagnosis may have on the developing child's behavior and on the behavior of significant others in the diagnosed child's environment.

Other developmental psychologists suggest that differential diagnosis is of secondary interest, with primary emphasis being on the origins and time course of a disturbance (Sroufe & Rutter, 1984). Still others suggest that classification is nothing more than "an essential framework for understanding the processes of normal and abnormal development" (Garber, 1984, p. 31), which should be viewed as a challenge for developmental psychopathologists. Even those developmentalists who believe that classification is possible do not embrace current systems as feasible vehicles, however.

Disenchantment with classification stems from a growing awareness that children are developing much more rapidly than adults, and consequently the extent to which measurement on any one occasion adequately portrays their "typical" functioning is necessarily limited. In other words, the developmental tasks at any one point on the continuum are often very different from those encountered only a few months later, especially in early childhood. Thus the difficulties that a child may encounter and the ways in which these difficulties are manifested can substantially vary across relatively brief amounts of time. A developmentally sensitive classification system would describe the child's current rather than typical problematic functioning, and would integrate this description with consideration of current levels of functioning in other areas, as well as with the child's expected developmental level. Some examples of such classification schemes are presented in the final portion of this chapter.

In any case, developmental psychopathology offers some new conceptualizations and insights into children's dysfunctional behavior, many of which have already been described in this chapter. We will attempt a brief summary of these ideas here. First, developmental psychopathologists view the child as an evolving, active, dynamic force, inextricably tied to significant others in the environment. As a result, proponents of this approach focus on children's functioning within relevant ecological contexts, particularly the child–parent relationship. Developmental psychopathologists also emphasize children's competency rather than dysfunction. Furthermore, because development is regarded as cumulative, deficiency or acquired maladaptive responding at any level is thought to influence subsequent development.

Admittedly, the processes that underlie development are complex. Diagramming the multiple relationships between early biopsychosocial development and subsequent competencies and dysfunctional behaviors would result in an intricate web of connections. For example, early social attachment to the caretaker may influence not only later social behavior but also later motor and cognitive development. To complicate matters further, development does not always involve linear change, even within the same modality. For example, parallel play precedes interactive play but parallel play does not resemble the later developing interactive play in terms of its observable components. As mentioned earlier, behavior that is acceptable and normal at one developmental level can be viewed as pathological at another level. Carlson and Garber (1986) made this point succinctly: "Enuresis and fears of monsters under one's bed mean something very different at age 22 than they do at age 2" (p. 412). Finally, even within a given age, an isolated behavior may not be pathological. It is the constellation of certain behaviors that defines pathology (Achenbach, 1980).

In addition to these conceptual issues in diagnosis, developmental psychopathologists also have focused on the more pragmatic issues of assessment and measurement. Because children typically do not present themselves as needing assistance and do not have a clear view of the "patient" role, they begin the diagnostic process in a different way than do adults (Kovacs, 1986). Limitations in both language and cognition for the most part render adult-oriented diagnostic tools clearly inappropriate for children. Therefore, we consider next some of the problems inherent in employing adult-based measures with children and identify several diagnostic instruments that are more developmentally appropriate.

DIAGNOSTIC INSTRUMENTS

Adult-oriented diagnostic tools most often rely on structured or semistructured interview and pencil-and-paper self-report measures. In contrast, assessment methods for infants and small children cannot be language based. As a result, observation of the child is the most frequently employed vehicle with very young children. Most measures depend on eliciting problematic behavior in representative situations created in the clinic to mimic common environmental situations in the home, or having a person familiar with the child's current typical behavior to provide the ratings. As children acquire some verbal ability, familiar activities such as play may be used not only to draw out typical behaviors but also to examine intrapsychic processes such as affect and self-esteem. For still other children, interviews specifically structured for children can be employed, as can modified self-report and projective instruments. In addition, other sources of information have been viewed as central to child diagnosis. The more traditional interview and pencil-and-paper measures are still employed with significant others, such as parents and teachers, who are able to report on the child's overt behavior and apparent affect.

It is not possible to do justice to the broad area of assessment here; instead, we describe one or two representative examples of differing types of assessment procedures to illustrate the developmentally specific nature of these methods. Because assessment instruments for use with infants are least like familiar adult diagnostic tools, and because they are not covered elsewhere in this text (or most psychopathology texts), we give them the most focus here. As the child's developmental level largely determines the appropriateness of each assessment method, we have grouped such strategies in terms of major developmental periods.

Infants

Observation: Newborn Period

Based on the Brazelton Neonatal Behavioral Scale (Brazelton, 1973), the Assessment of Preterm Infants' Behavior (APIB) is a behavioral measure for systematically documenting the infant's behavioral organization within six discrete subsystems: physiology, motor organization, state organization, interactive ability, attention, and self-regulation (Als & Brazelton, 1981). Through a series of graded interactions with a highly trained examiner, the degree of structure and support necessary to elicit the infant's best performance is noted. Auditory, visual, and tactile stimuli are utilized to challenge the infant's ability to integrate reactions to the stimuli. Rather than calculating one global score, the infant's progress within each subsystem is rated, which allows diagnosis of problems within any given subsystem as well as an overall assessment of behavioral organization.

Observation: 3 to 5 Months

The face-to-face paradigm is a method of assessing the early communication processes that occur between the infant and mother (Tronick, Als, & Adamson, 1979). The 3-minute interaction is usually videotaped and can be scored on a 13-point scale from 1—"against the interaction" (in which infant protests or parent becomes angry) to 12—"involved in the interaction" (scored as "high euphoria"). These data are coded on the basis of facial expressions, vocalization, eye direction, head position, body position, and limb position of both the mother and the child (Als, 1980). Although the test–retest reliability and the validity of this measure continue to be explored, it is clear how such specific data could be used to diagnose early interactional difficulties as well as to suggest specific necessary strategies for intervention.

Observation: 9 Months to 1 Year

Many investigators have suggested that the child's attachment to the caretaker in infancy is the most important developmental task, and that secure attachment predicts later emotional health. The most frequently studied infant assessment paradigm is the Ainsworth Strange Situation (Ainsworth, Blehar, Water, & Walls, 1978). During this assessment, the infant goes through eight 3-minute episodes of increasing stressfulness. The infant and the mother are introduced into an unfamiliar room, joined by an unfamiliar female stranger, the mother leaves the infant with the stranger, and then they are reunited, while the stranger leaves. Then the mother leaves the infant alone, the stranger reenters, and then the stranger leaves as the mother reenters. The Strange Situation is thought to provide a valid assessment of the infant's level of attachment to the parent. Infants are traditionally classified as either A (insecure–avoidant), B (secure), or C (insecure–resistant). Recently, a D (disorganized or disoriented) classification has been suggested (Main, Kaplan, & Cassidy, 1985) to classify infants who show simultaneous signs of secure and insecure attachment. In addition, some systems break down these groupings even further to reflect more specific gradations of attachment. In general, the "B" baby seeks proximity to the mother, is quickly comforted by her presence, and disrupts normal exploration or play in her absence, reinstituting such activity upon her return. Recent reviews suggest that early sensitive, responsive interaction with the mother predicts later secure attachment (Goldsmith & Alansky, 1987) and that "B" infants seem more competent than non–"B" infants, with both adults and peers (Lamb, 1987). However, both reviews stress the low level of these relationships, the need for further replication, and the desirability of using additional measures of attachment.

The Assessment of Older Infant Behavioral Organization (Als & Brazelton, 1978) utilizes a similar paradigm in which infant and parent play with a hopping, wind-up kangaroo (this task has also been called the "kangaroo box"). The play ends when the parent places the toy in a plexiglass box. Then the parent sits with a "still face," motionless, for 6 minutes. The parent then plays with the infant again. This task assesses reciprocal play, the child's ability to retrieve the toy in the parent's behavioral (if not actual) absence, and the child's response when emotionally reunited with the parent. Thus not only attachment but initiative and motor, cognitive, affective, and social organization can be measured in such interactions. Details of even more elaborated measures of problem solving and attachment used for clinical purposes are available (e.g., Gaensbauer & Harmon, 1981).

Parent Measures

There are a variety of differing measures used with infants' parents. Some ask the parent to rate the infant on various parameters or to report on current behaviors. For example, the Revised Infant Temperament Questionnaire (Carey & McDevitt, 1978) asks parents to rate their infant 4 to 8 months old on 95 behavioral items according to frequency of occurrence and on nine global temperament ratings. Infants can be classified as difficult (withdrawing, poor adaptability, intense, negative, arrhythmic), easy (approaching, adaptable, relaxed, and rhythmic), slow to warm up (inactive, mildly adaptive, negative), or intermediate. Extremes in temperament in infancy are thought to predict later forms of maladjustment and to provide cues for special caretaker intervention (Carey & McDevitt, 1978).

Other parent measures focus on the risk of dysfunctional parenting. For example, the 101-item Parenting Stress Index asks parents to rate their children on items that assess child characteristics such as adaptability, demandingness, and moodiness, and to rate themselves on parent characteristics such as depression, sense of competence, and social isolation and situation factors such as demographic variables and stressful life events (Burke & Abidin, 1978). This inventory can be used not only for screening purposes but as an indication of where intervention is needed.

Some structured parental interview and direct observation of parenting strategies have also been used. For example, the Home Observations for Measurement of the Environment (HOME) examines six areas, including maternal responsibility, punishment, organization of the environment, play materials, maternal involvement, and opportunity for stimulation (Caldwell & Bradley, 1979). A trained observer uses a scale from 0 to 3 to rate 45 differing items drawn from these areas. Data suggest that these measures may predict later psychosocial adjustment (Minde & Minde, 1986).

Preschool Age

Diagnostic Nursery

The Diagnostic Nursery Program (Karp, Herzog, & Weinberg, 1985) exemplifies a broad, multivariate approach to the classification of problem preschoolers. This eight-session program includes an intake appointment, six weekly 90-minute diagnostic sessions, and a final parent conference. During the intake, the parents give a detailed history of the child and their description of the problem. The child is seen in a traditional diagnostic play interview in which play is used as a vehicle for assessing emotional expression as well as a sample of typical interaction behavior. Then, if indicated, the child is enrolled in 6 weeks of the children's play group to assess relevant problems further. Once a week, four to six children play in the nursery school setting. The children are supervised by a clinician and a student intern who are alert to the maladaptive behavior reported by the parents and are trained to try a variety of different interventions to assess their effectiveness in altering the target behavior. The child's general interactions with the peers and adults are noted as well.

The parents initially separate from the children and then observe a portion of the session through a one-way mirror. After this observation, parents participate in a diagnostic group led by a psychiatric social worker. In this group, parental expectations, recognition of the problem, and desire and ability for change are assessed. The child, in turn, goes directly from each of the six group sessions to an individual evaluation by a psychiatrist, an educational psychologist, and, if necessary, a speech and language specialist. During the final session, all of the information obtained during the program is integrated and discussed with the parents.

As noted earlier, this program exemplifies many techniques used with young children and it provides a broad basis for diagnosis. Karp and colleagues (1985) reported on 40 children who had completed the program and had been diagnosed using DSM-III criteria. The majority of these children (85%) were found to have emotional (including adjustment) disorders. Other diagnoses included developmental (40%), physical (20%), behavioral (8%), and intellectual (5%) disorders.

Structured Playroom

In contrast to the diagnostic nursery's general applicability, many diagnostic systems using formal group work and play situations focus more on specific behavioral problems. For example, Milich, Loney, and Roberts (1986) describe the use of a structured playroom to diagnose hyperactive boys. The boys were exposed to two 15-minute playroom observations during free play and restricted, academic activity. During free play, four tables containing identical sets of toys were present, and the child was told he could play with any toys he wished. Then worksheets were placed on three of the tables and the child was charged with remaining seated and completing as many worksheets as possible. There were unfamiliar toys on the first table, and the child was told not to play with these toys.

During free play, the number of times the child crossed a grid, vocalized, fidgeted, shifted attention, or was on task was noted. During the academic task, two additional behaviors were observed: touching forbidden toys and worksheet items completed. This task has been shown to differentiate hyperactive from aggressive and normal boys, and demonstrated impressive stability across time periods up to 2 years (Milich et al., 1986).

In general, play is an excellent vehicle for establishing communication with the preschool child. Several authors have written about more dynamic aspects of play, both as diagnostic (A. Freud, 1946) and therapeutic (Axline, 1947) tools, and others have urged that the clinical interpretations of children's play must be tempered with knowledge of normal development of play behaviors (e.g., Elkind, 1982). Music, art, puppetry, and many other expressive modalities can also be used as communication vehicles with preschool children. These techniques can be applied to older children as well, but older children are also capable of participating in more advanced diagnostic strategies.

School-Age Children

Interviews

A great deal has been written on adapting the diagnostic interview, a common tool of classification with adults, for use with children (e.g., Bierman, 1983; Furman, 1980; Kanfer, Eyberg, & Krahn, 1983; Kovacs, 1986; Palmer, 1970, 1983; Wenar, 1982). In general, these articles have emphasized matching the complexity of the interview to the child's current linguistic and cognitive abilities. For example, techniques such as open-ended questions and the use of silence, strategies that are often useful with adults, can confuse a child. Also, questions involving memory for remote events or judgments concerning specific intervals of time are inappropriate for younger children whose memory and time estimation skills are more limited. Recently, several highly structured interview techniques have been developed for use with children, including the Structured Pediatric Psychosocial Interview (Webb & Van Devere, 1980), the Diagnostic Interview for Children and Adolescents (Herjanic & Campbell, 1977), and the Child Assessment Schedule (Hodges, Kline, Fitch, McKnew, & Cytryn, 1981). Such interviews use developmentally appropriate language, phrase questions so the child's memory, judgment, or linguistic abilities are not strained, and typically last under an hour so that the child's attention span is not exceeded. Some interviews have more sophisticated parallel parent forms worded in the third person to obtain the perspective of parents on their children's functioning. A common conclusion regarding child interviews is that, although diagnoses based on the child interview alone are probably less valid for most diagnoses than those based on the parent form alone, both are needed to obtain the most psychometrically sound diagnoses of child psychopathology (Hodges, McKnew, Burbach, & Roebuck, in press). Given that a separate chapter in this text discusses diagnostic interviews, they will not be considered further here.

Self-Report Inventories

Use of self-report inventories was popular three decades ago, and recently there has been a renewed interest in this format. Like the diagnostic interview, self-report formats are linguistically based vehicles that focus on obtaining information about relatively specific internal structures. They parallel adult measures in this respect, and are most appropriate for older children who not only are verbally proficient but are capable of making the precise judgments concerning affect, motivation, and beliefs that these instruments require.

Obviously, where possible, it is preferable to get direct evidence on such internal data rather than inferring it from behavior. Thus for questions on affect, cognition, or beliefs, self-report data are most valuable. Self-report inventories in current use tend to be more specific than general and are often derived from adult forms. For example, the Children's Manifest Anxiety Scale (CMAS) was created in 1956 by Casteneda, McCandless, and Palermo and was modeled on the adult Taylor Manifest Anxiety Scale. The CMAS was revised by Reynolds and Richmond in 1978, and currently taps anxiety stemming from common childhood encounters with stressors (e.g., parents, principals, thunderstorms). Similarly, the Children's Depression Inventory (Kovacs & Beck, 1977) was modeled after the adult Beck Depression Inventory and includes measures of common depressive symptoms.

Use of self-report instruments with children presumes not only linguistic and cognitive competence but also the child's willingness to engage in the task and to give valid answers (Achenbach, 1982). Evidence for the utility, reliability, and validity of children's self-report inventories has been scarce. Some, like the Children's Manifest Anxiety Scale, do not correlate well with ratings by teachers (Wirt & Broen, 1956) or psychiatrists (Hafner, Quast, Speer, & Grams, 1964), while others, like the Children's Depression Inventory, tend to be strongly related to clinicians' ratings (Kovacs, 1979). Future research on the value of children's self-report inventories is needed to reveal how best to structure and use this format.

Projective Techniques

The use of ambiguous stimuli to encourage the projection or elicitation of unconscious material has been a staple in adult diagnosis for years. In general, most projective instruments used with children involve the downward extension of adult instruments. For example, Ames, Metraux, and Walker (1977) present developmental norms for the Rorschach inkblot test, and Bellak and Bellak (1974) constructed the Children's Apperception Test as a companion to the adult-based Thematic Apperception Test. A few projective techniques for children, such as the Draw-A-Person (Machover, 1949) or House-Tree-Person tests, were not extended downward from adult inventories, and therefore are the exception to the rule.

The use of projective tests with children is based on the premise that children's interpretations of ambiguous material can yield evidence of personality organization, specific personality characteristics, mental disorder, or specific syndromes of psychiatric dysfunction (Gittelman, 1980). Although they do not exceed the skills of school-age children, it appears that such projective methods are particularly unreliable and incapable of discriminating disturbed children to a clinically significant degree (Gittelman, 1980). Consequently, projective instruments appear inappropriate for use in the diagnostic classification of children based on current research evidence.

Summary

A variety of differing types of measures are viewed as developmentally appropriate for children at different periods in the life cycle. Early methods attempt to assess relatively global aspects of the infant's functioning, such as ability to sustain attention or to regulate emotionality. This is most appropriate at an undifferentiated level of development. Later observations during the preschool years focus on more sophisticated abilities, such as interactive play behaviors and the ability to engage in a structured group task. Diagnostic play at a later point utilizes both overt behavior and children's emerging verbal skills to describe their own emotions. As children increasingly become more adultlike in cognitive and verbal abilities, the diagnostic tools that can be appropriately used more closely approximate those employed with adults, although adjustments in instrument length, complexity, and language must be made to ensure fit with children's level of competency.

We began this discussion by noting that the field of developmental psychopathology has made important contributions to the array of diagnostic tools currently available. As our discussion demonstrates, the need for developmentally specific tools has been perceived as greater with younger children. However, tools relevant to children at each age level could benefit from a more developmental approach. It is incumbent on future researchers to consider both the clinical and developmental ramifications of an instrument when constructing and validating tools to diagnose child psychopathology. Most current tools, particularly those used with school-age children, have been designed for use with traditional classification systems, which may explain the relative neglect of developmental variables. In our final section, we briefly review the attributes of classification systems that are instead based on developmental theory.

Developmental Models of Classification

Piaget's theory of cognitive development is perhaps the best-known overspanning developmental theory. It epitomizes some of the unique aspects of existing developmental theories in its emphasis on an active, dynamic child who accumulates experiences during qualitatively different periods of development. It is not surprising that many theorists have employed Piaget's model as a framework for creating developmentally appropriate methods of classifying psychopathology. There are, of course, some difficulties encountered when integrating Piaget's model with concepts of psychopathology. First, Piaget's theory focuses specifically on cognitions rather than emotions. Second, Piaget's analyses concern relatively active organisms in interaction with relatively passive objects (Riegel, 1978). Therefore, the structure and much of the content of Piaget's theory are not directly applicable to an interpersonal reality. Similarly, Piaget's theory does not describe the executive direction or motivation behind the evolution of cognitive structures. To Piaget, cognition spontaneously unfolds in a prewired, genetic plan. This does not leave room for a concept of "ego" or self, which seems central to conceptualizing many forms of psychopathology.

Despite these difficulties, many exciting links between Piaget's theory and conceptualizations of psychopathology have been forged. Anthony (1957) was one of the first to suggest the application of Piagetian concepts to child psychodiagnosis, and Wolff's (1960) monograph "The Developmental Psychology of Jean Piaget and Psychoanalysis" followed. Recently, developmentalists have described intriguing applications of Piagetian concepts. For example, Elkind (1982) has linked Piaget's (1971) view of reflective abstraction to the acquisition of pathology and to its alleviation in psychotherapy. Piaget suggested that reflective abstraction was the way in which the child formed logical operations and altered his or her own quality of thought. Through direct action on the environment, the child abstracted from and experienced basic truths (such as conservation of matter). Although figurative learning (such as memorizing a telephone number) could be easily forgotten, learning acquired through reflective abstraction was viewed as more permanent, as the very way in which the child thought about the world was altered by reflective abstraction.

Elkind (1982) argued that the child may engage in reflective abstraction through the actions of highly significant others, such as parents, as well as from his or her own actions. If this were true, it would explain many inexplicable aspects of child behavior. For example, children often employ grammatical rules even when such rules exceed their cognitive abilities. The use of such rules demonstrates more than simple modeling, as the child often applies the rules in a novel way (e.g., as when a child says "the horse hoofed me" although never having heard an adult articulate such a phrase). Reflective abstraction of others' actions could explain the child's acquisition of the rule before cognitive mastery of the basis for the rule. If some pathological beliefs or values were acquired in this fashion, they would be relatively impervious to change through normal intellectual vehicles, because reflective abstractions involve alterations in cognitive structures in childhood, upon which later structures are built. This viewpoint would also suggest that a strong psychotherapeutic relationship (posited by many to be the common denominator of different therapy forms: Frank, 1985; Patterson, 1973) would be useful in altering such beliefs and values. If reflective abstraction occurs only from highly significant others, then the therapist may be one of the few sources of more adaptive beliefs and values. Some theorists label this exchange of values and beliefs *transference*. In any case, our discussion illustrates the use of a Piagetian vehicle to explicate the internalization of maladaptive cognitive structures.

Block (1982) similarly utilized Piagetian concepts of assimilation, accommodation, and equilibration to explain certain psychopathological defense mechanisms and to explore psychological resiliency as a developmental phenomenon. To Piaget, disequilibration described the power that propelled cognitive development. Disequilibration resulted in intense intellectual activity to restore equilibrium by incorporating the experience into the current schemes (assimilation) and altering current schemes better to fit the experience (accommodation). Block suggests that disequilibration results in a disruption of the typical perceptual–cognitive–response sequence, which leads to anxiety and a sense of helplessness and dissatisfaction with one's coping abilities. In normal development, the next step is effective resolution through accommodation. However, in the development of psychopathology, effective accommodation may not take place. The struggle to evolve a new accommodative scheme can result in dysphoric arousal. If the arousal cannot be endured, rather than creating a new accommodation, the individual may return, perseveratively, to assimilative efforts. The individual may even regress by denying or removing the environmental messages that contradicted current schemes and caused the disequilibrium. Thus Block explains how adaptive development can stop and be replaced by hysterical reactions or regression.

Greenspan's (1979) monograph provides one of the most detailed integrations of psychodynamic and Piagetian theory. Greenspan and Lourie (1981) extended the discussion on integration by describing an application of a developmental structuralistic approach to the classification of infants and children. They argued that such an approach adds an extra dimension to traditional classification methods by focusing on the individual's unique strategies of processing, organizing, integrating, and differentiating information. Specifically, Greenspan and Lourie outline six stages of development. They posit four parameters within each stage of assessment, including: (1) range and depth of experiences appropriate to that stage; (2) stability of experiential organization; (3) resilience to stress; and (4) unique individual characteristics. Categorization of the child would involve placing current activities and abilities on a continuum of adaptive to pathological for each parameter. They give several compelling examples of the application of this classification system within early infancy.

Tanguay (1984) summarized the model described by Greenspan and his associates (Greenspan, 1979; Greenspan & Lourie, 1980; Greenspan & Porges, 1984) and reaffirmed the strength of such a classification system. However, he argued for an even more comprehensive system of classification based on neuropsychological and developmental literature. First, he suggested that the component elements of "personality" should be identified. (These would include but not be limited to affect, language, attention, cognition, perception, and motor functioning.) Then diagnosis would refer not only to the level of development within each component but also to the typical, naturally occurring intercomponent relationships. Retardation could be viewed as slowed development across categories, for example, whereas various forms of psychopathology could be manifested by dissociated development across categories. The pattern of development within each area would give the clearest information about etiology and treatment, and thus would yield the most useful diagnosis.

Finally, Cicchetti and Schneider-Rosen (1986) described an organizational approach to psychopathology that extends many of the ideas already described. This approach is built on Werner's (1948) orthogenetic principle, which postulates that development involves increasing differentiation and hierarchical integration. Within this framework, it is the organization of behavior rather than its frequency or duration that determines the degree to which the behavior is considered adaptive or pathological. Organization can be multiply determined by genetic, cognitive, affective, behavioral, and social factors, and refers to the individual's ability to interact competently with the environment. Organization of social and emotional behavior, for example, begins in an undifferentiated state in which self and caretaker are perceived as one. Later, attachment and a differentiated sense of self develop, as the child produces new organizations. Processes such as language and perspective taking generate additional organizations. Each level of organization predisposes (although it does not entirely determine) later organization, and general environmental or biological factors that may enhance or impede organization can make the organism either more resilient or more vulnerable to maladaptive as opposed to adaptive organizations. Like Tanguay's (1984) model, the organizational approach presumes multiple relevant and interlocking contributory factors that determine the organization of behavior at any one point in time. Although not intended to produce classifications per se, the organizational approach suggests that diagnosis would most profitably consist of a description of the current organization of cognitive, affective, and social structures.

Significantly, none of the developmental models discussed in this section is described as having a complete diagnostic system in place. Indeed, it is explicitly noted that it would be premature to attempt to replace traditional classification schemes with these models. However, each approach offers insight concerning the potential for important developmental contributions to future diagnostic systems.

CONCLUSION

Classic developmental research and recent investigations within developmental psychopathology offer important, fresh perspectives to the diagnosis of child psychopathology. It is not enough to agree that children differ from adults and thus deserve their own diagnostic nomenclature. If the presumptions of a static background and of a single set of standards for psychopathology are applied to reformulations of child diagnosis, the problems inherent in traditional classification systems will remain. The greatest promise for a reliable, valid, and useful diagnostic system for diagnosing child psychopathology lies in combining expertise in classification and psychopathology with a sound knowledge of normal and abnormal development. Fortunately, the exciting body of literature reviewed here suggests that the beginnings of such combinations are currently under way.

REFERENCES

Abraham, K. (1927). *Selected papers of Karl Abraham.* New York: Brunner/Mazel.

Achenbach, T.M. (1974). *Developmental psychopathology.* New York: Wiley.

Achenbach, T.M. (1980). DSM-III in light of empirical research on the classification of child psychopathology. *Journal of the American Academy of Child Psychiatry, 19,* 395–412.

Achenbach, T.M. (1982). *Developmental psychopathology* (2nd ed.). New York: Wiley.

Adler, A. (1916). *The neurotic constitution.* New York: Moffat.

Agras, W.S., Chapin, H.N., & Oliveau, D.C. (1972). The national history of phobia. *Archives of General Psychiatry, 26,* 315–317.

Ainsworth, M., Blehar, M., Waters, E., & Walls, S. (1978). *Patterns of attachment.* Hillsdale, NJ: Erlbaum.

Als, H. (1980). Infant individuality: Assessing patterns of very early development. In J. Call & E. Galenson (Eds.), *Proceedings of the First World Congress on Infant Psychiatry*. New York: Basic.

Als, H., & Brazelton, T.B. (1978). *Stages of early infant organization*. Paper presented at the meeting of the American Cleft Palate Association, Atlanta.

Als, H., & Brazelton, T.B. (1981). A new model of assessing the behavioral organization in preterm and fullterm infants. *Journal of the American Academy of Child Psychiatry*, *20*, 239–263.

American Psychiatric Association. (1980). *Diagnostic and statistical manual of mental disorders* (3rd ed.). Washington, DC: Author.

American Psychiatric Association. (1987). *Diagnostic and statistical manual of mental disorders* (3rd ed., rev.). Washington, DC: Author.

Ames, L.B., Metraux, R.W., & Walker, R.N. (1977). *Adolescent Rorschach responses: Developmental trends from ten to sixteen years* (rev. ed.). New York: Brunner/Mazel.

Anthony, E.J. (1957). The significance of Jean Piaget for child psychiatry. *British Journal of Medical Psychology*, *30*, 20–34.

Axline, V. (1947). *Play therapy*. Boston: Houghton Mifflin.

Bellak, L., & Bellak, S.S. (1974). *Children's Apperception Test* (6th and rev. ed.). Larchmont, NY: C.P.S.

Bierman, K.L. (1983). Cognitive development and clinical interviews with children. In B.B. Lahey & A.E. Kazdin (Eds.), *Advances in clinical child psychology* (Vol. 6). New York: Plenum.

Block, J. (1982). Assimilation, accommodation, and the dynamics of personality development. *Child Development*, *53*, 281–295.

Bowlby, J. (1951). Maternal care and mental health. *World Health Organization Monograph*, *No. 2*. London: Her Majesty's Stationery Office.

Bowlby, J. (1980). *Attachment and loss: III. Loss, sadness, and depression*. New York: Basic.

Brazelton, T.B. (1973). *Neonatal Behavior Assessment Scale*. Spastic's International Medical Publications. London: Heinemann; Philadelphia: Lippincott.

Burke, W.T., & Abidin, R.R. (1978). *The development of a parenting stress index*. Paper presented at the annual convention of the American Psychological Association.

Caldwell, B.M., & Bradley, R.H. (1979). *Home observation for measurement of the environment*. Little Rock: University of Arkansas Press.

Cantwell, D.P. (1980). The diagnostic process and diagnostic classification in child psychiatry—DMS-III. *Journal of the American Academy of Child Psychiatry*, *19*, 345–355.

Carey, W.B., & McDevitt, S.C. (1978). Revision of the infant temperament questionnaire. *Pediatrics*, *61*, 735–739.

Carlson, G.A., & Garber, J. (1986). Developmental issues in the classification of depressed children. In M. Rutter, C.E. Izard, & P.B. Read (Eds.), *Depression in young people: Clinical and developmental perspectives*. New York: Guilford.

Casteneda, M., McCandless, B.R., & Palermo, D.S. (1956). The children's form of the Manifest Anxiety Scale. *Child Development*, *27*, 317–326.

Cicchetti, D. (1984). The emergence of developmental psychopathology. *Child Development*, *55*, 1–7.

Cicchetti, D., & Schneider-Rosen, K. (1986). An organizational approach to childhood depression. In M. Rutter, C.E. Izard, & P.B. Read (Eds.), *Depression in young people: Clinical and developmental perspectives*. New York: Guilford.

Crowther, J.H., Bond, L.A., & Rolf, J.E. (1981). The incidence, prevalence, and severity of behavior disorders among preschool-aged children in day care. *Journal of Abnormal Child Psychology*, *9*, 23–42.

Douglas, J.W.B. (1975). Early hospital admission and later disturbances of behaviour and learning. *Developmental Medicine and Child Neurology*, *17*, 456–480.

Elkind, D. (1982). Piagetian psychology and the practice of child psychiatry. *Journal of the American Academy of Child Psychiatry*, *21*, 435–445.

Evans-Jones, L.G., & Rosenbloom, L. (1978). Disintegrative psychosis in childhood. *Developmental Medicine & Child Neurology*, *20*, 462–470.

Frank, J.D. (1985). Therapeutic components shared by all psychotherapies. In M. Mahoney & A. Freeman (Eds.), *Cognition and psychotherapy*. New York: Plenum.

Freud, A. (1946). *The psycho-analytical treatment of children*. New York: International Universities Press.

Freud, S. (1905). *Three essays on the theory of sexuality*. London: Hogarth.

Furman, W. (1980). Promoting social development: Developmental implications for treatment. In B.B. Lahey & A.E. Kazdin (Eds.), *Advances in clinical child psychology* (Vol. 3). New York: Plenum.

Gaensbauer, T.J., & Harmon, R.J. (1981). Clinical assessment in infancy utilizing structured playroom situations. *Journal of the American Academy of Child Psychiatry*, *20*, 264–280.

Garber, J. (1984). Classification of childhood psychopathology: A developmental perspective. *Child Development*, *55*, 30–48.

Gelfand, D.M., & Peterson, L. (1985). *Child development and psychopathology*. Beverly Hills: Sage.

Gittelman, R. (1980). The role of psychological tests for differential diagnosis in child psychiatry. *Journal of the American Academy of Child Psychiatry*, *19*, 413–438.

Goldsmith, H.H., & Alansky, J.A. (1987). Infant temperament and maternal predictors of attachment: A meta-analytic review. *Journal of Consulting & Clinical Psychology*, *55*, 805–816.

Greenspan, S.I. (1979). Intelligence and adaptation, an integration of psychoanalytic and Piagetian developmental psychology. *Psychological Issues Monograph 47/48*. New York: International Universities Press.

Greenspan, S., & Lourie, R.S. (1981). Developmental structuralist approach to the classification of adaptive and pathological personality organizations: Infancy and early childhood. *American Journal of Psychiatry*, *138*, 725–735.

Greenspan, S.I., & Porges, S.W. (1984). Psychopathology in infancy and early childhood: Clinical perspectives on the organization of sensory and affective thematic experience. *Child Development*, *55*, 49–70.

Hafner, A.J., Quast, W., Speer, D.C., & Grams, A. (1964). Children's anxiety scales in relation to self, parental, and psychiatric ratings of anxiety. *Journal of Consulting Psychology*, *28*, 255–258.

Hartmann, H. (1939). *Ego psychology and the problem of adaptation*. New York: International Universities Press.

Herjanic, B., & Campbell, W. (1977). Differentiating psychiatrically disturbed children on the basis of a structured interview. *Journal of Abnormal Child Psychology*, *5*, 127–134.

Hodges, K., Kline, J., Fitch, P., McKnew, D., & Cytryn, L. (1981). The child assessment schedule: A diagnostic interview for research and clinical use. *Catalogue of Selected Documents in Psychology*, *11*, 56.

Hodges, K., McKnew, D., Burbach, D.J., & Roebuck, L. (in press). Diagnostic concordance between the Child Assessment Schedule and the Kiddie-SADS in an outpatient sample using lay interviewers. *Journal of the American Academy of Child Psychiatry*.

John, R., Mednick, S., & Schulsinger, F. (1982). Teacher reports as a predictor of schizophrenia and borderline schizophrenia: A Bayesian decision analysis. *Journal of Abnormal Psychology*, *91*, 399–413.

Kanfer, R., Eyberg, S.M., & Krahn, G.L. (1983). Interviewing strategies in child assessment. In C.E. Walker & M.C. Roberts (Eds.), *Handbook of clinical child psychology*. New York: Wiley.

Karp, N.A., Herzog, E.P., & Weinberg, A.M. (1985). The diagnostic nursery: A new approach to evaluating preschoolers. *Journal of Clinical Child Psychology*, *14*, 202–208.

Kovacs, M. (1979). *Interim information on the Children's Depression Inventory*. Unpublished manuscript, Western Psychiatric Institute and Clinic.

Kovacs, M. (1986). A developmental perspective on methods and measures in the assessment of depressive disorders: The clinical interview. In M. Rutter, C.E. Izard, & P.B. Read (Eds.), *Depression in young people: Clinical and developmental perspectives*. New York: Guilford.

Kovacs, M., & Beck, A.T. (1977). An empirical-clinical approach toward a definition of childhood depression. In J.G. Schulterbrandt & A. Raskin (Eds.), *Depression in childhood: Diagnosis, treatment and conceptual models*. New York: Raven.

Lamb, M.E. (1987). Predictive implications of individual differences in attachment. *Journal of Consulting & Clinical Psychology*, *55*, 817–824.

Lefkowitz, M.M., & Burton, N. (1978). Childhood depression. *Psychological Bulletin*, *85*, 716–726.

Loeber, R. (1982). The stability of antisocial and delinquent child behavior: A review. *Child Development*, *53*, 1531–1446.

Machover, K. (1949). *Personality projection in the drawing of the human figure*. Springfield, IL: Charles C Thomas.

Main, M., Kaplan, N., & Cassidy, J. (1985). Security in infancy, childhood, and adulthood: A move to the level of representation. In I. Bretherton & E. Waters (Eds.), *Growing points of attachment theory and research* (pp. 66–104). *Monographs of the Society for Research in Development*, *50* (Serial No. 181).

Masterson, J.F. (1967). The symptomatic adolescent five years later: He didn't grow out of it. *American Journal of Psychiatry*, *123*, 1338–1345.

Matthews, K.A., & Angulo, J. (1980). Measurement of the Type A behavior pattern in children: Assessment of children's competitiveness, impatience–anger, and aggression. *Child Development*, *51*, 466–475.

Milich, R., Loney, J., & Roberts, M.A. (1986). Playroom observations of activity level and sustained attention: Two-year stability. *Journal of Consulting & Clinical Psychology*, *54*, 272–274.

Minde, K., & Minde, R. (1986). *Infant psychiatry: An introductory textbook*. Beverly Hills: Sage.

Palmer, J.O. (1970). *The psychological assessment of children.* New York: Wiley.

Palmer, J.O. (1983). *The psychological assessment of children* (2nd ed.). New York: Wiley.

Patterson, C.H. (1973). *Theories of counseling and psychotherapy* (2nd ed.). New York: Harper & Row.

Phillips, L., Draguns, J.G., & Bartlett, D.P. (1975). Classification of behavior disorders. In N. Hobbs (Ed.), *Issues in the classification of children.* San Francisco: Jossey-Bass.

Piaget, J. (1971). *Biology and knowledge.* Chicago: University of Chicago Press.

Rescorla, L.A. (1986). Preschool psychiatric disorders: Diagnostic classification and symptom patterns. *Journal of the American Academy of Child Psychiatry, 25,* 162–169.

Reynolds, C.R., & Richmond, B.O. (1978). What I think and feel: A revised measure of children's manifest anxiety. *Journal of Abnormal Child Psychology, 6,* 271–280.

Riegel, K.F. (1978). *Psychology, mon amour.* Boston: Houghton Mifflin.

Robins, L. (1966). *Deviant children grown up.* Baltimore: Williams & Wilkins.

Robins, L.N. (1978). Sturdy childhood predictors of adult antisocial behavior. *Psychological Medicine, 8,* 611–622.

Roff, M., & Ricks, D. (Eds.). (1970). *Life history research in psychopathology* (Vol. 1). Minneapolis: University of Minnesota Press.

Rolf, J., & Read, P.B. (1984). Programs advancing developmental psychopathology. *Child Development, 55,* 8–16.

Rutter, M. (1965). Classification and categorization in child psychiatry. *Journal of Child Psychology & Psychiatry, 6,* 71–83.

Rutter, M. (1986). The developmental psychopathology of depression: Issues and perspectives. In M. Rutter, C.E. Izard, & P.B. Read (Eds.), *Depression in young people: Clinical and developmental perspectives.* New York: Guilford.

Rutter, M., & Garmezy, N. (1983). Developmental psychopathology. In P.H. Mussen (Ed.), *Handbook of child psychology* (Vol. 4). New York: Wiley.

Rutter, M., Quinton, D., & Liddle, C. (1983). Parenting in two generations: Looking backwards and looking forwards. In N. Madge (Ed.), *Families at risk.* London: Heinemann.

Rutter, M., & Shaffer, D. (1980). DSM-III: A step forward or back in terms of the classification of child psychiatric disorders? *Journal of the American Academy of Child Psychiatry, 19,* 371–394.

Rutter, M., Tizard, J., Yule, W., Graham, P., & Whitmore, K. (1976). Isle of Wight studies, 1964–1974. *Psychological Medicine, 6,* 313–332.

Santostefano, S. (1971). Beyond nosology: Diagnosis from the viewpoint of development. In R.E. Rie (Ed.), *Perspectives in child psychopathology.* New York: Aldine-Atherton.

Sroufe, L.A., Fox, N., & Pancake, V. (1983). Attachment and dependency in developmental perspective. *Child Development, 54,* 1615–1627.

Sroufe, L.A., & Rutter, M. (1984). The domain of developmental psychopathology. *Child Development, 55,* 17–29.

Tanguay, P.E. (1984). Toward a new classification of serious psychopathology in children. *Journal of the American Academy of Child Psychiatry, 23,* 373–384.

Thomas, A., & Chess, S. (1972). Development in middle childhood. *Seminars in Psychiatry, 4,* 331–341.

Tronick, E., Als, H., & Adamson, L. (1979). Mother-infant face-to-face communicative interaction. In M. Bullowa (Ed.), *Before speech.* Cambridge: Cambridge University Press.

Tyson, R.L. (1986). The roots of psychopathology and our theories of development. *Journal of the American Academy of Child Psychiatry, 25*, 12–22.

Victor, J.B., & Halverson, C.F., Jr. (1976). Behavior problems in elementary school children: A follow-up study. *Journal of Abnormal Child Psychology, 4*, 17–29.

Webb, T.E., & Van Devere, C.A. (1980, July). *Interviewing methodology for psychological factors in pediatrics: A search for attributes.* Paper presented at the meeting of the Association for Care of Children in Hospitals, Dallas.

Weiner, I.B. (1972). *Child and adolescent psychopathology.* New York: Wiley.

Wenar, C.L. (1982). *Psychopathology from infancy through adolescence.* New York: Random House.

Werner, H. (1948). *Comparative psychology of mental development.* New York: International Universities Press.

Wirt, R.D., & Broen, W.E. (1956). The relation of the Children's Manifest Anxiety Scale to the concept of anxiety as used in the clinic. *Journal of Consulting Psychology, 20*, 482.

Wolff, P.H. (1960). The developmental psychologies of Jean Piaget and psychoanalysis. *Psychological Issues Monographs, No. 5.* New York: International Universities Press.

CHAPTER 24

Diagnostic Interviews for Children
and Adolescents

HELEN ORVASCHEL

A comprehensive evaluation of child psychopathology must assess many domains of behavior. These domains include the child's physical well-being, developmental level, intellectual functioning, family structure, culture, interaction, and psychiatric history, as well as the child's psychological–psychiatric symptomatology. In light of the vast array of information required, no single assessment measure can be expected to met all the needs of the practitioner or the research investigator. For the evaluation of behavioral symptomatology, however, several reliable methods are now available for information gathering and classification of child psychopathology. In fact, structured and semistructured psychiatric interviews are an important tool in the diagnostic assessment of children, and their use has become increasingly common during the past decade.

The development of diagnostic interviews has, in part, paralleled the trend toward the use of specified criteria symptoms (DSM-III, RDC) in both adult and child psychiatry (APA, 1980; Spitzer, Endicott, & Robins, 1978). While such diagnostic instruments are most frequently used by researchers, they provide advantages for the clinician as well. The use of these assessment tools enables the clinician systematically to evaluate the signs and symptoms of disorder, without regard to any preestablished biases. Such a procedure ensures a more complete and frequently more accurate assessment of psychopathology due to the reduction of information variance (Spitzer et al., 1978). It also enables the practitioner to reach a diagnostic formulation using a methodology similar to that of the researcher, allowing for better comparability between science and practice.

There are, of course, a number of reasons for the initiation of a child diagnostic evaluation, and the choice of the assessment tool should be guided by the purpose of the evaluation. The clinician interested in determining the focus of treatment may be more concerned with a child's areas of functional impairment than with specific diagnostic criteria. Initial and follow-up evaluations concerned with the measurement of treatment efficacy require symptom severity ratings that can be assessed over time. Research involving large-scale epidemiologic population surveys may be guided in instrument selection by the practical need of using lay interviewers, while other research endeavors will be more concerned with specific clinical questions. Instrument selection must, therefore, be based on the needs of the investigators, the questions they wish to address, the diagnostic categories of interest, research design issues, and the realistic limitations of the investigation or evaluation endeavor.

This chapter describes three structured and two semistructured diagnostic interviews available for use with child and adolescent populations. Of the five interviews, three are symptom oriented and two are syndrome oriented. Symptom-oriented interviews are organized according to subjects of assessment (e.g., school, friends, activity levels, sleep, etc.). The subjects are ordered according to the developers' interpretation of the "natural flow" for a clinical interview. Therefore, specific behaviors within categories generally cut across different syndromes. Symptoms relevant to particular diagnostic categories are clustered after the interview is completed, by computer-derived algorithms and/or by clinician-determined diagnosis.

Syndrome-oriented interviews are organized according to diagnostic categories. This format is more amenable to lifetime assessment and to skips out of some interview sections. Decisions on structural organization are a function of developers' preference and users' needs. Both types have been accepted without difficulty by patients and clinicians.

The interviews presented should be viewed not as competing with one another but as alternatives offered to clinicians and researchers with varying needs for assessment tools. The interviews were developed originally for different purposes, and each has strengths and weaknesses that must be considered. The interviews selected for review here also have much in common. All are well designed and cumulatively represent considerable progress in the field of child and adolescent diagnostic assessment. Their structure and format are based on extensive empirical experience with, primarily, clinically referred populations. They all assess behaviors that provide diagnoses according to DSM-III or DSM-III-R criteria (APA, 1980, 1987) and they all use parent (or primary caretaker) and child informants. Finally, they all have psychiatric data available that show good test–retest and/or interrater reliability, and all have face and content validity.

SYMPTOM-ORIENTED INTERVIEWS

Diagnostic Interview Schedule for Children

The NIMH Diagnostic Interview Schedule for Children (DISC) was developed by Anthony Costello, Craig Edelbrock, Mina Dulcan, Robert Kalas, and Sheree Klaric, under contract to the Division of Biometry and Epidemiology of the National Institute of Mental Health. The initial version of the DISC was written by Keith Conners, Barbara Herjanic, and Joaquim Puig-Antich and was similar in structure to the Diagnostic Interview for Children and Adolescents (DICA). Subsequent changes by Costello and his colleagues resulted in the version currently available (Costello, Edelbrock, Dulcan, Kalas, & Klaric, 1984). The DISC is a highly structured interview designed primarily as a survey instrument for use in large-scale epidemiologic research. It can be administered by clinicians or trained lay interviewers and requires no clinical judgment. The DISC is appropriate for use with children 6 to 17 years old, while its parallel, the DISC-P, is administered to the parents about the child. It takes approximately 50 to 70 minutes to administer to each informant (Costello et al., 1984).

The wording and order of questions on the DISC are completely specified and the interview structure is explicit. Items are to be asked as written and the line of inquiry has been predetermined. Therefore, a "yes" to a particular item may be followed by one series of questions and a "no" may be followed by another series of questions, but the choice of follow-up is indicated in the interview and the examiner need make no other choices. Items are precoded and questions are rated as "not true" (0), "somewhat" or "sometimes true" (1), and "very" or "often true" (2), or "no" (0)/"yes" (2). Questions on duration and onset are included for some behaviors and categories of disorder. Severity of problems is based on quantitative symptom scores or by summing the $0-1-2$ response codes for each item. Symptoms are rated primarily for the past year. Parents and children are interviewed separately. A training manual is available that provides a general interviewing guide and specific instructions on administering the DISC.

The DISC contains 264 items and the DISC-P contains 302 items. The structure is symptom oriented with questions organized according to subjects (i.e., family, school, friends, etc.). The interview begins with some general questions about the child's family and proceeds to cover the behaviors and symptoms needed to assess most Axis I DSM-III categories of disorder. Algorithms are available for obtaining computer-derived diagnoses based on DISC interview data. Questions provide information on the following DSM-III categories of disorder: attention deficit disorder (and hyperactivity), oppositional disorder, conduct disorder (all subtypes), alcohol abuse and dependence, other substance abuse and dependence, major depression, dysthymic disorder, cyclothymic disorder, mania, anorexia nervosa, bulimia, enuresis, encopresis, separation anxiety, avoidance disorder, overanxious disorder, phobic disorder, panic disorder, obsessive–compulsive disorder, schizophrenic disorder, and psychosexual disorders. The DISC-P contains questions for the following additional disorders: elective mutism, stereotyped movement disorder, pervasive developmental disorders, and dissociative disorders.

Data available on the DISC include test–retest and interrater reliability, parent–child agreement, and comparisons with clinicians' diagnoses. Test–retest reliability for parent reports on 243 clinically referred children ranged from .44 to .86 with an average intraclass correlation of .76. The reliability of behavior–conduct problems was somewhat higher than for affective–neurotic problems (Edelbrock, Costello, Dulcan, Kalas, & Conover, 1985). Reliability of parent interviews for DSM-III diagnoses ranged from .35 to .81 with an average kappa of .56 (Edelbrock, Costello, Dulcan, Conover, & Kalas, 1986). Test–retest reliability for child reports ranged from .28 to .78 with an average correlation of .62. Again, reliability was higher for behavior–conduct symptoms (.69) than for affective–neurotic symptoms (.57).

Reliability was also found to increase with the child's age for most symptom areas (.43, .60, and .71 for children aged 6 to 9, 10 to 13, and 14 to 18, respectively) (Edelbrock et al., 1985; Edelbrock et al., 1986).

Interrater reliability for symptom scores ranged from .94 to 1.00 with an average correlation of .98 (Costello et al., 1984). Parent–child agreement for 299 clinically referred children ranged from .04 to .68 with an average correlation of .27. Agreement was higher for questions concerned with overt behavior ($r = .42$) than for questions on affect ($r = .19$). Parent–child agreement was also associated with the age of the child (.10, .27, and .35 for children 6 to 9, 10 to 13, and 14 to 18, respectively) (Edelbrock et al., 1985). Diagnoses based on the DISC and the DISC-P showed poor agreement with diagnoses based on clinicians' standard assessments. The reasons for these poor agreement rates are as yet unclear. Results of DISC interviews did correlate significantly with clinicians' ratings of adaptive functioning and with parent, teacher, and child ratings of children's problem behaviors, social functioning, school performance, peer relations, and self-concept (Costello et al., 1984).

The DISC has potential for use in large-scale epidemiologic research requiring lay interviewer administration. Rates of test–retest and interrater reliability are available for large samples of clinically referred children and have been high. Comprehensive computer algorithms and data dictionaries are available for generating diagnoses according to DSM-III criteria. No gradations of severity are available on positively rated symptoms, although many items contain a "1" code meaning "somewhat or sometimes." Investigators may wish to calculate change on the basis of the total number of problem behaviors reported at different points in time. Diagnoses are derived separately from parent and child interviews. Therefore, investigators must contend with discrepant diagnoses based on different informants. Resolution of these problems must be considered along with the advantages of using this assessment instrument.

Children's Assessment Schedule

The Children's Assessment Schedule (CAS) was developed by Kay Hodges at the University of Missouri (currently Duke University Medical Center) in collaboration with Leon Cytryn and Donald McKnew of the National Institute of Mental Health. The interview was designed to facilitate rapport while systematically collecting comprehensive clinical information (Hodges, Kline, Stern, Cytryn, & McKnew, 1982). In its current form, the CAS is a semistructured psychiatric interview designed for clinical or research assessments. When used by clinicians, information can be qualitatively analyzed to determine a diagnosis and treatment plan. For research purposes, investigators may derive a total score of problems or symptoms, separate scores for specific content areas, or scores for symptom complexes similar to many DSM-III diagnostic categories. The CAS is appropriate for use with children 7 to 16 years old, with a parallel form for use with parents (P-CAS). Administration time is approximately 45 to 60 minutes for each informant. Parents and children are interviewed separately, but no method of resolving discrepant information is specified by the author.

The CAS comprises three parts. Part 1 is the semistructured interview composed of approximately 75 questions about school, friends, activities and hobbies, family, fears, worries, self-image, mood, somatic concerns, expression of anger, and symptoms of thought disorder. Items are grouped according to what the author refers to as natural topics of conversation so that the child experiences the interview as a discussion about various areas of his or her life. The time frame of the interview is current or recent past (last 6 months). Items are rated as positive, negative, ambiguous, not applicable, or no response. Part 2 of the CAS allows the interviewer to record information on the onset and duration of positive symptoms of Part 1. In the third section of the interview, the interviewer rates 53 observational items.

A manual accompanying the CAS is available. The manual discusses each of the interview's content areas, provides suggested probes for items, identifies problematic issues in scoring, defines terms, suggests guidelines for establishing interrater reliability with the CAS, and offers a good overview of general interviewing techniques. The manual also provides information on various methods of scoring the interview, including the specification of items needed for obtaining a number of DSM-III diagnoses. The diagnostic categories covered by the CAS are attention deficit disorder (and hyperactivity), conduct disorder (all subtypes), oppositional disorder, separation anxiety, avoidant disorder, overanxious disorder, phobic disorder, obsessive–compulsive disorder, major depression, dysthymic disorder, manic episode, cyclothymic disorder, anorexia nervosa, bulimia, enuresis, encopresis, panic disorder, generalized anxiety disorder, schizoid disorder, psychotic disorder, substance abuse disorder, sleepwalking disorder, and sleep terror disorder.

Data available on the CAS include interrater reliability and discriminant and concurrent validity. Agreement among interviewers for items ranges from .44 to .82, with a total CAS correlation of .90. Kappa coefficients for items ranged from .47 to .61 (Hodges, McKnew, Cytryn, Stern, & Kline, 1982). The CAS was reported to discriminate inpatients, outpatients, and controls on the basis of total scores and individual category scores. Correlations were reported to be significant between child interviews and CBCL scores obtained from mothers, while child scores on a depression and an anxiety self-report were moderately correlated with CAS symptom complexes on affect. Concordance between results on the CAS and the K-SADS-E (Orvaschel, Puig-Antich, Chambers, Tabrizi, & Johnson, 1982) ranged from moderate to high agreement, with the exception of overanxious disorder. Kappa coefficients were better when information from parent and child was combined (.59 to .60), and better for parents alone than for child alone. Agreement for conduct disorder was reported to be good for both informants (Hodges, McKnew, Burbach, & Roebuck, in press).

Overall, the CAS provides a standardized method for obtaining information on a broad range of child behaviors relevant to many Axis I DSM-III categories of disorder. The interview format is fairly structured but written primarily for clinician administration. While organization of the interview is symptom oriented, a scoring system for deriving diagnoses is provided. No gradations of severity are available on positively rated items, but treatment effects may be estimated on the basis of a reduction of total number of symptoms. In addition, the manual accompanying the

CAS is well written and provides many useful guidelines for the administration and interpretation of this interview and for interview techniques in general. The resolution of discrepant findings between parent and child interviews is not discussed and remains an area of practical clinical importance.

Interview Schedule for Children

The Interview Schedule for Children (ISC) was developed by Marika Kovacs. The first version was constructed in 1974 for a research project on childhood depression. Since that time, it has undergone numerous revisions and additions as a result of psychometric testing, extensive experience, and expanded research needs. The remaining discussion of the ISC refers to the version currently used and its accompanying addenda.

The ISC is a semistructured psychiatric interview designed primarily for research assessments of childhood depression. Administration of the interview requires an experienced clinician trained in its use and familiar with the DSM-III diagnostic criteria. The ISC is appropriate for use with children 8 to 17 years old. Mothers are interviewed about their children and children are then interviewed directly by the same clinician. Interviews with children take approximately 45 to 60 minutes and interviews with parents between 90 and 120 minutes. A follow-up ISC is also available to assess change over time (Kovacs, 1983).

The ISC comprises the core interview and the addenda. The addenda provide questions that assess additional symptoms necessary for determining DSM-III criteria and categories of disorder not included in the core interview. The ISC begins with an unstructured interview focusing on an overview of the child's problems, the history of the complaints, and their duration. Following this, the interviewer inquires about the presence and severity of 43 symptoms of psychopathology and records a global rating of the child's functional impairment. Also included in this section of questioning are additional items asking if certain symptoms are recorded as positive. The remaining questions that constitute the approximately 100 items in the core interview include ratings on psychotic symptoms and developmental milestones. The interviewer also rates 12 observational items (e.g., pressure of speech), records his or her clinical impressions, any DSM-III diagnoses, their duration, and duration of symptoms, and then dictates a summary. Addenda items include questions relevant to most other Axis I DSM-III categories of disorder and several Axis II diagnoses. In the core ISC interview, information on the following DSM-III disorders is obtained: conduct disorder (all subtypes), dysthymia, major depression, mania (and hypomania), adjustment disorder with depressed mood, schizophrenia, schizoaffective disorder, obsessive–compulsive disorder, separation anxiety disorder, phobic disorder, substance abuse (drugs and alcohol), and enuresis and encopresis. Additional Axis I disorders assessed in the addenda include attention deficit disorder (and hyperactivity), avoidant disorder, oppositional disorder, overanxious disorder, and panic disorder. Axis II categories covered in the addenda include borderline, compulsive, histrionic, schizoid, and schizotypal personality disorders.

Most items in the core ISC are rated on an 8-point scale, with specific anchor points indicated for scoring level of severity. Behaviors assessed in the addenda are rated as present or absent only. For most symptoms, ratings reflect behavior for the past 2 weeks. Acting-out behavior is assessed for the past 6 months, while mental status is rated for "current" and examiners' observations and impressions are rated on the basis of interview behavior. The follow-up ISC allows the recording of symptom ratings between interviews and for the past 2 weeks. It also includes "interim ratings" that reflect any significant changes in the severity of acting-out behaviors.

The ISC is symptom oriented and precoded. Specific questions are provided for each of the items to be rated. Interviewers have considerable discretion regarding the order of behaviors they assess and the extent of questioning needed to determine a particular rating. Items are rated on the basis of mothers' reports, children's reports, and clinicians' overall evaluation from both informants. Diagnoses are based on the clinicians' summary ratings and are generally verified by consensus of the clinicians involved in the evaluation. The ISC interview is accompanied by instructions on its administration and a description of the clinical rules developed to ensure reasonable decision making and uniformity of diagnoses (Feinberg & Kovacs, 1983).

Data available on the ISC include interrater reliability and parent–child agreement. Interrater reliability was ascertained for interviews of 35 clinically referred children. Intraclass correlations of corated symptoms ranged from .64 to 1.0. Agreement on observational items ranged from .53 to .96, and the correlation for ratings of current disorder was .86. Parent–child agreement for 75 clinically referred children ranged from .02 to .95 for symptoms and .32 to .86 for syndromes, with an average correlation of .61. Variability in parent–child agreement was generally a function of the internality versus externality of the symptoms assessed (Kovacs, 1983).

In summary, the ISC is a semistructured, symptom-oriented psychiatric interview that provides a systematic procedure for assessing most Axis I and several Axis II DSM-III categories of disorder. Severity ratings are provided for depressive symptomatology and for a number of additional areas of behavior. A follow-up version of the ISC is also available to record change over time. Diagnoses are based on an integration of information from parent and child informants and are a function of consensual clinical judgment. Experienced and well-trained clinicians are required for the administration of the ISC.

SYNDROME-ORIENTED INTERVIEWS

Diagnostic Interview for Children and Adolescents

The Diagnostic Interview for Children and Adolescents (DICA) was developed at Washington University by Herjanic and Welner. The 1981 version of the DICA was modeled after the Diagnostic Interview Schedule (Robins, Helzer, Crougan, & Ratcliff, 1981) and is designed to assess child psychopathology according to

DSM-III criteria (Welner, Reich, Herjanic, & Amado, in press). Discussion of the DICA will refer to the 1981 version unless otherwise specified.

The DICA is a structured diagnostic interview designed for use in clinical and epidemiologic research. It can be administered by clinicians or trained lay interviewers and requires no clinical judgment on the part of the interviewer. The DICA is appropriate for use with children 6 to 17 years old, while its parallel, the DICA-P, is administered to the parent about the child. It takes approximately 60 to 90 minutes to administer to each informant.

The DICA and DICA-P comprise three parts. Part 1, the same for both instruments, is a joint interview with the parent and child, introducing the interview and obtaining baseline and general demographic information. Following these initial 19 questions, parent and child are separated and interviewed individually by different interviewers. Part 2 of the child interview comprises 247 questions, grouped according to category of disorder. The items ask about symptoms for the following disorders: attention deficit disorder (and hyperactivity), oppositional disorder, conduct disorder (all types), tobacco dependence, other substance abuse and dependence, major depression, adjustment disorder with depressed mood, mania, separation anxiety disorder, overanxious disorder, phobic disorder, obsessive–compulsive disorder, anorexia nervosa, bulimia, somatization disorder, enuresis, encopresis, and psychotic symptoms. The interview also includes questions about menstruation (for girls), gender identity, sexual experience and abuse, and psychosocial stressors.

Part 3 of the DICA provides the interviewer an opportunity to rate eight categories of observational items. Part 2 of the DICA-P is the same for the parent as for the child but is written in the third person (i.e., "Does he . . . ?"). Part 3 of the DICA-P asks the parent about pregnancy complications, the child's infancy and early development, stuttering, medical history, siblings of the child, and additional diagnostic information about the child that is best obtained from the parent (e.g., autism, elective mutism, pica, stereotyped movements, and avoidant disorder).

Symptoms on the DICA are generally rated as present or absent, and no severity scoring of positive symptoms is available. Questions on duration, onset, and offset of disorders are included. Questions are phrased in the present tense for all children. If a child is on medication for a behavioral or emotional problem, the interviewer may determine whether a problem was present before the medication. Children 12 or older may be asked whether a particular problem was true in the past, if it is not present now. Therefore, some information on past psychiatric symptoms is obtained. All items are precoded, and computer-derived diagnoses are possible.

Data available on the DICA include parent–child agreement on items and diagnostic categories, test–retest reliability, and diagnostic comparisons between interviews and charts. Parent–child agreement on items, calculated with the kappa statistic, ranged from 0 to .87 (Herjanic & Reich, 1982). According to the authors, items with high agreement between informants were objective, concrete, and serious, while low-agreement items required judgment or were subject to misinterpretation. Diagnostic agreement between parents and children was also quite varied, but tended to show more disagreement than agreement on earlier versions of the interview (Reich, Herjanic, Welner, & Gandhy, 1982). On the more recent version of the

DICA, an increase in mother–child agreement was noted (Welner et al., in press). Test–retest reliability has thus far been quite high, while comparisons of DICA diagnoses with chart diagnoses have been more moderate. These rather preliminary validity data must await more extensive testing, since chart comparisons are not generally the best standard against which to compare research interview assessments.

The DICA is a well-written syndrome-oriented diagnostic interview, with considerable value in clinical and epidemiologic research. Much of the interview structure and phrasing has been the product of sound research and thoughtful development. Its lay interviewer administration capability is an additional asset for many types of research programs. However, the DICA's dicthotomous scoring of items as positive or negative and its lack of symptom severity ratings result in a less sensitive measure of change in follow-up assessments requiring the evaluation of treatment. In addition, diagnoses are derived separately for parent and child interviews and no method for aggregating information from both is provided. Therefore, clinicians must contend with discrepant diagnoses and difficult data-analytic decisions. These disadvantages must be weighed against the advantages of other aspects of this diagnostic assessment instrument.

Schedule for Affective Disorders and Schizophrenia for School-Age Children (Kiddie-SADS)

The Kiddie-SADS is currently available in two forms, the Present Episode (K-SADS-P) and the Epidemiologic Version (K-SADS-E). The K-SADS-P was developed by Joaquim Puig-Antich and William Chambers as a children's version of its adult counterpart (SADS) (Endicott & Spitzer, 1978). The interview was originally constructed as a diagnostic instrument for the assessment of ongoing episodes of psychiatric disorder in pediatric treatment studies of childhood depression. The original version of the K-SADS was constructed in 1977 and was revised in 1978. A 1983 revision was developed on the basis of reliability data reported for the 1978 version and incorporated 6 years of experience with the interview. The latest and fourth version of the K-SADS-P is dated November 1986 and incorporates changes in line with the most recent version of the DSM (APA, 1987).

In its current form, the K-SADS-P is a semistructured psychiatric interview designed for clinical or research assessments. Administration of the interview requires a trained clinician experienced in child psychiatric assessment. The K-SADS is appropriate for use with children 6 to 17 years old. Mothers (or primary caretakers) are interviewed about their children and children are interviewed directly by the same interviewer. It takes approximately 60 minutes to administer to each informant.

The K-SADS-P comprises three parts. The first part of the interview is relatively unstructured. The informant is asked to identify all presenting problems and symptoms so that the interviewer can obtain and record the chronological picture of the ongoing episode, its mode of onset, and its duration. The child's treatment history is then recorded and the informant is asked to identify the time during the current episode or during the previous year (whichever is shortest) when symptoms were the most severe. The second part of the K-SADS includes questions on approximately 200 specific symptoms or behaviors relevant to most Axis I DSM-III-R diagnoses. Information on the following DSM-III-R disorders is obtained: major depression, manic disorder, other affective disorders (i.e., minor depression, dysthymia, hypomania, cyclothymia), anorexia nervosa, bulimia, panic, separation anxiety, phobias, obsessive–compulsive disorder, generalized anxiety (overanxious) disorder, conduct disorder, schizophrenia, schizophreniform disorder, brief reactive psychosis, paranoid disorder, schizoaffective disorder, and schizoptypal disorder. Additional behaviors that are rated include depersonalization, derealization, impulsivity, unstable interpersonal relationships, and identity disturbance. Part 3 of the K-SADS includes seven observational items rated by the interviewer and a rating on the children's version of the Global Assessment Scale. Information on age of onset and duration of disorder(s) is also recorded.

Most items on the K-SADS are rated on a 6- or 7-point range of severity, with specific criteria indicated for scoring levels. Most symptoms are rated twice. The first rating is for symptom severity during the worst period of the present episode. The second rating records symptom severity during the previous week. The second rating is used for comparison when investigators wish to assess change (e.g., following completion of a treatment trial or at specified intervals during a research protocol).

The K-SADS-E is designed to assess past and current episodes of child and adolescent psychopathology (Orvaschel et al., 1982). The fourth revision of the K-SADS-E, dated February 1987, was developed by Helen Orvaschel and Joaquim Puig-Antich and also incorporates changes in line with the DSM-III-R. The K-SADS-E includes all the categories of affective, anxiety, psychotic, and eating disorders mentioned for the K-SADS-P, as well as sections for attention deficit, oppositional, conduct, alcohol use, drug use, and other psychiatric (psychotic and nonpsychotic) disorders, tobacco use, and suicidal behavior. Each section begins with a brief description of the category of disorder covered and then continues with screen questions or specific symptom items. For each category of disorder, information is obtained on chronology, treatment, impairment, and severity, providing data on age of onset, offset, duration, and number of episodes, as well as type and length of treatment and functional impairment.

Administration of both the K-SADS-P and the K-SADS-E requires an interview with the parent first, followed by an interview with the child. Responses are recorded separately for each informant on an accompanying scoring sheet. The same clinician interviews both informants and records summary ratings for all items on the basis of information from parent, child, and any additional sources of data available. Discrepancies between parent and child responses are resolved during the course of the interview. Summary ratings reflect the interviewer's best clinical judgment of the presence and degree of symptomatology reported. The final diagnostic assessment of the child is based on the clinician's summary ratings, which also become the standard against which to measure change.

The K-SADS-P is organized primarily according to diagnostic category, while the K-SADS-E is completely syndrome oriented. Both interviews provide sample questions for all the items to be rated. These sample questions have been found most helpful with previous child interviews and are provided as a guide to the clinician. The presence of these questions is not intended to limit the interviewer, who should feel free to ask whatever is necessary to arrive at an accurate rating of each specific item. Both instruments are intended for use only by individuals trained in the psychiatric assessment of children and adolescents. The K-SADS-E does not assess levels of symptom severity (only category severity), making it less sensitive to the measurement of change or treatment effects than the K-SADS-P. Users of the present episode version who require information on past psychiatric history or assessment of categories of disorder not covered should supplement their assessment with the K-SADS-E.

Data available on the K-SADS-P include test–retest reliability, mother–child agreement, interrater reliability, and sensitivity of ratings due to pharmacologic treatment. Agreement between raters for individual symptoms and major diagnostic syndromes on the second version of the K-SADS-P ranged from .65 to .96. Comparisons following imipramine treatment of depressed children indicated K-SADS ratings to be sensitive to changes due to drug trials (Puig-Antich et al., 1978). Mother–child agreement for the K-SADS-P and K-SADS-E versions has ranged from −.08 to 1.0, with most items and syndromes in the acceptable range (>.50) (Chambers et al., 1985; Orvaschel et al., 1982). Test–retest reliability of depressive symptoms ranged from .28 to .88, with the vast majority of ratings over .50. Items relevant to the diagnosis of depression scored between .63 and .81 on test–retest and had internal consistency ratings between .65 and .84. Test–retest for conduct disorder was .89 and for psychotic symptoms ranged from .10 to .53. Anxiety diagnoses also demonstrated low test–retest reliability. Preliminary data on the validity of retrospective assessment of depression with an earlier version of the K-SADS-E provided good diagnostic agreement (kappa = .86) (Orvaschel et al., 1982).

The K-SADS-P and K-SADS-E are semistructured psychiatric interviews that provide a standardized method for obtaining and recording behaviors necessary for the assessment of most Axis I DSM-III (and DSM-III-R) categories of disorder. The K-SADS-P version allows for severity ratings to be recorded for most symptoms and is particularly useful for clinical intake assessments and for the measurement of treatment effects. The K-SADS-E version provides for a lifetime assessment of psychopathology and covers a broader range of psychiatric disorders, specifically, those requiring past history or chronology of behavior.

The psychiatric interviews reviewed were designed for different purposes, and each has its merits and deficiencies. Nevertheless, the use of a structured or semistructured psychiatric interview will provide a more reliable and often more comprehensive assessment of psychopathology. As has been noted, however, these instruments should be supplemented with additional evaluation material relevant to diagnostic formulation and treatment recommendations. The use of instruments such as those reviewed in this chapter should add to the overall quality of the psychiatric assessment of the child, but is not a substitute for other appropriate clinical assessments.

REFERENCES

American Psychiatric Association. (1980). *Diagnostic and statistical manual of mental disorders* (3rd ed.). Washington, DC: Author.

American Psychiatric Association. (1987). *Diagnostic and statistical manual of mental disorders* (3rd ed., rev.). Washington, DC: Author.

Chambers, W.J., Puig-Antich, J., Hirsch, M., Paez, P., Ambrosini, P.J., Tabrizi, M.A., & Davies, M. (1985). The assessment of affective disorders in children and adolescents by semi-structured interview: Test-retest reliability of the K-SADS-P. *Archives of General Psychiatry, 42*, 696–701.

Costello, A.J., Edelbrock, C., Dulcan, M.K., Kalas, R., & Klaric, S. (1984). *Report on the NIMH Diagnostic Interview Schedule for Children (DISC)*. Washington, DC: NIMH.

Edelbrock, C., Costello, A.J., Dulcan, M.K., Conover, N., & Kalas, R. (1986). Parent–child agreement on child psychiatric symptoms assessed via structured interview. *Journal of Child Psychology & Psychiatry, 27*, 181–190.

Edelbrock, C., Costello, A.J., Dulcan, M.K., Kalas, R., & Conover, N. (1985). Age differences in the reliability of the psychiatric interview of the child. *Child Development, 56*, 265–275.

Endicott, J., & Spitzer, R.L. (1978). A diagnostic interview: The SADS. *Archives of General Psychiatry, 35*, 837–853.

Feinberg, T.L., & Kovacs, M. (1983). *Research diagnosis in a study of the depressive disorders in childhood: The formulation of clinical decision making*. Unpublished manuscript.

Herjanic, B., & Reich, W. (1982). Development of a structured psychiatric interview for children: Agreement between child and parent on individual symptoms. *Journal of Abnormal Child Psychology, 10*, 307–324.

Hodges, K., Kline, J., Stern, L., Cytryn, L., & McKnew, D. (1982). The development of a child assessment interview for research and clinical use. *Journal of Abnormal Child Psychology, 10*, 173–189.

Hodges, K., McKnew, D., Burbach, D.J., & Roebuck, L. (1987). Diagnostic concordance between two structured interviews for children using lazy interviewer: The Child Assessment Schedule and the Kiddie-SADS. *Journal of the American Academy of Child Psychiatry, 26*, 654–661.

Hodges, K., McKnew, D., Cytryn, L., Stern, L., & Kline, J. (1982). The Child Assessment Schedule (CAS) Diagnostic Interview: A report on reliability and validity. *Journal of the American Academy of Child Psychiatry, 21*, 468–473.

Kovacs, M. (1983). *The Interview Schedule for Children (ISC): Interrater and parent–child agreement*. Unpublished manuscript.

Orvaschel, H., Puig-Antich, J., Chambers, W., Tabrizi, M.A., & Johnson, R. (1982). Retrospective assessment of child psychopathology with the Kiddie-SADS-E. *Journal of the American Academy of Child Psychiatry, 21*, 392–397.

Puig-Antich, J., Blau, S., Marx, N., Greenhill, L.L., & Chambers, W. (1978). Prepubertal major depressive disorders: A pilot study. *Journal of the American Academy of Child Psychiatry, 17*, 695–707.

Reich, W., Herjanic, B., Welner, Z., & Gandhy, P.R. (1982). Development of a structured psychiatric interview for children: Agreement on diagnosis comparing child and parent interview. *Journal of Abnormal Child Psychology, 20*, 325–336.

Robins, L.N., Helzer, J.E., Crougan, J., & Ratcliff, K.S. (1981). National Institute of Mental Health Diagnostic Interview Schedule. *Archives of General Psychiatry*, *38*, 381–389.

Spitzer, R.L., Endicott, J., & Robins, F. (1978). Research Diagnostic Criteria. *Archives of General Psychiatry*, *35*, 773–782.

Welner, Z., Reich, W., Herjanic, B., & Amado, H. (in press). Parent-child agreement, reliability and validity studies of the Diagnostic Interview for Children and Adolescents (DICA). *Journal of the American Academy of Child Psychiatry*.

CHAPTER 25

Epidemiology and Child Diagnosis

ELIZABETH J. COSTELLO AND RICHARDEAN BENJAMIN

This is a chapter for readers interested in the following topics:

What is epidemiology?
What can epidemiology contribute to the study of child psychiatric diagnosis?
What is the current state of knowledge about the epidemiology of child psychiatric disorders?
What issues should child psychiatric epidemiology address next?

WHAT IS EPIDEMIOLOGY?

"Epidemiology is concerned with patterns of disease occurrence in human populations and of the factors that influence these patterns" (Lilienfeld & Lilienfeld, 1980, p. 3). Traditionally, epidemiology was concerned with infectious diseases, an understandable focus since these have been some of the major afflictions of humankind in the past (Mausner & Bahn, 1974). Now that such epidemics are no longer so threatening to western communities, we can see a shift toward concern with diseases of a chronic nature. The epidemiology of child psychiatric disorders represents an aspect of this trend.

The Tripartite Model

The epidemiologist searching for patterns of disease occurrence looks at the interaction of three types of factor: the *agent*, the *host*, and the *environment*. Agents, or etiological factors, may be of many kinds, for example, bacterial, chemical, or mechanical. Among the few identified agents of child psychiatric disorders are niacin, phenylalanine, and lead. Some agents of psychiatric disorder appear to be genetically determined structural faults, for example, in the relative levels of various neurotransmitters that are essential parts of the organism. In addition, life events have been viewed by some as agents, precipitating the onset or recurrence of psychiatric disorder in people made vulnerable by environmental or host factors (e.g., Brown & Harris 1978). However, in child psychiatric disorders, as in other chronic diseases, it is the exception to find single identifiable agents of disease. *Host factors* are generally defined as those aspects of the individual that influence exposure, susceptibility, or response to agents of disease. These include genetic factors, age, sex, ethnicity, immunological history, comorbidity, and patterns of behavior, which could include eating and exercise habits, drug and alcohol use, and utilization of environmental resources. In psychiatric illness the distinction between agent and host may sometimes be difficult to make. The third part of the system consists of *environmental factors*, which influence the extent to which the host is exposed to, or susceptible to, an agent. These factors may be physical, biological, or socioeconomic. For example, poor children in urban environments are at greater risk of exposure to environmental lead than are rural children.

The agent–host–environment model has proven to be a very powerful organizing principle for directing epidemiological research for more than a century. The role of the epidemiologist, according to this model, is to integrate information collected by a diversity of specialists—geneticists, microbiologists, physicists, physicians, psychologists, sociologists, and so on—and study its interaction in relation to a specific disease. The research strategy in studying risk factors for disease is to establish the prevalence of the disease in the community and then to examine the extent to which its occurrence varies as a function of a particular risk factor. For example, how does the individual's sex influence the probability of developing a major depressive episode? Or, is an environmental disaster such as the Three Mile Island nuclear accident associated with an increase in anxiety disorders among children in the area? Since risk factors do not exist in isolation, the next stage is to examine the relative risk of disease in persons with different patterns of risk factors. For example, it appears that the ratio of girls to boys with major depressive disorders is 1:1 in the prepubertal years, but closer to 3:1 in late adolescence; the relative risk associated with age is different for males and females. Gradually, it becomes possible to define the group or groups within the population who are at highest risk for a given disorder; their "risk profile," or position on a range of risk factors, is associated with the highest prevalence rate. A study of these risk profiles may in turn suggest etiological hypotheses to be tested using clinical trials, intervention studies, or other quasi-experimental methods of hypothesis testing. Thus epidemiology uses a three-stage attack on a given problem. The first stage, which is largely descriptive, leads to a second, hypothesis-generating stage, in which etiological links are derived, to be tested in the third, hypothesis-testing stage.

WHAT CAN EPIDEMIOLOGY CONTRIBUTE TO THE STUDY OF CHILD PSYCHIATRIC DIAGNOSIS?

Confronted with an epidemiologically derived risk profile for a given disease, clinicians may often be tempted to retort, "I could have told you that!" It does not require a large community study, they may say, to tell one that girls are more likely to have emotional disorders and boys more likely to have conduct problems. However, it cannot be assumed that patterns observed in clinical settings are true of the population as a whole. The role of epidemiology is, as outlined earlier, essentially one of integration, and this includes integrating clinical knowledge with information obtained from community sources, to address such questions as:

Is the risk profile for a given disorder in the community the same as that seen in the clinic?

It is possible, for example, that the sex or social class risk ratio for a given disorder seen in a clinic may have to do with selection factors influencing referral rather than, or as well as, the distribution of the disorder in the population (Berkson, 1946)? Population-based studies are necessary to answer this question.

Will a given treatment work outside the specific clinic setting in which it is developed? It sometimes happens that a clinical intervention is successful in meeting the needs of the subgroup of people with a disorder who seek treatment, but fails to address the problem when used in the community. Attempts to reduce neonatal mortality rates by increased prenatal care for teenage mothers, for example, have only limited success unless they extend out from medical centers to reach the people whose life-style both puts them at high risk *and* reduces the probability that they will seek prenatal care. One of the functions of the epidemiologist is to help direct interventions to where they are most needed, according to the available evidence derived from patterns of agent–host–environment interactions. In child psychiatry, for example, studies of families with a history of depressive disorder are beginning to direct attention to a group of children who may be at particularly high risk for a range of psychiatric disorders (e.g., Keller et al., 1986).

Can data from clinical and community studies be combined to yield new etiological hypotheses? For example, the clinician may be aware that psychiatric problems are more common in children coming from disturbed families in poor, urban environments; a study using epidemiological methods has shown that, although the proportion of disturbed families was higher in an urban than a rural setting, *within disturbed families* the rate of child psychopathology was the same in the country as in the town (Rutter, 1982). Findings of this sort are important in focusing attention on certain etiological mechanisms rather than others, which can then be tested in intervention studies.

WHAT IS THE CURRENT STATE OF KNOWLEDGE ABOUT THE EPIDEMIOLOGY OF CHILD PSYCHIATRIC DISORDERS?

Background and Methodological Issues

In the United States, the origin of child psychiatric epidemiology can be found in concern about delinquency. It coincided with what Kanner (1960) called the second period in the history of child psychiatry, when the nineteenth century's philanthropic, protective, adult-oriented approach to children and their problems gave way to an era of concern with community development as a way of tackling children's problem behavior. It is in this period that we see the expansion of juvenile courts, guidance clinics, foster homes, and education for the mentally retarded and handicapped. It is also a time when psychologists were developing new methods to study normal child development. Concern about the amount of deviance in the community was a natural extension of this work. It quickly became apparent that large-scale community surveys were necessary for the purposes of both science and administrative action. Only in this way was it possible to provide reliable data about the characteristics of the child population at different phases of development and estimate the number of children likely to require special care (Shepherd, Oppenheim, & Mitchell, 1971).

Early studies frequently used as sources of information questionnaires completed by teachers (e.g., Wickman, 1924) or parents (e.g., Long, 1941), or searches of clinic records (e.g., Ackerson, 1931). Children were rarely used as sources of information about their own problems. The existence of disorder was generally assessed by summing the questionnaire responses to produce a general scale of "maladjustment" rather than specific diagnoses. Child psychiatry at that time provided little guidance about how childhood psychopathology should be classified: the earliest *Diagnostic and Statistical Manual* of the American Psychiatric Association, for example, had only two categories for childhood disorders (APA, 1952). At this time, when the "disease" concept was not generally seen as a useful way of conceptualizing the emotional and behavioral problems of childhood, the host–agent–environment model of epidemiological research had little to offer.

Following the pattern of adult psychiatric research, there has been a movement in the past two decades toward exploring the usefulness of the disease-based model of childhood mental disorder. This movement has brought with it several shifts of focus:

Away from "mental health" toward "mental illness"

Away from general indices of "maladjustment" toward specific disorders

Away from questionnaires alone toward multiple methods of collecting information, including interviews and observations

Away from reliance on a single source of information (usually the teacher) toward multiple sources, including the children themselves

Away from nonscheduled interviews toward highly scheduled formats

Away from concern only with psychosocial risk factors toward a biopsychosocial approach emphasizing family genetic factors and biological markers

Away from a static view of childhood psychopathology toward a concern with the impact of growth and development on risk for various disorders

Many of these changes—toward a disease-based approach to mental illness, greater specificity in diagnosis, and a concern with the role of biological predictors—run parallel to developments in clinical psychiatry and psychology. Other changes, such as the use of more structured methods of inquiry and multiple informants, arise out of the search for diagnostic validity and reliability. These issues, which had less urgency when global "maladjustment" measures were used, have become acute with the move toward discrete diagnostic categories. The problem became critical in the United States in 1980 with the introduction of DSM-III (APA, 1980), which elaborates on Section V of the International Classification of Diseases (ICD) (World Health Organization, 1977) and includes more than 80 different Axis I disorders applicable to children.

Issues of reliable and valid diagnosis are of course a problem for clinical psychiatry in general, but they are of particular concern to epidemiologists, for two reasons. First, the low base rate of most psychiatric disorders in the community, compared with their prevalence in a hospital or clinic, makes errors of estimate particularly likely and misleading, as Shrout, Spitzer, and Fleiss (1987) have demonstrated. Second, when epidemiological researchers are engaged in a community study looking for cases that are not known to a clinician, they have to deal with the issue of "What is a case?" (Wing, Bebbington, & Robins, 1981). How can they be sure that the individual really has the disorder in question? This is a particular problem in child psychiatric epidemiology. Children rarely refer themselves for psychiatric evaluation, and the relationships among psychopathology, family and school tolerance for—or sensitivity to—deviant behavior in the child, and referral for diagnostic evaluation can be very complex.

As we defined epidemiology at the beginning of this chapter, it is concerned with both description and etiological hypotheses; that is, with *rates of disorder* and with *factors* that may either increase or decrease the rate in a particular segment of the population. In order to establish a rate, two figures are needed: the *number of cases* (the numerator) and the size of the *population at risk* (the denominator). It will be clear that rate estimates are crucially influenced by the choice of the denominator; to take an obvious example, the prevalence of conduct disorder among children seen in a child guidance clinic is likely to be much higher than the prevalence found when the population at risk is a random community sample, since the population of child guidance children (the denominator) has already been selected for reasons that increase the probability of disorder. Equally, rates are affected by the criteria used to define the "cases" (numerator), and by extension, by the method of collecting the data used to make a diagnosis. The most generally accepted standard of validity of diagnoses made in a community study is the extent to which clinical assessments of the same children would result in the same diagnoses. For this reason, current epidemiological studies have tended to adopt interview methods that come as close as possible to clinical assessments.

What information, then, should an epidemiological study report, so that the reader can draw conclusions about prevalence rates of specific disorders, and possible risk factors? The preceding discussion indicates the following minimum:

The criteria used to make a diagnosis (numerator)

The population at risk (denominator)

The sampling methods used, including criteria for inclusion and exclusion, the compliance rate, and possible biases caused by differential response rates

The rates of all relevant risk factors (e.g., age, sex) among noncases as well as cases

In addition, it is important to know who the informant or informants are and, if information is available from more than one source, to know how data have been combined to reach the diagnosis. This may seem to be a simple and obvious set of requirements. Unfortunately, it is rare to find a published study that provides these basic facts.

Recent Studies of Prevalence and Risk Factors

The European literature on the epidemiology of child psychopathology has recently been reviewed (Rutter & Sandberg, 1985), as has research preceding the adoption of DSM-III (Earls, 1979; Gould, Wunsch-Hitzig, & Dohrenwend, 1980; Links, 1983; Yule, 1981). This chapter will concentrate on studies appearing since 1980 and using the diagnostic framework of DSM-III. At this point in time there are no studies of prevalence and risk factors following DSM-III-R (APA, 1987), given its very recent publication. As a background against which to evaluate current research, we briefly review the findings of the series of epidemiologic studies of child psychiatric disorder carried out in the 1960s and 1970s by Rutter and his colleagues. These studies set the standard for careful sampling and research, reliable instrumentation, and good clinical assessment of children. Diagnoses were made using only six ICD categories, whereas studies using DSM-III have the opportunity not only to use the very large range of diagnoses included in that taxonomy, but also to make fine distinctions among, for example, six subtypes of conduct disorder. In practice, however, rates based on these fine-grained categories are rarely sufficently reliable to be useful. All the studies reviewed here use methods that bear some relation to clinical assessment. That is, they produce categorical diagnoses, using detailed interviews with parent, child, or both, or else questionnaires whose diagnostic validity has been reasonably well established in relation to clinical assessments of the same children. Studies that provide only rating scale data without reference to diagnosis are not included in this review.

The Isle of Wight and Associated Studies

In the 1960s Rutter and his colleagues carried out a study of the prevalence of child psychiatric disorder in the population of 10- and 11-year-olds with homes on the Isle of Wight, a small rural island off the south coast of England. The authors used a two-stage design, in which the entire population at risk was surveyed using relatively inexpensive questionnaires for rating by parents and teachers, and a sample was selected for detailed evaluation, based on the questionnaire scores. A cutoff point for the questionnaire ratings had previously been established based on comparisons of scores from normal children with those of children referred to child guidance clinics (Rutter, Tizard, & Whitmore, 1970). All children scoring at or above the cutoff point on either form were selected for interview. Other high-risk groups were also selected for interview: all children who had been before a juvenile court or on probation or in a local authority children's home during the previous year. A small group of low-scoring children was also interviewed. A higher proportion of high-risk (i.e., high-scoring) subjects than low-risk subjects was selected to increase the reliability of the prevalence estimates. Population prevalence estimates were made by weighting the rates for high- and low-risk samples according to the sampling fractions used.

Interviews were conducted by psychiatrists who were carefully trained in the use of the specific semistructured interviews designed for the study. The interviews' test–retest reliability had previously been demonstrated (Graham & Rutter, 1968; Rutter & Graham, 1968). Parent and child were interviewed separately, and the results combined to produce the diagnosis. Rutter and his colleagues used this or a similar study design again in the Isle of Wight to follow up the original sample (Graham & Rutter, 1973) and in a further study of 10-year-olds, comparing another group of island children with a sample going to school in an inner London borough (Rutter, Cox, Tupling, Berger, & Yule, 1975; Rutter et al., 1974).

Table 25.1 shows the prevalence rates reported for various samples using the ICD diagnostic categories and the two-stage methodology described. The first study of 10- and 11-year-olds, in which diagnosis was based on interviews with mothers and children, found a prevalence rate of 6.3%, made up mainly of neurotic disorder (2.2%), antisocial disorder (2.1%), and mixed neurotic–antisocial disorder (1.4%). However, the replication published 5 years later estimated almost twice this prevalence (12% ± 2.6%). This may be because mothers were interviewed in greater detail than in the first study, or it may be a cohort effect, or both. Reinterviews of the first sample 4 years later also produced considerably higher rates (21% ± 2.3%), but once again there were differences in the methodology (teachers were interviewed). The biggest increase was in neurotic disorders, which increased from 2.2% to 12.9%. A fourth study, of 10-year-olds living in an inner urban area, yielded the highest rates of all these studies (25.4% ± 3.9%). It is not possible to obtain population prevalence estimates for specific disorders from these last three samples, as rates are given for the deviant group only (i.e., those scoring above the cutoff points on the screening questionnaires), and in some cases are not based on all sources of information. Conclusions drawn from these studies have been generally accepted and confirmed by other studies using the same measures in different populations: that the rate of clinically significant psychiatric disorder in prepubertal children in the community is 12% or more, increasing with age (especially emotional disorders), and in inner urban areas (see, e.g., Connell, Irvine, & Rodney, 1982).

Studies Using DSM-III

A number of detailed interviews have been developed for epidemiological use in conjunction with DSM-III. These are reviewed in detail elsewhere in this volume. Some, such as the Diagnostic Interview Schedule for Children (DISC) (Costello, Edelbrock, Kalas, Kessler, & Klaric, 1982), are designed so that trained nonclinicians can be used as interviewers; others, such as the K-SADS (Puig-Antich & Chambers 1978), require that interviewers be experienced psychiatric clinicians who are also trained to administer the interviews. Diagnoses may be based on computer algorithms that combine symptom, duration, and intensity data to generate diagnoses, or they may be made by clinicians. They may be made separately from the interview with parent or child, or they may aggregate the information from both, using formal rules or clinical judgment. Some studies use a two-stage design similar to that of the Isle of Wight studies (e.g., Bird et al., 1987; Costello, Edelbrock, Costello, Dulcan, & Brent, 1986). Others use a hybrid design in which the whole population at risk is interviewed, but questionnaires are used to obtain additional information from other sources, such as teachers or parents (e.g., Anderson, Williams, McGee, & Silva, 1987).

The largest of the DSM-III-based studies is one carried out in Canada using the resources of the Canadian Census Bureau to evaluate a probability sample of 2679 children (Offord et al., 1987). In this study diagnostic rates are based on the questionnaire responses; psychiatric interviews carried out on 194 children were for validation purposes only. To make a survey of such large numbers feasible, Offord and colleagues used the Child Behavior Checklist (CBCL) (Achenbach & Edelbrock 1983), adding items required to provide the information needed to make four diagnoses: conduct disorder, hyperactivity, emotional disorder, and somatization disorder. Hyperactivity corresponds to the DSM-III diagnosis of attention deficit disorder with hyperactivity, emotional disorder combines elements of the DSM-III categories of overanxious disorder, affective disorder and obsessive-compulsive disorder, and somatization refers to physical symptoms without evident organic cause" (Boyle et al., 1987). Criteria were based as clearly as possible on DSM-III. As Table 25.2 shows, Offord and colleagues estimated that 18.1% of children suffered from one or more disorders, according to parental reports. Emotional disorders were the most common and conduct disorders the least. The rate of hyperactivity (6.2%) is in marked contrast to the 0.1% reported by Rutter and colleagues (1970).

The other four large community studies discussed here all used the structured interviews that make up the Diagnostic Interview Schedule for Children (DISC: Costello et al., 1982), one for the child (DISC-C), and one for parents about their child (DISC-P). In 1971 a longitudinal study began in Dunedin, New Zealand, taking as its subjects a large representative sample of children born during a single year in the city's only obstetric hospital. Measures of health, development, and behavior have been taken every 2 years from age 3. When the children were 11, a full psychiatric interview was carried out on 792 of the children by a child psychiatrist using the DISC-C (Anderson et al., 1987). Unfortunately, only the children, not the parents, were interviewed, but information from parental and teacher quesionnaires was incorporated into the diagnostic process. Four levels of diagnosis were established: *strong pervasive* (meets criteria on the basis of two or more sources of information); *situational* (meets criteria from one source of information); *weak pervasive* (meets criteria only if two or more sources are combined); and *no diagnosis*. Data for strong pervasive and situational diagnoses are given in Table 25.2. The Dunedin study found that 7.3% of the diagnoses made were strong pervasive, 6.1% were situational, and 4.2% weak pervasive. There were interesting differences across diagnoses; the majority (60%) of overanxious disorders were weak pervasive, all simple phobias and social phobias were situational, and the majority of attention deficit disorders (66%) were strong pervasive. In general,

TABLE 25.1. Prevalence Rates of Psychiatric Disorder in Children, from Studies by Rutter and Colleagues

Study	Informants	Sample	Neurotic/ Emotional Disorder	Antisocial Disorder/ Disturbance of Conduct	Mixed Disorder	Other Disorders
Isle of Wight, 1970	Child (interview), parent (questionnaire, interview), teacher (questionnaire)	$N = 432/2193^a$; age 10–11	2.2%	2.1%	1.4%	0.6%
Isle of Wight, 1975	Parent (interview), teacher (questionnaire)	$N = 237/1279$; age 10	$(1.6\%)^b$	(2.2%)		(0.5%)
Inner London, 1975	Parent (interview), teacher (questionnaire, interview)	$N = 265/1689$; age 10	(3.2%)	(3.5%)		(1.6%)
Isle of Wight, 1976	Child (interview), parent (questionnaire, interview), teacher (questionnaire, interview)	$N = ?/2303$; age 14–15	12.9%	2.1%	5.8%	(0.5%)

[a] N = interviews/screens.
[b] Rates in parentheses apply to deviant sample only.

One or More Diagnoses	Excluded	Selected for Interview if		Refusal Rate
6.3%	Children in private schools unless paid for by local authority	(a) score ≥ 9 on teacher scale (b) score ≥ 13 on parent scale		Not specified
		(c) attended child guidance clinic, juvenile court, probation office, or in long-term care during previous year, $N = 15$.		
		(d) 146 children not selected by (a), (b), or (c) chosen at random		
12% ± 2.6%	Children at private schools unless local authority paid fees	(a) score ≥ 9 on teacher scale (10.6%) (104/136 selected at random). (b) every 12th screened child ($N = 107$).		8% (9.7% of deviants, 5.6% of nondeviants)
25.4% ± 3.9%	All immigrant families (25.9% of population)	(a) score ≥ 9 on teacher scale (19.1%) (139/322 selected at random). (b) every 16th screened child ($N = 106$).		8.4% (10.7% deviants, 4.4% of nondeviants)
21% ± 2.3%	Children in private schools unless paid for by local authority	(a) score ≥ 9 on teacher scale (b) score ≥ 13 on parent scale (c) charged with offenses, on probation, attended a psychiatric service or a special school for maladjusted children during past year.	$N = 304$	Not specified
		(d) had some significant disorder at age 10–11 ($N = 126$)		
		(e) 200 children not selected by (a)–(d), chosen at random.		

TABLE 25.2.   Prevalence Rates of DSM-III Diagnoses in Nonclinic Samples

Study	Informants	Sample	Attention Deficit Disorder (± Hyperactivity)	Oppositiona Disorder
Anderson and colleagues (1987)	Child (interview), parent (checklist), teacher (checklist)	N = 782, age 11	6.7%	5.7%
Bird and colleagues (in press)	Child (interview), parent (interview)	N = 777, age 4–16	10.1%	9.7%
Cohen and colleagues (1987)	Child (interview), parent (interview)	N = 752, age 9–19	4.3%	6.6%
Costello and colleagues (1986)	Child (interview), parent (interview)	N = 789, age 7–11	2.2%	6.6%
Earls (1982)	Child (observation), parent (interview)	N = 100, age 3	2.0%	4.0%
Offord and colleagues (1987)	Parent (checklist), teacher (checklist)	N = 2679, age 4–16	6.2% ("Hyperactivity")	N/A

behavioral problems were the most common disorders in this sample, which may have to do with using two adult sources of information (parent and teacher).

A two-stage survey of children in Puerto Rico has recently been carried out to estimate the prevalence of maladjustment in children 4 to 16 years old on the island. Using a two-stage design, Bird and colleagues (1987) obtained CBCLs from parents of 777 children, representing a 1:900 multistage probability sample of the population. Teacher report forms and, for children 12 to 16 years old, youth self-report forms, providing information closely similar to that provided by the CBCL, were also obtained, together with much family and demographic information. The sample for the second stage of the study consisted of 20% of the screened sample, selected at random, together with all children scoring above the published cutoff scores on either the parent or the teacher screening questionnaire; a total of 386 children. Each was interviewed by one of a team of eight psychiatrists, using the Diagnostic Interview Schedule for Children. The same person interviewed the child's parent and also assigned a score on the Children's Global Assessment Scale (CGAS) (Shaffer et al., 1983) to the child. The CGAS provides a measure of overall impairment, and in this study was incorporated into the diagnostic process. The psychiatrist made a diagnosis using DSM-III criteria based on the data from both interviews, and prevalence estimates were calculated by defining as a "case" a child who met these criteria *and* had a low CGAS score. The aim in using this decision rule was to include in the prevalence estimates only children whose psychiatric disorder was associated with a level of functional impairment that made some form of mental

Conduct Disorders (All Types)	Separation Anxiety	Overanxious Disorder	Simple Phobia	Depression, Dysthmia	Enuresis	One or More Diagnoses
3.4%	3.5%	2.9%	2.4%	1.8%	N/A	17.6%
1.5%	4.8%	N/A	2.3%	5.9%	4.8%	18.0% ± 3.4%
5.4%	5.4%	2.7%	N/A	1.7% (major depression)	N/A	20.6%
2.6%	4.1%	4.6%	9.2%	2.0%	4.4%	22.0% ± 3.4%
0.0%	5.0%	N/A	N/A	0.0%	N/A	14.0%
5.5%		9.9%	("Emotional disorder")		N/A	18.1%

health care desirable. The prevalence estimates shown in Table 25.2 present a picture of a high level of disturbed behavior in this sample, especially of conduct disorder and attention deficit disorders.

Two recently completed studies of children in the United States have also used the DISC. In two counties of New York State, Cohen and colleagues assessed a multistage probability sample of 752 children aged 9 to 19, as part of a longitudinal study of childhood psychopathology (Cohen, O'Connor, Lewis, & Malachowski, 1987). Parent and child were interviewed separately, but the data were combined to reach a diagnosis. Within each group of symptoms relevant to a particular DSM-III disorder (adapted where necessary to comply with the March 1986 revision of those criteria) a child was given a diagnosis if (1) the "core" symptom for that disorder was present, and (2) the child's total symptom score was two standard deviations above the population mean, as estimated from the study sample. The prevalence rate for one or more disorders is increased in this sample by the high rates of alcohol and tobacco dependence recorded in the children over 13, as Table 25.2 shows.

A recent two-stage study of children 7 to 11 years old using the DISC (Costello et al., 1986) is of more limited generalizability, because the population from which its sample was drawn consists of children attending a pediatric primary care clinic. Although most children in the United States do visit their pediatrician at least once during the course of a year, some do not, and it is not clear whether the two groups have different rates of psychopathology (Costello, 1986). Also, the study was carried out in a health maintenance organization, whose enrollees tend to be drawn from the middle socioeconomic groups, with few members from either the lowest or the highest groups. This is, however, the only other large American sample on which DSM-III prevalence estimates are currently available. The diagnostic rates given in Table 25.2 are based on the interviews with the parents and children, and do not incorporate any information from teachers. Taking as the criterion a diagnosis derived from one or both interviews, 22.0% of the sample had one or more disorders. The lower rate of "antisocial" disorders, such as conduct disorders and attention deficit disorders, is probably due to the absence of teachers' information. A higher rate of situational than of pervasive disorders is found in this as well as the Dunedin study; only 3.6% of children received a strong, pervasive diagnosis, showing a low level of agreement between parents and children.

Earls (1982) has used DSM-III criteria to diagnose psychiatric problems in 3-year-olds in a small rural community. The sample is small, and the method of making diagnoses from written case summaries is not ideal. However, this study provides some rare information about specific disorders in young children. Separation anxiety and oppositional disorder were the most common problems reported by parents in this age group, as Table 25.2 shows.

In addition to these general surveys, there is a group of studies using standard instruments and DSM-III criteria to establish the prevalence of a small group of disorders, usually depressive disorders. McCracken and colleagues (1986) used a section of the DISC to estimate the prevalence of depressive disorders in a sample of 149 children 9 years old. The children in this sample reported twice the rate of major depressive disorder indicated by their parents, 2.7% compared with 1.3%, and the level of agreement between the two was not high. Earlier, Kashani and colleagues had used part of the K-SADS for the same purpose with the Dunedin sample (Kashani et al., 1983). Unfortunately, only the children were interviewed on that occasion. The authors found 1.8% of children with major depression and 2.5% with minor depression. Kashani and Carlson (1986) interviewed 150 children 14 to 16 years old in Columbia, Missouri, using the Diagnostic Interview for Children and Adolescents (DICA) (Herjanic & Campbell, 1977) and its parallel parent version (DICA-P) to make DSM-III diagnoses of major depressive disorder, dysthymic disorder, and anxiety disorder. Combining major depressive and dysthymic disorder produced rates of 4.7% in boys and 3.3% in girls.

Community studies are an expensive and unreliable method of estimating the prevalence of very rare diseases. With a few exceptions (e.g., Burd, Kerbeshian, Wikenheiser, & Fisher, 1986, for Tourette's syndrome; Crisp, Palmer, & Kalucy, 1976, for anorexia nervosa; Kendell, Hall, Hailey, & Babigian, 1973; Lotter, 1966, for autism), prevalence estimates for rare disorders are based on clinic samples or children in special schools. This can produce valid estimates when all cases come to the attention of medical or educational services, but can be unreliable if there are community cases that escape public notice.

This brief review of the few published community studies using DSM-III criteria shows rates of disorder that are higher than those found in the first Isle of Wight study, but within the range found in later studies. Despite the variability in instruments used and methods of aggregating data from different sources, consistent and disturbingly high 17.6% to 22.0% prevalence rates for significant psychiatric disorder emerge from all these studies.

Risk Factors

Table 25.3 summarizes information from the studies discussed earlier, on how a range of host and environmental factors increases or decreases the prevalence estimates. Looking first at age, the studies that cover a wide age range show increasing rates of disorder with age; those with a narrower age range do not show this effect. However, there are differences in the prevalence rates of specific disorders by age. Among the emotional disorders, levels of separation anxiety and phobias tend to fall with age, while depression and dysthymia increase. Among the behavioral disorders, oppositional disorders decrease, but conduct disorders increase.

The effect of *sex* on prevalence estimates appears with remarkable consistency across these studies. The ratio of boys to girls is between 0.5 and 0.9 to 1 for emotional disorders and between 1.2 and 4.3 to 1 for behavioral problems, giving overall a roughly equal sex ratio. The exceptions to this pattern are a boy:girl ratio of 5.4:1 for depression/dysthymia and 1.7:1 for overanxious disorder in the Dunedin sample. However, in the latter cases the numbers are very small. For both emotional and behavioral problems, the difference between the sexes in prevalence rates appears to increase with age.

The increased prevalence found in *urban areas* is possibly an artifact of the concentration of children with various types of family problems in urban areas (Rutter, 1975). Unfortunately, few studies provide information about the effect of family problems on rates of different disorders. Graham and Rutter (1973) provide this information for their sample of 14- and 15-year-olds, but only for those with high screen scores, so one cannot be sure whether whole population estimates would be similar. Offord and colleagues (1987) found more problems overall, and more emotional problems in urban children, but rates of conduct disorder were similar in both types of settings. Costello and colleagues (1986) compared suburban with inner urban children and found an excess of behavioral (but not emotional) problems in urban children. The final column of Table 25.3 gives a brief summary of some other factors that have been found to increase the risk of psychopathology. In addition to the effects of individual stressors, which are much as would be predicted, some studies have found interesting interactions among stressors that could generate hypotheses for future study. For example, Rutter and colleagues (1974) report that marital discord or a broken home is associated in their sample with higher rates of conduct disorder than of emotional disorder, whereas the opposite is true of the association with mental disorder in the mother. Costello and colleagues (1986) found that both types of stressors were associated with higher rates of both emotional and conduct disorders. Rutter and colleagues found no effect of father's occupational status; Costello and colleagues replicated this finding for white children only. Black children in this sample were more likely to have conduct disorders if they came from lower rather than higher socioeconomic backgrounds.

TABLE 25.3. Factors Influencing Risk for Psychiatric Diagnosis

Study (age range)	Age			Sex			Urban–Rural			Other Factors That Increase Risk
	Emotional	Behavioral	Any	Emotional	Behavioral	Any	Emotional	Behavioral	Any	
Rutter et al. (1970, 1975, 1976) (age 10–15)	$Y < O$	$Y = O$		$B = G$	$B > G$		$U < R$	$U > R$	$U > R$	Not living with both natural parents. Parents' poor or broken marriage Mental disorder in mother Children with persistent disorder more likely to be boys, to have been in care, not to be living with both natural parents

510

Study	Age	Sex	Urban/rural/suburban	Risk factors
Anderson et al. (1987) (age 11)		$B > G$ $B > G$ $B > G$	$U = R$	Low socioeconomic status
Bird et al. (in press) (age 4–16)	$Y < O$	$B > G$ $B > G$	$U = S$	Family history of psychiatric treatment; Child's high life stress score; School report of problems
Cohen et al. (1987) (age 9–19)	$Y > O$ $Y < O$ $Y < O$	$B < G$ $B > G$ $B = G$	(urban–suburban) $U = S$ $U > S$	
Costello et al. (1987) (age 7–11)	$Y = O$ $Y = O$ $Y = O$	$B < G$ $B > G$ $B = G$	$U > R$ $U = R$ $U > R$	
Offord et al. (1987)	$Y = O$ $Y < O$ $Y < O$	$B < G$ $B > G$ $B = G$	$U > R$ $U = R$	Family dysfunction; Family medical or psychiatric problems; Child's chronic health problem; Child's early developmental problem

Key: Y = younger; O = older; B = boys; G = girls; U = Urban; R = rural; S = suburban.

WHAT ISSUES SHOULD CHILD PSYCHIATRIC EPIDEMIOLOGY ADDRESS NEXT?

The current state of knowledge about the epidemiology of child psychiatric diagnosis is clearly very incomplete. In particular, prevalence rates for the various disorders, usually the foundation stone on which etiological hypotheses are built, have emerged from this review as highly variable, although methodological improvements are narrowing the range of variability. However, this review has revealed some order as well as much disorder in the data, and the patterns that emerge suggest the direction in which future research could most usefully go.

The clearest message is that it is possible to see consistent patterns of risk factors across studies, even when they differ considerably in the reported prevalence of a given disorder. Thus the distribution of the major diagnostic categories across the sexes and social classes, for example, is similar in almost all the studies that report such data. This suggests that, rather than becoming obsessed with the search for the perfectly "valid" diagnosis, it makes more sense to concentrate research efforts on identifying patterns of risk that suggest possible causal mechanisms. Even in the absence of known agents, relationships among environment, host, and disease, if reliably established, suggest some causal hypotheses.

A particularly interesting and almost unexplored aspect of risk factors for childhood psychiatric disease is the effect of growth and development on the risk for a given disorder. For example, why is it that the first episode of conduct disorder rarely occurs in late adolescence, and the prognosis for recidivism is much worse in early onset cases (Loeber, 1985)? Why is there apparently no sex difference in prepubertal rates of depression, but a marked female preponderance among depressives in late adolescence? Future studies must be designed to capture the effect of development on risk factors if they are to make a useful contribution to our understanding of why some children develop psychiatric disorders and others do not.

Another development with promise for the future is a renewed interest in mental health, as well as mental illness. Family genetic and life event studies have focused attention on groups of children who are at high risk for psychiatric disorder in the short or long term. Yet clearly some children survive and are perhaps even strengthened by the rigors of the environment in which they grow up. Why do they survive, and what can be learned from these children that could help others? The concept of *resilience* (Rutter 1985) encompasses such questions and is giving rise to some new research strategies.

Two further developments are crucial if epidemiology is to contribute fully to the development of a valid, reliable nosology of child psychiatric disorder. First, increased attention must be paid to the other axes of classificatory systems for which these have been developed—DSM-III or the WHO multiaxial system for the International Classification of Disease (Rutter, Schaffer, & Shepherd, 1975). Clinicians make considerable use of information about the child's intellectual development, health, family and school environment, and current level of functioning in reaching a diagnosis. Community studies could increase the validity of their diagnoses by paying greater attention to the way in which clinical judgment incorporates such data.

Second, agreement must be reached on how information from a range of sources and assessment instruments is best aggregated in making a diagnosis. For example, should different weight be attached to information from parent and child depending on whether one is assessing conduct disorder or depression? Anderson and colleagues' (1987) method of distinguishing among strong pervasive, situational, and weak pervasive diagnoses is one promising approach.

Most children with psychiatric problems are never seen by a mental health professional (Costello, 1986). We are still a long way from knowing the full extent of this hidden morbidity and from estimating its cost in present and future suffering. We are equally far from having a clearly specific risk profile for most diagnoses, from which testable etiological hypotheses could be derived. Perhaps this review has illustrated, however, that epidemiological methods and approaches can clarify the questions that need to be asked and suggest some ways of answering them.

REFERENCES

Achenbach, T.M., & Edelbrock, C. (1983). *Manual for the Child Behavior Checklist*. Burlington, VT: University Associates in Psychiatry.

Ackerson, L. (1931). *Children's Behavior Problems* (Vol. I). Chicago: University of Chicago Press.

American Psychiatric Association (1952). *Diagnostic and statistical manual of mental disorders*. Washington, DC: Author.

American Psychiatric Association (1980). *Diagnostic and statistical manual of mental disorders* (3rd ed.). Washington, DC: Author.

American Psychiatric Association (1987). *Diagnostic and statistical manual of mental disorders* (3rd ed., rev.). Washington, DC: Author.

Berkson, J. (1946). Limitations of the application of fourfold table analysis to hospital data. *Biometrics, 2*, 47–53.

Bird, H.R., Canino, G., Rubio-Stipec, M., Gould, M.S., Ribera, J., Sesman, M., Woodbury, M., Huertas-Goldman, S., Pagan, A., Sanchez-Lacay, A., & Moscoso, M. (in press). Estimates of the prevalence of childhood maladjustment in a community survey in Puerto Rico. *Archives of General Psychiatry*.

Boyle, M.H., Offord, D.R., Hofmann, H.G., Catlin, G.P., Byles, J.A., Cadman, D.T., Crawford, J.W., Links, P.S., Rae-Grant, N.I., & Szafmari, P. (1986). Ontario Child Health Study I. Methodology. *Archives of General Psychiatry, 44*, 826–831.

Brown, G.W., & Harris, T. (1978). *Social origins of depression: A study of psychiatric disorder in women*. London: Tavistock.

Burd, L., Kerbeshian, J., Wikenheiser, M., & Fisher, W. (1986). A prevalence study of Gilles de la Tourette syndrome in North Dakota school-age children. *Journal of the American Academy of Child Psychiatry, 25*, 552–553.

Cohen, P., O'Connor, P., Lewis, S., Velez, N., & Malachowski, B. (1987). A comparison of the agreement between DISC and KSADS-P interviews of an epidemiological sample of children. *Journal of the American Academy of Child Psychiatry, 26*, 262–267.

Connell, H.M., Irvine, L., & Rodney, J. (1982). The prevalence of psychiatric disorder in rural school children. *Australia & New Zealand Journal of Psychiatry, 16*, 43–46.

Costello, E.J. (1986). Primary care pediatrics and child psychopathology: A review of diagnostic treatment and referral practices. *Pediatrics, 78*, 1044–1051.

Costello, E.J., Edelbrock, C., Costello, A.J., Dulcan, M.K., & Brent, D. (1986). *The diagnosis and management of child psychopathology in an organized primary care setting: Final report.* (Contract #278-83-0006 (DB)). Rockville, MD: National Institute of Mental Health.

Costello, A.J., Edelbrock, C., Kalas, R., Kessler, M.K., & Klaric, S.A. (1982). *National Institute of Mental Health Diagnostic Interview Schedule for Children.* Bethesda, MD: National Institute of Mental Health.

Crisp, A.H., Palmer, R.L., & Kalucy, R.S. (1976). How common is anorexia nervosa? A prevalence study. *British Journal of Psychiatry, 128*, 549–554.

Earls, F. (1979). Epidemiology and child psychiatry: Historical and conceptual development. *Comprehensive Psychiatry, 20*, 256–269.

Earls, F. (1982). Application of DSM-III in an epidemiological study of preschool children. *American Journal of Psychiatry, 139*, 242–243.

Gould, M.S., Wunsch-Hitzig, R., & Dohrenwend, B.P. (1980). Formulation of hypotheses about prevalence, treatment and prognostic significance of psychiatric disorders in children in the United States. In B.P. Dohrenwend, M.S. Gould, B. Link, R. Neubauer, & R. Wunsch-Hitzig (Eds.), *Mental illness in the United States: Epidemiological estimates.* New York: Praeger.

Graham, P., & Rutter, M. (1968). The reliability and validity of the psychiatric assessment of the child: II. Interview with the parent. *British Journal of Psychiatry, 114*, 581–592.

Graham, P., & Rutter, M. (1973). Psychiatric disorder in the young adolescent: A follow-up study. *Proceedings of the Royal Society of Medicine, 66*, 1226–1229.

Herjanic, B., & Campbell, W. (1977). Differentiating psychiatrically disturbed children on the basis of a structured interview. *Journal of Abnormal Child Psychology, 10*, 307–324.

Kanner, L. (1960). Child psychiatry: Retrospect and prospect. *American Journal of Psychiatry, 117*, 15–22.

Kashani, J.H., & Carlson, G.A. (1986). *Prevalence of depression in a community sample of adolescents.* Presented at the Annual Meeting of the American Academy of Child and Adolescent Psychiatry, Los Angeles.

Kashani, J.H., McGee, R.O., Clarkson, S.E., Anderson, J.C., Walton, L.A., Williams, S., Silva, P.A., Robins, A.J., Cytryn, L., & McKnew, D.H. (1983). Depression in a sample of 9-year-old children. *Archives of General Psychiatry, 40*, 1217–1223.

Keller, M.B., Beardslee, W.R., Dorer, D.J., Lavori, P.W., Samuelson, H., & Klerman, G.R. (1986). Impact of severity and chronicity of parental affective illness on adaptive functioning and psychopathology in children. *Archives of of General Psychiatry, 43*, 930–937.

Kendell, R.E., Hall, D.J., Hailey, A., & Babigian, H.M. (1973). The epidemiology of anorexia nervosa. *Psychological Medicine, 3*, 200–203.

Lilienfeld, A.M., & Lilienfeld, D.E. (1980). *Foundations of epidemiology*. New York: Oxford University Press.

Links, P.S. (1983). Community surveys of the prevalence of childhood psychiatric disorders: A review. *Child Development, 54*, 531–548.

Loeber, R. (1985). Patterns and development of antisocial child behavior. *Annals of Child Development, 2*, 77–116.

Long, A. (1941). Parents' report of undesirable behavior in children. *Child Development, 12*, 43–62.

Lotter, V. (1966). Epidemiology of autistic conditions in young children: I. Prevalence. *Social Psychiatry, 1*, 124–137.

Mausner, J.S., & Bahn, A.K. (1974). *Epidemiology*. Philadelphia: Saunders.

McCracken, J., Shekim, W., Kashani, J.H., Beck, N., Martin, J., Rosenberg, J., & Costello, A. (1986). *The epidemiology of childhood depressive disorders*. Paper presented at the Annual Meeting of the American Academy of Child and Adolescent Psychiatry, Los Angeles.

McGee, R., Silva, P.A., & Williams, S. (1984). Behavior problems in a population of seven-year-old children: Prevalence, stability and types of disorder—A research report. *Journal of Child Psychology & Psychiatry, 25*, 251–259.

Offord, D.R., Boyle, M.H., Szatmari, P., Rae-Grant, N.I., Links, P.S., Cadman, D.T., Byles, J.A., Crawford, J.W., Munroe Blum, H., Byrne, C., Thomas, H., & Woodward, C.A. (1987). Ontario Child Health Study: II. Prevalence of disorder and rates of service utilization. *Archives of General Psychiatry, 44*, 832–836.

O'Leary, K.D., Vivian, D., & Nisi, A. (1985). Hyperactivity in Italy. *Journal of Abnormal Child Psychology, 13*, 485–500.

Puig-Antich, J., & Chambers, W. (1978). *The Schedule for Affective Disorders and Schizophrenia for School-Aged Children*. New York: New York State Psychiatric Institute.

Rutter, M. (1967). A children's behaviour questionnaire for completion by teachers: Preliminary findings. *Journal of Child Psychology & Psychiatry, 8*, 1–11.

Rutter, M. (1982). Surveys to answer questions. *Acta Psychiatrica Scandinavica* (Suppl. 296), *65*, 64–76.

Rutter, M. (1985). Resilience in the face of adversity: Protective factors and resistance to psychiatric disorder. *British Journal of Psychiatry, 147*, 598–611.

Rutter, M., Cox, A., Tupling, G., Berger, M., & Yule, M. (1975). Attainment and adjustment in two geographical areas: I. The prevalence of psychiatric disorder. *British Journal of Psychiatry, 126*, 493–509.

Rutter, M., & Graham, P. (1968). The reliability and validity of the psychiatric assessment of the child: I. Interview with the child. *British Journal of Psychiatry, 114*, 563–579.

Rutter, M., Graham, P., Chadwick, O.F.D., & Yule, W. (1976). Adolescent turmoil: Fact or fiction? *Journal of Child Psychology & Psychiatry, 17*, 35–36.

Rutter, M., & Sandberg, S. (1985). Epidemiology of child psychiatric disorder: Methodological issues and some substantive findings. *Child Psychiatry & Human Development, 15*, 209–233.

Rutter, M., Shaffer, D., & Shepherd, M. (1975). *A multiaxial classification of child psychiatric disorders*. Geneva: World Health Organization.

Rutter, M., Tizard, J., & Whitmore, K. (1970). *Education, health and behavior*. London: Longmans.

Rutter, M., Yule, B., Quinton, D., Rowland, O., Yule, W., & Berger, M. (1975). Attainment and adjustment in two geographical areas: II. Some factors accounting for area differences. *British Journal of Psychiatry, 126*, 520–533.

Shaffer, D., Gould, M.S., Brasic, J., Ambrosini, P., Fisher, P., Bird, H., & Aluwahlia, S. (1983). Children's Global Assessment Scales (CGAS). *Archives of General Psychiatry, 40*, 1228–1231.

Shepherd, M., Oppenheim, A.N., & Mitchell, S. (1971). *Childhood behavior and mental health*. London: University of London Press.

Shrout, P.E., Spitzer, R.L., & Fleiss, J.L. (1987). Quantification of agreement in psychiatric diagnosis revisited. *Archives of General Psychiatry, 44*, 172–177.

Werner, E.E., Burman, J.M., & French, F.E. (1971). *The children of Kauai*. Honolulu: University of Hawaii Press.

Wickman, E.K. (1928). *Children's behavior and teachers' attitudes*. New York: Commonwealth.

Wing, J.K., Bebbington, P., & Robins, L.N. (1981). *What is a case?* London: Grant McIntyre.

World Health Organization. (1977). *Manual of the international classification of diseases, injuries, and causes of death* (9th ed.). Geneva: Author.

Yule, W. (1981). The epidemiology of child psychopathology. In B.B. Lahey & A.F. Kazdin (Eds.), *Advances in clinical child psychology*. New York: Plenum.

CHAPTER 26

Psychiatric Diagnosis and Behavioral Assessment in Children

MICHEL HERSEN AND CYNTHIA G. LAST

It is only in the last few years that behavioral assessors have considered the possibilities of integrating their evaluative strategies under the more embracing umbrella of the psychiatric diagnostic scheme (e.g., Hersen, 1988; Hersen & Bellack, in press; Hersen & Turner, 1984; Kazdin, 1983; Nathan, 1981; Nelson, 1987; Taylor, 1983). Prior to such calls for integration, behavioral assessors and psychiatric diagnosticians had conducted their empirical studies in isolation from one another, although there now is a tacit understanding that each of the empirical camps stands to benefit from the work of the other. It is of particular interest that the concern for integrating findings from behavioral assessment and psychiatric diagnosis has emanated from the behavioral psychologists, not the psychiatrists. The one exception to this is Taylor (1983), who, of course, is a behavioral psychiatrist.

There are several reasons why behavioral assessors now speak of the need to integrate their findings with those of their psychiatric counterparts. The *first* is that target behaviors in behavioral assessment do not always present a full picture and/ or complexity of the problem under study (cf. Hersen, 1988; Kazdin, 1983; Nathan, 1981). The *second* is related to the *first*, in that psychiatric diagnosis often presents a more communicative summary statement of the patient than that designated by specific targets selected for modification via behavioral assessment. Even more robust, however, is the combination of diagnosis and clinically identified problems as a guide to treatment (see Longabaugh, Stout, Kriebel, McCullough, & Bishop, 1986). The *third* reason is more concerned with the politics and pragmatics of diagnosis. That is, despite several attempts to develop behavioral diagnostic schemes (see Adams, Doster, & Calhoun, 1977; Cautela, 1973; Goldfried & Sprafkin, 1976; Kanfer & Saslow, 1965), none has been widely accepted by the community of clinicians, researchers, third-party payers, or governmental agencies. Thus behavioral assessors cannot ignore the third edition of the *Diagnostic and Statistical Manual of Mental Disorders* (DSM-III) (APA, 1980) and its recent revision (DSM-III-R) (APA, 1987). It is a necessity in order to communicate effectively with other professionals in the field. *Fourth*, as has been shown on several prior occasions (Hersen, 1988; Hersen & Bellack, 1988; Hersen & Turner, 1984), there is no incompatibility between use of behavioral assessment and psychiatric diagnosis. And *fifth*, behavioral assessors increasingly are looking at the reliability and validity of child psychiatric diagnoses (e.g., Last, Francis, Hersen, Kazdin, & Strauss, 1987; Last, Hersen, Kazdin, Finkelstein, & Strauss, 1987). Moreover, some behavioral assessors now are involved in the development of semistructured and structured interview schedules for use in reliability and validity studies in the diagnostic field (e.g., development of the Anxiety Disorders Inventory Schedule by DiNardo, O'Brien, Barlow, Waddell, & Blanchard, 1983), an activity that previously was carried out only by psychiatric researchers.

In considering the parallel developments of child psychiatric diagnosis and child behavioral assessment, we should note that there is a relatively long tradition for the latter, dating back to the pioneering efforts of Watson and Rayner (1920), Jones (1924), and Holmes (1936). Although there was a subsequent hiatus, the child behavioral assessment movement took full force in the late 1950s and early 1960s and has continued to flourish and expand (cf. Ollendick & Hersen, 1984). By contrast, child psychiatric diagnosis was given almost no attention in DSM (APA, 1952), with most children and adolescents of that era receiving a diagnosis of adjustment disorder, no classification whatsoever, or downward revisions of adult diagnoses (Kazdin, 1983; Ollendick & Hersen, 1983). This state of affairs is, nonetheless, consistent with the prevailing historical view that children were miniature adults.

With the emergence of DSM-II (APA, 1968), there was some recognition that there were unique features in child psychopathology, with a category entitled "Behavior Disorders of Childhood and Adolescence" included. Subsumed under this new rubric were six subcategories, including hyperkinetic reaction, withdrawing reaction, overanxious reaction, runaway reaction, unsocialized reaction, and group delinquent reaction.

Only in 1980, with publication of DSM-III (APA, 1980), were childhood and adolescent disorders fully acknowledged. In DSM-III five major types of childhood categories appeared: intellectual, behavioral, emotional, physical, and developmental. Subsumed within these five major categories were individual disorders and their subtypes (e.g., anxiety under *emotional*, with subtypes of separation anxiety disorder, overanxious disorder, and avoidant disorder).

Thus, until relatively recently, in the area of childhood diagnosis there were few possibilities for the integration of the behavioral and psychiatric diagnostic systems, especially since childhood diagnosis was accorded so little importance and attention. The primary purpose of this chapter, therefore, is to examine how such integration may be implemented. However, before doing so we will detail the inherent value of classification, improvements in DSM-III and DSM-III-R for child diagnosis, criticisms of DSM-III and DSM-III-R for child diagnosis, the unique contribution of behavioral assessment, and the increased scope of behavioral assessment. Finally, when discussing the strategies for integration, we will look at how motor measurements may lead to refinement and precision in making diagnoses, describe a two-tier system of evaluation, and take a peek at future applications.

THE VALUE OF CLASSIFICATION

To some it may appear ironic that anywhere in a book on the psychiatric diagnosis of children a section justifying the value of classification should appear. Indeed, classification is at the cornerstone of any scientific endeavor, including the description and categorization of child psychopathology. As earlier argued by Adams and colleagues (1977), "Classification is the basis of any science because it is the process of identification of a phenomenon so that events can be measured and communication can occur between scientists and professionals" (p. 47). In its absence, of course, only chaos can exist. However, we must underscore that behavior therapists have a long history of eschewing the need for psychiatric labeling in favor of selecting direct targets for modification. Hersen (1976) has detailed the historical determinants for the behaviorists' rather extreme position on this issue. Included in their reasoning were the notoriously poor reliability and validity of the DSM-I and DSM-II diagnostic schemes and the absence of a relationship between selection of a diagnostic label and subsequent treatment. But with the attendant improvements in DSM-III and DSM-III-R, many of the arguments against the use of diagnosis no longer have as much merit.

Let us now consider in a bit more detail the several purposes served by psychiatric classification. The *first* of these, already mentioned, refers to *organization*. Even the most ardent critics of child psychiatric diagnosis are cognizant of the numerous variants of abnormal behavior in children and adolescents. And simply listing the behaviors without an encompassing umbrella would only result in confusion and disorganization. Thus a primary function of a diagnostic scheme is to present the disparate data in a coherent and meaningful fashion that is both reliable and valid.

A *second* function of diagnosis is to facilitate rapid *communication* among professionals and ancillary personnel working with children and adolescents. When, for example, contrasting separation anxiety to major depression, the clinician is aware of the specific behaviors and symptoms (present in the child for a designated time interval) that comprise the particular disorder. Such knowledge of a specific constellation of behaviors and symptoms permits a considerable amount of communication in a shorthand fashion (i.e., a summary statement about the child). Although this was not the case with DSM and DSM-II, a *third* function of diagnosis (at least at the theoretical level) is to enable the clinician to identify the most appropriate *treatment strategies*. In DSM-III and DSM-III-R, with the delineation of clear criteria for making the diagnosis, there is some rapprochement between diagnosis and treatment (see Taylor, 1983), which has always been one of the hallmarks of the behavioral approach (Hersen, 1976). As diagnostic categories, subcategories, and specific treatments are refined, we undoubtedly will see continued attempts to improve the linkage between diagnosis and treatment, although the ideal isomorphic relationship may never be fully attained.

A *fourth* general function of psychiatric diagnosis has related to the *legal status* of our patients. Perhaps more of a concern with adults, diagnosis has had major legal implications with respect to whether patients are considered fiscally and psychologically competent and whether they are hospitalized against their will (i.e., committed). Although specific behaviors often dictate the use of legal commitment (i.e., suicidality, homicidal intent, psychosis leading to deteriorated self-care), the particular diagnostic label attached to the patient will have some effect on the court's decision.

And *fifth*, increasingly in the last decade the particular diagnosis given to a patient will determine whether the case provider is *reimbursed* by a third-party payer for services rendered, and at what level. As should be obvious, such a system does not always lead to the clinician arriving at the most accurate diagnosis, since the payment factor can be conceptualized as a confounding variable that clouds the diagnostic picture.

IMPROVEMENTS IN DSM-III AND DSM-III-R FOR CHILD DIAGNOSIS

Despite the numerous criticisms of DSM-III (e.g., Hersen & Turner, 1984; McLemore & Benjamin, 1979; McReynolds, 1979; Rutter & Shaffer, 1980; Schacht & Nathan, 1977), before, during, and subsequent to its publication, we must agree with Rutter and Shaffer (1980) that it is "a landmark in the history of systems of psychiatric classification" (p. 371). In considering DSM-III, Rutter and Shaffer not only have highlighted its numerous problems but also have indicated how it surpasses its two predecessors from a general perspective and, specifically, as it relates to childhood psychopathology. Let us detail these seven positive features in turn.

First, and foremost, DSM-III and its successor (DSM-III-R) assume a descriptive or phenomenological stance that is fully atheoretical in nature. This in itself has served to facilitate communication across the inevitable theoretical boundaries. *Second* is the thrust of the system to avoid "labeling" people by recognizing that it is the disorders that are being classified. *Third*, and probably most innovative, is the multiaxial approach that considers: (1) specific clinical syndromes; (2) diagnosis of personality disorder; (3) the patient's medical status; (4) the severity of recent psychosocial stressors; and (5) the global assessment of the patient's psychological, social, and occupational functioning, both currently and in the past year. Thus a most comprehensive portrayal of each patient is painted. The *fourth* feature applies to childhood diagnosis, in that DSM-III has the most comprehensive categorization of child psychopathology. *Fifth* is the provision of precise diagnostic criteria to enhance reliability and validity and to ensure accurate differential diagnostic appraisals. In theory, at least, the diagnostic endeavor now should have a more scientific understructure. *Sixth* is the explicit recognition that psychosocial stressors (Axis IV) have bearing on the development, elicitation, and prolongation of some psychiatric conditions. And *seventh* is the awareness of the originators of DSM-III that there are residuals of childhood disorders into adulthood, although criteria for such residuals are not terribly precise at this point in time. To underscore how much better DSM-III is than its two predecessors (referred to by Begelman, 1975, as "twice-told tales"), Kazdin (1983) states that "DSM-III represents an elaboration of childhood and adolescent disorders and reflects a quantum leap from DSM-II in the attention accorded the populations" (p. 81). But at this juncture let us consider the other side of the coin and look at the perceived failings of DSM-III as applied to children. Unfortunately, DSM-III-R does not represent a vast improvement in this respect over DSM-III.

CRITICISMS OF DSM-III AND DSM-III-R FOR CHILD DIAGNOSIS

Rutter and Shaffer (1980) have identified for us seven basic shortcomings of DSM-III. The *first* is concerned with the extension of the Research Diagnostic Criteria (Feighner et al., 1972) to childhood diagnosis. The problem here is that on an a priori basis criteria have been developed for conditions that indeed may not exist (cf. Hersen & Bellack, 1988; Kazdin, 1983). For example, only recently have there been any empirical data in support of the controversial category of overanxious disorder (cf. Last, Hersen, Kazdin, Finkelstein, & Strauss, 1987). Indeed, as a consequence of these data, this category has been retained in DSM-III-R. As noted by Rutter and Shaffer (1980), "the point is that if criteria are pulled out of the air for conditions not yet adequately validated, it is almost inevitable that some of the rules will prove to be inappropriate even before the manual has been printed" (p. 388).

Second is the fact that each of the diagnostic categories does not have very specific criteria (e.g., developmental reading disorders) and *third* is that a number of the criteria are not practicable (e.g., the notion that attachments in reactive attachment disorder must be made by the eighth month of life). As clearly documented by Rutter and Shaffer (1980), this is contrary to the extant research evidence.

Fourth, it is pointed out that some of the criteria underscore "unwarranted etiological assumptions" (Rutter & Shaffer, 1986). *Fifth*, there is a problem for categorizing disorders that *do not* fit any of the particular criteria in any of the listed categories. *Sixth*, Rutter and Shaffer (1980) rightfully indicate that the manual is contradictory, in that for some conditions there are necessary criteria while for others several criteria out of a given number are required to establish the diagnosis. This, of course, is compounded by the fact that elsewhere in the manual the criteria are referred to as guides, subject to one's clinical expertise. The *seventh* critique, related to all others, concerns the educational value of the manual. Rutter and Shaffer (1980) cogently argue:

> It is a function of the manual to make any adequate differentiation between these statements which represent the summary of decades of research and those which are no more than spitting in the wind. The introduction to the manual does make it clear that much of the description relies solely on clinical judgment. That is fair enough,

but surely it is not asking too much to provide some indication of the degree of empirical support for the statements given. Without that indication, it provides a rather unsatisfactory educational look which is likely to mislead as often as it enlightens. (p. 392)

UNIQUE CONTRIBUTION OF BEHAVIORAL ASSESSMENT

Long before the development and publication of the Research Diagnostic Criteria (cf. Feighner et al., 1972), behavioral assessors devised both simple and complex coding schemes to faciliate the precise observation of behavior in naturalistic and analogue settings (for historical overviews see Hersen & Bellack, 1976; Ollendick & Hersen, 1984). Indeed, child behavioral assessors were among the first clinicians to pinpoint behaviors by operationalizing their descriptions, thus enabling independent judges to achieve high interrater agreement (more than 80%) and high reliability ($r = .80$ and greater). The pages of the *Journal of Applied Behavior Analysis* are replete with examples of sophisticated technologies for assessing and categorizing the behaviors of retarded, autistic, impulse-disordered, organically impaired, conduct-disordered, fearful, psychotic, and even normal children functioning in classroom settings.

Pinpointing and reliably coding motoric behaviors has been a hallmark of the behavioral movement right from its inception. As noted in prior publications tracing the historical developments of behavioral assessment (Hersen, 1976; Nelson, 1983), the insistence on a scientific approach to evaluation undoubtedly arose as a reaction to the growing disillusionment with traditional assessment, including the ubiquitous use of the projective tests and the very unclear relationship between diagnosis and treatment. Although it is costly at times to carry out and a bit cumbersome as to the numbers of raters required, behavioral assessors in general, and child behavioral assessors in particular, underscored the importance of the direct observation of behavior. That is not to say that behavioral assessors are uninterested in the cognitions and physiological responses of their clients and patients. Quite to the contrary, the tripartite assessment, incorporating motoric, cognitive, and physiological channels, has received much attention in the behavioral literature (see Hersen, 1973; Lang, 1968). However, the measuring and recording of simple and complex behaviors of their clients and patients represent one of the most unique and prescient contributions of the behavioral assessors to the field of evaluation. Much credit is due to the behaviorists for demonstrating the feasibility of such assessment and for elaborating its highly refined technology.

A third unique contribution of the behavioral assessors has been the repeated demonstration of the linkage between assessment and treatment (one of the primary failings of the DSM and DSM-II schemes). Following the dictates of the operant tradition, pinpointed behaviors selected for modification were evaluated very carefully over extended time periods in single-case analyses. In the prototypical A–B–A–B single-case analysis (Hersen & Barlow, 1976), the controlling effects of treatment B are clearly documented by introducing, removing, and reintroducing treatment following initial baseline assessment A. Although statistical analyses are available for confirming such controlling effects (Kazdin, 1984), when clinical effects are large and meaningful, the results are portrayed graphically in striking fashion. Not only are there demonstrations of the controlling effects of treatments over selected specific targets (often of the motoric channel), but the concurrent effects of treatments in other motoric behavior can be seen as well as collateral changes in cognitive and physiological responses. In the more complicated analyses, multiple targets have been assessed across motoric, physiological, and cognitive channels (see Van Hasselt, Hersen, Bellack, Rosenblum, & Lamparski, 1979).

But in spite of its obvious contribution to the field of assessment, the analysis of motoric behavior in formal single-case designs has had greater pragmatic application in research than clinical settings. In short, some of our more elaborate coding schemes to evaluate clients and patients are too difficult to implement in clinical settings where personnel are scarce. Considering these limitations, Nelson (1981) has recommended alternatives, such as self-ratings, card sorts, clinic observation, behavioral byproducts, self-ratings, and questionnaires. Although the targets suggested by Nelson are a bit different, the recommendation for using behavior-analytic procedures holds.

INCREASED SCOPE OF BEHAVIORAL ASSESSMENT

In the earlier days of behavioral assessment (e.g., in the 1960s and even into the early 1970s) there was a certain insularity of the field, in that relatively little attention was paid to the other empirical currents in evaluation. From historical and political vantage points, this is fully understandable given that behavioral assessors had to stake their territory, in a manner of speaking. Indeed, a certain amount of breast beating typifies the development of a new empirical discipline, irrespective of its theoretical roots. However, in the more recent writings of enlightened behavioral assessors (Hersen, 1988; Hersen & Bellack, 1988; Kazdin, 1985; McFall, 1986; Nelson, 1983; Patterson & Bank, 1986), recognition of some of the shortcomings of how behavioral assessors have operated has been clearly articulated.

First, we now acknowledge that singular targets slated for modification do not do justice to the richness and complexity inherent in human interaction (cf. Hersen, 1981; Kazdin, 1985). A more comprehensive picture of the intricate interrelationships among outcome measures is certainly required. To do so, behavioral assessors of the future will need broadened vision and understanding of the seminal contributions from other disciplines.

Second, we must incorporate the contributions of developmental psychology, especially in child behavioral assessment, so that the most relevant targets are selected for treatment. The critical role of the developmental stages of childhood and adolescence cannot be ignored if the treatments are to have social relevance (Edelbrock, 1984; Harris & Ferrari, 1983). *Third*, behavioral assessors will have to give greater thought to the use of intelligence tests within the behavioral analysis (Nelson, 1980). *Fourth*, and related to the *third* concern, behavioral assessors have much to gain by learning about neuropsychology, and how neuropsychological assessment impacts on behavioral assessment and subsequent treatment for organically impaired populations. *Fifth*, although surface behavior may be identical in several patients, there may be different etiological differences that result in an identical symptom picture (cf. Hersen, 1981; Michelson, 1984, 1986; Wolpe, 1986a, 1986b). The implications for treatment here are enormous, especially since the cause of the disorder needs to be considered with care if we are to attain our cherished goal of a precise behavioral analysis. And *sixth*, given the numerous significant studies in biological psychiatry and behavioral medicine, the biological underpinnings of overt behavior also must be given close scrutiny in the contemporary behavioral analysis.

Hersen and Bellack (1988) elsewhere stated that the field of behavioral assessment is at a "crossroads," given the criticisms from within and without, and the improvements in DSM. We feel that if the field of behavioral assessment is to avoid stagnation in the future a new and broadened empirical thrust will be required. Otherwise, it may suffer the fate of its predecessor (projective testing) and fall into increasing obscurity.

STRATEGIES FOR INTEGRATION

There now have been a number of calls for integrating DSM-III and behavioral assessment that have appeared in press (Hersen, 1988; Hersen & Bellack, 1988; Hersen & Turner, 1984; Kazdin, 1983; Maser, 1984; Nathan, 1981; Nelson & Barlow, 1981; Taylor, 1983; Tryon, 1986). For example, Maser (1984) states:

> There seems to be no a priori reason why the criteria symptoms in the DSM-III should not include direct measures of behavior. Behavioral testing has been used so little either for reaching a DSM-III diagnosis or for validating existing diagnosis that it can hardly be known if it has value for these purposes at all. (p. 404)

In spite of these generalized concerns about the integration of diagnosis and behavioral assessment, to our knowledge, at this time, there is only one formal proposal outlined that clearly articulates how this might be accomplished. Tryon (1986) has carefully delineated how *motor activity measurements* (i.e., the motoric channel of behavioral assessment) can be used to improve the precision of the diagnostic criteria that appear for many of the categories in DSM-III. A good example in child psychiatric diagnosis is attention deficit hyperactivity disorder. This diagnostic entity currently has eight hyperactivity criteria included, with several related to accelerated motor activity ("difficulty remaining seated, excessive jumping about, running in classroom, fidgeting, manipulating objects, and twisting and wiggling in one's seat" [APA, 1987, p. 50]). Yet in other disorders certain behaviors may be decelerated (e.g., psychomotor retardation in major depression).

Many of the criteria in DSM-III and DSM-III-R include such terms as *increase*, *excessive*, *more*, *decrease*, and *slowed down*. But without proper behavioral referents, they are quite imprecise. On the other hand, if behavioral norms for activity were to be developed in observational coding schemes, we would have available to us a strategy to make such diagnostic appraisals with greater precision, clarity, and reliability. We fully agree with Tryon (1986) that "we need bench marks and ultimately norms for patient and normal populations if we are to develop an empirical basis for rendering diagnoses using activity measurements" (p. 65). Given our methodological sophistication and technology available, including telemetric measuring devices, development of such norms and coding schemes is feasible, even as patients and subjects are interacting daily in their natural environments.

Another possibility to integrate psychiatric diagnosis and behavioral assessment is to use the two approaches to evaluation in complementary fashion. In this conceptualization behavioral assessment is the *idiographic* approach and the DSM-III-R represents the *nomothetic* approach. That is, once a particular diagnosis has been established following DSM-III-R criteria, a behavioral analysis is carried out to determine the specific targets for either behavioral or pharmacological intervention. In so doing we have the advantage of the summary statement of diagnosis and the precision of relating specific targets to specific treatments in single-case strategies. As we have argued previously, behavioral assessment and psychiatric diagnosis are not incompatible (Hersen & Bellack, 1988; Hersen & Turner, 1984).

Finally, in the near future we foresee the validation of the specific criteria of many of the DSM diagnoses by monitoring patient behaviors in their natural environments. Although a most laudable goal, in the past this has not always been possible due to the intrusive effects of observers. However, now that we have the scientific technology to obtain telemetric readings of physiological and motor responses (see Agras, 1986), the prior barriers to success have been lifted. Consider, for example, the possibility of having children and adolescents phobic of school confront their fears (attend classes) while wired to a Holter monitor, and then correlating their cognitive, motoric, and physiological responses. Considerable accurate information would then result, permitting a more precise assessment and consequently a more precise treatment.

SUMMARY

The objective of this chapter has been to consider the relationship of psychiatric diagnosis and behavioral assessment in children. In so doing we first examined the value of classification, followed by an analysis of the improvements in child diagnosis as a result of DSM-III. We then examined some of the major criticisms of DSM-III and DSM-III-R in general and in particular as to child psychiatric diagnosis. Next we looked at the unique contribution of behavioral assessment, considering its historical context, and recognized how in recent times the scope and vision of contemporary behavioral assessors have widened. Six modifications of the practice of behavioral assessment were outlined. In the last section of the chapter we talked about the strategies for integrating psychiatric diagnosis and behavioral assessment. These include: (1) the use of motor assessment to refine and make more precise the behavioral referents in child psychiatric diagnosis; (2) the use of psychiatric diagnosis for molar assessment and subsequent behavioral assessment to select specific targets; and (3) the futuristic use of telemetry in the child's natural environment to gain a better understanding of motoric and physiological responses as they relate to cognitions for specific diagnostic categories.

REFERENCES

Adams, H.E., Doster, J.A., & Calhoun, K.S. (1977). A psychologically based system of response classification. In A.R. Ciminero, K.S. Calhoun, & H.E. Adams (Eds.), *Handbook of behavioral assessment.* New York: Wiley.

Agras, W.S. (1986, November). *So where do we go from here?* Presidential address to the Twentieth Annual Meeting of the Association for Advancement of Behavior Therapy, Chicago.

American Psychiatric Association. (1952). *Diagnostic and statistical manual of mental disorders.* Washington, DC: Author.

American Psychiatric Association. (1968). *Diagnostic and statistical manual of mental disorders* (2nd ed.). Washington, DC: Author.

American Psychiatric Association. (1980). *Diagnostic and statistical manual of mental disorders* (3rd ed.). Washington, DC: Author.

American Psychiatric Association. (1987). *Diagnostic and statistical manual of mental disorders* (3rd ed., rev.). Washington, DC: Author.

Begelman, D.A. (1975). Ethical and legal issues in behavior modification. In M. Hersen, R.M. Eisler, & P.M. Miller (Eds.), *Progress in behavior and modification* (Vol. 1). New York: Academic.

Cautela, J.R. (1973, December). *A behavioral coding system.* Presidential address to the seventh annual meeting of the Association for Advancement of Behavior Therapy, Miami.

DiNardo, P.A., O'Brien, G.T., Barlow, D.H., Waddell, M.T., & Blanchard, E.B. (1983). Reliability of DSM-III anxiety disorder categories using a new structured interview. *Archives of General Psychiatry, 40,* 1070–1074.

Edelbrock, C. (1984). Diagnostic issues. In T.H. Ollendick & M. Hersen (Eds.), *Child behavioral assessment: Principles and procedures.* New York: Pergamon.

Feighner, J.P., Robins, E., Guze, S.B., Woodruff, R.A., Winokur, G., & Munoz, R. (1972). Diagnostic criteria for use in psychiatric research. *Archives of General Psychiatry, 26,* 57–63.

Goldfried, M.R., & Sprafkin, J.M. (1976). Behavioral personality assessment. In J.T. Spence, R.C. Corron, & J.W. Thibaut (Eds.), *Behavioral approaches to therapy.* Morristown, NJ: General Learning Press.

Harris, S.L., & Ferrari, M. (1983). Developmental factors in child behavior therapy. *Behavior Therapy, 14,* 54–72.

Hersen, M. (1973). Self-assessment of fear. *Behavior Therapy, 4,* 241–257.

Hersen, M. (1976). Historical perspectives in behavioral assessment. In M. Hersen & A.S. Bellack (Eds.), *Behavioral assessment: A practical handbook.* New York: Pergamon.

Hersen, M. (1988). Behavioral assessment and psychiatric diagnosis. *Behavioral Assessment, 10,* 107–121.

Hersen, M., & Barlow, D.H. (1976). *Single-case experimental designs: Strategies for studying behavior change*. New York: Pergamon.

Hersen, M., & Bellack, A.S. (1988). DSM-III and behavioral assessment. In A.S. Bellack & M. Hersen (Eds.), *Behavioral assessment: A practical handbook* (3rd ed.). New York: Pergamon.

Hersen, M., & Turner, S.M. (1984). DSM-III and behavior therapy. In S.M. Turner & M. Hersen (Eds.), *Adult psychopathology and diagnosis*. New York: Wiley.

Holmes, F.B. (1936). An experimental investigation of a method of overcoming children's fears. *Child Development, 7*, 6–30.

Jones, M.C. (1924). A laboratory study of fear: The case of Peter. *Journal of Genetic Psychology, 31*, 308–315.

Kanfer, F.H., & Saslow, G. (1965). Behavioral diagnosis. *Archives of General Psychiatry, 12*, 529–538.

Kazdin, A.E. (1983). Psychiatric diagnosis, dimensions of dysfunction, and child behavior therapy. *Behavior Therapy, 14*, 73–99.

Kazdin, A.E. (1984). Statistical analyses for single-case experimental designs. In D.H. Barlow & M. Hersen (Eds.), *Single case experimental designs: Strategies for studying behavior change*. New York: Pergamon.

Kazdin, A.E. (1985). Selection of target behaviors: The relationship of the treatment of focus to clinical dysfunction. *Behavioral Assessment, 7*, 33–47.

Lang, P.J. (1968). Fear reduction and fear behavior: Problems in treating a construct. In J.M. Schlien (Ed.), *Research in psychotherapy* (Vol. 3). Washington, DC: American Psychological Association.

Last, C.G., Francis, G., Hersen, M., Kazdin, A.E., & Strauss, C.C. (1987). Separation anxiety and school phobia: A comparison using DSM-III criteria. *American Journal of Psychiatry, 144*, 653–657.

Last, C.G., Hersen, M., Kazdin, A.E., Finkelstein, R., & Strauss, C.C. (1987). Comparison of DSM-III separation and overanxious disorders: Demographic characteristics and patterns of comorbidity. *Journal of the Academy of Child & Adolescent Psychiatry, 26*, 527–531.

Longabaugh, R., Stout, R., Kriebel, G.M., McCullough, L., & Bishop, D. (1986). DSM-III and clinically identified problems as a guide to treatment. *Archives of General Psychiatry, 43*, 1097–1103.

Maser, J.D. (1984). Behavioral testing of anxiety: Issues, diagnosis, and practice. *Journal of Behavioral Assessment, 6*, 397–409.

McFall, R.M. (1986). Theory and method in assessment: The vital link. *Behavioral Assessment, 8*, 3–10.

McLemore, C.W., & Benjamin, L.S. (1979). Whatever happened to interpersonal diagnosis: A psychological alternative to DSM-III. *American Psychologist, 34*, 17–33.

McReynolds, W.T. (1979). DSM-III and the future of applied science. *Professional Psychology, 10*, 123–132.

Michelson, L. (1984). The role of individual differences, response profiles, and treatment consonance in anxiety disorders. *Journal of Behavioral Assessment, 6*, 349–367.

Michelson, L. (1986). Treatment consonance and response profiles in agoraphobia: The role of individual differences in cognitive, behavioral and physiological treatments. *Behaviour Research & Therapy, 24*, 263–275.

Nathan, P.E. (1981). Symptomatic diagnosis and behavioral assessment: A synthesis. In D.H. Barlow (Ed.), *Behavioral assessment of adult disorders*. New York: Guilford.

Nelson, R.O. (1980). The use of intelligence tests within behavioral assessment. *Behavioral Assessment, 2*, 417–423.

Nelson, R.O. (1983). Behavioral assessment: Past, present, and future. *Behavioral Assessment, 5*, 195–206.

Nelson, R.O. (1987). DSM-III and behavioral assessment. In M. Hersen & C.G. Last (Eds.), *Issues in diagnostic research*. New York: Plenum.

Nelson, R.O., & Barlow, D.H. (1981). Behavioral assessment: Basic strategies and initial procedures. In D.H. Barlow (Ed.), *Behavioral assessment of adult disorders*. New York: Guilford.

Ollendick, T.H., & Hersen, M. (1983). A historical overview of child psychopathology. In T.H. Ollendick & M. Hersen (Eds.), *Handbook of child psychopathology*. New York: Plenum.

Ollendick, T.H., & Hersen, M. (Eds.). (1984). *Child behavioral assessment: Principles and procedures*. New York: Pergamon.

Patterson, G.R., & Bank, L. (1986). Bootstrapping your way in the nomological thicket. *Behavioral Assessment, 8*, 49–73.

Rutter, M., & Shaffer, D. (1980). DSM-III: A step forward or back in terms of the classification of child psychiatric disorders. *Journal of the Academy of Child Psychiatry, 19*, 371–394.

Schacht, T.E., & Nathan, P.E. (1977). But is it good for psychologists: Appraisal and status of DSM-III. *American Psychologist, 32*, 1017–1025.

Taylor, C.B. (1983). DSM-III and behavioral assessment. *Behavioral Assessment, 5*, 5–14.

Tryon, W.W. (1986). Motor activity measurements and DSM-III. In M. Hersen, R.M. Eisler, & P.M. Miller (Eds.), *Progress in behavior modification* (Vol. 20). Orlando: Academic.

Van Hasselt, V.B., Hersen, M., Bellack, A.S., Rosenblum, N., & Lamparski, D. (1979). Tripartite assessment of the effects of systematic desensitization in a multi-phobic child: An experimental analysis. *Journal of Behavior Therapy & Experimental Psychiatry, 10*, 51–56.

Watson, J.B., & Rayner, R. (1920). Conditioned emotional reactions. *Journal of Experimental Psychology, 3*, 1–14.

Wolpe, J. (1986a). Individualization: The categorical imperative of behavior therapy practice. *Journal of Behavior Therapy & Experimental Psychiatry, 17*, 145–153.

Wolpe, J. (1986b). The positive diagnosis of neurotic depression as an etiological category. *Comprehensive Psychiatry, 27*, 449–460.

PART 4

Future Directions

CHAPTER 27

Future Directions in Child Psychiatric Diagnosis

JUDITH L. RAPOPORT

It is daunting to predict the future, and all the more so at the conclusion of a comprehensive volume summarizing the general methodological and more specific issues in child psychiatry. The message remaining, I think, is that diagnosis is a process that will not and should not ever gel into a "true" system, and so we must avoid taking arbitrary stands on questions such as dimensionality versus categorical measurement on particular subcategories. Multivariate factors will always be with us, and major new etiological discoveries will not make them less useful. Finally, we need to worry more about reliability and consistency between classification systems as international research should be expanded, but will depend on compatible schemes.

DIMENSIONS VERSUS CATEGORIES

Eisenberg (1986) has provided us with excellent examples of the arbitrariness of "correct" categories and of the dangers of commitment to caseness versus continuum approaches to diagnosis. Disease definitions change historically as they are influenced by new ideas and new observations. This is, of course, not any more true for psychiatry than for other specialties. In general medicine, it is clear that many individuals are carriers of infectious agents that produce febrile illness in patient A without any symptoms in subject B. Thus even with a defined etiological agent, other factors known and unknown may be the most important, or as important as the presence of the causative agent. Today, the most important predictors of infection with tuberculosis are psychosocial. Years before the discovery of the tubercle bacillus, the mortality rate from tuberculosis in the United Kingdom fell, probably because of the improvement in nutrition and living conditions. This is not to disparage the biological role of the tubercle bacillus or the advances in public health understanding of the disease. But a diagnostic system that includes factors for risk, prognosis, and treatment should be a multiaxial system.

It is also clear that subcategories that once seemed final "truth" have proved to be far more complex as biological research progresses. Cooley's anemias, for example, now comprise an array of more than 50 genetic disorders that can be separated by complex laboratory and clinical measures. Furthermore, individuals can now be identified as carriers of a gene that conveys risk to offspring, but the carrier may be asymptomatic.

The point is that dichotomous thinking about etiology will always be a mistake, with disservice to clear thinking and to patient care, and that medical insights will not necessarily reduce the complexity of a diagnostic system.

It is also hopeful that the controversy between caseness and continuum among psychiatrists and psychologists seems to be lessening. There are disorders where continuous measures may be helpful and others where a particular constellation of features has been uniquely predictive. It should be clear by now to most readers that we need both approaches and also that the debates have not been fruitful.

Here, too, the new biology is probably not going to solve this question. The most interesting biobehavioral correlative research on the role of brain serotonin in human behavior already escapes categorical definition. Postmortem studies of human brains, and of cerebrospinal fluid (CSF) serotonin from brain postmortem studies and CSF 5HIAA, have supported a role for this monoamine in aggression and suicide (Asberg et al., 1981). This well-replicated biological correlate holds across a variety of disorders including antisocial personality disorder, major depression, and suicide. Moreover, unpublished data indicate that CSF 5HIAA also will correlate with personality measures of impulsivity within diagnostically normal groups of students (D. Schalling, personal communication, 1986). It seems probable that an impulsivity factor is most salient here that would be handled best by dimensional rather than categorical measures.

Continuous measures, such as height and IQ, are most useful within the middle range of values, while at the extremes they provide more fertile ground for seeing distinct diagnostic entities. Thus, for example, the correlates are quite different between mild and severe mental retardation. Similarly, there are several unique diagnostic subgroups of dwarfs, or of patients with extremely tall stature, which are not likely to be found across the middle range of height. The best answer will likely be a mix rather than a choice of one approach over another.

Within child psychiatry, studies of attention deficit disorder suggest that continuous measures may be quite as useful as more discrete ones for identifying high-risk groups. However, other measures (age of onset, pervasiveness, family pathology) also seem important for prediction of outcome and of associated features. Within the complex spectrum of childhood affective disorders, it is clear that the seemingly milder dysthymic disorder may be more ominous than isolated single episodes of major affective disorder. A dimensional approach alone would miss issues such as chronicity that seem to be crucial. On the other hand, important ratings of severity can be missed without a quantitative approach to symptoms, and are particularly useful in treatment.

RELIABILITY, DSM-III, AND ICD-9

Child psychiatric diagnosis has urgent needs for everyday clinical application and for academic research. In spite of substantial progress in measurement, diagnosis, and classification of childhood psychopathology, there are major unresolved problems. A most basic problem is the deplorable lack of reliability outside research settings. This difficulty is illustrated by data from a collaborative cross-national diagnostic study that has just been completed between the Child Psychiatry Branch at the National Institute of Mental Health and the Institute of Psychiatry in London (Prendergast et al., in press).

In this study, 41 case histories were diagnosed both by U.S. and U.K. research teams and by panels of about 20 clinicians in London and in Washington, D.C. The use of written case materials focused attention on differences between diagnostic scheme and clinician training, and helped avoid the differences that could arise from different material being extracted from the same interview. Reliabilities of diagnosis from this case history study are given in Table 27.1.

The clinician panels consisted of senior child psychiatrists on both sides of the Atlantic who were well versed in their respective diagnostic schemes and who taught the use of these schemes to their respective trainees. The case histories were addressing the area of disruptive behavior disorders and so most of the cases were grade school boys with either emotional disorders or conduct disorder–hyperkinetic syndrome. As can be seen, agreement was equally poor for both clinician panels and the ICD-9 and DSM-III (APA, 1980) diagnostic schemes. Only the research teams achieved adequate reliability, and that was after lengthy training and discussion.

At least we can say from this exercise that training can improve reliability. It is also unfortunately true that neither the DSM-III nor ICD-9 is sufficiently operationalized

TABLE 27.1.   Agreement about the Presence or Absence of Individual Diagnoses

	Research Teams	U.K. Clinical Panel	U.S. Clinical Panel
	Kappa I[a]	Kappa II[b]	Kappa II[b]
ICD-9			
Hyperkinetic syndrome	.77	.30	.34
Conduct disorder	.60	.28	.20
Emotional disorder	.62	.39	.29
DSM-III			
Attention deficit disorder	.83	.29	.30
Conduct disorder	.80	.33	.27
Emotional disorder			
(excluding oppositional)	.74	.33	.27
Oppositional disorder	.40	.05	.07

[a]Fleiss, 1984, p. 218.

[b]Kappa II is an index of rater agreement for multiple raters and two categories (Fleiss, 1984, p. 227).

Source: Prendergast et al., in press.

to let us assume adequate reliability even among hand-picked academicians, many of whom have participated in research and teaching in this very area.

Prendergast and colleagues' (in press) study addressed differences between ICD-9 and DSM-III, and now the first draft of ICD-10 has just been circulated. As DSM-III-R (APA, 1987) has reached its final version, we need to anticipate the differences between the systems, as these will create or ameliorate issues in cross-national research and communication at any level across cultures.

A number of differences across schemes should be recognized, and will probably be the focus of future studies. A few of these differences between the ICD-10 and DSM-III-R should be mentioned. ICD-10 has both clinical and research criteria; this is the first time any official classification scheme has attempted to do so. In addition, while in theory ICD-10 *can* be multiaxial, it is not officially multiaxial. Thus it will be extremely important to know how ICD-10 is being used at a given center, because as ICD-10 urges a single diagnosis, only a multiaxial approach will determine whether other disorders are noted at all in that system.

While the major classifications are broadly similar between the two schemes, there are a number of subcategories that differ and may make for problems in international exchange. For example, ICD-10 has a subcategory within pervasive developmental disorders for hyperkinetic disorders associated with stereotyped movements. This may clarify research considerably as it undoubtedly will be used for a number of moderately and severely retarded subjects, but there is no counterpart in DSM-III or DSM-III-R. The subcategories of conduct disorder, a problem in any classification, are also different in ICD-10. While retaining the socialized and unsocialized categories, ICD-10 has a category of conduct disorders confined to the family context. Emotional disorders have two subcategories for which there is no exact counterpart in DSM-III-R, namely, social sensitivity disorder and sibling rivalry disorder. A new category, disorders of social functioning, contains elective mutism and two new categories, reactive attachment disorder and attachment disorder of childhood (disinhibition type).

None of these differences is insurmountable, but future research efforts need to clarify areas particularly where differences exist to bring the two schemes even closer together.

The U.S.–U.K. cross-national study of Prendergast and colleagues also demonstrated that there are considerable differences across diagnostic schemes in their ability to handle different types of cases. ICD-9, which permits only one diagnosis per child, created the most dissension in mixed cases. The crucial distinction between conduct disorder and hyperkinetic syndrome, for example, which created considerable disagreement when ICD-9 was used, did not occur with DSM-III when both diagnoses were permitted. DSM-III suffered particularly with respect to oppositional disorder and with respect to subtypes of conduct disorder and attention deficit disorder where agreement was poor for subtypes even within the research teams.

What was particularly interesting was the examination of reliability with respect to the agreement on presence or absence of individual symptoms. Here, too, it was clear that disagreement did not stem from disagreement about whether or not a child was, for example, restless, inattentive, or sad. It seemed that the scheme employed and physician training were both major contributors to the diagnostic process.

The results of this study were discouraging because they do not even begin to take into account the other sources of variability such as variation in a patient over time, or differences in interpretation of phenomena.

It is clear that emotional disorders and conduct disorders account for most of the diagnostic decisions made in child psychiatry. These large categories have been well validated, leaving the next wave of research the harder task of subcategorization. A number of variables, such as family history, age of onset, duration, pervasiveness, and severity, will all need to be taken into consideration in addition, of course, to presenting pattern of behavior.

DEVELOPMENTAL DISABILITIES

One surprising omission in the present volume is a section on diagnosis of specific developmental disorders (pervasive developmental disorders are covered). There are numerous issues that still remain with these disorders, and I will address them in particular—because they are not covered elsewhere in this handbook, not because they are in so much more trouble than other disorders! As with all the other diagnoses, there are basic questions about how severe a disability should be in order to be considered pathological, and about how finely to subcategorize.

There are not sufficient standardized data or widespread use of any test materials that permit adequate scoring across appropriate age levels for many patients to specify degree of impairment. DSM-III-R has added a new specific developmental disorder, motor skills disorder, to the group. This disorder is of considerable interest in that its correlates may be with anxious, withdrawn behavior within the school-age population (Henderson, 1987). Because of the association of neurological "soft signs" in childhood with anxiety disorder in adolescence (Shaffer et al., 1985), this disorder will in all probability be more widely recognized in the next decade.

As with the other developmental disorders, it seems unlikely that all of the subgroups will remain over time. For example, the usefulness of "cluttering" under developmental language disorders will need to be established. However, in view of the powerful association between the developmental disorders and virtually all of the Axis I behavioral syndromes, this research should be closely tied to child psychiatric research and not left to other specialties.

BIOLOGICAL VALIDATION AND PEDIATRIC PSYCHOPHARMACOLOGY

It had been hoped that advances in biological child psychiatry would significantly advance treatment as well as more refined diagnostic approaches. While there are exciting advances in brain imaging techniques, genetics, and psychopharmacology, there are not yet any changes that will radically alter the way we go about making diagnoses. It seems as if biological studies of autism are most likely to provide such a new change, as the fragile-X syndrome has illustrated the heterogeneity of this group of children, with multiple, probably biological, underlying causes. Even here, however, the presence of the fragile-X chromosome may be associated with autism, retardation, or even, in rare cases, normality. Thus chromosomal abnormality remains an important but not sufficient factor to account for the presence of autism.

At one time it was hoped that pediatric psychopharmacology would provide the diagnostic specificity that was lacking in phenomenological approaches (Gittelman-Klein, Spitzer, & Cantrell, 1978). However, this has not proved to be the case. The stimulants appear to be useful for a wide spectrum of hyperactive, aggressive, and possibly even autistic children (when given in small doses), and will not pharmacologically "dissect" the syndromes. While intriguing findings continue to appear, their diagnostic specificity is lacking. One novel study, that of Flament and colleagues (1985), suggests that clomipramine may have a unique antiobsessional action in adolescents with obsessive–compulsive disorder. Considerably more work is expected on this poorly understood disorder from a biological perspective. Whether or not it should be an anxiety disorder and its relationship to depression remain key questions.

Biological and cognitive measures need to be studied in new ways to be more informative about diagnostic correlates. Future studies need to examine these measures (e.g., attentional tasks, platelet imipramine binding) in whole populations that include both referred and nonreferred subjects. It is not clear, for example, whether any cognitive disability is specific for attention disorder. Studies that compare cognitive or biological markers between patients and normal controls will be less informative than studies that use these markers across a variety of populations in community-based samples. It would be most intriguing to see whether different varieties of "inattention" can be separated by cognitive measures that will correlate differently with depression, hyperactivity, and high risk for schizophrenia.

A lack in child psychiatric diagnosis, also not covered in this volume, is research with preschool populations. At the simplest level, there are no satisfactory structured interviews with the preschool child, although some preliminary studies of a brief play interview have been carried out (Stephens, Bartley, Rapoport, & Burg, 1980) in which some play behaviors (e.g., aggression toward peers, separation problems) showed significant correlation with parent and teacher reports, while others (mood and attention span) did not. As preschool behavior problems have been shown to persist into school years (Richman, Stevenson, & Graham, 1982), this is of considerable importance for future diagnostic and prevention research.

REFERENCES

American Psychiatric Association (1980). *Diagnostic and statistical manual of mental disorders* (3rd ed.). Washington, DC: Author.

American Psychiatric Association (1987). *Diagnostic and statistical manual of mental disorders* (3rd ed., rev.). Washington, DC: Author.

Asberg, M., Bertilsson, L., Rydin, E., Shalling, D., Thoren, P., & Traskman-Bendzi, L. (1981). Monoamine metabolites in cerebrospinal fluid in relation to depressive illness, suicidal behavior and personality. *Advances in the Bio-Sciences*, *31*, 257–271.

Eisenberg, L. (1986). When is a case a case? In M. Rutter, C. Izard, & P. Read (Eds.), *Depression in young people: Developmental and clinical perspectives*. New York: Guilford.

Flament, M., Rapoport, J., Berg, C., Sceery, W., Kilts, C., Mellstrom, M.B., & Linnoila, M. (1985). Clomipramine treatment of adolescent obsessive compulsive disorder: A controlled trial. *Archives of General Psychiatry*, *42*, 977–983.

Fleiss, J. (1984). *Statistical methods for raters and proportions*. New York: Wiley.

Gittelman-Klein, R., Spitzer, R., Cantrell, D. (1978). Diagnostic classifications and psychopharmacological indications. In J. Werry (Ed.), *Pediatric psychopharmacology: The use of behavior modifying drugs in children*. New York: Brunner/Mazel.

Henderson, S.E. (1987). The assessment of "clumsy" children: Old and new approaches. *Journal of Child Psychology & Psychiatry*, *28*, 511–527.

Prendergast, M., Taylor, E., Rapoport, J., Bartko, J., Donnelly, M., Zametkin, A., Ahearn, M., Dunn, G., & Wieselberg, M. The diagnosis of childhood hyperactivity: A U.S.–U.K. Cross-National Study of DSM-III and ICD-9. *Journal of Child Psychology & Psychiatry*, in press.

Richman, N., Stevenson, J., & Graham, P. (1982). *Preschool to school: A behavioral study*. London: Academic.

Rutter, M., & Tuma, A.H. (1987). Epilogue-diagnosis and classification: Some outstanding issues. In M. Rutter, A.H. Tuma, & I. Lann (Eds.), *Assessment, diagnosis and classification in child and adolescent psychopathology*. New York: Guilford.

Rutter, M. (1986). Child psychiatry: Looking 30 years ahead. *Journal of Child Psychology & Psychiatry*, *27*, 803–840.

Shaffer, D., Schonfeld, I., O'Connor, P., Stockman, C., Trautman, P., Shafer, S., & Ng, S. (1985). Neurological soft signs: Their relationship to psychiatric disorder and intelligence in childhood and adolescence. *Archives of General Psychiatry*, *42*, 342–351.

Stephens, R., Bartley, L., Rapoport, J.L., & Burg, C. (1980). A brief preschool playroom interview: Correlates with independent behavioral reports. *Journal of the American Academy of Child Psychiatry*, *19*, 213–224.

Author Index

Subject Index